MECHANISMS
OF MEMORY

MECHANISMS OF MEMORY

J. DAVID SWEATT

Division of Neuroscience
Baylor College of Medicine
Houston, Texas

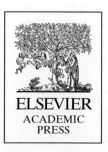

ELSEVIER
ACADEMIC
PRESS

AMSTERDAM • BOSTON • HEIDELBERG • LONDON
NEW YORK • OXFORD • PARIS • SAN DIEGO
SAN FRANCISCO • SINGAPORE • SYDNEY • TOKYO

Academic Press is an imprint of Elsevier

Academic Press
An imprint of Elsevier
525 B Street, Suite 1900, San Diego, California 92101-4495, USA
http://www.academicpress.com

Academic Press
84 Theobald's Road, London WC1X 8RR, UK
http://www.academicpress.com

Library of Congress Catalog Card Number: 2003107470

International Standard Book Number: 0-12-678957-6

Cover art: Cellular Complexity, J. David Sweatt, Acrylic on canvas, 2002.

PRINTED IN CHINA
03   04   05   06   07   7   6   5   4   3   2   1

How small the cosmos (a kangaroo's pouch would hold it), how paltry and puny in comparison to human consciousness, to a single individual recollection, and its expression in words!

Vladimir Nabokov–from *Speak, Memory*

*I have had the great good fortune to marry
a most creative, intelligent, caring,
and beautiful woman. The mysteries
of memory pale in comparison
to the mysteries of Kim.*

Contents

Foreword

In 1967, the neuroscientist E. Roy John published *Mechanisms of Memory*, a substantial 468-page survey of how the brain learns and remembers. Now, in 2003, the neuroscientist J. David Sweatt has written a book about memory under the same title. A consideration of the differences between the two books provides a dramatic picture of the progress that has been made in recent years. Indeed, it is striking how dissimilar the two books are, beyond the title. Building from the techniques and tools available at the time, Roy John emphasized work at a global, structural level of analysis: for example, the problem of localization of function, representation of information in assemblies of neurons, and electrophysiological correlates of learning and memory. One chapter discussed how macromolecules might be important for memory storage, but the first studies of protein synthesis inhibition and memory had been done only a few years earlier, and molecular techniques were not available to take the problem further.

David Sweatt's comprehensive book shows not only that much has happened since the 1960s, but that the field has been revolutionized. Consider the range of discoveries, tools, and ideas that are part of contemporary memory research, but which were absent altogether in the 1960s: the development of *Drosophila* and *Aplysia* as model systems for studying the genetics and the synaptic changes underlying behavioral memory, the discovery of LTP, the concept of multiple memory systems, and an entire new discipline that is delineating the biochemistry and molecular biology of short-term and long-term neural plasticity. As one of the very few books available that surveys learning and memory from molecules to behavior, *Mechanisms of Memory* (vintage 2003) provides a welcome and readable treatment of these extraordinary developments. Progress in the neuroscience of behavior follows a slower, more gradual course than molecular biology or biochemistry, but across the time spanned by these two books about the mechanisms of memory, the progress is breathtaking.

Larry R. Squire
March, 2003

Preface

This book is primarily intended for advanced undergraduates, graduate students, and researchers interested in learning and memory. After a brief introduction to the basics of learning and memory at the psychological level, the book will describe current understanding of memory at the molecular and cellular level. Particular emphasis will be on the hippocampus and its role in declarative and spatial learning, although examples from other anatomical and behavioral systems will also be used. As the book overall progresses from chapter to chapter, I will deliberately move from well-established facts and background, to a description of current work and thinking in the area, to at last what should be clearly labeled speculation.

In my opinion, this book is appropriate for use in advanced undergraduate and graduate-level learning and memory courses, courses that typically are based in Psychology, Biology, and Neuroscience Departments at the University and Medical School levels. I hope that it provides a nice foundation for thinking about the molecular underpinnings of synaptic plasticity and information storage. However, the book is primarily targeted to active researchers (at all stages of their career development) in the learning and memory fields.

One goal of the book is to begin to embrace the complexity of mechanisms of learning and memory at the molecular level. Some who work on the cellular processes of learning and memory seem to want to ignore this complexity, deny its existence, or throw up their hands in frustration and imply that the problem is insoluble. I share none of these viewpoints. My hope in this book is to begin to organize a framework of thinking about synaptic plasticity and memory at the molecular level—one which recognizes and begins to incorporate this extreme biochemical complexity into our thinking about memory. I note that building these models is at a relatively early stage, but one thing the reader hopefully will take from the book is some perspective on where we stand at present and where the future may lie.

Most of us have seen the large and complex schematic diagrams summarizing intermediary metabolism. Hundreds of discrete and highly regulated enzymatic steps are necessary for the relatively basic function of converting glucose into ATP. How can memory be any less complex than that at the molecular level? Human learning and memory is likely the most highly evolved and sophisticated biological process in existence. In my view, the ultimate molecular understanding of learning and memory will make processes such as intermediary metabolism seem simple in comparison. This book represents one first step at beginning to put together the complex puzzle of the molecular basis of memory.

While a strong case can be made that the molecular basis of memory will of necessity be quite complex at the biochemical level, a more difficult argument arises as to whether understanding these processes is even really important. Is it molecular stamp collecting? If all the nervous system really cares about is the firing of action potentials, isn't the underlying biochemistry really just housekeeping? A second point that I want to try to make with this book is that understanding the underlying molecular basis *is* important. Where possible, I will try to utilize examples illustrating that various molecular processes are being used for information processing; information processing that occurs at a level independent of patterns of action potential firing. Also, I want to highlight that action potentials and neurons *per se* are incapable of *storing* information. That is because all biological processes are subserved by biochemical phenomena. This book is written from the perspective that, in the limit, neurons are bags of chemicals and the fundamental unit of information storage is the molecule.

This book seeks to take the reader from a basic background of learning theory and synaptic physiology, to a detailed discussion of the biochemical mechanisms of long-term changes in synaptic function and information storage, to a discussion of the molecular basis of learning and memory disorders. Themes that are highlighted include:

- Genes and gene regulation in memory formation.

- The role of long-term changes in synaptic function in memory.

- Does Long Term Potentiation = Memory?

- Multimodal signal integration at the molecular level and its role in cognition as related to memory.

- Learning disorders with a focus on mental retardation syndromes.

- Memory disorders with a focus on Alzheimer's Disease.

- The biochemical basis of cellular information processing.

- Biochemical mechanisms for information storage.

A few comments concerning references are in order. There have been many thousands of publications in the fields that are covered by this book. The chapters covering LTP biochemistry, which is the area that the book covers in the greatest detail, are drawn from about 900 primary publications. Some single paragraphs in these sections summarize work from about 50 different research papers. In writing the book, I had to make a decision – I could write sentences like "Postsynaptic calcium is known to be involved in LTP induction: blocking a rise in postsynaptic calcium blocks LTP induction, elevating postsynaptic calcium elicits synaptic potentiation, and a rise in postsynaptic calcium has been shown to occur with LTP-inducing stimulation." Or I could write sentences like "X *et al.*, Y *et al.*, and Z *et al.* showed that injecting calcium chelators postsynaptically blocked LTP induction, P *et al.*, Q *et al.*, and Z *et al.* showed that …." The latter type of sentence, the historical narrative, obviously has a more scholarly tone and gives appropriate credit to X *et al.*, etc. However, it rapidly leads to bloated verbiage that is much more difficult to read. Taking all this into consideration, I decided to handle the citations in the following way. At the end of each chapter is a section titled "References," which is a little different from the typical list of references in terms of its content. It is not exhaustive. "References" is the short list of papers that were the principal papers I used in preparing the chapter, and there is a distinct bias toward citing reviews that I feel are particularly lucid and informative. In a real sense, the references are my list of recommended readings for further information. The cited reviews are a place where readers looking for more detailed references can find citations to the extensive list of primary literature. I apologize in advance to the many researchers whose primary papers I have not cited directly.

I strongly encourage anyone with any complaint, correction, criticism or suggested addition to e-mail me (david@cns. neusc.bcm.tmc.edu). Constructive criticism is the only means by which the content of the book may be improved in the future. So, when John Lisman wants to fire off a scathing critique of my inadequate representation of his work, I encourage him to send me an e-mail so that I can take his comments into consideration in future writing efforts. I want to emphasize that I encourage everyone to do this. I want the post-doc who spent two years optimizing assays for measuring protein kinase activation, so that they could measure an LTP-associated increase in CaMKII, to be able to e-mail me and get at least some recognition for their effort. In cases like this it is likely to be helpful to send me the relevant citation and a few sentences describing its significance and relevance. The overall goal of encouraging this sort of interaction is to allow a means for dynamically correcting and updating the book content.

Finally, I am more than happy to share Powerpoint files containing the figures from the book with anyone who would like to use them for teaching purposes, etc. An e-mail to the above address will suffice to get that particular ball rolling.

David Sweatt

Acknowledgments

Only one set of eyes can be the first to read any book. In the case of *Mechanisms of Memory*, those eyes belonged to Sarah Brown. Sarah was much more than a reader, however—she was a colleague, collaborator, and contributor in the making of the book. Her contributions were so numerous and diverse that they constitute a gestalt. A mere listing will only detract from an acknowledgment of her contributions. I *will* note specifically that Sarah executed all the many figures for the book, bringing a discerning and creative approach to that artistic endeavor. Each picture is worth a thousand thank-you's. Just as only one set of eyes can be the first to read a book, only one person can be listed first in the acknowledgments. My first and foremost acknowledgment goes to Sarah Brown.

I thank my many colleagues and collaborators from whom I have learned much over the years. I especially thank my former students and post-docs, from whom I have learned much more than I ever taught.

I also thank my editor Johannes Menzel for his infectious enthusiasm for the book project and numerous suggestions to help improve the book, as well as his associate Cindy Minor for her help and input on many aspects of the book. The anonymous reviewers of the book proposal and the anonymous readers of the near-final manuscript also deserve recognition for their contributions in making the book better—they made many useful suggestions that I incorporated into the text. I also thank John Assad, Sara Copeland Shalin, Dan Johnston, Eric Klann, and Eric Roberson specifically for reading all or various sections of the first draft of the book and providing feedback and numerous constructive comments.

Finally, I thank the good citizens of the town of Austin, Minnesota, for sharing their beautiful public library with me. I wrote the entirety of Chapter Ten sitting near the back windows, looking out over the Mill Pond. I spent many hours there, pondering and writing about the complexities of gene regulation and their relationship to learning and memory. When I was ready to take a break, I walked up the block to the Tendermaid, sustaining myself with one of their unique hamburgers and delicious milkshakes. There is no finer place to write a book chapter than Austin, Minnesota during the week of the July 4th holiday.

It has not escaped my attention that two particular citizens of Austin, Donna and Bill Strifert, deserve special thanks for their creative contributions to helping this book become a reality.

MECHANISMS
OF MEMORY

———

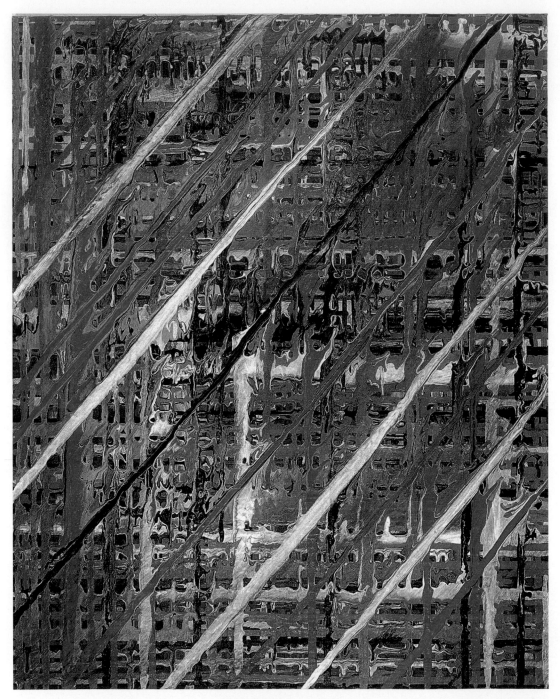

Multiple Memory Systems
J. David Sweatt, Acrylic on canvas, 2002

Introduction

The Basics of Psychological Learning and Memory Theory

I. INTRODUCTION

My father grew up during the Great Depression. When he was in the sixth grade, his father died of cancer, and my dad dropped out of school so that he could go to work and help support his mother and siblings. Despite having only an elementary school education, my father was fortunate enough to soon be able to go to work for the Western of Alabama Railroad, at the age of 15 as a carmen's apprentice. He worked a good union job for that railroad for the next 45 years, first as a railroad coach carpenter and then as a diesel engine mechanic. My father had a lifelong yearning for the education that had been denied him owing to his circumstances. From a very young age I remember him telling me to "get an education, that's the way out." He instilled in me a concrete understanding that learning is an opportunity, and that in a very tangible way that knowledge is power.

Shortly before I received my Ph.D. from Vanderbilt University, I had a realization. I realized that, like my father before me, I was likely to spend the rest of my life working on a single thing, so whatever that thing was, it had better be interesting to me. I asked myself the question: "What is the most interesting thing in the world?" For me, the answer to that question was to understand learning and memory. In retrospect, this answer might not be surprising given my father's lifelong emphasis on the importance of learning as an opportunity to be vigorously pursued. From that point on, I have undertaken a course of laboratory investigation aimed at trying to understand learning and memory.

Knowledge really is power, and learning is the tool we use to get it. For that reason, humans have evolved extremely sophisticated mechanisms for learning new information and storing it for subsequent recall. This book will describe recent laboratory findings that have begun to scratch the surface of the amazingly complex phenomenon of learning and memory, focusing on their cellular and molecular bases.

An understanding of the cellular and molecular basis of learning and memory of course requires a firm foundation of understanding the behavioral processes these mechanisms subserve. This first chapter serves as an introduction to the basics of learning and memory, its theory and terminology. It will provide you with the fundamental terms most psychologists use to describe the types and forms of learning and memory that we will be discussing throughout the book.

What is learning? Before we can begin to discuss categorizing types of learning and memory effectively, it is useful to define both of the terms we will be using extensively throughout this book: learning and memory. Both of these terms are so widely used and implicitly understood that there is a great temptation to say "learning is when you learn something and memory is when you remember it." This type of definition obviously is not going to take us very far.

Upon serious reflection, we can clearly see that neither learning nor memory will be easy to define, and indeed learning and memory psychologists continue to debate these definitions to this day. Thus, I am delivering the caveat that the definitions I

have chosen to use, even though they are derived from the literature, are not universally accepted. I define learning as the acquisition of an *altered* behavioral response due to an environmental stimulus. In other words, learning is when an animal changes its behavior pattern in response to an experience. Note that what is defined is a *change* in a behavior from a preexisting baseline. I am not defining learning as a response to an environmental stimulus, but rather as an *alteration* in that response due to an environmental stimulus. An animal has a baseline response, experiences an environmental signal, and then has an altered response different from its previous response. This I define as learning (see Figure 1).

Memory is defined as the storage of the learned item, which of course must be subject to recall by some mechanism.

I like these definitions because at heart I am an experimentalist, and these are clear functional definitions that lend themselves to experimental application. An experimentalist must be able to observe something (and ideally measure it) in order to be able to test a hypothesis. The definitions of learning and memory that I use derive directly from the experimentalist mindset. This practical orientation is at once both a strength and a weakness for the definitions—their ready application in practice leads to limitations for their use in theory.

Learning: The acquisition of an altered behavioral response due to an environmental stimulus.

Memory: The processes through which learned information is stored.

Recall: The conscious or unconscious retrieval process through which this altered behavior is manifest.

FIGURE 1 Definitions of learning, memory, and recall.

For example, one criticism of the definition of learning that I (and many others) use is that it is too narrow. If someone learns my name and stores it as a perfectly legitimate memory, that learned item may never be manifest as an altered behavioral output on their part. This is a completely valid theoretical criticism and a limitation to the definition. My only rebuttal is that in order for you to ever prove to me that such a memory exists, you would need to demonstrate an altered behavioral output on the part of the person involved. For example, they would need to respond with "David" instead of "I don't know" when you showed them my picture. This is really more of a practical Catch-22

than a logical rebuttal, however, and it is certainly clear that the definition does not adequately cover every type of memory. I will leave for other authors the discussion of whether memories are in fact quantum Schroedinger's Cats that don't exist until recalled (a discussion some would take quite seriously).

At the other end of the spectrum is the criticism that the definition is too broad. It certainly covers many types of alterations in behavior such as simple sensitization and habituation, which most people would not consider to be "real" learning (this is illustrated in Box 1). Nevertheless, a considerable body of literature is available indicating, and most researchers in the

---

BOX 1

LEARNING IN A PLANT? "SENSITIZATION" IN THE VENUS' FLYTRAP

Our functional definition of learning is: a change in an animal's behavioral responses as a result of a unique environmental stimulus. This broad definition is useful in that it encompasses various nonassociative forms of learning such as sensitization and habituation, but the breadth of the definition can be criticized. This can be illustrated by a consideration of "sensitization" in the Venus' flytrap plant.

Although plants are not thought of as expressing behavior in the same sense as an animal, plants can and do respond to environmental stimuli. We are all familiar with the phototactic responses of plants as, for example, they turn to follow the sun, their foliage changes in response to cooling weather, and the petals of certain flowers, close at night. These types of responses, however, are really more akin to reflexive, nonlearned behaviors in animals.

One intriguingly complex, multicomponent response of a plant to an environmental stimulus is exhibited by *Dionaea muscipula*, commonly known as the Venus' flytrap. This carnivorous plant, indigenous to the peat bogs of the Carolinas in the southeastern United States, supplements its nutrition by capturing and digesting insects. *Dionaea* trap insects when they land in one of the plant's V-shaped leaves, which closes on the hapless victim like a miniature steel bear trap.

The triggering mechanism for closure of the trap warrants our attention. Each half of the V-shaped trap has on its inward facing surface three trigger hairs. Mechanical stimulation of these hairs elicits closure of the trap. To eliminate "false alarms," *Dionaea* has evolved a mechanism whereby stimulation of a single trigger hair is insufficient to cause the trap to close. Two hairs must be

Continued

BOX 1—cont'd

LEARNING IN A PLANT? "SENSITIZATION" IN THE VENUS' FLYTRAP

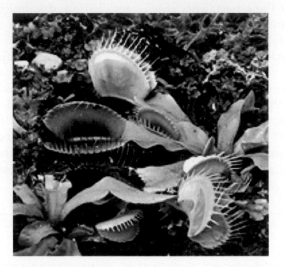

stimulated in succession (or simultaneously) to trigger a trapping response. Thus, in one circumstance, stimulating a particular trigger hair will give no response, whereas stimulating the same trigger hair will in another instance, depending on recent history, give trap closure. This is clearly an example of an altered response that depends on a prior environmental stimulus. In a sense, the mechanical stimulation of the first trigger hair could be viewed as analogous to "sensitizing" the plant, so that it will respond to the mechanical stimulation of the second hair. Photo courtesy of Muriel Weinerman, NY Botanical Gardens.

field agree, that many simple forms of behavioral modification qualify as learned responses. These forms of simple, nonassociative learning are described in the next section.

This broad, umbrella-like definition of learning covers so many different types of behavioral modifications that some sort of organizing principle and attendant nomenclature are necessary. Even though there is no universally accepted version of this at present, most contemporary experimentalists who work on learning utilize some variation of a system promulgated by Larry Squire and Eric Kandel (1–3). I will use their system as a starting point and would be remiss if I did not credit their many significant and influential contributions in this area. However, I note that there are some significant differences between their published framework and my own, so that I don't saddle them with responsibility for any inadequacies on the part of my framework.

A. Categories of Learning and Memory

I divide learning into two broad classes—unconscious learning and conscious learning. I also introduce a "recall"

Hierarchical Organization of Memory

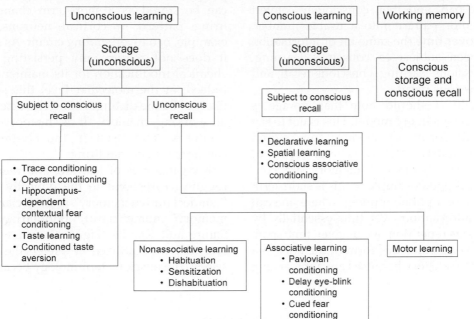

FIGURE 2 Hierarchical organization of memory. Short- and long-term memory is subject to being learned by either conscious or unconscious processes. Similarly, memory can be recalled either consciously or unconsciously. Many forms of simple learning such as motor learning, simple associative conditioning, and non-associative learning can be learned and recalled unconsciously. More complex forms of learning typically involve conscious processes. Short-term working memory is listed as a separate category because it is essentially entirely conscious and not stored for more than a few seconds.

term (see Figure 2), and apply conscious and unconscious to it as well. Thus, any type of memory (with one exception, which is discussed later) falls into one of four categories: unconscious learning with unconscious recall, unconscious learning subject to conscious recall, conscious learning subject to unconscious recall, and conscious learning subject to conscious recall. Specific examples are listed in Figure 2 for illustrative purposes, and for the rest of this chapter and in Chapters 2 and 3 we will cover many specific examples in each category.

I like the nomenclature summarized in Figure 2 because it emphasizes that any given memory event comprises three components: learning, storage, and recall. An item or event is learned, stored for some period of time, and recalled. Highlighting

these three components is necessary, in my opinion, because each corresponds to a distinct molecular and cellular set of events.

It also is important to note that the category for the learning, memory, and recall of a specific bit of information is not static over time, but instead is subject to change. Consider, for example, the learning and recollection of a phone number that becomes familiar with repetition. You first look up the number in the phone book and consciously store and recall the number. Over time, you repetitively punch in the number, and it is subject to being learned unconsciously as a motor pattern and recalled unconsciously in the same way. After a while, however, a thoroughly familiarized phone number can become difficult to recall in a direct, conscious fashion. Many times I have seen friends "recall" a familiar phone number by pretending to punch it out on a touch-tone phone pad, and then consciously convert the motor pattern into a usable number. Thus over time the same bit of information has been subject to conscious learning, unconscious learning, conscious recall, and unconscious recall.

Finally, I should note that storage is unconscious in my model. This is not to say that all forms of memory are stored unconsciously—clearly several forms of short-term "working" memory are conscious. A good example of this is short-term storage of a phone number, where one can store information over time essentially by conscious repetition over a given time span. However, I place this form of memory in a separate category because I am approaching

memory from a cellular and molecular perspective (see Figure 2). Working memory can be stored as a short-term change in firing pattern in cortical neurons, for example, in a reverberating circuit. As such, it does not require any persisting biochemical modification for its maintenance. Indeed, at the molecular level this seems likely to be the distinguishing characteristic of working memory. It is memory that cannot sustain itself in the absence of continuing neuronal firing.

My categories of learning and memory roughly correspond to the typically used "nondeclarative memory" and "declarative memory" nomenclature popularized by Squire and Kandel (Figure 3) and widely accepted and utilized. I prefer the conscious/unconscious terminology because it

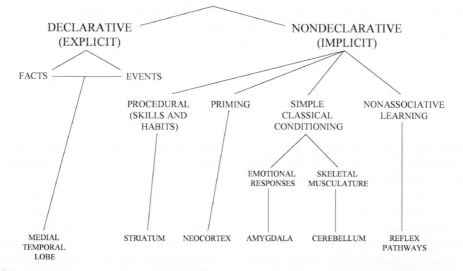

FIGURE 3 Subdivisions of human memory and associated brain regions. Human memory is typically divided into declarative and nondeclarative types, also known as explicit and implicit memory, respectively. In addition to various types of memory described in the text, priming is also listed. Priming is unconscious memory formation. For example, if one hears or reads a word, for a period of time afterward one is more likely to use that word in conversation or in a word completion task. This occurs even if no conscious memory for having heard the word is formed. Chart adapted from Milner, Squire, and Kandel (13).

This type of chart, which subdivides memory into several, separately identified components distills the modern concept of *multiple memory systems*. It is now clear that different anatomical structures in the brain are involved in different types of memory formation. Moreover, the different systems can operate as parallel processors that function independently. This allows multitasking, with conscious and unconscious memory systems operating simultaneously and increasing the overall "memory throughput" of the central nervous system. I highly recommend reading *From Conditioning to Conscious Recollection* by Eichenbaum and Cohen (4) for a more thorough treatment of the multiple memory systems concept.

emphasizes the cognitive differences between the two forms more effectively, in my mind. In addition, I like these terms because they tend to highlight the intrinsic role of learning and memory in cognition in general. Finally and most importantly, I prefer this terminology because it semantically separates the learning from the memory from the recall – an important mindset to adapt as we seek to understand behavioral events in molecular terms.

B. Memory Exhibits Long-Term and Short-Term Forms

As has been emphasized by Eric Kandel, Jim McGaugh, and many others (see reference 4), almost all forms of memory can be either short-lasting or long-lasting. With only a few exceptions (see Box 2), the duration of the memory for a learned event depends on the number of times an animal experiences a behavior-modifying stimulus.

BOX 2

NONGRADED ACQUISITION OF MEMORY: FOOD AVERSION AND IMPRINTING

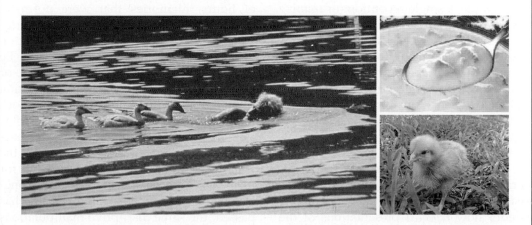

While most forms of long-term memory exhibit graded acquisition, some types of learning are so critical to an animal's survival that extremely robust learning mechanisms have evolved to subserve them. One striking example of this is *conditioned food avoidance*. Generally, if an animal consumes a novel foodstuff that subsequently causes sickness, even after a single such experience the animal will exhibit a lifelong aversion to that particular food. For animals in the wild, the survival value of this type of learning is obvious, but the phenomenon can have unintended consequences. For example, I once got food poisoning after eating a bowl of New England clam chowder; to this day, even the sight of a can of New England clam chowder on the grocery store shelf is enough to send me scurrying to the next aisle. This is a textbook case of conditioned food avoidance—being from Alabama, I had never had clam anything until that day. I certainly will fastidiously avoid future clam encounters of any kind.

Continued

BOX 2—cont'd

NONGRADED ACQUISITION OF MEMORY: FOOD AVERSION AND IMPRINTING

Although I have not personally experienced it, hatchling chicks exhibit a robust form of learning termed *imprinting*. A newborn bird will develop a strong, long-lasting affinity for whatever it sees in the first hour after hatching. In one famous example, a group of young geese imprinted on the experimental ethologist Konrad Lorenz. In experimental situations, chicks will even imprint on inanimate objects such as red boxes or dolls. Of course, in the wild this type of learning serves a useful purpose, as hatchlings will almost always first see their mother and imprint upon her. The chicks will then stick close by the mother as she guides and protects them through the perilous fledgling period. Photo of chick courtesy of Reuben Clements.

For example, a single repetition (or *training trial*) may elicit a memory that lasts only a few minutes, whereas repeated stimulations will likely result in memory lasting hours to days. Repeated presentations of multiple training trials can elicit memory lasting for even more prolonged periods, up to the lifetime of the animal. Thus, the acquisition of memory is a *graded* phenomenon (see Figure 4).

One exciting area of contemporary learning research is to try to understand the basis for this attribute. It is intriguing to wonder how *repeated* presentations of the identical environmental stimulus can *uniquely* elicit a long-lasting behavioral alteration, especially when one considers that the behavioral output (e.g., enhanced responsiveness) is identical in the short- and long-lasting forms. This phenomenon is still fairly mysterious at present for the various mammalian systems that we will be discussing; however, at several points in subsequent chapters, I will describe current thinking in this area.

Long-term memory also has the general attribute that it undergoes a period of *consolidation*. Decades ago, researchers discovered that, for a period of time after the training period, generally on the order of hours, memories that were normally destined to become long-term memories were susceptible to disruption. Disruption of nascent long-term memories can be brought about by trauma, for example, or in a more refined manipulation application of inhibitors of protein synthesis can block memory consolidation (Figure 5). Thus it is clear that some set of molecular processes is occurring for some period of time after the training trial, which are necessary for memory to be established as truly long-lasting. After the critical time window has passed, the same disruptive manipulations have no effect on memory storage. Aside from the insight that protein synthesis inhibitors can block memory consolidation, not much is known concerning the specific molecular underpinnings of this fascinating process. Studies of the cellular and molecular mechanisms contributing to the consolidation of hippocampus-dependent long-term memory will be an area of emphasis in Chapters 6–9 and Chapter 12 of this book.

There has been a resurgence of interest in the consolidation phenomenon lately because several groups have reported that previously stored memories are subject to disruption in certain circumstances.

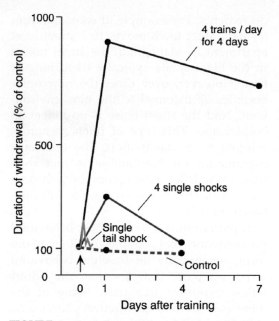

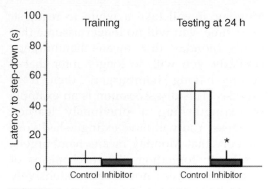

FIGURE 4 Graded acquisition of memory. Multiple training trials typically result in more robust and long-lasting memory formation. In this case, sensitization of the gill-withdrawal reflex was measured by quantitating the duration of gill withdrawal in response to a slight touch (duration of withdrawal, Y-axis). Delivery of a tail shock to the animal elicits sensitization, an increase in the magnitude of the protective gill withdrawal reflex (see Box 3 and text). Increasing the number of training trials (tail shocks) increases both the duration of the memory (days of duration) and the magnitude of the learned response. Adapted with permission from Kandel (14). Copyright 2001 American Association for the Advancement of Science.

FIGURE 5 Protein synthesis inhibitors block consolidation of long-term memory. Inhibitors of protein synthesis typically block the ability of learned information to be consolidated into a long-lasting form. In this experiment rats were trained in a step-down avoidance paradigm (see Chapter 2). Animals are placed on an elevated platform in the middle of an electric grid and receive a mild foot shock when they step down from the platform. On the training day, animals that received a saline infusion (CONTROL) or the protein synthesis inhibitor anisomycin (INHIBITOR) both quickly step down from the platform (latency to step-down, Y-axis). Twenty-four hours later, the control animals exhibit a much longer latency to step-down, indicating that they have learned to avoid the electrified floor. Animals treated with protein synthesis inhibitor have not consolidated their memory for the step-down training and exhibit a short latency to step-down just as they did on the first day. Additional experiments (not shown) have demonstrated that anisomycin treatment immediately after training is also effective at blocking memory consolidation, indicating that consolidation is a post-training phenomenon (5). Adapted from reference 5. Copyright 2001 National Academy of Sciences, USA.

Specifically, for some types of memory an event already learned and stored in long-term memory is selectively subject to disruption when it is recalled. The basic experimental observation is that while protein synthesis inhibitors do not wipe out stored memory, the same protein synthesis inhibitor treatment will disrupt memory if the subject is simultaneously required to recall the information (see references 5 and 6). Thus, pairing protein synthesis inhibitors with a behavioral task requiring information recall can lead to a selective loss of a previously stored memory from long-term stores. The intriguing but still ill-defined process underlying this

observation is currently referred to as *reconsolidation* of memory.

Finally, to round out our terminology, we need to introduce two terms related to the loss of memories: *extinction* and *forgetting*. Forgetting is woefully familiar to most of us, and its basis is essentially unexplored. Extinction is the specific erasure of a memory in response to an environmental stimulus. Extinction has largely been studied in the context of reversal of learning. For example, if your cafeteria serves hamburgers every Monday, you will over time learn that the cafeteria always serves hamburgers on Monday. If at some later point they quit serving hamburgers on

Monday, it will take a while to readjust. Over time, you will no longer assume that if it's Monday that means hamburgers; similarly, you will no longer infer that if you're having hamburgers then it is Monday. This disassociation is an example of extinguishing a previously learned response. You will have extinguished your memory that Monday means hamburgers. Similar to forgetting, the mechanisms of extinction have not been extensively studied. One intriguing speculation is that the reconsolidation mechanism may be involved in some cases, the thinking being that perhaps reconsolidation is the process that has evolved to allow specific erasure of previously learned material, by opening up a period of susceptibility upon recall (5, 6).

II. UNCONSCIOUS LEARNING

A. Simple Forms of Learning

In this section, we will explore several "simple" (i.e., nonassociative) forms of learning. Keep in mind that even those forms of learning that exhibit themselves in a fairly straightforward manner at the behavioral level involve elaborate underlying cellular and molecular machinery. In this section, we will emphasize that several forms of nonassociative learning are exhibited by animals, including: *habituation*, *dishabituation*, and *sensitization* (see Figure 6). These forms of learning involve altered responses to a single stimulus and do not necessitate the animal forming any association between one environmental stimulus and another; that is, these forms of learning are nonassociative. They also can occur unconsciously (see Figure 2), generally requiring neither conscious perception of environmental stimuli nor conscious recall of information.

Perhaps the simplest form of learning in existence is habituation. When an animal is repeatedly presented with an innocuous environmental stimulus, over time the animal's response to that stimulus

decrements. For example, if someone from a small, quiet town moves to a street-level apartment in Manhattan, the street noises in the big city are typically disturbing at first. However, over time, the newcomer becomes accustomed to the new environment, and the street noise is no longer so bothersome. This type of phenomenon is referred to as habituation. The teleologic explanation for habituation is that over time animals learn to ignore environmental stimuli that carry no unique informational content.

Habituation is a very robust behavioral phenomenon that exhibits itself in many forms—essentially all baseline behavioral responses more complex than the purest reflex responses habituate. Some of the more well-studied habituation phenomena experimentally are habituation of the *Aplysia californica* gill-and-syphon defensive withdrawal response and habituation of reflexive leg-lifting in *Drosophila*. Habituation is also frequently encountered outside the laboratory setting; in particular,

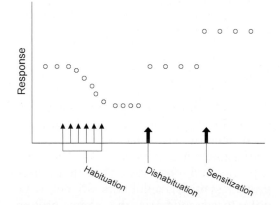

FIGURE 6 Some simple nonassociative forms of learning. Habituation, dishabituation, and sensitization are illustrated. Each circle represents a hypothetical response to an environmental stimulus. Habituation is a decrease in response (arbitrarily defined in this schematic example) with repeated presentation of the stimulus. Dishabituation is a recovery to normal baseline response when the animal receives a different environmental stimulus. Sensitization is an increase in the magnitude of the response above the original baseline.

it is frequently observed by teachers in the classroom lecture environment.

After a response is habituated, if you present another, unique stimulus, *dishabituation* can occur. For example, even after becoming habituated to street noises, if one is expecting a visitor to be dropped off at their doorstep, street noises may once again become noticeable. It is worth noting that dishabituation is a useful tool to distinguish habituation from fatigue. A habituated response can be overcome by a dishabituating stimulus; however, a decreased response due to fatigue cannot.

Animals can also learn to become hyper-responsive to an environmental stimulus, a phenomenon known as *sensitization*. Sensitization is defined as an increased response over and above the normal baseline response, that occurs in response to an environmental signal. Sensitizing stimuli typically can elicit an augmentation in response from either a nonhabituated or a habituated starting point. In the second scenario, a component of the increased responsiveness must, by definition, then be described as dishabituation (see Figure 6).

Keep in mind that in some ways the definitions of habituation, dishabituation, and sensitization are arbitrary. In the natural setting, animals are constantly modifying their behaviors in response to the ongoing barrage of environmental signals. Thus, it is difficult to determine what a "baseline" response is outside of a stringently controlled experimental setting.

All of these nonassociative forms of learning can exhibit themselves in either short- or long-term forms. The duration of the memory for a learned event depends on the number of times an animal experiences a behavior-modifying stimulus. For example, a single sensitizing stimulation may elicit sensitization that lasts only a few minutes, whereas repeated stimulations will likely result in sensitization lasting hours to days (see Figure 1.4, for example). Repeated presentations of multiple training trials can elicit sensitization lasting for weeks.

One exciting area of contemporary neurobiological research is to try to understand the basis for short- and long-term nonassociative learning. Starting in the 1960s, the mechanisms underlying habituation and sensitization began to be worked out at the cellular and biochemical level. Part of this watershed of new understanding of the basis of learning and memory came about as a result of the insight to capitalize on easily studied, simple forms of learning in special preparations that lent themselves to experimental investigation at the cellular level. In particular, the work of Eric Kandel (Figure 7) and his colleagues allowed enormous progress in our understanding of the cellular basis of behavior in general, and learning and memory specifically. Kandel and his colleagues—Jimmy Schwartz, Vince Castellucci, Jack Byrne, Tom Carew, and Bob Hawkins, along with many others—have used the simple marine mollusk *Aplysia californica* (Figure 8) to great effect to study the behavioral attributes and cellular and molecular mechanisms of learning and memory.

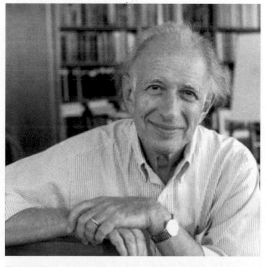

FIGURE 7 Dr. Eric Kandel. Kandel is a University Professor at Columbia University and Nobel Prize-winner who led pioneering studies on the cellular basis of learning and memory. Reprinted with permission.

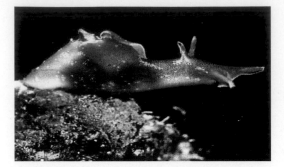

FIGURE 8 *Aplysia californica. Aplysia,* a nudibranch mollusk found in the cool waters off the coast of Calfornia, is popularized for its use in studies of simple forms of learning and memory. Photo courtesy of Dr. John Byrne, UT Houston.

A few words about the particulars of the *Aplysia* model system are appropriate at this point because we will refer to this system at later points in the book. Much (but by no means all) of the work in *Aplysia* has been geared toward understanding the basis of sensitization in this animal. *Aplysia* has on its dorsum a respiratory gill and siphon complex, which is normally extended when the animal is in the resting state. Lightly touching the gill or siphon (or experimentally squirting it with a Water-Pic) elicits a *defensive withdrawal reflex* in order to protect the gill from potential damage. This defensive withdrawal reflex can undergo both habituation (by repeated light stimuli) and sensitization. Sensitization occurs when the animal receives an aversive stimulus, for example a modest tail-shock experimentally or a predatory nip in the wild (see Box 3). After sensitizing stimulation, the animal exhibits a more robust, longer-lasting gill-withdrawal in response to the identical light touch or water squirt. Acquisition of this sensitization response is graded; repetitive sensitizing stimuli can give sensitization lasting minutes to hours (one to a few shocks) or weeks (repeated training trials over a few days) (see Figure 4). We will return to the *Aplysia* system in the later chapters of the book, where we

---

BOX 3

APLYSIA IN ITS NATURAL HABITAT

Given the popularity of *Aplysia* as an experimental system, one might be tempted to think of *Aplysia* as being indigenous to the aquaria of neurobiology labs. However, the most widely studied *Aplysia* species, *californica*, lives in the cool Pacific waters off the California coast. *Aplysia* spends its time in the tidal and near-coastal zones, where it feeds on a diet of seaweed. Except for the buffeting of the ocean waves and currents (and, one must assume, the occasional curious SCUBA diver), *Aplysia* lead a fairly peaceful existence. They are unsavory to fish and have very few natural predators; however, *Aplysia* can serve as prey to certain types of sea anemones. When an *Aplysia* is seriously perturbed, it exhibits its most dramatic behavioral response—inking.

Aplysia possess an ink gland and can release a cloud of viscous purple ink, similar to that of the well-known octopus. Although the precise function of the inking is unknown, two popular ideas are that the ink may either contain noxious compounds to help ward off predators or serve to camouflage the animal from potential attackers. A strong aversive stimulus such as one that elicits inking by *Aplysia* also results in sensitization of the animal. For some period of time after inking, an animal will exhibit enhancement of its baseline defensive withdrawal responses. This ethologically relevant form of behavior modification is the basis for laboratory study of sensitization in *Aplysia*. Figure adapted from Walters and Erickson, reference 15.

BOX 3—cont'd

APLYSIA IN ITS NATURAL HABITAT

Aplysia Inking

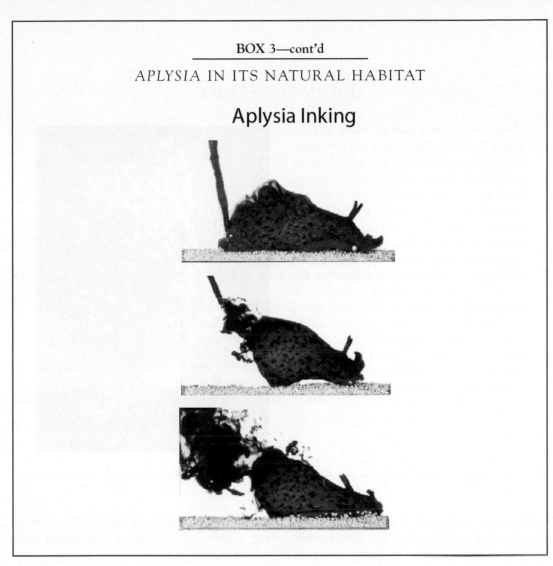

BOX 4

HERMISSENDA: THE GOOD-LOOKING ONE IN THE FAMILY

Even a dedicated neurobiologist would be hard-pressed to describe *Aplysia* as aesthetically attractive, but another popular invertebrate species used in studies of learning and memory is a clear winner in any molluscan beauty contest. With its bright coloration and striking profile, *Hermissenda* is the closest thing to a poster child available among the invertebrate species commonly studied by neurobiologists.

Continued

BOX 4—cont'd

HERMISSENDA: THE GOOD-LOOKING ONE IN THE FAMILY

Hermissenda is not just all looks and no brains, however. This system has been used to study the cellular and molecular basis of a particular form of associative learning exhibited by the animal. *Hermissenda* are normally phototactic; that is, they will move toward a lighted area. However, if the animal is trained that light predicts an upcoming aversive stimulus, in this case turbulence in the water surrounding the animal, the normal phototactic response is suppressed. The laboratories of Dan Alkon and Terry Crow have been instrumental in discovering the neuronal circuitry, cellular physiology, and molecular mechanisms underlying this form of associative conditioning. Image copyrighted by Mike Johnson. Used with permission.

will discuss several of the biochemical mechanisms underlying the short- and long-term modification of this behavioral response.

B. Unconscious Learning and Unconscious Recall

Motor learning, skills, and habits are the classic examples of unconsciously learned and unconsciously recalled memories. Walking is a good example. Walking is an extremely complex task involving intricate motor movements, which we generally perform automatically and with great facility. We learned to walk unconsciously as small children, and if anything trying to exert conscious control over our walking as adults likely leads to an awkward gait.

Another example of unconscious learning is learning to play an instrument such as the guitar or piano, at least as concerns the motor components. Repetition allows the development of finely tuned motor patterns that can be recalled without conscious thought. Learning of the motor components also occurs without much conscious control, although certainly there is conscious involvement when the initial motor patterns are beginning to be laid down. Even in this case, though, one does not consciously work out the pattern of firing of individual muscles; indeed, by and large, we don't have very much control over the contraction of single muscles and are not really conscious of them as single units. When we learn to play an instrument, a multitude of complex muscle contractions and hand movements are taking place completely below the level of conscious thought.

While complex unconscious processes go into the initial establishment of learned motor patterns, in some cases such as speech and walking, there is probably also a complicated interaction of developmental processes with signals generated in response to environmental stimuli. As mentioned earlier, in early stages of many types of motor learning, there is conscious involvement, the need for which disappears over time as part of the learning process. The circuitry and cellular mechanisms underlying motor learning are quite complex, involving the motor cortex, basal ganglia including the neostriatum, and cerebellum. We will not deal much with mechanisms of motor learning in this book. However, in later chapters, we will touch briefly on some forms of cerebellar synaptic plasticity, which is probably relevant to some forms of motor learning.

The site of memory storage for most types of motor memory are not clear but, of course, in some way, must involve or have access to the principal circuits that mediate the behavioral motor pattern, such as the motor cortex, basal ganglia, and spinal cord motor neurons. A discussion of these systems is not within the scope of this book, so I refer the reader to any of a number of good reviews and textbooks dealing with this area (Chapter 13 of reference 4 is a good place to start).

Some motor memories are subject to limited conscious recall, but in most cases trying to replay a motor memory with too much conscious control simply messes things up. This is likely a component of the common "choking" component of sports, although stress-induced release of modulatory neurotransmitters, which affect performance, is also certainly a factor. It is interesting that the unconscious aspect of motor recall has made it into popular sports lingo. When athletes are at the top of their game, they are typically referred to as being "unconscious."

C. Unconscious Learning and Subject to Conscious Recall

The forms of learning we have talked about so far are nonassociative. In habituation, sensitization, and the like, nothing is learned about the relationship or association of one event with another. We next move on to a more complex form of learning where a predictive relationship is learned—an animal learns that one environmental stimulus reliably predicts another.

An important set of nomenclature in this area arose out of the pioneering work of Ivan Pavlov. Pavlov and his co-workers studied *associative conditioning* of the salivary response of dogs—studies indeed so classic that the terms *classical conditioning* and *Pavlovian conditioning* are now used synonymously with associative conditioning. Pavlov knew, as does anyone that has ever owned a dog, that when a dog is presented with a food stimulus, a strong salivatory response is elicited (see Figure 9). This is a natural response, of course, and this salivation is referred to as the *unconditioned response* (UR), and correspondingly the food stimulus is referred to as the *unconditioned stimulus* (US). Pavlov's breakthrough realization, which he subsequently

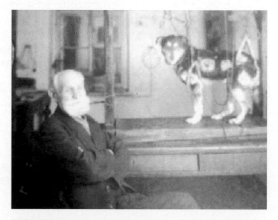

FIGURE 9 Ivan Pavlov and one of his canine subjects. Pavlov pioneered the study of associative conditioning, studying modification of reflex responses in dogs. Image courtesy of the Alan Mason Chesney Medical Archives of the Johns Hopkins Medical Institutions.

rigorously documented and studied, was that he could train dogs to associate a neutral stimulus, such as the ringing of a bell, with the food stimulus. Over time, the dog would form an association between the bell and the food, and Pavlov found that the bell alone would ultimately cause a salivatory response just like the food did. The bell-elicited salivation was termed the *conditioned response* (CR), and correspondingly the bell tone was termed the *conditioned stimulus* (CS) (Figure 10).

In associative learning, an animal learns the predictive value of one stimulus for another, in Pavlov's example the reliability of a tone for predicting a subsequent food presentation. This type of learning is profoundly important for survival in any natural environment and, for this reason, has been robustly selected for in animal evolution. Stated another way, associative learning allows the neural encoding of cause-and-effect relationships. The stable formation of a memory trace, such that an accurate record of cause-and-effect relationships is available for future reference, provides such a pronounced competitive

advantage that this form of learning is typically quite vigorous.

The importance of this last point cannot be overstated! Nature has selected for a robust capacity of nervous systems to accurately reflect one of the principal physical laws that govern the real world: cause and effect. Thus, nervous systems of all sorts have evolved, to the best of their capacity, sophisticated and robust circuit, cellular, and molecular mechanisms to encode these types of information.

Generally, associative learning is quite reliable—obviously the accuracy of storing cause-and-effect relationships is of paramount importance and has been selected for evolutionarily. This is one significant factor in the popularity of studying associative learning experimentally—the learned behaviors are observable, relatively rapidly acquired, and reliably expressed. However, this is not to say that associative learning is flawless. Numerous examples exist in the literature and anecdotally of animals having mislearned associations. For example, one of my colleagues who works with Macaque monkeys had a

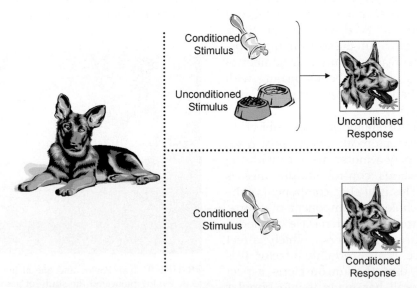

FIGURE 10 Pavlovian associative conditioning of the canine salivary response. Repeated pairings of an auditory cue with food causes the animal to learn the predictive value of one for the other. See text for details.

monkey who learned that certain visual stimuli predicted the subsequent arrival of a food reward. However, the animal also "learned" that it was necessary to wave his hand in an idiosyncratic way in order for the food reward to be delivered. Of course, in reality, the hand movement was entirely superfluous to the task and the reward delivery. B. F. Skinner recorded several similar circumstances in training pigeons in associative learning tasks, where in some cases elaborate but unnecessary motor patterns were executed before the animal pecked an object to receive a food reward. Skinner termed these behaviors "superstitious" behaviors, a somewhat loaded term that is anthropomorphic but not without appeal. Regardless of the terminology, it is clear that these are examples of associative learning gone awry. Presumably what has happened is that, early on in the training, the animal has erroneously associated some movement on their part with the food reward and formed a lasting but inaccurate memory that executing the movement is necessary to receive the reward. I bring up these examples as indications of the robustness of associative memory, but with the interesting twist, that as with all robust systems, there is an attendant possibility of error-proneness.

Against this backdrop, it is then interesting to consider that associative learning depends on two attributes of the environmental stimuli—*contiguity* and *contingency*. Contiguity refers to the property of the stimuli occurring co-incidentally, that is overlapping in time or one immediately after the other in time. This captures Nature's rule of cause and effect. Environmental stimuli generally are perceived simultaneously with or immediately after the events that cause them. Contingency refers to the ordering of the stimuli—that one stimulus consistently precedes the other in onset. This captures the predictive value of one event for the other; that is, in nature the cause will always precede the

effect. In the examples of mislearning in the previous paragraph, the animals presumably misrepresented contiguous stimuli as also being contingent.

We will return to contiguity and contingency in subsequent chapters as we delve into the molecular underpinning of learning. This is one of the areas where molecular studies have begun to yield great insight into the molecular mechanics of unique biochemical events that can be triggered by stimuli that are contiguous—close to each other in time or overlapping in time. Also, much new insight is being gained into how molecular systems can deal with the issue of order-of-pairing, that is contingency. In my mind, these examples are where the best case can be made for the beginnings of an understanding of the molecular basis of cognition.

The issue of contiguity in associative conditioning raises a consideration of two basic types of classical associative conditioning—delay conditioning and trace conditioning (see Figure 11). The type of classical associative conditioning we have discussed so far is referred to as delay conditioning. This term derives from the typical timing of this type of associative

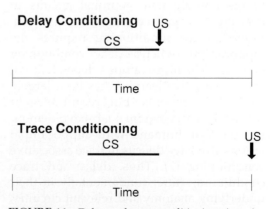

FIGURE 11   Delay and trace conditioning. Associative conditioning falls into two broad categories—delay conditioning and trace conditioning. In trace conditioning, an intervening time interval is introduced between the termination of the CS and the onset of the US. Trace conditioning involves the hippocampus.

conditioning protocol experimentally. For example, if one is training an animal to learn that a tone predicts a food reward using a delay conditioning protocol, the tone is started and maintained continuously until the food reward is presented. Thus, the onset of the CS is followed by a delay before the onset of the US. With delay conditioning, the CS and US are contiguous and overlapping—in other words, the animal receives a US simultaneously with a CS after the CS has been presented continuously for some delay period.

Trace conditioning refers to a conditioning protocol where the CS is presented, terminated, and followed after some intervening period by the US. The CS and US never overlap in time and are temporally contiguous in the sense that they are presented closely in time but never simultaneously. The term "trace" arises from the fact that some memory trace for the CS must be preserved over time so that it can subsequently be associated with the US.

The distinct use of the two terms "delay conditioning" and "trace conditioning" may seem like the typical scientific hypersemanticism because the two protocols seem so similar. However, the reasonably subtle alteration of introducing a brief intervening time-span between CS and US brings entirely new neuronal circuits to bear on the cognitive processing involved. Indeed, trace conditioning requires the hippocampus, whereas delay conditioning does not. The hippocampus-dependence of trace associative learning has been largely studied in rodents, but recent elegant studies in Larry Squire's lab have demonstrated that humans with hippocampal lesions also have deficits in trace associative conditioning (7). Thus, delay and trace conditioning differ fundamentally in their underlying anatomy and relevant circuitry, so much so that they indeed are quite different forms of learning. For this reason, making the reasonably small move from delay conditioning to trace conditioning progresses us from one category of learning to another entirely.

The recall of trace conditioning has mapped onto it a temporal component as well. Re-experiencing the CS after trace conditioning has occurred allows for conscious recollection of the US, during the "trace" period. For example, let's say that I am trained that a tone preceeds a foot shock by 5 seconds. During testing, when I hear the tone, I have 5 seconds during which I am expecting the foot shock to be delivered. Because of this aspect, I have chosen to use trace conditioning as the first example of learning that can occur unconsciously but can be subject to conscious recall (see Figure 2).

We will explore trace conditioning and similar forms of learning subject to conscious recall at many places in this book. Before proceeding to the cellular and molecular details, however, I will review the remaining major categories of learning from a behavioral perspective.

D. Operant Conditioning

Pavlov's dogs were passive participants in their learning experience. That did not have to do anything beyond perceiving the environmental stimulus, after which natural reflex took over and an unconscious salivatory response occurred. This type of learning is distinct from learning paradigms where a voluntary motor response is elicited. Conditioning where the animal is required to execute a motor response is referred to as *operant conditioning*. It is important to bear in mind that the distinction is a practical one based in experimentation. Operant conditioning simply refers to the fact that the experimenter is quantitating a voluntary movement (not a reflex) as the behavioral output indicating that learning has occurred. The examples I used earlier, where monkeys or pigeons were required to push a lever or peck a button are examples of operant conditioning. Over the years, scientists have debated whether operant conditioning will use different mechanisms from classical associative conditioning, and whether operant and classical conditioning should really be considered as distinct categories. At this point, we don't have the final answer to this question, but suffice it to say that it appears that there is no compelling reason to think that operant conditioning will require unique cellular or molecular mechanisms—likely the differences will be confined to the types of neuronal circuitry involved.

E. Currently Popular Associative Learning Paradigms

Two associative learning paradigms that are used extensively in the modern study of learning are conditioned fear (8, 9) and conditioned taste aversion (10). In both paradigms, animals learn an association between a neutral conditioned stimulus and an aversive unconditioned stimulus. Both serve as powerful examples of classical, Pavlovian conditioning, and both result in robust, long-lasting memory after even a single CS-US pairing. These two behavioral paradigms are also accommodating to researchers because the neuroanatomical pathways underlying the learning are fairly well established.

One specific example of fear conditioning involves the delivery of an innocuous acoustic cue (CS) paired with a mild foot shock (US) within a novel environment (see Figure 12). When tested 24 hours after training, rats, mice and other rodents exhibit marked fear, measured by freezing behavior or other reflex fear responses, in response to representation of either the context (*contextual fear conditioning*) or the auditory CS delivered in a different context (*cued fear conditioning*). Both cued and contextual fear conditioning have been shown to be dependent upon the amygdala, whereas contextual fear conditioning also involves the hippocampus. I will return to these two forms of learning in the next chapter where I discuss rodent behavioral models of learning in more detail.

TRAINING

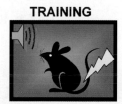

•Animal is placed in novel context
•Hears a tone
•Receives foot shock

CONTEXTUAL TEST

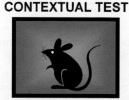

•Animal is returned to same context
•Test for freezing behavior

CUED TEST

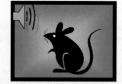

•Animal is placed in modified context
•Hears a tone
•Test for freezing behavior

FIGURE 12   Fear conditioning. Fear conditioning is a form of associative conditioning in which an aversive, fear-evoking stimulus is paired with a novel environmental cue. A wide variety of environmental stimuli can be used for fear conditioning, including places (contexts), auditory dues, visual cues, and odors. Adapted from a figure by Joel Selcher.

Conditioned taste aversion is another form of associative learning; in this case, an animal learns to associate the novel taste of a new foodstuff (CS) with subsequent illness (US) resulting from the ingestion of some toxic agent (see Figure 13). The adaptiveness of this form of learning should be apparent; by preventing subsequent ingestion of poisonous foods, survival is greatly enhanced. This is obviously a form of learning that is not very forgiving of multiple trials; not surprisingly, animals learn after a single pairing of novel taste and toxin to avoid that taste in future encounters.

One interesting aspect of conditioned taste aversion learning is the long CS-US interval. Unlike other associative conditioning paradigms such as fear conditioning or eye-blink conditioning, where the CS-US interval is typically on the order of seconds, with conditioned taste aversion the system can tolerate delays of hours between the CS taste and the US toxin. This suggests that there are cellular and biochemical events initiated by the taste stimulus alone that are likely to be long-lasting. Indeed, novel tastes alone trigger memory formation automatically, as can be measured by increased food consumption upon re-presentation of a foodstuff (Figure 13). This phenomenon is referred to as attenuation of neophobia, which we will return to shortly (11).

Finally, comparing and contrasting fear conditioning with conditioned taste aversion raises a final general attribute of associative conditioning, referred to as *salience*. We discussed earlier that contingency and contiguity are two hallmarks of associative conditioning, and "salience" is a

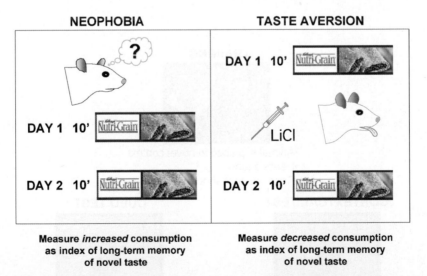

Behavioral Procedures Used to Assess Novel Taste Learning

Measure *increased* consumption as index of long-term memory of novel taste

Measure *decreased* consumption as index of long-term memory of novel taste

FIGURE 13 Taste learning. Taste learning is a robust and automatic form of learning in animals. The two types of assessments generally used to evaluate taste learning are attenuation of neophobia, in which an animal learns that a taste is not dangerous, and conditioned taste aversion, in which an animal learns that a given taste is dangerous. These can be measured experimentally by giving a single exposure to a novel food on Day 1 (10 minutes of Nutri-Grain bar in this case) and monitoring the animal's response to re-presentation of that same stimulus 24 hours later (Day 2). If the animal finds the new food to be nonaversive, consumption of the food will be increased—attenuation of neophobia. If an aversive stimulus is paired with the novel food (e.g., a lithium chloride injection), then the animal will exhibit a decreased consumption of the food on Day 2—conditioned taste aversion. See text and Chapter 2 for additional details. Diagram courtesy of Mike Swank.

term used to refer to the third general property. Salience refers to the fact that animals do not, in general, learn to associate conditioned stimuli and unconditioned stimuli that are not typically paired in their natural environment. For example, nausea-inducing stimuli are by far much more robust producers of taste aversion than are generic painful stimuli that may robustly support other types of aversive conditioning. Similarly, pairing nausea with visual stimuli or auditory cues is not very effective at aversive conditioning to these stimuli. Clearly, evolution has operated to select for robust learning of associations that can occur in the natural environment. We describe this condition in terms of the stimulus being *salient* to the animal; in other words, the stimulus is likely to be pertinent to the animal under the given condition.

Thus, in general, it is not the case that unconscious associative learning operates such that any two environmental signals can be associated. This likely arises from a combination of factors. First, there is a degree of anatomical specialization in the central nervous system (CNS) such that particular functions are parsed out into particular areas. Thus, as a practical matter the central processing of two environmental stimuli may never "touch" each other in the brain and, therefore, can never be associated. In this instance, the stimuli "touching" each other can be taken quite literally in that some anatomical cross-connection must be made. Conversely, for any association to take place, the underlying neural circuits processing the environmental information must be able to connect anatomically. It is only possible to draw an associative learning circuit if the two stimuli being paired impinge upon each other at some point.

This seems like a statement of something that is intuitively obvious. However, my point here is that there is no such thing as an anatomical connection in the brain. There are only *molecular* connections. If associative learning requires that two information-processing circuits connect with each other, this connection must of necessity utilize molecular and chemical processes. A description of these types of processes, in particular molecular mechanisms that can contribute to associative events, is a central theme of later chapters of this book.

Overall, we have seen in this section that various models of associative conditioning have transitioned us from unconscious processes to conscious processes. Many associations can be learned unconsciously and expressed unconsciously. However, various types of associative learning begin to recruit conscious processes as well. Even though they are learned unconsciously, they can be recalled consciously. As a generalization, the transition involves recruitment of the hippocampus into the learning process. In the following section, we will move on to even more complex forms of learning that also depend on the hippocampus.

III. CONSCIOUS LEARNING—SUBJECT TO CONSCIOUS AND UNCONSCIOUS RECALL

A. Declarative Learning

Human declarative learning is what we typically think of when we think of "learning." This is the conscious acquisition of new facts, or the formation of memories for events that occur in our lives, that are available for subsequent recall at will. The extent to which you remember what you read in this book will depend upon the processes of conscious declarative learning. Of course, the extent to which you remember this book will also depend on a large number of other factors, such as motivation, attention, and level of arousal. Thus, human declarative learning, and likely most analogous forms of learning in animals, is subject to a wide variety of modulatory factors.

For example, particularly robust memory for single events is typically referred to as "flashbulb" memory in humans. Most Americans have shared several examples of this type of memory, the most recent example being the terrorist destruction of the Twin Towers in New York City. Like most people, I remember vividly how I learned of the attacks, and I am sure I will never forget seeing live on television the second tower collapse. Flashbulb memories are usually associated with a high state of arousal or a high level of emotional valence—an example of the strong modulatory influences to which learning is subject to.

As are the other types of conscious learning we will discuss in this section, declarative learning is dependent upon the hippocampus. In later sections of the book we will return to the importance of modulatory influences on hippocampus-dependent learning and discuss some likely molecular mechanisms underlying this effect.

It is difficult to model declarative learning in nonhuman animals because the behavioral output for these types of memories is actually quite subtle. In most cases, it is not even clear what the relevant types of learning might be in lower animals. In part for this reason, most of what we know about declarative learning comes from human studies, in particular studies of patients with hippocampal lesions.

Because I am largely focusing on studies in rodents in this book, I am not going to go into much detail on these important and interesting human studies. Moreover, there have been many excellent reviews of these types of studies and their relationship to learning and memory theory (see references 1, 2, 4, 12, and 13). Suffice it to say for our purposes that a number of classic studies of humans with hippocampal lesions led to the dissociation of declarative from nondeclarative forms of memory in humans.

Declarative memory is that type of memory that is lost when a human suffers hippocampal damage—this includes the capacity to form memories for facts, names, places, and personal experiences (Figure 3). Hippocampal damage results in *anterograde amnesia* for these types of memories; that is, there is a loss of the capacity to form new memories. Old memories (> about 1 year) are largely spared (i.e., there is relatively little *retrograde* amnesia). Nondeclarative forms of memory such as sensitization, motor learning, and delay classical conditioning are spared in humans with hippocampal lesions.

It is difficult to imagine a rodent model for declarative memory, but there is one potentially parallel type of learning in rodents that I will mention briefly. Because toxic plants and other poisonous foodstuffs coexist with most animals, conditioned taste aversion evolved to protect animals from poisoning themselves out of the gene pool. However, avoidance of something that is toxic is not possible if it has been ingested in lethal quantities, so a supplementary behavior has also evolved to protect animals from toxic foods. *Neophobia* is the characteristic fear of novel foods, and ensures that animals ingest only small quantities, as if to sample the food to determine if it is safe to eat. If the animal develops illness, a conditioned taste aversion results, and this foodstuff will be avoided on future encounters. If no illness results, and assuming the food is reasonably palatable, animals will increase their intakes on subsequent exposures. This is readily demonstrated in the laboratory. When rats or mice are presented with highly palatable solutions of novel tastes such saccharin or sucrose, they will consume small amounts on the first exposure; on subsequent exposures, the animals consume more (Figure 13). This attenuation of neophobia is a behavioral measure of memory for the novel taste and is part of a process of familiarization to the formerly novel taste. There is a fairly clear consensus that the insular cortex is the primary site of learning and memory for novel tastes, so this form of learning is clearly not strictly analogous to human declarative learning.

However, it does depend on the cerebral cortex as its storage site, as is likely in human declarative memory. Furthermore, it is reasonably analogous to a human learning a "fact," in this case what something tastes like, and having that information available for conscious recall.

Finally, declarative learning is generally associative, although not in the sense of classical associative conditioning where a cause-and-effect relationship is learned. Most declarative learning does not take place in a cognitive vacuum, but items are typically learned in the context of other related facts or objects. A good example is learning someone's name. Learning a name is a declarative learning event certainly, and you can list off the names of all the people you know well as a reiteration of a list of "facts." However, each name also serves as a descriptor of an individual and is associated with that person, their face, their house, and so on. This type of multiple association for learned facts (i.e., declarative learning) is the rule rather than the exception. It is likely that most declarative learning occurs as learning something within a variety of contexts (i.e., other facts or places with which the fact is associated). I stress this point because it is important to keep it in mind as we begin to explore the molecular basis for declarative learning. Certainly, many of the molecular mechanisms that are discovered as subserving what we have defined as *associative* conditioning may translate directly as mechanisms for declarative learning. Stated more strongly, at this point, it is appropriate to hypothesize that associative molecular mechanisms will be part of the molecular infrastructure of declarative learning.

B. Spatial Learning

Another example of hippocampus-dependent learning in both humans and lower animals is spatial learning. Obviously animals must learn to navigate their environment and learn to associate particular places with particular items or events. This type of learning has been the classically defined learning system in which the hippocampus is involved. A wide variety of different studies have shown that molecular or anatomical lesions of the hippocampus lead to spatial learning deficits in both humans and lower animals. Also, direct measurements of a wide variety of molecular and physiologic changes have been shown to correlate with spatial learning. Much of this behavioral literature for humans and lower animals has been nicely covered in recent texts by Squire and Kandel (1) and Eichenbaum and Cohen (4), so I will not reiterate the details here.

In the next chapter, I will delve in more detail into rodent learning paradigms that probe spatial learning, such as the Morris water maze and contextual learning. In fact, much of this book deals with hippocampus-dependent learning, synaptic plasticity, and molecular regulation. This book will be strongly biased toward hippocampal synaptic plasticity and hippocampus-dependent learning and memory for several reasons. We have the most detailed understanding of the pertinent molecular mechanisms of hippocampal synaptic plasticity, and, of course, this book is focused on trying to understand memory at that level. Even though it may seem conterintuitive, I am also focusing on hippocampus-dependent memory formation because these memory processes are the least understood at the cellular and circuit levels.

Compared to the amygdala and cerebellum, for example, our understanding of the hippocampal neuronal circuit in mediating behavior is rudimentary. For me this is not a negative, but rather the hippocampus becomes a great frontier to be explored. The hippocampus and associated cortices are involved in conscious learning and memory. This is in contrast to the better-understood amygdala and cerebellum, where the systems operate in simpler and in most cases *unconscious* learning. Understanding the hippocampus, including its associated circuitry and molecular and cellular function, is likely to give us the greatest insights into higher-level cognitive function. This is the most appealing aspect of studying the hippocampus and a principal reason for the focus of this book on hippocampal processes.

IV. FINAL NOTE—WILL MOLECULAR STUDIES CHANGE THE WAY WE THINK ABOUT LEARNING BEHAVIOR?

Finally, a comparison and contrast of behavioral learning studies with biochemical learning studies is in order. The advent of new technologies has made it possible to measure distinct biochemical changes in particular brain regions in the CNS in response to environmental stimuli. The behavioral parts of these studies typically are based on behavioral protocols established over time to study learning and memory. The general design of the experiments is to use an established behavioral paradigm such as associative conditioning to measure some biochemical change in the brain. This approach has great appeal of course because one can do parallel experiments to control for the training protocol eliciting learning and memory formation. One also can perform additional parallel experiments where, for example, one can show that blocking the molecular change with an inhibitory drug leads to a disruption of the learning or memory.

Doing these types of studies based on the long-standing behavioral literature leads to an interesting problem, however. These types of behavioral studies have well-established behavioral control experiments that go along with them. For example, consider cued fear conditioning. In this paradigm, you give the animal a pairing of noise cue preceding foot shock. The animal of course learns that the noise (conditioned stimulus, CS) predicts the foot shock (unconditioned stimulus, US). The foot shock elicits a behavioral response,

freezing (unconditioned response, UR), and after training the noise (CS) then elicits the same response (conditioned response, CR). One type of behavioral control experiment that you typically do along with this conditioning protocol is "backward pairing," where you give CS and US identically except with a reverse order. In this case, re-presentation of the CS (noise) does not cause the conditioned response (freezing) behaviorally—the animal has not learned that the noise predicts the foot shock because it in fact does not. Thus, with this experiment, you demonstrate that the conditioned response is specifically elicited only when the animal receives paired training in the correct order and can eliminate possible alternative explanations such as a general arousal effect of sensitization.

But now consider the same experiment where one is measuring a learning-associated molecular change in the nervous system. You pair noise and foot shock in that order and observe some specific molecular change in the brain—in this thought experiment, the animal uses this molecular mechanism to store the information that noise predicts foot shock. You do the "backward pairing" control where you give foot shock and then noise and observe the same molecular change. Does this mean that the animal is not using this mechanism for information storage? No. Perhaps the animal is using this same molecular mechanism to store the information that foot shock predicts noise.

I use this example to illustrate that it is not straightforward to map control experiments developed for behavioral studies measuring a behavioral output onto behavioral studies measuring a molecular output in the brain. In measuring behavioral outputs, we use the animal itself as a filter— can nicely design my experiment to measure a behavior that is selectively expressed in response to one environmental stimulus and not another. We do not have this luxury in looking at molecular events triggered in the nervous system. Anytime learning of any sort occurs, it will be reflected as a set of molecular changes in the animal's nervous system.

Moreover, the molecular mechanisms for learning one type of contingency are likely to be the same ones used for learning any other type of contingency. Most of the types of control experiments done in learning studies using a behavioral index of learning are likely to lead to the animal learning a variety of different things, it's just that none of them lead to the behavioral output being measured. Nevertheless, all those many things the animal is learning are being encoded in meaningful molecular changes in their nervous system.

I raise these issues to make several points. First, molecular studies of learning and memory using the behaving animal are at a very early stage—in fact only relatively few such studies have been published (at least in mammalian systems). Advancing into this area, and similarly for studies using real-time brain imaging, will require some rethinking of how to design appropriate controls when there is experimentally such an all-encompassing read-out. We will not necessarily be able to map the tried-and-tested behavioral control paradigms directly onto these new systems. Second, this may necessitate some reevaluation of learning and memory terminology in general, with molecular aspects taken into consideration. For example, it is difficult to apply the terms CS, US, CR, and UR in a molecular study (measuring molecular changes in the brain in response to environmental stimuli) in a way that is strictly analogous to their application to behavioral studies. Even though a CS that gives no UR behaviorally can be selected, it is likely that every CS gives an UR at the molecular level in the nervous system. In the limit, this rethinking may have to extend to the definitions of learning and memory as well. We started the chapter by defining learning and memory in behavioral terms. It is certainly premature at this point, but in the future it may be necessary to refine the definitions to take molecules into consideration.

References

1. Squire, L. R., and Kandel, E. R. (1999). *Memory: from mind to molecules*. New York: Scientific American Library: Distributed by W. H. Freeman and Co.
2. Eichenbaum, H. (2001). "The hippocampus and declarative memory: cognitive mechanisms and neural codes." *Behav. Brain Res.* 127:199–207.
3. Kandel, E. R., and Squire, L. R. (2000). "Neuroscience: breaking down scientific barriers to the study of brain and mind." *Science* 290:1113–1120.
4. Eichenbaum, H., and Cohen, N. J. (2001). *From conditioning to conscious recollection : memory systems of the brain*. New York: Oxford University Press.
5. Vianna, M. R., Szapiro, G., McGaugh, J. L., Medina, J. H., and Izquierdo, I. (2001). "Retrieval of memory for fear-motivated training initiates extinction requiring protein synthesis in the rat hippocampus." *Proc. Natl. Acad. Sci. USA* 98:12251–12254.
6. Nader, K., Schafe, G. E., and LeDoux, J. E. (2000). "The labile nature of consolidation theory." *Nat. Rev. Neurosci.* 1:216–219.
7. Clark, R. E., and Squire, L. R. (1998). "Classical conditioning and brain systems: the role of awareness." *Science* 280:77–81.
8. LeDoux, J. E. (2001). Synaptic self : how our brains become who we are. New York: Viking.
9. Quirk, G. J., Repa, C., and LeDoux, J.E. (1995). "Fear conditioning enhances short-latency auditory responses of lateral amygdala neurons: parallel recordings in the freely behaving rat." *Neuron* 15:1029–1039.
10. Berman, D. E., and Dudai, Y. (2001). "Memory extinction, learning anew, and learning the new: dissociations in the molecular machinery of learning in cortex." *Science* 291:2417–2419.
11. Swank, M. W., and Sweatt, J. D. (2001). "Increased histone acetyltransferase and lysine acetyltransferase activity and biphasic activation of the ERK/RSK cascade in insular cortex during novel taste learning." *J. Neurosci.* 21:3383–3391.
12. Eichenbaum, H. (1999). "The hippocampus and mechanisms of declarative memory." *Behav. Brain Res.* 103:123–133.
13. Milner, B., Squire, L. R., and Kandel, E. R. (1998). "Cognitive neuroscience and the study of memory." *Neuron* 20:445–468.
14. Kandel, E. R. (2001). "The molecular biology of memory storage: a dialogue between genes and synapses." *Science* 294:1030–1038.
15. Walters, E. T., and Erickson, M. T. (1986). "Directional control and the functional organization of defensive responses in Aplysia." *J. Comp. Physiol. A.* 159:339–351.

Lashley Maze
J. David Sweatt, Acrylic on canvas, 2002

Rodent Behavioral Learning and Memory Models

I. INTRODUCTION

The study of learning and memory requires the development and use of experimental model systems that can be utilized both to characterize the fundamental behaviors associated with memory and to explore the underlying mechanisms. In this chapter, we will transition from the abstract discussion of the last chapter into a discussion of real-life systems used experimentally and will focus on *behavioral* model systems for the study of learning and memory. We will limit our discussion to rodent model systems, particularly those involving rats and mice, because essentially all the cellular and molecular studies that comprise the rest of the book utilized rats and mice. We also will focus largely on learned behaviors that involve the hippocampus, although some other paradigms will also be described briefly. Thus, this chapter sets the stage for the next chapter, where we will begin to discuss examples of hippocampal cellular plasticity that have been extensively studied and that are hypothesized to be involved in hippocampus-dependent learning and memory.

Our current understanding is based on a foundation laid many years ago. During the beginning and middle of the last century, studies by a number of experimental psychologists led to an explosive advancement of our understanding of the basics of learned behaviors. Classic studies by Pavlov, Skinner, and Lashley, to name a few who used nonhuman models, laid the foundation for much of modern laboratory memory research. These studies even received a reasonable degree of public recognition—there's a line from a Rolling Stones song that goes "Girl, when you call my name, I salivate like Pavlov's dog." How many experiments have ever reached that level of popular recognition? These studies have reached the level of iconism; running rats through mazes is now symbolic in the public eye of neuroscience studies in general.

Of course, rat maze learning is but the tip of the iceberg of modern rodent behavioral research. In this chapter, we will discuss a number of specific examples of contemporary rodent behavioral paradigms used to study learning and memory. In reviewing these models, it is important to always keep in mind that when we do a memory experiment at least three things are happening with the animal: they are learning (forming a memory), they have generated a stable record of the event (a memory), and they are recalling the memory in order to produce a detectable read-out. The complexity of these several processes is in many ways obscured by the apparent simplicity of the learning behaviors themselves.

II. BEHAVIORAL ASSESSMENTS IN RODENTS

A. Fear Conditioning

One popular behavioral model system with which to study learning and memory is a robust learning paradigm that capitalizes on the capacity of mammals, including rodents, to associate environmental cues with a mild aversive stimulus. This type of learning, generally called fear conditioning, is an example of classical associative conditioning similar to Pavlovian conditioning. Some aspects of the neuronal circuitry underlying this behavior have been worked out and it is clear that the amygdala is involved in memory formation in this behavior (see references 1 and 2 for example). In addition, the fear-conditioning paradigm has been quite fruitful of late as a model in which to study molecular mechanisms underlying learning and memory, as we will return to repeatedly in this book. One final reason for the high level of enthusiasm for pursuing this behavioral paradigm is its potential relevance as a model system for human anxiety disorders.

Cue-Plus-Contextual Fear Conditioning

A typical fear conditioning experiment proceeds as follows. Animals are placed in a fear-conditioning apparatus for about 2 minutes, then a 30-second acoustic CS (tone or preferably white noise, but light cues can also be used) is delivered. During the last 2 seconds of the tone, a mild foot shock (US) is applied to the floor grid. This pairing protocol can be repeated with a brief intervening period (e.g., 2 minutes) between pairings. The stimulus strength and number of training pairs are typically chosen based on pilot experiments to optimize learning without overtraining the animals. When trained in this fashion, the animals learn at least two things. One thing they learn is that the training chamber is bad news; that is, that the context in which they are trained is a place to be feared. Another thing that they learn is that the noise or light CS predicts an upcoming foot shock, and thus it also is to be feared. These two components of the learning are referred to as contextual and cued fear conditioning, respectively (see Figure 1).

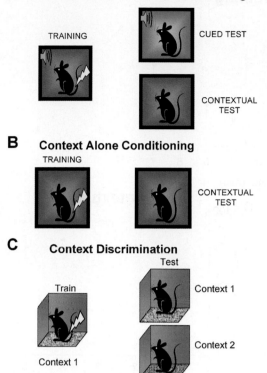

A Cue-Plus-Contextual Fear Conditioning

TRAINING

CUED TEST

CONTEXTUAL TEST

B Context Alone Conditioning

TRAINING

CONTEXTUAL TEST

C Context Discrimination

Test

Train

Context 1

Context 2

Context 1

FIGURE 1 Variants of fear conditioning in rodents. See text for details.

Cued Fear Conditioning

Cued fear learning is assessed by quantitating the amount of fearful behavior exhibited by the animal following re-presentation of the CS, when the CS is presented in a different context from that in which the training took place. This use of a different context is important to isolate the cued conditioning from the contextual conditioning: a variation is to habituate the animal to the fear-conditioning apparatus before presenting the CS-US pairing (see reference 3 for example).

Increased fearful behavior upon later re-presentation of the CS is an indication of the animal having formed a lasting association between the CS cue and the fear-evoking stimulus. To assess cue learning, animals are placed in a context different from the training context (e.g., novel odor, cage floor, and visual cues or alternatively a context similar the the home cage) and baseline behavior is measured for a few (e.g., 3) minutes. Then the acoustic CS is presented for about 3 minutes, and learning is assessed by measuring fearful behavior every 5 seconds (see Figure 2).

To assess short-term cue learning, the animals are typically placed in the non-training context 1–2 hours following the completion of the training session and fear assessed in response to re-presentation of the acoustic or light CS. Long-term cue learning can be tested 24 hours to several weeks later.

How does one assess the fearful behavior indicative of learning? There are two basic ways to assess fear in rodents: freezing and startle potentiation. Freezing is a stereotyped immobile posture exhibited by rats and mice when they are fearful; it is readily recognizable to a trained human observer. In this case, the scorer of the behavioral experiments should, of course, be blind in reference to whether the animal is a control or an experimental. The other variation for assessing fear in rodents is measuring fear-associated potentiation of their normal startle response, which can be quantitated automatically using a variety of devices. Potentiation of the animal's normal startle response to a loud noise, by re-presentation of the CS (light for example) is one of the standard indices of cue-evoked fear. Anyone who has ever watched a Hollywood "slasher" movie is familiar with fear potentiated startle.

Contextual Fear Conditioning

To assess contextual learning, the animals are placed back into the training context post-training and scored for fear behavior for a short period of time, typically a few minutes to minimize extinction of their fear of the context (see Figures 1–3). Similar to cued fear conditioning, contextual fear conditioning exhibits short-term and long-term forms.

It also is possible to train animals using a context-alone variant (see Figures 1 and 3).

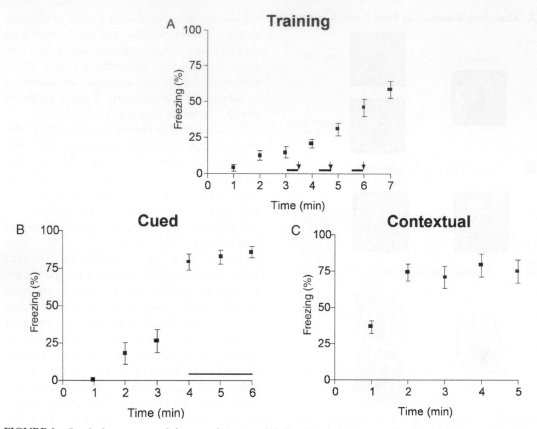

FIGURE 2   Cued-plus-contextual fear conditioning. (A) Freezing behavior on the day of training. The white noise CS is presented for the three periods of time underlined. Foot shocks are presented at the arrows. Stereotyped freezing posture is scored visually and expressed as percent of time spent freezing. (B) Freezing in response to CS presentation on day 2 after training. For these experiments the animals are in a different context than that in which they were trained. The period of white noise (CS) presentation is indicated by the line. (C) Freezing in response to replacement in the training context. The animal is placed in the context at $t = 0$. All panels: Results shown are for C57Bl6 animals, mean ± SEM for $n = 10$ animals. Freezing is scored every 5 seconds and averaged over 1-minute epochs. Data from Weeber et al. (5).

The procedures are essentially the same as the context-plus-cued paradigm, but no visual or auditory cue is delivered when the animal is trained. With this procedure, the animal learns to fear the training context—upon re-placement into the training context the animal exhibits marked freezing.

There is good evidence indicating that contextual fear conditioning is hippocampus-dependent, mostly based on lesioning studies, selective infusion of pharmacological agents into the hippocampus, and animals genetically engineered to have

hippocampal deficits. However, the point of the hippocampal dependence of contextual fear conditioning is still somewhat controversial. A certain amount of controversy is perhaps not surprising given the ill-defined nature of the "context." Generally what is meant by context is a multimodal representation of the training environment. Of course, an individual animal may simply be associating a single aspect of the training environment with the foot shock, in essence converting contextual conditioning into cued conditioning for a

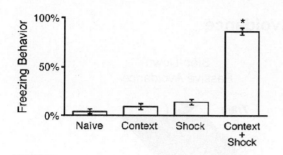

FIGURE 3 Contextual fear conditioning in rats. Rats were placed in the fear-conditioning chamber for 2 minutes, then a 1-second shock (1.5 mA) was delivered to the floor grid. This protocol was repeated for a total of five shocks with 2 minutes between each shock. Following the fifth shock, the subject remained in the training chamber for 1 minute and was removed to its home cage. Results shown are an assessment of fear conditioning 24 hours after training. Freezing behavior was measured every 10 seconds for 5 minutes, 24 hours after exposure to the contextual fear conditioning paradigm. One control group of animals ("Context") was exposed to the conditioning chamber for the same amount of time as the fear conditioned group but did not receive any shocks. A second control group ("Shock") was shocked (5 sec, 1.5 mA) immediately upon placement into the conditioning chamber and immediately removed. "Naïve" animals were not exposed to the fear-conditioning chamber, nor did they receive an electric shock. Exposing animals to the contextual fear-conditioning paradigm significantly enhanced freezing behavior in animals 24 hours after training that paired the context and electric shock, but did not affect freezing behavior of animals that received either the context or shock alone, relative to naïve animals (Fig. 4A; F[3,24] = 226.6, p < 0.0001). Data from Levenson et al. (15).

single visual or olfactory cue in the training apparatus. To help get around this problem, a variant of contextual fear conditioning called *context discrimination* has been developed (4). In this variant, an animal is tested in the training environment and also in another environment that shares some of the same cues as the training environment. The testing thus allows one to determine if the animal has learned to distinguish two similar environments from each other. The available evidence indicates that context discrimination is very sensitive to hippocampal deficits.

In experiments where one is looking for learning deficits in an experimental animal, a variety of behavioral control experiments are necessary to bolster any conclusion that animals are deficient in learning or memory versus simply having derangements of normal sensory or motor function. A wide variety of these experiments are described in the last section of this chapter. However, one simple control is to monitor animals during the training phase of fear conditioning, for example by assessing the freezing of the animal in response to presentation of the foot shock (see Figure 2). Normal animals exhibit a freezing response to foot shock presentation. Normal freezing by an experimental animal during training indicates that they are able to at least sense the foot shock and to freeze normally.

As an additional control in experiments where a learning deficit is indicated, one can undertake a retraining experiment. Thus, you simply retrain the same animals that exhibited a learning deficit using a more vigorous training protocol in order to assess whether they are capable of fear conditioning at all. The goal in retraining experiments is to control for the potential confound that an apparent fear-conditioning deficit is simply due to an inability of experimental animals to exhibit the freezing or fear-potentiated startle that is quantitated as an index of learning. With retraining or overtraining, if the animal ultimately learns, you can conclude that at least they are capable of exhibiting the learned behavior. It is also reasonable to infer that they are capable of sensing the environmental stimuli, although one possible explanation for a necessity for overtraining is that the animal has sensory deficits.

Passive avoidance training can also be used as a "control" for cued fear conditioning, although it also is a learning model in its own right as well. In this test (see the next section and Figure 4), animals learn to suppress their normal dark-seeking reflex because their entry into a dark chamber is paired with a foot shock. This control is

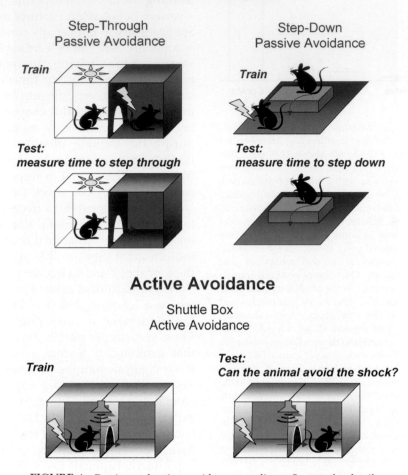

FIGURE 4   Passive and active avoidance paradigms. See text for details.

particularly appealing because it can be set up to use the identical aversive sensory stimulus (foot shock) as cued fear conditioning. Passive avoidance is not as well suited as a control for contextual fear conditioning because both tasks are likely to involve the hippocampus and share some underlying mechanisms, although manipulations have been found that can lead to selective deficits in passive avoidance versus contextual fear conditioning (see reference 5 for example).

In summary for this section, fear conditioning is a robust form of classical conditioning exhibited by rodents. Cued conditioning can be used as an index of general associative learning that is amygdala-dependent but hippocampus-independent. Context-dependent conditioning is a variant to assess a likely hippocampus-dependent form of learning. The initial responses of the animal during and immediately after the training period also serve as a good screen for sensory responses to the foot shock and for the ability of the animal to exhibit fearful behavior.

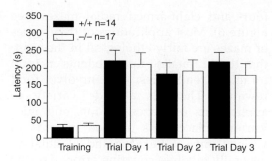

FIGURE 5   Passive avoidance. This test utilizes the natural tendency for mice to retreat from a lighted area to darker area during the training session. Upon entering the dark area, a mild foot shock is given, and learning is assessed as the avoidance of the dark area following the training session. Passive avoidance was tested by measuring step-through latencies from a lighted compartment to a dark compartment when the animals are re-placed into the avoidance chamber. Results are shown as step-through latency during trial sessions 1, 2, or 3 days following training for PKCβ deficient mice (□) or wildtype mice (■), mean ± SEM. Data from Weeber et al. (5). Both control and knockout animals successfully learned to avoid the darkened half of the chamber.

B. Avoidance Conditioning

In the passive avoidance learning test, rodents learn to suppress their natural tendency to seek out dark areas over well-lit areas after being exposed to the pairing of a mild foot shock with the animals' passage into the dark area from the well-lit one. One typical variation is referred to as the *step-through passive avoidance task* (see Figures 4 and 5). Animals are placed in a conditioning chamber separated into two compartments, one illuminated (e.g., by a 75-W light bulb) and one dark. The two sides are separated by a guillotine-type partition. On the training day, animals are placed into the illuminated side of the conditioning apparatus and the amount of time it takes to move into the dark compartment, called the step-through latency, is measured. Once a subject has passed into the dark chamber, the partition is lowered and the animal receives a foot shock through the grid floor. After 10 seconds in the dark compartment, the animal is removed and returned to its home cage. Various periods of time later, each animal is tested for associating the darkened chamber with the foot shock by measuring their step-through latency upon re-placement into the lit side of the conditioning chamber.

Another variation of passive avoidance is referred to as *step-down avoidance*. During one-trial step-down avoidance training, animals are placed on an elevated platform and given a mild foot shock when they step off the platform onto the grid below. Memory is then assessed by the latency to step off the platform following training. Both step-down avoidance and step-through avoidance learning are subject to disruption with hippocampal lesions.

Much more elaborate avoidance conditioning paradigms that involve active avoidance on the part of the animal have also been developed. Because specific directed behavior on the part of the animal is required, active avoidance is, of course, an example of operant conditioning. In one popular active avoidance paradigm, an apparatus called a *shuttle-box* is used. In the shuttle-box paradigm animals are trained to move from one side of the apparatus to the other in order to avoid foot shock. The trigger for movement can be linked to various CS cues such as light or sound, or the animal can simply learn that it must periodically change sides within a given time period. Interestingly, several different types of operant learning such as active avoidance in a shuttle box are actually enhanced by hippocampal lesions.

C. Simple Maze Learning

The study of maze learning in rodents has always played a prominent role in experimental psychology, so much so that in some ways it can be considered the archetypal experiment in the field. From a historical perspective, this can be illustrated nicely by Karl Lashley's use of maze learning in his studies to try to find the anatomical locus of the engram—the engram being defined as the finite locus for memory storage in the central nervous system. Lashley undertook a number of studies of maze learning in rats and of memory storage for previously learned mazes. His basic experiment was to induce lesions of the cerebral cortex and evaluate the subsequent effects on learning and memory in rats learning or remembering the location of food rewards in mazes of increasing complexity. These pioneering studies were some of the first studies to illustrate the complexity of learning and memory, for Lashley found that no single cortical locus for learning or memory could be found using this approach. At best, memory loss could be related in a general sense to the extent of the lesioned area. These studies ultimately led to the currently held view that complex memories are held in (or at least accessed by) broadly distributed loci in the central nervous system.

Fast-forwarding to the current day, a wide variety of mazes containing food rewards are still gainfully employed in behavioral studies of rodent learning and memory. Popular variations include "T"-shaped mazes of various sorts, and four- and eight-armed radial mazes (see Figure 6). Most applications of these types of mazes are fairly ethological in the sense that they capitalize upon rodents' natural foraging tendencies and involve food rewards. There is a wide variety of applications of mazes for rats and mice learning placements of food rewards in various limbs of the maze, and quantitation generally involves counting errors (i.e., the animal entering places in the maze where they should know, based on prior experience, that no food is available). Also, manipulating the delay period between training and testing is commonly used to parse short-term memory from long-term memory, and variations in the use of distal spatial cues can assess the role of this type of information in the learning process.

Overall, maze learning has been widely used to probe for the role of the hippocampus in rodent learning and memory, using a wide variety of types of lesions to the CNS. Also, maze learning has lent itself well to studies where hippocampal cellular responses are recorded *in vivo* in real time as the animal learns and remembers. Using these approaches along with others, hippocampal "place cells"

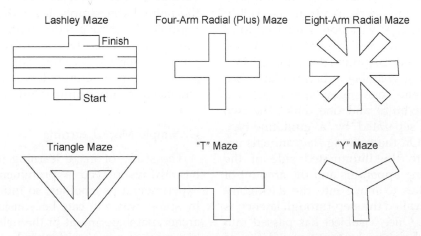

FIGURE 6   Types of mazes. A few representative types of rodent mazes are shown for illustrative purposes. Most of these mazes are used in conjunction with food rewards located at specific positions in the maze.

(i.e., hippocampal pyramidal neurons that fire specifically when an animal occupies a specific spatial location) have been identified. We will return to behaviorally identified patterns of hippocampal neuron firing later when we discuss neuronal firing patterns that are capable of eliciting long-lasting changes in synaptic function in the hippocampus. Various types of maze learning and attendant insights from *in vivo* recording during maze learning have recently received sophisticated treatment by Eichenbaum and Cohen (6), so I refer the reader to this text for more detailed discussion. We also will discuss these experiments in more detail in the next chapter.

D. Spatial Learning

The Morris Maze

Richard Morris has developed a "water" maze that is now a classic test of spatial learning in rodents (7). The Morris water maze is a hippocampus-dependent spatial learning task in which mice or rats are required to learn to locate an escape platform in a pool of water, using visual cues surrounding the maze (see Figure 7). The basic set-up is a circular shallow pool full of opaque water with an escape platform hidden just under the surface of the water so that it is not visible to the animal. Animals are placed in the pool at either constant or varying starting positions and forced to swim because the water is just deep enough that they cannot touch the bottom. Similarly, the walls of the pool are high enough that they cannot climb out. Rodents, while they are generally good swimmers, of course prefer to be on a stable platform out of the water. In initial training trials, by random chance most animals bump into the hidden platform and can thus escape the water. Those who don't find the platform by luck (usually swims are limited to a 1-minute duration) are retrieved from the water by the experimenter and manually placed on the platform.

For the *hidden platform version* of the task, a typical training protocol generally consists of two blocks of four training trials a day with an interblock interval of approximately 1 hour (see Figure 8). Subjects are released into the pool from 1 of 4 starting positions, and the location of the platform remains constant throughout training. The training is given for about 6 consecutive days. Time to find the escape platform is measured. Mice and rats display significant improvement in their performance in locating the hidden platform over the several blocks of training trials (Figure 8A), as assessed by the animals' *escape latencies* (i.e., the time taken to locate the escape platform).

To determine if animals are using a spatial learning strategy to locate the escape platform, they are subjected to "probe" trials after training (see Figure 8B, C). In the probe test, the platform is removed, and animals are allowed to search the pool for 60 seconds. Quadrant

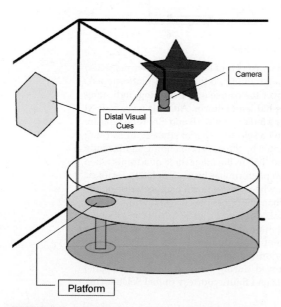

FIGURE 7 Morris water maze. The basic components of the Morris water maze system include visual cues on the walls, a monitoring camera, a pool with opaque water, and a hidden platform.

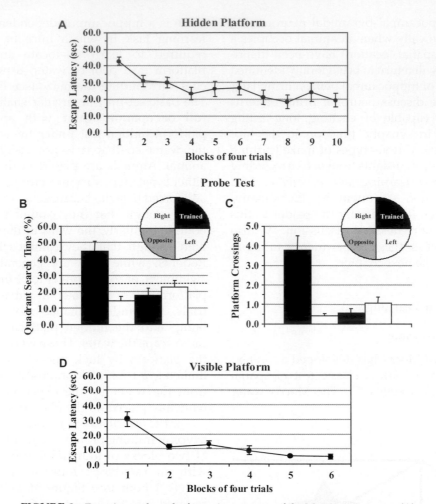

FIGURE 8   Experimental results for various aspects of the Morris water maze. (A) Average escape latency was assessed during training on the hidden platform task. Performance for mice (n = 13) improved over the course of the training, indicating learning of the task and the location of the hidden platform. Animals were trained using ten blocks of four training trials, over a 5-day period. (B and C) Probe tests are used to assess whether the animal has used a selective spatial strategy in learning the task. A selective search strategy is indicated by the subject spending significantly more time searching in the trained quadrant than in the other three quadrants when they are placed in the tank, after the hidden platform has been completely removed (see text). The subject also crosses the area where the platform had been during the training sessions significantly more often than they cross the corresponding areas in the other quadrants. During the probe trials on days 4 and 5, mice (n = 13) spent significantly more time searching in the trained quadrant (B) and crossed the platform area in the trained quadrant more frequently than in any of the alternate quadrants (C). (D) Average escape latency during training on the visible platform task. Performance for mice (n = 5) improved during training in this nonspatial variant of the Morris water maze task. Data and figure courtesy of Joel Selcher (16).

search time and platform crossings are assessed to characterize a subject's search behavior during the probe trial. The quadrant search measure is obtained by conceptually dividing the pool into four equal quadrants and then measuring the amount of time that the subject spends searching in each quadrant. The platform crossing measure is the number of times a subject crosses the exact place where the platform had been located during training. For comparison, the number of times a subject crosses the equivalent location in the other quadrants is determined. Animals that have learned the (now presumed) location of the underwater platform spend significantly more time searching in the trained quadrant than in each of the other three quadrants (Figure 8B). They also cross the place where the platform had been located during training significantly more often than the corresponding place in the other quadrants (Figure 8C). Thus, animals that have learned the location of the platform selectively search in the correct quadrant.

Modern automated monitoring systems also allow the acquisition of additional control data during the probe trials. For example, one can monitor the swimming behavior of each animal during the probe trials to determine general mobility. Thus, one can assess total path length and swim velocity for individual mice (see Figure 9).

It is generally held that data acquired during the probe trial is the best indicator of the animals using a spatially biased search strategy to locate the platform during training and performance. Data acquired during training (i.e., measurement of escape latencies) may be less informative and in some instances can be dissociated from the performance during the probe trail.

To control for motivational factors and perceptual and motor abilities, animals are tested in the *visible platform version* of the Morris water maze task (Figure 8D). In this variant of the task, the escape platform is clearly indicated by placement of a visible

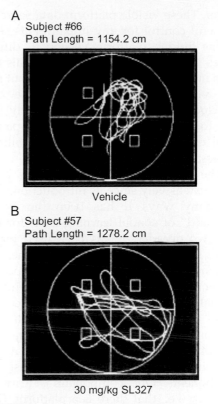

A
Subject #66
Path Length = 1154.2 cm

Vehicle

B
Subject #57
Path Length = 1278.2 cm

30 mg/kg SL327

FIGURE 9 Path tracking in the probe test. Representative probe trial of a mouse in the Morris water maze task. (A) The swim path trace shown here provides an excellent example of a selective search. This particular subject was trained with the platform located in the northeast quadrant. During the probe trial, this mouse spent 56% of the time in the correct quadrant and crossed the exact area where the platform had been nine times. Adult male 129S3/SvImJ mice (formerly 129/Sv-$^{+p+Tyr-c+Mgf-SlJ}$/J; Jackson Laboratory, Bar Harbor, ME) were used in these experiments and those in Figure 8. (B) The path of an animal whose learning during training was blocked with an inhibitor of Mitogen Activated Protein Kinase (MAP Kinase) activation. The animal swims randomly throughout the tank. Data and figure courtesy of Joel Selcher (16).

colored marker directly above the escape platform, and the location of the platform remains constant throughout training. Training typically consists of two blocks of four trials a day for 3 consecutive days. Escape latencies are determined for each trial, and animals quickly learn to swim to the marked platform in order to escape the water. These visible platform data serve as a useful control for any impairments seen in the hidden platform version. If differences in controls versus experimentals are seen in the hidden platform version but not the visible platform version, one can conclude that the difference is likely not due to changes in motivation to escape the pool or to changes in the motor abilities necessary to execute the task.

The Morris water maze task has been used extensively since its introduction, and in many ways it has been the "gold standard" of spatial learning tasks for the last two decades. It has been used many times in order to probe the involvement of specific anatomical structures and specific molecules in hippocampus-dependent spatial learning. It is important to keep in mind that Richard Morris himself has demonstrated that the task overall is cognitively quite complex and can be experimentally dissociated into at least two components. One component is learning the task (i.e., that there is a platform, that spatial cues are relevant). A second component is learning the specific location of the escape platform. Some types of lesions can lead to a loss in an animal's ability to learn the task, while not affecting the ability of the animal to learn a specific platform location, for example. These considerations do not limit the utility of the task but rather point out the importance of considering the complexity of the task when interpreting the resulting data. For example, a deficit may not be the result of a deficit in spatial learning per se but rather in learning the parameters of the task. Of course, this caveat applies to learning tasks in general; it's just that this aspect has been best explored with the Morris water maze.

The principal practical limitations of the water maze are that it requires a fairly large dedicated room, it is messy (in the housekeeping sense), and the training and testing periods are fairly long. Thus, in contrast to a single-training-trial task such as fear conditioning, there is no temporally well-defined period of learning. This can present some practical difficulties when trying to design experiments using drug administration, or where one is trying to measure learning-associated biochemical or physiological changes.

Another practical limitation to the water maze is that it is a fairly rigorous and demanding task physically for the animals under study. This consideration is most pronounced when undertaking experiments on old or otherwise infirm animals. However, in these circumstances, an alternative is available, commonly referred to as the *Barnes maze*.

The Barnes Maze

Carol Barnes has had a long-standing interest in aging-related memory decline and developed a circular hole-board maze task to use as an assessment of spatial learning (8). This task is applicable in circumstances where the strength and stamina of the animals under study may be limiting because it involves only mild locomotor activity. In addition, the measured parameter is errors, not time to complete the task, so the speed at which the animal completes the task is not a factor.

The Barnes maze is essentially a well-lit round table with many holes around the periphery (see Figure 10). Rodents find open, well-lit spaces aversive and they will search around the platform trying to find a safe, dark haven. All the holes around the periphery but one lead simply to a drop-off to the floor. However, one hole leads to an escape chamber, that is a darkened box secured under the hole. Upon locating this hole animals will enter the chamber to escape the lit surface.

The spatial learning in the task involves visual cues placed on the four walls around the table top. The escape hole is always located in a constant place relative to these spatial cues, and much like the water maze the animal must use these cues to learn the location of the escape hole. Performance can be quantitated in its simplest form by

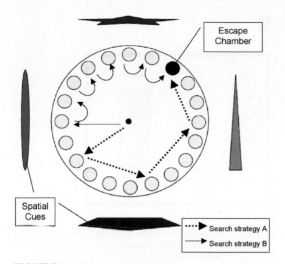

FIGURE 10 Diagram of the basic components of the Barnes maze. Animals learn to locate an escape chamber using visual cues placed on the walls of the room. Learning is assessed as a decrease in the number of errors an animal makes in locating the escape chamber.

simply counting the number of errors an animal makes before it finally finds the escape hole. An error is of course defined as an attempt to enter a nonescape hole. In one of the first examples of the use of this task, aged rats displayed impairment in the rate of acquisition of spatial memory involving navigation around the circular platform (8).

E. Taste Learning

Taste learning and *conditioned taste aversion* are fascinating behavioral phenomena that have only relatively recently begun to be studied mechanistically in rodents. One reason for being interested in these forms of learning is that they are clearly cortex-dependent and may represent the closest rodent homologue to high-order human learning of factual information. Regardless of whether this last speculation is correct, taste learning is without a doubt one of the most robust and ethologically relevant forms of rodent learning currently under study.

Conditioned Taste Aversion

Conditioned taste aversion is a form of associative learning; in this case, an animal learns to associate the novel taste of a new foodstuff (CS) with subsequent illness (US) resulting from ingestion of some nausea-inducing agent. As we discussed in the last chapter, the adaptiveness of this form of learning is clear; by preventing subsequent ingestion of sickening foods, survival is enhanced. For this reason, evolution has selected for robust learning under these conditions, and animals learn after a single pairing of a novel taste with a nausea-inducing agent to avoid that taste in the future. This single-trial learning is also quite robust in that there can be a rather long delay—often measured in hours—between the novel taste and toxin.

A typical conditioned taste aversion paradigm is to pair a novel taste with intraperitoneal injection of a malaise-inducing agent such as LiCl (see Figure 11). Pairing intake of a novel taste with LiCl significantly suppresses subsequent intake of that taste either as a solid food or in drinking water. In these experiments, the effect of LiCl is typically compared to NaCl injected controls.

Conditioned taste aversion is selective for novel tastes. If an animal has experienced a taste previously, it is no longer successful in serving as a CS in conditioned taste aversion. Behavioralists term this phenomenon *latent inhibition*. A "latent" memory for the taste is formed, inhibiting subsequent formation of an association with the toxic agent. Again, ethologically, this makes sense—if a foodstuff has been previously tried and found nonaversive, it should thereafter be taken out of consideration as a toxic agent. This aspect of taste learning is particularly fascinating and still mysterious.

The implications of latent inhibition of taste aversion are twofold. First, somewhere in the taste processing centers of the CNS is a novelty detector, a system that is

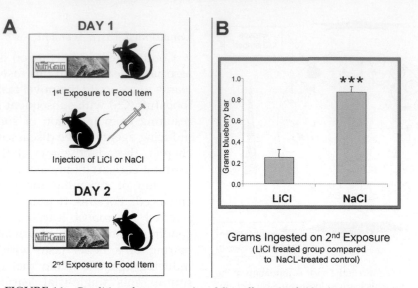

FIGURE 11   Conditioned taste aversion. Mice all received 10-minute access to blueberry bar, a novel taste stimulus, followed by injection of LiCl or NaCl. Pairing of solid novel food with LiCl, which produces nausea, produces a conditioned taste aversion (CTA). CTA is indicated by the observation that mice injected with LiCl following access to the blueberry bar consume significantly less than NaCl-injected controls when tested for food consumption 24 hours later (***$p < .001$ by one-way ANOVA). Data and figure courtesy of Mike Swank (9).

able to tag a taste as something that the animal has never before experienced. If you take a few minutes to consider this, it will become apparent what a conundrum this is. How can you know that something is an unknown? Is there a recorded list somewhere in the brain that contains every taste ever experienced by the animal, against which every subsequent taste is compared throughout the animal's lifetime? Or is there a system present that has a pre-arranged matrix of every conceivable potential taste combination that an animal will ever experience, from which tastes are scratched off after they are first experienced? It is food for thought, so to speak. The second implication is that every novel taste experience is a learning experience. Automatically when a taste is first experienced if forms a memory trace that is perpetuated for the lifetime of the animal. This second consideration brings us to our

next form of taste learning—novel taste learning and neophobia.

Novel Taste Learning and Neophobia

Neophobia is the characteristic fear of novel foods and ensures that animals ingest only small quantities of new foodstuffs. If no illness results upon consumption of the new food, and assuming the food is reasonably palatable, animals will increase their intakes on subsequent exposures. This is readily demonstrated in the laboratory. When rats or mice are presented with highly palatable solutions of saccharin or sucrose, they will consume small amounts on the first exposure; on subsequent exposures, the animals drink more. In these types of experiments, animals are usually maintained on water deprivation so that they are motivated to drink.

Michael Swank recently developed a variation of this procedure that uses solid food in nondeprived mice (see reference 9 and Figure 12). In developing a novel taste learning paradigm Michael found that Kellogg's Nutri-Grain blueberry breakfast bars are readily consumed by rodents and that consumption of this food is easy to measure. During a single 10-minute exposure to the novel blueberry bar, mice will consume around 200–300 mgs (see Figure 12). On subsequent exposures, the mice will double their intakes, thus demonstrating an attenuation of the initial neophobia. This attenuation of neophobia is a behavioral measure of memory for the novel taste.

One very appealing aspect of these simple taste learning paradigms is that the learning is robust and automatic. The learning is a simple single-trial experience (simply exposure to a novel taste) that results in lifelong memory. Also, there is a fairly clear consensus that the insular cortex is the primary site of learning and memory for novel tastes, so the relevant brain region

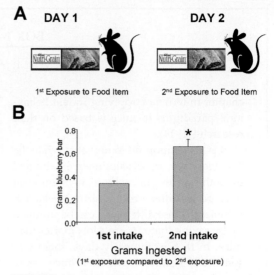

FIGURE 12 Neophobia. Neophobia during first access to a novel solid food is attenuated on second exposure. Mice were given ten-minute access to a novel taste, Nutri-Grain blueberry bar, and intakes were recorded. Ten-minute intakes on the second day are significantly higher, demonstrating attenuation of neophobia through familiarization. (*$p < .05$ by one-way ANOVA). Data and figure courtesy of Mike Swank (9).

BOX 1

OF MICE AND RATS

Rats have been the prototype animal for learning studies, although recently great effort has been expended to adapt these procedures to mice. This is because the recent advent of transgenic mouse technologies has generated substantial optimism concerning the development of murine models for human learning disorders and memory dysfunction, as well as optimism for their application to understanding the basic molecular mechanisms of memory itself. Moreover, the potential applicability of transgenic animal approaches in mice gives great promise for the discovery of new gene products involved in behavior in general. Against this backdrop, it has been important to develop standardized protocols for behavioral characterization of transgenic animals that are widely adaptable for laboratory use. Jean Wehner at the University of Colorado and my colleague Richard Paylor here at Baylor College of Medicine have been leaders in adapting the historically used rat behaviors into the modern situation of mouse characterization, and much of what is described in this

Continued

BOX 1—cont'd

OF MICE AND RATS

chapter in terms of applying rodent behavioral paradigms in mice is based on their research (11–14).

It is also important to note that while the behaviors we are discussing are exhibited by both rats and mice, there are significant interspecies differences in learning behavior. In general, these differences can be summed up by saying that rats are a lot smarter than mice. In fact, in the early days, there was some discussion of whether mice could even learn to perform some of the standard rat behavioral paradigms, although fortunately this concern was unfounded.

Finally, it is important to point out that, in addition to interspecies differences, there are appreciable interstrain differences in learning behavior. Learning in outbred

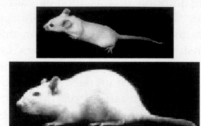

strains of rats and mice is typically much more robust than that in inbred strains. Additionally, different inbred strains of rats and mice have different, specific deficits that affect their learning and memory. Many of these differences are described by Crawley *et al.* (11).

---

in rodents has also been identified. While taste learning has not been nearly as extensively studied as the spatial learning tasks described previously, these types of paradigms hold great promise for future use. They represent one of the most tractable experimental models for measuring cortically dependent learning in rodents.

III. MODERN EXPERIMENTAL USES OF RODENT BEHAVIORAL MODELS

Having briefly described several of the basic rodent learning paradigms in common use, we now turn our attention to thinking about their application in cellular and molecular studies. By way of introduction to this topic, I think it is useful to step back and review the basics of

experimental design. In the next section we will consider the basics of hypothesis testing. We then will proceed to considering how the fundamentals of experimental design are applied in the modern era in extending behavioral studies into the cellular and molecular realm.

A. The Four Basic Types of Experiments

In general there are four basic types of experiments that any scientist can perform. I refer to them as *block, measure, mimic,* and *determine* experiments. I have found this categorization a useful mnemonic device throughout my career as a scientist, and, at the risk of sounding overly pedantic, I strongly encourage any young scientist who reads this book to incorporate them into their thinking about experimental design. For example, every time I write or review a paper I ask whether the investigation has included all these different types of experiments. Especially when writing or reviewing grant applications, where multiyear projects are proposed to test a hypothesis comprehensively, I cross-check myself and others on whether all of these approaches (if technically possible) have been applied to the problem at hand. It is important because what we do as scientists is test hypotheses, and the testing of any hypothesis is much stronger if a variety of independent lines of evidence are available to support the conclusions reached.

What follows is a brief description of each of these four types of experiments.

The determine "experiment" is not really an experiment at all. The determine approach is to perform a basic characterization of the system or molecule at hand independent of any experimental manipulation whatsoever. Examples of this type of pursuit are determining the amino acid sequence of a protein, sequencing a genome, determining the crystal structure of an enzyme, or determining the structure of the DNA double helix. Determinations of this sort are not experiments in that no manipulation of the system is attempted—to do an experiment you tweak the system to see what happens. If you mutate a residue in a protein and see what effect that has on the structure, then you have done an experiment. The basic determination of the structure is not an experiment in and of itself.

Determinations are some of the most satisfying laboratory pursuits to undertake because these are the rare types of studies where definitive data can be obtained. An amino acid sequence is what it is—you get to use unambiguous words like "identical" (versus indistinguishable or similar) and "determined" (versus concluded or inferred) when describing gene and amino acid sequences. There's slightly more ambiguity in determining protein structures and anatomical structures, but in general this pales in comparison to the ambiguity of a

conclusion made on the basis of an experimental manipulation. The down side of determinations is that, as a practical matter, they are viewed as boring unless they involve lots of expensive equipment. It's very difficult to get a grant review study section to recommend approval of a basic anatomical characterization, for example, because no experimental testing of a hypothesis is involved. In modern biomedical research, hypothesis testing is *de rigueur*. In rodent behavioral systems, which are the topic of this chapter, most of the basic behavioral characterization has already been done. However, there is a growing recognition that more sophisticated and detailed basic characterizations, and the development of new rodent behavioral models for human mental disorders, is necessary for the next stage of progress in this field.

Block, *measure*, and *mimic* are experiments, and they are all specific types of approaches to test different predictions of a hypothesis. For the following discussion we will take the simple case of testing the hypothesis "A causes C by activating B" (see Figure 13).

The *mimic* experiment tests the prediction that "if B causes C, then if I activate B artificially I should see C happen as a result." An example that we will return to later is: if I hypothesize that a particular protein kinase causes synaptic potentiation, then applying a drug that activates that protein kinase should elicit synaptic

Hypothesis: A → B → C

Experiment	Prediction
• Determine	• None (**A** makes **C** happen)
• Block	• Blocking **B** should block **A** causing **C**
• Mimic	• Activating **B** should cause **C**
• Measure	• **A** makes **B** happen

FIGURE 13   The four basic types of experiments. See text for discussion.

potentiation. The mimic terminology arises from the fact that you are trying to mimic with a drug (etc.) an effect that occurs with some other stimulus, potentiation-inducing synaptic stimulation in this example. The principal limitation of the mimic experiment is that B may be able to cause C but that in reality A acts independently of B to cause the same effect. B causing C and A causing C may be true, true, and unrelated.

At the current state of understanding and experimental sophistication, mimic experiments are just about impossible to execute in the context of mammalian learning and memory. This is because an enormous amount of fundamental understanding of the system is necessary, along with the capacity for very subtle manipulation, in order for the experiment to work. For example, suppose I hypothesize that a synaptic potentiation underlies learning. In theory, the mimic experiment is to put an electrode in the brain, cause synaptic potentiation, and then the animal will have an altered behavior identical to that caused by a training session. Of course, doing this experiment requires that I know exactly which synapses to potentiate so that I can selectively achieve the right behavioral output—this is beyond the level of understanding for essentially all mammalian behaviors at this point.

The *measure* experiment tests the prediction that "A should cause activation of B." Using our example of kinases in synaptic potentiation, the measure experiment predicts that the potentiating stimulus should cause an increase in the activity of the kinase. This is, of course, determined by measuring the activity of the kinase as directly as possible, hence the measure terminology. The measure experiment has been applied in a variety of different ways in the memory field, ways that we will discuss at various points throughout the book including looking for anatomical, physiologic, and molecular changes in the nervous system in association with learning. The principal theoretical limitation of the measure experiment is that it is correlative. One can show that A causes activation of B, but that does not demonstrate that activation of B is necessary for C to occur.

Which brings us to the *block* experiment. The block experiment tests the prediction that "if I eliminate B, then A should not be able to cause C." In our working example, this means that a kinase inhibitor should block the ability of the potentiating stimulus to cause potentiation. At present, the vast majority of investigations into mechanisms of memory involve this approach, and we will make many references to this type of experiment throughout the book. Specific examples include anatomical lesions, drug infusion studies, and genetic manipulations. The principal theoretical limitation of the block experiment is that it does not distinguish whether *activation* of B is necessary for C, versus whether the *activity* of B is necessary for C. For example, suppose that B provides some tonic effect on C that is necessary for it to occur. Inhibiting B will block the production of effect C when in fact A never has any effect on B whatsoever. In behavioral terms for learning experiments, this is referred to as a *performance deficit*—the animal is simply unable to execute the behavioral read-out necessary to exhibit the fact that they have learned.

In summary, then, the mimic experiment tests sufficiency, the block experiment tests necessity, and the measure experiment tests whether the event does in fact occur. Each type of experiment has its strengths and weaknesses. Positive outcomes in testing each of these three predictions for any hypothesis makes for clear, strong support of the hypothesis.

B. Using Behavioral Paradigms in Block and Measure Experiments

The behavioral paradigms I have been discussing in this chapter have, by and large, been used in two ways in the modern era. The first application is as a stimulus in measure experiments. The second is as a read-out in blocking experiments. We will return to the specific results of several of these various experiments in Chapter 9. However, for our present purposes, I would like to describe briefly some examples of the use of behavioral paradigms in these two types of experiments. This is because the specific examples will help to introduce some refinements of the procedures that are necessary for some applications, and also to introduce some of the sorts of behavioral control experiments that are used to shore up the conclusions reached in executing the experiments.

Using Behavioral Paradigms as a Stimulus in Measure Experiments

In measure experiments, the behavioral paradigms we have reviewed are used to train the animal using a set of defined and optimized environmental signals that are known to elicit learning and memory. The behavioral read-out of the learned behavior is really only used as confirmation that the animal has learned—it is, in essence, control data that the procedure has been effective. What is really of interest in these types of experiments is determining what has gone on inside the animal's CNS while or after it learned. A variation that has great potential for future use is to monitor events occurring when the animal recalls a memory, but that type of experiment has received scant attention so far.

There are several prominent examples of great successes in measuring physiologic changes in the brain with behavioral training paradigms. The best-established paradigm is measuring alterations in hippocampal pyramidal neuron firing with rodent spatial learning. These elegant experiments use implanted recording electrodes to monitor neuronal responses *in vivo* in the behaving animal. As described previously, these experiments led to the identification of hippocampal "place" cells and variations thereof. The Eichenbaum, Wilson,

McNaughton, Tonegawa, and Kandel laboratories have all made significant use of this approach and I will review a number of their findings in Chapters 3 and 9.

Somewhat of a "holy grail" experiment in learning and memory has been to obtain data demonstrating that long-term potentiation of hippocampal synaptic transmission occurs with learning in rodents. To date, this approach has met with only limited success as pertains to the hippocampus. However, there have been landmark findings in this area from the LeDoux and Shinnick-Gallagher laboratories, utilizing fear conditioning and amygdala recordings of synaptic transmission. We will return to these observations later, in Chapter 9, with a review of the data supporting a role for long-term potentiation in learning.

Finally, while the search for alterations in hippocampal synaptic transmission with learning has been somewhat frustrated, there actually have been nice demonstrations of alterations of hippocampal neuron excitability that occur with learning. Both the Wilson and Disterhoft laboratories have found alterations in hippocampal pyramidal neuron excitability with spatial learning and trace eye-blink conditioning, respectively. These alterations, for which there is indirect and direct evidence suggesting involvement of altered potassium channel function, will be addressed in more detail in Chapter 3.

These studies all involve cellular changes, but what about molecular changes triggered in association with the behavioral paradigms we have been discussing? There have been fewer experiments looking at molecular changes in association with learning, and we will be discussing changes in kinase activity with learning in subsequent chapters. For our purposes here, I will limit my discussion to one set of studies in order to give a specific example of the approach.

In a sophisticated series of studies, Soren Impey and Dan Storm and co-workers produced a transgenic mouse line that allowed read-out of increased transcription

BOX 2

EYE-BLINK CONDITIONING

During classical associative learning, an animal is taught to associate a neutral conditioned stimulus (CS) with an aversive unconditioned stimulus (US). Classical conditioning of the eye-blink response in rabbits uses the association of a neutral stimulus such as tone or light with a nociceptive stimulus, such as an airpuff delivered to the eye or a periorbital shock. Re-presentation of the CS results in an eye-blink conditioned response (CR) in anticipation of the US. Trace eye-blink conditioning (CS followed by an intervening time delay) is a hippocampus-dependent form of associative learning, while delay conditioning (no intervening time delay) is hippocampus-independent. An elegant series of studies has implicated a role for long-term depression (LTD) in the cerebellum in eye-blink conditioning. Additional sophisticated studies have also mapped much of the relevant neuronal circuitry underlying this behavior. We will return to these studies in more detail in later chapters, where we discuss the general role of synaptic plasticity in learning and memory.

| Corneal Air Puff Elicits Eye-Blink Response | Corneal Air Puff Given with Tone | Tone Given Alone Elicits Eye-Blink Response |

BOX 2   Eye-blink conditioning in rabbits. Animals are trained in a Pavlovian conditioning paradigm to learn that a tone predicts a puff of air to the eye surface. Over time, the animals learn to blink in response to the tone alone. See text for additional details.

and translation of genes downstream of the CyclicAMP Response Element (CRE) DNA regulatory element (see reference 3 and Figure 14). A variety of prior "block"-type studies in a variety of model systems suggested that the CRE transcriptional pathway was involved in long-term memory. However, no mammalian behavioral model system had yet demonstrated that environmental signals associated with learning led to alterations in CRE-mediated gene expression. Impey and Storm undertook a "measure" study to assess this issue directly. They found that training for contextual fear conditioning or passive avoidance led to significant increases in CRE-dependent gene expression in the hippocampus. Auditory-cue fear conditioning, which is amygdala-dependent, was associated with increased CRE-mediated gene expression in the amygdala but not in the hippocampus. These studies demonstrated that behavioral conditioning activates the CRE transcriptional pathway in specific areas of the brain associated with specific learning behaviors—a fine example of applying the "measure" experiment in a behavioral paradigm.

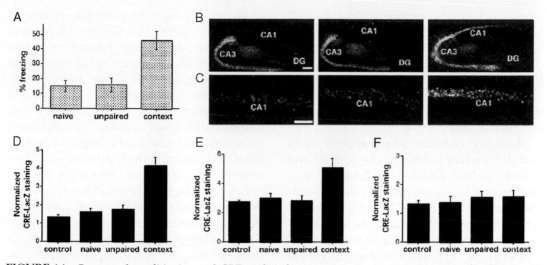

FIGURE 14 Contextual conditioning and CRE-mediated gene expression in mice transgenic for CRE-Lac Z. (A) Summary of associative learning (contextual fear conditioning) measured 8 hours after training. Mean percentage of time spent freezing in the conditioning chamber is depicted for naive, unpaired control and context-trained mice (naive, $n = 7$; unpaired, $n = 8$; context-trained, $n = 23$; naive versus context and unpaired versus context, $p < .0005$). (B) In these experiments hippocampal CRE-mediated gene expression was assessed using Lac Z expression (see text). (B) Low-magnification confocal images show CRE-regulated Lac Z immunostaining in hippocampal slices from representative naive, unpaired, control, and context-trained mice. Scale bar represents 500 mm. (C) Higher-magnification images of the CA1 region from representative naive, unpaired control and context-trained mice. Scale bar represents 100 μm. (D) Quantification of Lac Z immunostaining in area CA1 (unhandled control, $n = 5$; naive control, $n = 8$; unpaired control, $n = 8$; context-trained, $n = 23$; naive versus context and unpaired versus context, $p < .001$; $p > .3$ for comparisons between control groups). (E) Quantitative analysis of Lac Z immunostaining in area CA3 (unhandled control, $n = 5$; naive, $n = 8$; unpaired, $n = 8$; context trained, $n = 12$; naive versus context, $p < .01$; unpaired versus context, $p < .02$; $p > .5$ for comparisons between control groups). (F) Summary of Lac Z immunostaining in the dentate gyrus (control, $n = 5$; naive, $n = 8$; unpaired, $n = 8$; context trained, $n = 11$; naive versus context and unpaired versus context, $p > .3$). Figure adapted from reference 3, courtesy of Dan Storm.

I point out these studies in part because they are such an elegant combination of behavioral and transgenic animal approaches. However, I also like to use these studies to illustrate how assaying molecular changes using behavioral paradigms necessitates some rethinking of these paradigms because they have been historically developed using a behavioral perspective. One of the controls that is necessary in an experiment like the one described above is a foot shock alone control, where the animal experiences the foot shock under a condition where it does not associate the foot shock with a particular context. This allows you to demonstrate that the molecular change is not due to a direct sensory response to the shock, for example, but rather is selective for the condition where the animal is actually learning something. However, how do you keep the animal from learning to associate the foot shock with the place where it is shocked? One way to solve this problem is to repeatedly expose the animal to the place in which you will shock it, in the absence of foot shock. In other words, you habituate them to the shock environment prior to delivering the foot shock so that no unique association is made between the foot shock and that environment. Then you can deliver the shock alone in the absence of the animal learning an association. This procedure works quite well behaviorally, and the animal exhibits no fear conditioning to the shock environment. It also works in molecular studies like the one described earlier—no molecular changes in CRE-dependent gene expression occur in the hippocampus with an unpaired control like this.

However, consider what happens when you put a naïve animal in the context and deliver a foot shock—conditioning and changes in CRE-dependent gene expression both occur. Thus, in the "control," habituation to the context has made the hippocampus refractory to foot shock-induced molecular changes. This refractoriness of course must *itself* be mediated by some molecular change in the hippocampus (or its input pathways). Thus, the behaviorally straightforward "shock alone" control becomes the molecularly complicated "refractoriness to contextual learning" experimental sample. I want to make clear that this consideration in no way diminishes the legitimacy of the conclusions that Impey and Storm drew from their experiments. I use this simply as an example of the complexities involved in trying to transition from behavioral studies that use behavior as a read-out to behavioral studies that use cellular changes or molecules as a read-out.

We ran up against a similar puzzle in some experiments that Coleen Atkins and Joel Selcher did in my laboratory a few years ago (10). They were using contextual conditioning (context alone paired with foot shock) and contextual-plus-cued (context plus white noise auditory cue paired with foot shock) conditioning protocols and looked for changes in protein kinase activation in the hippocampus. They observed a significant activation of hippocampal Calcium/calmodulin-dependent Protein Kinase (CaMKII) that was selectively associated with the context-plus-cue conditioning paradigm (Figure 15). Why is there a unique hippocampal effect associated with the context-plus-cue paradigm versus the context alone paradigm? After all, in both paradigms the animal is learning to associate the identical context with the foot shock, and the cued component is not dependent on the hippocampus. We do not know the answer, but one interesting possibility is that the change is indicative of the animal having associated the noise cue with the context. Another possibility is that the CaMKII change is a manifestation of the animal having formed a unique multimodal association of cue, context, and foot shock. Again, I raise this point as an example of how we are likely to

Kinase	Contextual Conditioning			Cue and Contextual Conditioning		
	1 min	1 h	2 h	1 min	1 h	2 h
p42 MAPK	-9 ± 12 (8)	54 ± 27 (10)	-3 ± 9 (7)	-16 ± 5 (7)	83 ± 28 (14)	19 ± 8 (10)
p44 MAPK	-3 ± 5 (8)	18 ± 10 (11)	-5 ± 5 (8)	-3 ± 6 (7)	50 ± 21 (13)	13 ± 11 (10)
PKC	-7 ± 5 (8)	*25 ± 15 (11)	-5 ± 11 (7)	11 ± 23 (7)	25 ± 11 (12)	10 ± 11 (10)
α-CαMKII	-2 ± 7 (8)	7 ± 11 (11)	8 ± 10 (7)	-3 ± 16 (7)	13 ± 23 (14)	47 ± 20 (10)

FIGURE 15　Hippocampal protein kinase activation in fear-conditioning. Two different fear-conditioning paradigms were used, cued and cued plus contextual (see text). Protein kinase activation was assessed using phospho-selective antisera to measure kinase phosphorylation. Percent change in phosphorylation from control for each protein kinase is shown. Number of animals used are in parentheses. All protein phosphorylation measurements were normalized to corresponding protein kinase amounts. Shaded boxes are statistically significant. The asterisk (*) denotes a nonsignificant ($p = .1$) increase in autophosphorylated Protein Kinase C (PKC) 1 hour after contextual conditioning. Hippocampal CaMKII was selectively activated with cued-plus-contextual fear conditioning. Data courtesy of Coleen Atkins (10).

have surprises in store for us as we move from behavioral studies, where we select a particular behavioral output to measure and in essence use the animal as a filter, to molecular studies where molecular read-outs of a wide variety of different events are likely to occur.

Don't Forget Synapses are Made of Molecules

Finally, another variation of the measure experiment in learning is that there have been anatomical changes in various CNS regions, especially in the cerebral cortex, identified after raising animals in enriched environments. This approach was pioneered by Bill Greenough and has been extensively studied in his laboratory. A significant part of these anatomical changes in the fine structure of cortical neurons is presumed to be the result of (or at least influenced by) learning and memory during the growth of the animal. Among the changes identified are changes in synaptic density and dendritic morphology. Even though I am not going to elaborate further on these anatomical studies for now, I do wish to make one final point. It is important to bear in mind that these anatomical changes are of necessity subserved by molecular changes. The molecular events involved are not limited to the induction of these changes—their maintenance must also be a manifestation of molecular alterations. I will illustrate my point by reducing it to the simplest example. Suppose that there are 20% more synapses in an enriched environment brain due to a variety of learning events. If nothing else, this will require a steady-state increase in the rate of synthesis of all the proteins comprising those synapses because proteins are constantly turning over in the cell. This may seem like a simple feat to accomplish, but somewhere in those cells there must be some molecular mechanism(s) maintaining that increased net rate of synthesis. Once again, this adds a layer of molecular complexity to what

otherwise appears to be a straightforward application of behavioral approaches in a "measure" experiment.

Using Behavioral Paradigms as an Assay of Learning in Block Experiments

Block experiments are by far the most common use of rodent behavioral assessment paradigms. In these experiments, the behavioral paradigms we have reviewed are used to assess whether an animal has a learning or memory deficit when a particular process is blocked. The behavioral read-out of the learned behavior is used to assess whether the animal has learned. A "memory" variation commonly used is to assess animals behaviorally to determine if an experimental treatment causes a faster decrement of learned behavior over time. The three most common examples of experimental manipulations in the application of the block approach to behavior, roughly in historical order, are anatomical lesions, drug infusion studies, and, more recently, gene manipulation experiments. What is of interest in these types of experiments is determining what structures or molecules are necessary for an animal to learn, remember, and recall a learned event.

We will be returning to a great many specific examples of these types of experiments later, experiments that have implicated specific molecules and categories of molecules in learning and memory and synaptic plasticity. Thus, for the present, I will discuss these types of experiments only in general terms. Of course, there are a great many caveats in interpreting these types of experiments, and we will focus our discussion here on five general considerations that must be kept in mind. I review them here in general terms so that I can avoid repeating them throughout the book when we discuss specific experiments. They also lead us to the final section of the chapter where we will talk about a variety of behavioral assessments in rodents that are used as an adjunct to experiments designed specifically to look for learning and memory deficits (see references 11 and 12).

The first consideration in behavioral "block" experiments is that there may have been nonspecific effects of the manipulation, as is always the case with inhibitors or lesions of any sort. The drug may not be specific for the molecule of interest, the knockout animal may have not developed a normal CNS, or the anatomical lesion may have destroyed fibers of passage connected to distal brain regions. This limitation is practical in nature and, in general, has received a great degree of attention in the literature. The specifics also vary greatly depending on the specific experiment under consideration, so we will not address this point further for the present.

The second limitation is largely conceptual. In these behavioral learning experiments, you are training an animal using environmental signals and measuring at some later time point a complex behavioral read-out. Many things are occurring during the training, learning, memorizing, recalling, and execution of the read-out. It is fundamentally difficult with the basic experimental design employed to distinguish among effects on learning, memory, or recall. Imagine the simplest case where an animal has a molecular deficit throughout the experiment—it is clear that no conclusion can be drawn concerning whether the animal has a deficit in learning, memory, or recall.

Two basic variations of the experiment are used to try to begin to distinguish among these possibilities. A transient inactivation experiment, where a structure or molecule is inhibited for a limited period of time, allows one to begin to parse effects on learning/memory versus recall, for example. However, it is still difficult with the transient inactivation design to distinguish between effects on learning versus effects on early memory consolidation, for example. This brings us to the second variation, where memory is assessed at short time points versus long time points. If an animal with a molecular or anatomical deficit is able to perform normally at short time periods after training and has a selective deficit at longer time periods, this implies that learning has occurred but that there is a loss of longer-term memory. The principal limitation to this approach is that it assumes that the learning mechanisms for short-term memory are identical to the mechanisms used for long-term memory.

A third consideration that must be kept in mind in interpreting block experiments is that compensation may have occurred, acutely or chronically. For example, the loss of a brain structure or molecule may force the CNS to utilize an ancillary mechanism that is capable of doing the job, but that normally is never brought into play. From a hypothesis-testing perspective, this leads to a false negative result—we conclude that molecule or structure X is not necessary but in fact it *is* necessary under normal circumstances. The enormous plasticity of the CNS in general makes this a particularly bothersome concern. I will use Lashley's classic lesioning experiments to illustrate this point, precisely because they have been so important in shaping modern thinking about memory. Lashley trained rats in mazes and made post-training cortical lesions in order to try to localize the maze memory trace anatomically. Lashley observed that, by and large, no single lesion could erase a memory, but rather that maze performance declined in relation to the overall extent of cortical lesioning. Thus, Lashley concluded that memories likely are "distributed" throughout the cortex, and that there was no discrete memory trace. The caveat is that there may have been multiple, redundant, memory traces, and that only when the last one was destroyed was there an appreciable decline in maze perfomance. Unfortunately, very little can be done in the way of control experiments to address this general limitation clearly—for the most part, it must simply be left as a caveat to the interpretation.

The fourth and fifth overall considerations in interpreting block behavioral experiments are at least well-defined enough that control experiments can be brought to bear—these are *performance* deficits and *sensory processing* deficits. In hypothesis testing terms, both of these limitations lead to potential false positive results. In many of the types of memory paradigms we have been discussing, fairly sophisticated control experiments can be executed to rule out these limitations. However, the biology has to be working to the advantage of the experiments, and, of course, we have no control over that. One of my favorite examples is finding a selective deficit in contextual versus cued fear conditioning. If a lesioned animal performs normally in cued fear conditioning but has a deficit in contextual fear conditioning, one can make a reasonable interpretation that it can feel the foot shock (thus no sensory deficit for foot shock) as well as exhibit freezing behavior (no performance deficit in freezing). Another favorite is the selective effects on long-term versus short-term memory—if short-term memory is intact then it is reasonable to conclude that the lesioned animal both perceived the environmental stimuli and is capable of performing the necessary behavioral read-out of memory.

In many cases, however, the biology does not work to your advantage and these two types of sophisticated control experiments cannot be used. In that case then, more indirect measures must be employed to bolster the case that the experimental manipulation has not led to general deficits in overall health, motivation, perception, or motor performance. In the following section, I will briefly describe a number of behavioral assays that typically are used as controls in this situation. It's important to keep in mind that many of these behaviors are important behavioral tests in their own right, but that, for our purposes, I am simply presenting them in a context of their use as general control experiments for learning and memory assessments.

IV. CONTROL EXPERIMENTS

A. Open Field Analysis and Elevated Plus Maze Performance

Open field analysis is used to measure the level of spontaneous motor activity, exploratory behavior, and habituation of animals to an open area. Animals are placed in an open field chamber (e.g., 40 by 40 by 30 cm box) for 15 minutes in standard room-lighting conditions. Activity in the open field is typically monitored by light beams and photoreceptors on each side of the chamber and analyzed by a computer-operated optical animal activity system. With this test, general activity levels are evaluated by measuring of horizontal activity, vertical activity, and total distance traveled during a 10-minute test session in an open box in a lighted room (see Figure 16). These types of data are used to screen for hyperactivity, which can be a complication to the assessment of many different types of learned behaviors. The open field test also can be used to measure anxiety levels, as assessed by the center distance to total distance ratio. In the more general literature, this assessment is often used in conjunction with the Elevated Plus Maze as an anxiety index.

B. Rotating-Rod Performance— Coordination and Motor Learning

The rotating rod task is commonly used to assess two parameters related to cerebellar function. Initial trials are used to assess the animal's coordination. The amount of time an animal can stay on a rotating rod is an index of its general level of coordination. Obviously, motor coordination is an important component of most behavioral assessments of learning where complicated motor output is necessary for successful execution of a learned task. Mice

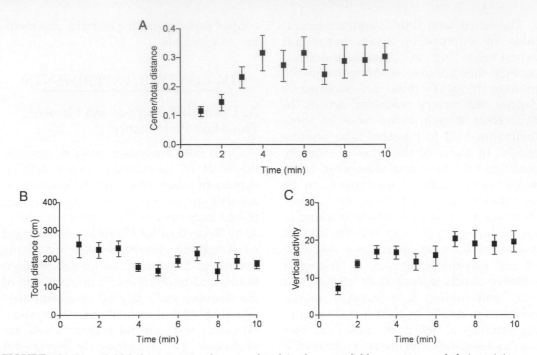

FIGURE 16 Open field behavior. Animals were placed in the open field apparatus, and their activity was monitored using automated recording equipment. (A) Total distance traveled per minute for a 10-minute period. (B) Vertical activity (number of rearings per minute) over a 10-minute period. (C) Ratio of center distance to total distance traveled for each minute over a 10-minute period. The data in panels A and B are taken as indices of general activity; the data in panel C are taken as an index of anxiety. Results shown are for C57Bl6 animals, mean ± SEM for n = 10. Data courtesy of Coleen Atkins (10).

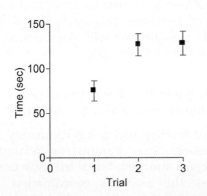

FIGURE 17 Rotating rod behavior. Total time the animals remained on the rotating rod was measured for each training period. Three training trials were given in a single day. The increase in time the animal remained on the rod is taken as an index of motor learning. Results shown are for C57Bl6 animals, mean ± SEM for n = 10 animals. Data courtesy of Coleen Atkins (10).

and rats also improve their performance with training (see Figure 17), which is an indicator of motor learning. Thus, motor skill acquisition can be assessed in its own right by determining the rate of improvement on the task upon repeated trials.

C. Acoustic Startle and Pre-Pulse Inhibition

Just like humans, mice and rats normally exhibit a startle response to a loud noise. Interestingly, if a modest noise is presented immediately preceding the loud noise, the startle response is significantly attenuated (see Figure 18) in all three species. This phenomenon is referred to as pre-pulse inhibition. In rats and mice pre-pulse inhibition can be used to assess the animal's general reflexes (startle), and it also serves as a very sensitive and quantitative assessment of the animal's hearing. Normal mice, for example, exhibit pre-pulse inhibition with a threshold around 70 dB, and reliably give quantitatively different responses to pre-pulses varying by only a few decibles (see Figure 18). Of course, hearing assessment is a critical control for cued fear conditioning, and pre-pulse inhibition can be used in this fashion. Pre-pulse inhibition is also used as an assessment of sensory-motor gating, which is deranged in schizophrenic patients. Thus, pre-pulse inhibition in rodents can also be used to model this aspect of schizophrenia.

D. Nociception

In many behavioral training paradigms, aversive sensory stimuli are utilized. It is important to note that it is almost universally the case that modest aversive stimuli are much more effective for training animals than are painful stimuli. In this

---

BOX 3

RODENT MODELS OF PAIN PLASTICITY

In humans, tissue injury results in persistently increased pain sensation to mildly noxious stimuli (hyperalgesia) and pain perception to normally non-noxious stimuli (allodynia). These two forms of sensitization clearly fit within the definition of learning developed in the first chapter—persisting behavioral modification in response to an environmental signal. However, in this case, one mechanism contributing to the altered behavior is persisting production of chemical signals locally at the site of damage, which is in a sense not a memory event but a persisting "environmental" signal. However, it is clear that there are also pain-associated central plastic changes that occur in the CNS that alter perception of constant environmental signals.

Rodent model systems have allowed the delineation of two main mechanisms underlying persistent pain sensitization after tissue injury. First, primary sensory afferents known as Aδ and C fibers conveying peripheral pain signals to the central nervous system become sensitized. Physiologically, this sensitization manifests as a lower stimulus intensity threshold for firing and possibly increased transmitter release in the primary sensory neurons. Second, the CNS changes its processing of signals received from the periphery such that mildly noxious stimuli are coded more intensely and non-noxious stimuli are coded as noxious.

Rodents behaviorally exhibit the sequelae of peripheral and central sensitization in a manner analogous to human behavior. Simple reflexive behavior, such as paw withdrawal, allows experimenters to quantify and study responsiveness to stimuli in rodents. Analogous to human sensations, rodents with tissue injury withdraw their paws when given non-noxious stimuli such as warm heat or a light brush. Therefore, rodents provide a model system to dissect out the molecular mechanisms of sensitization through biochemistry and physiology in correlation with simple behavioral assays.

One of the main loci for central sensitization is the spinal cord dorsal horn, the first relay station for pain signals arriving from the periphery. This sensitization involves

Continued

RODENT MODELS OF PAIN PLASTICITY

changes in the coding of noxious signals and minimally must involve a change in synaptic strength or neuronal excitability—an interesting parallel to mechanisms of synaptic plasticity that we will be discussing later in the book in context of learning and memory.

Thermal pain thresholds in rats and mice are determined using an apparatus known as a Hargreave's radiant heat apparatus. In this test, the animals are allowed to move freely in small enclosures on an elevated glass plate. After a 1-hour acclimitization period, radiant heat is applied locally to one paw via a visible light source. The animals are not restrained; thus, when they feel discomfort, they withdraw the stimulated paw. The latency from onset of the stimulus to paw withdrawal is recorded, as an index of sensory perception and sensitization.

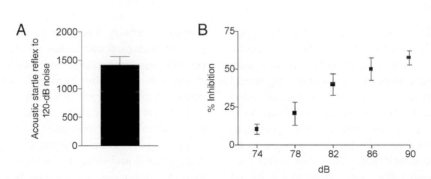

FIGURE 18   Acoustic startle and pre-pulse inhibition. (A) Acoustic startle in response to a 120-dB noise, assessed as the force exerted on an underlying footplate. (B) Effect of a pre-tone (sound intensity given in decibels) to diminish the magnitude of acoustic startle. Results are given as percent diminution of the force of the subsequent 120-dB startle response. Results shown are for C57Bl6 animals, mean ± SEM for n = 10 animals. Data courtesy of Coleen Atkins (10).

context it is of course important to have control data that animals are capable of normally perceiving aversive stimuli such as mild foot-shock. One test of nociception is assayed by placing the animals on a 55°C hotplate. Latency to lick the hind paw is measured (See Figure 19). In a similar test shock threshold sensitivity is measured by scoring animals for flinching, vocalizing and jumping behavior in response to 0.1-mA foot shock increments (typically 0–1.5 mA, delivered for 1 second long each).

E. Vision Tests—Light–Dark Exploration and Visual Cliff

In many learning tasks, visual perception is an important variable. Two common tests of vision are light-dark exploration and the "visual cliff." It is important to

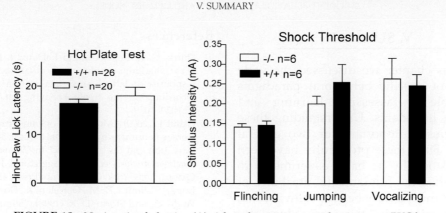

FIGURE 19   Nociception behavior. (A) A hot plate test was used to compare PKC beta knockout animals (□) versus wildtype (■) sensitivity to a noxious stimuli. Thermal nociception was measured on a 55°C hot plate as the latency to hind-paw lick. (B) As an additional control to the hot plate test, the shock threshold test was used to compare sensitivity to foot shock measured by the extent of flinching, jumping, or vocalizing to increasing foot shock intensities. Data courtesy of Coleen Atkins (5).

note that many inbred strains of rodents have poor vision and that in general rats and mice are not particularly "visual" creatures (limited stereopsis, for example). Overall, available visual tests for rodents are not very sensitive or sophisticated. One example of a visual task for rodents is light-dark exploration, which is used to asses an animal's ability to perceive light and dark. One typical variation consists of a polypropylene chamber (44 cm by 21 cm by 21 cm) unequally divided into two chambers by a black partition containing a small opening. The large chamber is open and brightly illuminated (800 lux), while the small chamber is closed and dark. Animals are placed into the illuminated side and allowed to move freely between the two chambers for 10 minutes—normal animals spend a majority of their time in the darkened chamber, as is expected for dark-preferring, nocturnal animals.

A second visual assessment paradigm is the visual cliff. In this task animals are placed on a see-through surface such as glass or plexiglass. This solid platform on one half has underneath it a solid surface and on the other half the air-space above the floor. Thus, a seeing animal perceives that one half of the chamber is a solid surface while the other half appears to be the open space above a large drop-off. Animals are placed on the "solid" surface and animals that can see rarely venture over the edge of the cliff. Non-seeing animals, of course, are unable to discern one area from the other as the tactile stimulus is a continuous smooth sheet.

The variety of control experiments described here can be combined into a general assessment battery consisting of open field test, rotating rod, acoustic startle, prepulse inhibition, hot plate, shock threshold, and visual assessment tasks. This battery of tests is quantitative and an excellent general screen for a wide variety of behaviors and sensory responses. Also typically included as control data are assessments of general physical parameters such as weight, temperature, coat appearance, and basic reflexes. Taken together, these tests serve as useful control experiments for experiments in which anatomical or molecular lesions are being used to probe for the role of specific structures or molecules in rodent behavioral learning and memory (11, 12).

V. SUMMARY

In this chapter we discussed the wide variety of specific behavioral paradigms applicable to assessing learning and memory in rodents. Understanding these procedures is important for two general reasons. First, these procedures have been used historically as basic experiments to characterize the fundamental attributes of learning and memory behaviorally. Second, in the modern era, these procedures are used in literally thousands of separate studies investigating the anatomical, cellular, and molecular basis of learning and memory. We will be discussing the results of many of these experiments in more detail throughout the rest of the book. Having a firm grasp on the basics of rodent behavioral paradigms is key to understanding the design, interpretation, and limitations of modern cellular and molecular investigations into memory formation in mammalian model systems. Thus, we have dedicated a reasonable amount of time to considering the design of these experiments, their attendant caveats, and the necessary control experiments that go along with them.

A second theme of this chapter has been the basics of hypothesis testing. We covered in an abstract sense the four fundamental types of experiments that scientists have available to them for testing various predictions of a hypothesis. We will return to these basic experimental types many, many times throughout this book. Although we will discuss them specifically as they pertain to studies of learning and memory and their attendant cellular and molecular mechanisms, mastery of the basic concepts of hypothesis testing is crucial for students whatever their ultimate field of endeavor. Working through their application in the context of learning and memory will undoubtedly be useful as a mental exercise, helpful beyond the specifics of their application in one scientific subdiscipline.

References

1. Quirk, G. J., Repa, C., and LeDoux, J. E. (1995). "Fear conditioning enhances short-latency auditory responses of lateral amygdala neurons: parallel recordings in the freely behaving rat." *Neuron* 15:1029–1039.

2. Cahill, L. (2000). "Modulation of long-term memory storage in humans by emotional arousal: adrenergic activation and the amygdala." In: *The amygdala: a functional analysis,* edited by Aggleton, J. P., 2nd ed. Oxford; New York: Oxford Univ Press; 425–445.

3. Impey, S., Smith, D. M., Obrietan, K., Donahue, R., Wade, C., and Storm, D. R. (1998). "Stimulation of cAMP response element (CRE)-mediated transcription during contextual learning." *Nat. Neurosci.* 1:595-601.

4. Frankland, P. W., Cestari, V., Filipkowski, R. K., McDonald, R. J., and Silva, A. J. (1998). "The dorsal hippocampus is essential for context discrimination but not for contextual conditioning." *Behav. Neurosci.* 112:863–874.

5. Weeber, E. J., Atkins, C. M., Selcher, J. C., Varga, A. W., Mirnikjoo, B., Paylor, R., Leitges, M., and Sweatt, J. D. (2000). "A role for the beta isoform of protein kinase C in fear conditioning." *J. Neurosci.* 20:5906–5914.

6. Eichenbaum, H., and Cohen, N. J. (2001). *From conditioning to conscious recollection : memory systems of the brain.* New York: Oxford University Press.

7. Morris, R. (1984)."Developments of a water-maze procedure for studying spatial learning in the rat." *J. Neurosci. Methods* 11:47–60.

8. Barnes, C. A. (1979). "Memory deficits associated with senescence: a neurophysiological and behavioral study in the rat." *J. Comp. Physiol. Psychol.* 93:74–104.

9. Swank, M. W., and Sweatt, J. D. (2001). "Increased histone acetyltransferase and lysine acetyltransferase activity and biphasic activation of the ERK/RSK cascade in insular cortex during novel taste learning." *J. Neurosci.* 21:3383–3391.

10. Atkins, C. M., Selcher, J. C., Petraitis, J. J., Trzaskos, J. M., and Sweatt, J. D. (1998). "The MAPK cascade is required for mammalian associative learning." *Nat. Neurosci.* 1:602–609.

11. Crawley, J. N., Belknap, J. K., Collins, A., Crabbe, J. C., Frankel, W., Henderson, N., Hitzemann, R. J., Maxson, S. C., Miner, L. L., Silva, A. J., Wehner, J. M., Wynshaw-Boris, A., and Paylor, R. (1997). "Behavioral phenotypes of inbred mouse strains: implications and recommendations for molecular studies." *Psychopharmacology (Berl)* 132:107–124.

12. Crawley, J. N., and Paylor, R. (1997). "A proposed test battery and constellations of specific behavioral paradigms to investigate the behavioral phenotypes of transgenic and knockout mice." *Horm. Behav.* 31:197–211.

13. Paylor, R., Baskall-Baldini, L., Yuva, L., and Wehner, J. M. (1996). "Developmental differences in place-learning performance between C57BL/6 and DBA/2 mice parallel the ontogeny of hippocampal protein kinase C." *Behav. Neurosci.* 110:1415–1425.

14. Paylor, R., and Crawley, J. N. (1997). "Inbred strain differences in prepulse inhibition of the mouse startle response." *Psychopharmacology (Berl)* 132:169–180.

15. Levenson, J., Weeber, E., Selcher, J. C., Kategaya, L. S., Sweatt, J. D., and Eskin, A. (2002). "Long-term potentiation and contextual fear conditioning increase neuronal glutamate uptake." *Nat. Neurosci.* 5:155–161.

16. Selcher, J. C., Atkins, C. M., Trzaskos, J. M., Paylor, R., and Sweatt, J. D. (1999). "A necessity for MAP kinase activation in mammalian spatial learning." *Learn. Mem.* 6:478–490.

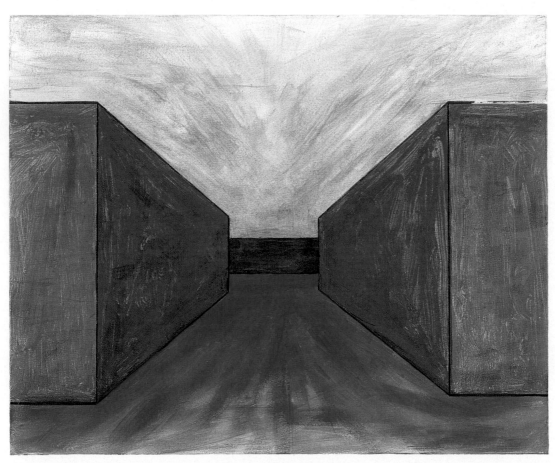

Lashley Maze—Rat's Eye View
J. David Sweatt, Acrylic on canvas, 2002

The Hippocampus Serves a Role in Multimodal Information Processing, and Memory Consolidation

I. INTRODUCTION

In the last chapter, we talked about rodent behavioral models in general, and touched on various examples of hippocampus-dependent learning and memory paradigms. In this chapter, we will delve into the role of the hippocampus in animal behavior in more detail, drawing specific examples from the literature for each of four categories of function. The first three categories involve the role of the hippocampus in information processing and cognition. Specifically, we will discuss how the hippocampus is involved in perceptual processing of information regarding *space*, *time*, and *relationships among objects*. The theme for the first part of this chapter, therefore, is that the hippocampus serves a role in multimodal information processing (see Figure 1).

The fourth function of the hippocampus that we will talk about is that it is required for *memory consolidation*, and we will address this in the final part of the chapter. This is the classic role of the hippocampus—to participate in the formation of long-term memories by helping to convert short-term sensory signals into long-term or permanently encoded memories. It is important to

Functions of the Hippocampus

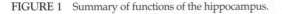

- Cognitive Processing:
    Space
    Time
    Relationships

- Memory Consolidation

FIGURE 1   Summary of functions of the hippocampus.

distinguish between memory consolidation and memory storage. The hippocampus generally does not store information for extended periods of time but rather serves as an intermediate-duration memory buffer that is involved in maintaining memories until they are transferred for more permanent storage in various regions of the cerebral cortex. This is referred to as consolidation of memories, that is, consolidation is the process by which memories are converted to very long-lasting forms.

Keep in mind that shorter-term memories undergo consolidation as well. The hippocampus is clearly involved in the consolidation of memories lasting from 24 hours to a lifetime, and it is also likely involved in the consolidation of memories of even shorter duration. This implies that there may be multiple hippocampus-dependent memory consolidation processes that subserve memories of various durations—this is an open question at this time.

Note that the first three functions (space, time, relationships) can conceptually be considered very differently from the fourth function (consolidation). The first three functions are related to real-time information processing, perception of environmental stimuli, and cognition in general. This information processing role of the hippocampus can be considered independently of the specific memory formation aspect of its role in memory consolidation. As a first approximation, it may be useful to think of the first three functions as what is going on *inside* the hippocampus on a minute-to-minute basis, while thinking of the memory consolidation function as what

happens to allow the hippocampus to later send its processed messages *outside* to other parts of the brain for long-term storage.

This overview of the four general functions of the hippocampus will prepare us for the next chapter, where we will begin to discuss synaptic plasticity in the hippocampal circuit and its attendant cellular physiology. This is in order to begin to explore how the hippocampus achieves its various functions as a signal integrator and as a cellular memory store for subsequent downloading of information to the longer-term storage areas of the cortex. In this chapter, we will talk about what the hippocampus does; in the next chapter and for most of the rest of the book, we will discuss current ideas about how it does it.

II. STUDYING THE HIPPOCAMPUS

If you are interested in studying the roles of the hippocampus in the behaving animal, how do you even begin to go about it? One approach is to remove the hippocampus or inactivate it and assess the cognitive and behavioral consequences of this experimental manipulation. These types of studies were the first to lead to an appreciation of the role of the hippocampus in memory consolidation (reviewed in reference 1). In fact, studies in a human patient, known as patient H.M., were breakthrough studies that led to the appreciation of the importance of the hippocampus in converting a short-lived memory into a long-lasting one (2). We will discuss this aspect of hippocampal function in the last section of the chapter.

A second approach to studying hippocampal function is quite different. If you want to know what is going on in the hippocampus of an animal that is learning, why not stick an electrode in its hippocampus and directly monitor the cellular firing pattern? This type of approach has been exploited to great effect of late, and in the next section we will talk about new and important insights into the role of the

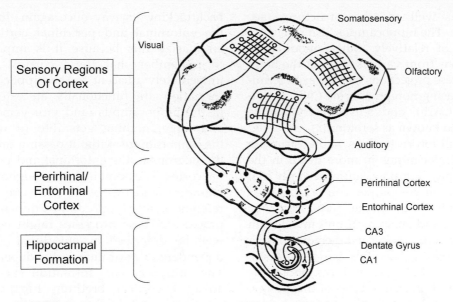

FIGURE 2 Hippocampal connectivity in the CNS. Illustration of the pathway from sensory perceiving regions of the cortex through the perirhinal and entorhinal cortices to the hippocampal formation. Figure adapted with permission from Squire and Lindenlaub (39).

hippocampus in the behaving animal that have been generated using these techniques.

A. Hippocampal Anatomy

First, an anatomical overview is helpful concerning the hippocampal structure, the inputs and outputs of the hippocampus, and the anatomy of the hippocampal formation and related structures in the context of the brain (see Figure 2). The hippocampus receives direct or indirect inputs from all the sensory areas of the cortex including the areas of the cortex involved in late stages of visual information processing, the auditory cortex, and the somatosensory cortex. The hippocampus also receives fairly direct input from the olfactory system via the olfactory bulb. Sensory information of these various sorts is funneled down to the hippocampus via the perirhinal and entorhinal cortices; these are the cortical areas in the immediate anatomical vicinity of the hippocampus near the rhinal fissure in the temporal lobe.

The outputs of the perirhinal and entorhinal cortices then project to the dentate gyrus and the hippocampus proper (these two are referred to jointly as the hippocampal formation). The hippocampus proper is also known in old-style anatomical nomenclature as Cornu Ammonis (Ammon's Horn, after the ram's horn-sporting Greek god) because of its shape. Indeed hippocampus is Greek for sea horse, which is a term coined by anatomists to describe the overall shape of the anatomical structure. The Cornu Ammonis terminology leads to four anatomical subdivisions of the hippocampus: areas CA1, CA2, CA3, and CA4, CA1 and CA3 being the largest and most easily identified. The principal neurons in the CA regions are called *pyramidal neurons* because of their shape—they comprise about 90% of all the neurons in the CA regions of the hippocampal formation. The output neurons of the hippocampus are the CA1 pyramidal neurons—their axons are glutamatergic, and information leaves the hippocampus proper via these axons. The axons of CA1 neurons project back to the entorhinal cortex as well as other structures (see Figure 3). The hippocampus also receives a number of relatively diffuse modulatory projections from various areas of the brain stem. These projections include axon terminals releasing norepinephrine (NE), acetylcholine (ACh), and 5-hydroxytryptamine (5HT, also known as serotonin).

We will return to the synaptic structure of the hippocampus in more detail in the next chapter. For now, suffice it to say that the hippocampus proper, comprising areas CA1–4, plus the dentate gyrus form one functional and anatomical unit involved in information processing and memory consolidation. Exactly how this happens is still mysterious, but current ideas about the cellular and molecular basis of this processing are, of course, the focus of this book.

Information goes out of the hippocampus and ultimately back up into the cortex, backtracking its way once again through the entorhinal and perirhinal cortices. I emphasize this because it is important to remember that these cortical areas immediately adjacent to the hippocampal formation are functionally an extension of the hippocampus (and vice versa). By and large, nothing gets into or out of the hippocampus without passing through the neurons in the entorhinal and perirhinal cortex. The point is that throughout the literature (and this book) there are many references to "hippocampus-dependent" processes. These processes might equally well be described as entorhinal cortex-dependent or perirhinal cortex-dependent. The hippocampal formation and its adjacent cortical brethren function in unison to execute the sophisticated cognitive and memory processing that is detailed here.

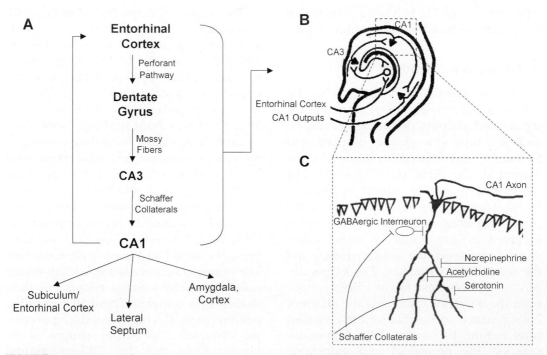

FIGURE 3 Hippocampal intrinsic circuit and output pathways. Schematic and illustration of the principal pathway through the hippocampus. (A) Schematic of the structures through which the sensory signal travels within the hippocampal formation. (B) A more realistic drawing of these structures (from reference 39 with permission). (C) The signaling that occurs in the area CA1 of the hippocampus, focusing on the cellular connections.

III. HIPPOCAMPAL FUNCTION IN COGNITION: THE HIPPOCAMPUS SERVES A ROLE IN INFORMATION PROCESSING—SPACE, TIME, AND RELATIONSHIPS

As just described, the roles of the hippocampus and associated cortices appear to be at least twofold. One role is to process information of a wide variety of sorts, which we will discuss in this section. The second general function, to serve to download information into the cortex for storage in a long-term fashion, we will deal with in the final section of this chapter.

The types of information that the hippocampus deals with, at least as a first approximation, can be divided into three different categories. First, the hippocampus deals with *space* (e.g., it is known to be involved in processing spatial information as described in the last chapter where we talked about hippocampus-dependent maze learning). Second, the hippocampus deals with *time* (e.g., with trace associative conditioning). Animals can learn associations that have no intervening time period between CS and US just fine without a hippocampus. However, introducing a delay period between the presentation of the CS and the presentation of the US brings the hippocampus into play. Thus, the hippocampus appears to be critical for allowing the animal to make an association between two stimuli separated in time. Finally, *complex associations* are hippocampus-dependent; the hippocampus is involved in an animal learning complex contingencies. For example, one specific type of learning of this sort that we will return to later is an animal learning how to predict whether or not a container labeled with a specific scent contains a hidden food reward, depending on recent experience. Learning these types of complicated associations and contingencies brings the hippocampus into play.

In the following sections we address specific examples for each of these categories, illustrating the categories with specific examples from the literature.

A. Space

When an animal is learning about spatial relationships and positions, it utilizes its hippocampus. Specific examples that we talked about in the last chapter include learning that a hidden platform is in a specific place (Morris water maze learning), learning that a specific place is a bad place (contextual fear conditioning), learning that one place is different from another (context discrimination), and learning the order of left/right turns to take in order to navigate a maze (e.g., the more complicated Lashley mazes).

What happens in the hippocampus when an animal is placed in a novel environment and learns about that environment? This is a question that has intrigued neuroscientists for decades, and many beautiful studies over the years have given us nice insights into a number of specific cellular phenomena that occur in the hippocampus when an animal is exploring and learning about a new environment. Most of these studies have used direct electrical recording of hippocampal electrical activity during exploration of a new environment.

Early studies in this area used electroencephalographic (EEG) recordings. EEG recording techniques allow the monitoring of the electrical activity of fairly large populations of cells, by monitoring the mild electric current that flows between and among active neurons as they fire, owing to the influx and efflux of cellular ions. Because EEG recording monitors populations of neurons, the technique is best at detecting the synchronous firing of groups of neurons.

Pioneering EEG studies identified and defined rhythmic firing in the hippocampus when an animal is exploring a novel environment (3). One pronounced example of this that has received much attention is rhythmic firing at the 4–8 Hz (4–8 per second) rate in rodent hippocampus. This type of rhythmic firing around the 5-Hz range is referred to as *theta frequency* firing, or more commonly as the theta rhythm (see Figure 4). The theta rhythm occurs during locomotion and exploration of a new environment, and many experiments have linked the theta rhythm firing with various spatial learning tasks. These initial studies indicated that specific patterns of neuronal firing in the hippocampus are correlated with spatial and contextual learning in animals.

But what is happening at the level of the firing of individual neurons? For example, suppose you put an animal in an open round field with visual cues in specific places and allow it to learn about its environment. What happens to the firing patterns of its hippocampal neurons? In classic studies, O'Keefe and Dostrovsky identified "place" cells in the hippocampus (4–6). In these experiments, the investigators recorded cell firing within the hippocampus by using implanted extracellular electrodes that could monitor the firing of single cells, referred to as single "units." Recording from neurons in the dorsal hippocampus, O'Keefe and Dostrovsky

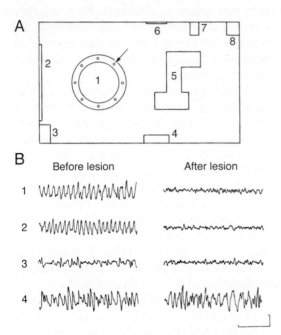

FIGURE 4 Theta pattern in hippocampal EEG. In this EEG study, electrodes were implanted to monitor the aggregate electrical activity in a population of neurons during exploration behavior. (A) Plan view of the testing room (5.5 m × 9.1 m). Contents: 1, circular maze; 2, elevated ventilating duct; 3, table; 4, animal cages; 5, test console, 6 door; 7, sink; 8, cabinet. Overhead fluorescent lights provide 330 lumen/m² of illumination at the level of the maze. (B) Recordings obtained during: 1, voluntary movement; 2, REM sleep; 3, still-alert; 4, slow-wave sleep. The recordings before and after a medial septal lesion was made which eliminated theta rhythm were from the same electrode. Time and voltage calibration: 1 second and 500 μV. Data and figure reproduced with permission from Winson (3). Copyright 1978 American Association for the Advancement of Science.

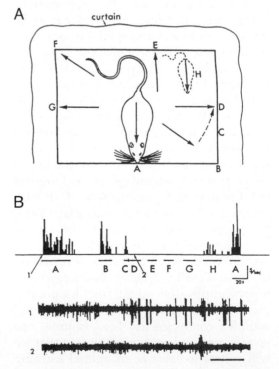

FIGURE 5 Place Cell firing patterns. (A) In the early place cell firing report from O'Keefe and Dostrovsky (4), place cells only fired in position A as shown in top diagram. (B) Histogram of firing at each location in the diagram and raw firing patterns during periods marked 1 and 2 in the histogram. Figure reproduced from O'Keefe and Dostrovsky (4). Copyright 1971, with permission from Elsevier Science.

discovered cells in the freely moving rat that fired only in a specific location within an open field or maze. They referred to these cells as "place cells" and coined the additional nomenclature of "place field" to describe the specific location in the environment where the cell selectively fires (see Figure 5).

Although place cells fire in a way that is highly correlated with the animal's position, these cells fire predominantly when the animal is moving in only one direction (Figure 6). The firing fields are very stable over days and months once established, and place fields are established reasonably quickly (see references 7 and 8), on the order of a few minutes to 1–2 hours (keep in mind that some consolidation process is likely involved). A given place cell can have more than one place field within an apparatus or in two apparati; in other words, a place cell is not exclusively linked to a specific location but may be called upon in connection with one location in one

environment and in connection with another location in another environment.

What are place cells? Place cells are hippocampal pyramidal neurons. The "unit" firing recorded in these early studies was a manifestation of action potential firing in pyramidal neurons in the CA regions of the hippocampus. We will return to these cells and their synaptic and biophysical properties in greater detail in the next two chapters.

The firing pattern is not absolute but relative; for example, place cell firing depends on the animal's perception of visual cues. This can be demonstrated fairly simply by rotating the cues clockwise or counterclockwise between testing trials for a given animal but keeping their position relative to each other constant. When the cues are rotated the place field for a given place cell stays constant in relation to the cues (see Figure 7) but is independent of the animal's absolute location. This experimental result eliminates the simplest explanation for place fields—the rat is not like a

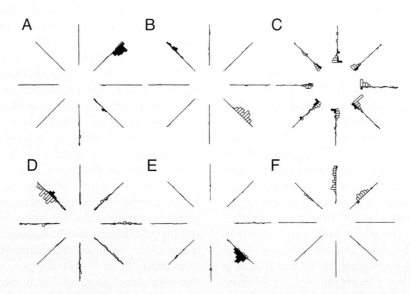

FIGURE 6 Direction selectivity in place cell firing. Typical directional "place fields" exhibited by pyramidal cells while rats move about the radial eight-arm maze. Arms are represented as pulled away from center to facilitate viewing. Spatial firing rates are broken down according to radial direction of motion (open and filled histograms represend outward and inward, respectively). Although, in extremely simplified visual environments, hippocampal cells are much more poorly directionally tuned, in most situations firing in the direction opposite to the preferred one is rarely significantly different from background. Data, figure, and legend reproduced with permission from McNaughton, Chen, and Markus (38).

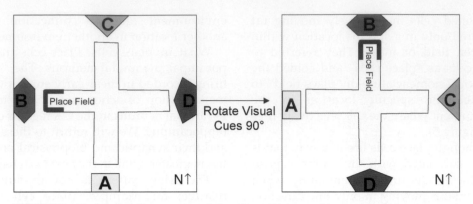

FIGURE 7   Place cells follow rotation of visual cues. Diagram of four-arm radial maze set-up. In this test, the maze remains stationary while the visual cues on the walls are rotated 90° clockwise. When the animal is placed in the first set-up the place field is in the arm closest to the cue marked B (the western arm before the rotation). When the cues are rotated, the place field is again in the arm closest to the cue marked B (the northern arm after the rotation). This indicates that the place field is determined by the animal's relationship to the distal visual cues, not the animal's absolute location in the room.

homing pigeon that can reference the earth's magnetic field for navigation.

But the rotated cues experiment has a much greater implication. Place cell firing is an example of cognition. The animal exhibits a specific cellular firing pattern in its hippocampus that depends upon its perception of the environment. The place cell firing is not dependent whatsoever on absolute position in space—it is dependent on the animal's perceived position, based on its interpretation of visual and other cues in the environment.

The place field is somewhat of an abstraction, in fact (9, 10). Suppose that you train an animal in a small circular chamber and allow place fields to develop. If you place the same animal in a much larger round chamber with the same relative visual cues, the place field stays constant relative to the cues, at least for a subset of place cells (see Figure 8). To me this is a mind-boggling example of cognitive processing—a direct demonstration that a cellular firing pattern can reflect a generalized construct, an abstract representation of the animal's environment.

Thus, place fields are manifest as a burst of action potential firing in a CA1 pyramidal neuron when an animal enters a *perceived* spatial location. Or, stated more precisely, place fields are manifest as a burst of action potentials when an animal enters what it perceives to be a particular spatial location. However, it is critically important to keep in mind that the ordering of this sentence may be exactly reversed. It is an equally valid interpretation, because the data are based on correlation, that the burst of action potential firing leads to the animal perceiving itself as being in a certain place. In other words, we might equally well say that an animal perceives itself to be in a particular location whenever a set of hippocampal place cells fires a burst of action potentials. As we learn more about the hippocampus, it will hopefully become more clear whether the hippocampus is "upstream" of spatial perception or "downstream" of spatial perception. In the limit we may find that it is exactly in the middle of spatial perception, (i.e., that place cell firing is *the* mechanism of spatial perception).

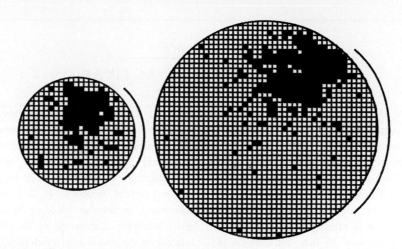

FIGURE 8   Place cells fire in a corresponding location in larger round chamber. Place field in original (left) and larger (right) circular open field is recorded from a hippocampal neuron of a rat searching for food. The larger open field maintains the same orientation in relation to the visual cue (black arc), which is the same size relative to the chamber as in the smaller version. The place field recorded from the rat is shown with black squares and was recorded first in the small chamber and then in the large chamber. The place fields are in the same position relative to the visual cue in each chamber, and also the place field is enlarged in the larger chamber. Data and figure reproduced with permission from Muller and Kubie (9).

BOX 1

ARC AND CELLULAR RE-ACTIVATION

"Immediate early genes" (IEGs) is a term that describes a diverse family of genes that have in common rapid regulation at the transcriptional level. Typically in neurons IEGs respond in an activity-dependent fashion within about 5–15 minutes of cellular stimulation. This rapid transcriptional response of a wide variety of genes clearly indicates the presence of signal transduction mechanisms that can quickly carry a signal from the neuronal cell surface to the nucleus.

IEGs code for proteins with a wide variety of cell functions. One major category is transcription factors, and the well-known transcription factors c-fos, c-jun, jun-B, and zif268 are indeed immediate early genes. This category of IEGs indicates that there

likely are secondary and tertiary waves of altered transcription in response to increased IEG expression and implies that activity-dependent alterations in neuronal gene expression are indeed likely to be quite complex and subject to elaborate control mechanisms. Along these lines, the term "immediate early gene" arises from early studies of transcriptional regulation in non-neuronal cells, where temporal waves of altered gene expression were observed and termed *immediate early*, *early*, and *late*.

Another category of IEGs code for cytoskeletal and structural proteins like Homer 1A, actin, and Arc (initially discovered as Activity-regulated gene 3.1, or Arg3.1). Work from Paul Worley and his collaborators Ozzie Steward, Carol Barnes,

Continued

BOX 1—cont'd

ARC AND CELLULAR RE-ACTIVATION

and Bruce McNaughton has demonstrated that Arc regulation is particularly interesting, and we will return to these studies in later chapters. Of course, in order to make an active product, all genes must be transcribed, processed into mRNA, and then translated into protein. Arc mRNA has the interesting attribute that it is rapidly transported into dendritic processes. In fact, the mRNA is selectively transported and compartmentalized to dendritic regions that have undergone recent excitation. There it participates in local protein synthesis, the net result of which is selective localization of Arc protein at synapses experiencing recent activity.

Like many other IEGs, Arc transcription is regulated in the brain in response to various types of environmental stimulation. Arc transcription is increased in specific pyramidal neurons in area CA1 within a

few minutes of exploration of a novel environment (see, for example, reference (31). This is most likely a molecular correlate to increased place cell firing and the establishment of place fields in hippocampal pyramidal neurons. In a study that combined molecular biology approaches with behavior, Guzowski et al. (31) capitalized on neuronal activity-dependent Arc expression to demonstrate that the same hippocampal pyramidal neurons that fire initially when place fields are established also fire when the animal is re-placed into the same context. In these studies Guzowski et al. used Arc as an activity-dependent molecular marker to track the activity of specific ensembles of pyramidal neurons over time, an elegant application of molecular approaches in the context of the behaving animal.

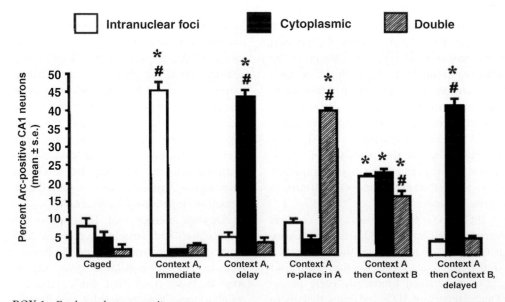

BOX 1   For legend see opposite page.

BOX 1—cont'd

ARC AND CELLULAR RE-ACTIVATION

BOX 1 Neuronal activity-dependent arc expression. Arc expression defines CA1 neuronal ensembles that encode distinct environments. Rats explored environments designated A and B. After being placed in context A, some groups of animals were placed back in A or placed in a different context (B). Arc expression in the nucleus □ or cytoplasm ■ was assessed. The time delay in Arc transport from nucleus to cytoplasm allows investigating whether the same cells are activated when an animal is re-placed in the same environment. "Double" staining means that Arc is found in both the nucleus and cytoplasm, indicating that the cell has been activated twice by the first and second exposures to context A. The distinct staining profiles seen in A/A and A/B groups demonstrate that the induction of Arc transcription in CA1 is highly specific to the nature of the behavioral experience. The A/ immediate, A/ delay and A/B/delay groups define the temporal properties of Arc expression. From each rat (n = 3 rats per group), 97–146 (mean, 120) neurons were counted; the total number of neurons analyzed for this experiment was 2,157. The percentage of positive cells for each staining profile was determined for each individual rat; reported values indicate the group mean. *$p < .002$ relative to caged controls, ANOVA with Scheffe post-hoc analysis. #$p < .05$ relative to the other two cell populations for that group by paired t-test. Data, figure, and legend reproduced from Guzowski, McNaughton, Barnes, and Worley (31), with permission from Nature Publishing Group.

BOX 2

SLEEP AND MEMORY CONSOLIDATION

One of the most interesting areas of current investigation into memory formation in general, and hippocampus-dependent memory formation specifically, are studies asking whether sleep is involved in memory formation (32–36). Specifically, current hypotheses from several groups posit that hippocampus-dependent memory consolidation *requires* sleep, or at least sleep-associated processes.

Sleep is, of course a mysterious process, so testing the role of sleep specifically is quite difficult (see reference 36). It is not sufficient to define sleep as a lack of consciousness, and indeed it is clear from monitoring CNS activity patterns that being unconscious is different from being asleep. In the modern era, sleep is specifically defined in the context of EEG patterns: several different specific stages of sleep have been defined including four progressive stages of "slow-wave" sleep and rapid eye movement (REM) sleep. I find it intriguing that REM sleep is associated with the same synchronized theta-frequency discharges in the hippocampus as are observed in exploring animals (see text). Thus, while "sleep" seems a fairly intuitive term, in fact the phenomenon is a very complex CNS circuit phenomenon, involving almost all areas of the brain, which is quite inconstant over the course of a single sleep episode. Thus, testing the hypothesis that sleep is required for memory is not straightforward. Moreover, sleep disruption

Continued

BOX 2—cont'd

SLEEP AND MEMORY CONSOLIDATION

obviously has a great number of secondary effects on disposition, attention, and motivation—further complicating attempts to approach the problem experimentally.

Nevertheless, there are a number of intriguing observations consistent with a role for sleep-associated neuronal activity in memory consolidation. Work in this area has come primarily from Bruce McNaughton, Carol Barnes, Matt Wilson, Gyorgi Buzsaki, and their respective colleagues. These investigators have shown sleep-associated reproduction of specific patterns of hippocampal pyramidal neuron firing: firing patterns that mimic firing patterns that the animal had established while awake and learning. In other words, it appears that the hippocampus and cortex are "replaying" episodic events while asleep as part of a process of consolidation of memory. In addition, there are a number of correlative studies suggesting that loss of these types of replay episodes causes memory dysfunction.

On the other hand, in the human literature there is not as much support for the idea of a necessity for sleep per se in memory consolidation. For example, patients with specific types of brain lesions or on certain types of medication never sleep or have profound disruptions of their sleep pattern (see reference 37). There also are a few examples of individuals who spontaneously lose the desire to sleep and are essentially insomniac for their entire remaining lifetime. These phenomena do not lead to any profound memory disruption, dissociating sleep from memory formation. However, given the ambiguity in defining sleep, it certainly is possible that insomniac individuals may have certain sleeplike patterns of CNS activity that functionally substitute for the lack of sleep.

Obviously, resolution of the issue of the role of sleep in memory formation will require much additional study. At this point, however, it looks like the answer could be fascinating.

This is the fundamental quandary of the cognitive neurobiologist, and it shows up over and over again in the contemporary literature in experiments involving monitoring of cellular firing (or functional Magnetic Resonance Imaging (fMRI) signals) in real time in response to environmental stimulation. Where does sensory processing end and cognition begin? How does cellular firing get translated into an abstract construct in the brain? The real potential of beginning to answer these types of questions, which really are the modern reformulation of the philosophical mind-body problem that has intrigued mankind

for millennia, is one of the best reasons I can think of to be particularly excited about being a neuroscientist in the contemporary era.

B. Time

The hippocampus is involved not only in processing of spatial information but also in what I will refer to, for lack of a better term, as processing temporal information. I do not necessarily mean that the hippocampus is involved in encoding time itself (which could also be true), but rather I am referring to the hippocampus being involved in temporally dependent learning such as trace associative conditioning and the ability to remember the order of events. Also, the hippocampus exhibits time- and experience-dependent alterations in its cellular firing properties. In this section, we will discuss a few examples of time-dependency of hippocampal function and information processing. We will start with an example of experience-dependent alterations in the behavior of hippocampal place cells as an example of changes in the hippocampus that occur with repeated environmental signals over time. In the next section, we will discuss the important role of the hippocampus in the formation of time-dependent associations, by and large using trace associative conditioning as our example.

We already discussed the impressive, rapid formation of hippocampal place fields when an animal is introduced into a new environment. These place fields are, of course, manifest as a burst of action potential firing in a CA1 pyramidal neuron when an animal enters a particular spatial location (or more precisely when an animal enters what it perceives to be a particular spatial location). What happens to place cell firing over time when the animal re-enters that same location? Are there time-dependent changes in place cell firing properties?

Recent work from the laboratories of Matt Wilson, Gyorgi Buzsaki, and Carol Barnes and Bruce McNaughton, along with several others, has given us clear answers to these two questions. There clearly are time-dependent changes in place cell firing properties that depend on the animal's experience (see Figure 9). Reentering the same place field repetitively over time leads to several pronounced effects on cellular firing patterns, at the level of the individual neuron. These changes are a clear example of experience-dependent changes in the firing properties of hippocampal pyramidal neurons, and, as described earlier, I use them to illustrate "time"-dependent information processing by the hippocampus.

Three specific examples of such cellular changes follow. One, with repeated reentry into the place field of a pyramidal neuron, there is an increase in the place cell's firing rate upon successive reexposure (11). Two, with reentry into a place field, there is a decrease in the latency of the time required for firing the first action potential in a place cell's burst of action potentials (11). Three, the extent of dendritic action potential attenuation decreases over time with experience in the place field (12, we will return to back-propagating action potentials in much more detail in later chapters). Thus, the first entry into a place sets up a hippocampal neuronal place field, but there are subsequent time- and experience-dependent changes in place cell action potential firing properties as well.

The mechanisms underlying this experience-dependent alteration in hippocampal pyramidal neuron properties is a subject of active investigation. In fact, we will return in later chapters to many details of the cellular and molecular mechanisms likely mediating these types of changes. For now, suffice it to say that intriguing mechanisms that could be contributing to these changes include activity-dependent changes in sodium or potassium channels in place cell neurons, changes in neuro-modulatory inputs (e.g acetylcholinergic or noradrenergic inputs) to the hippocampus, or activity-dependent synaptic plasticity within the hippocampus itself (12).

Memory for Real Time—Episodic Memory, Ordering, and the CS-US Interval

Experience-dependent changes in hippocampal place cell firing patterns only begin to scratch the surface of the involvement of the hippocampus in time-dependent encoding of information and temporal information processing. The hippocampus is necessary for a wide variety of different time-dependent learning tasks. I will briefly highlight a few examples here, but a common theme that is emerging in modern studies of hippocampal function is that the

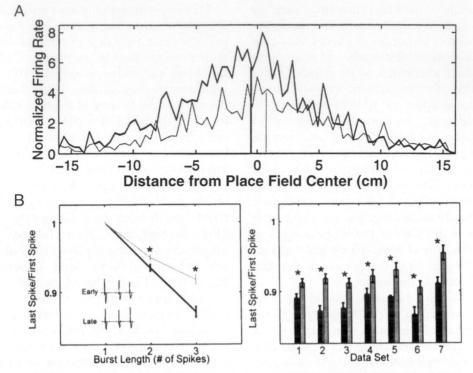

FIGURE 9   Experience-dependent changes in place cell firing. (A) Histogram of the total firing rate at various distances from the place field center during the first and the last visitation to the same place in an environment (light curve, visit 1; solid curve, visit 17; bin width = 0.41 cm, which corresponds to the resolution of the position tracking camera). Firing rates increase as the animal approaches the place field center. Data and figure from Mehta *et al.* (11). (B) Activity-dependent attenuation in spike amplitude is reduced with experience. The average (± SE) amplitude attenuation during high-frequency bursts for a population of simultaneously recorded cells is shown on the left. The amplitude of the last spike in a burst is expressed as a fraction of the amplitude of the first spike and is plotted as a function of the number of spikes in the burst. The black line plots the average attenuation for the animal's first 4 minutes in the environment, and the gray line plots the attenuation for the animal's last 4 minutes. The amount of attenuation is reduced with experience. On the right, the average attenuation for bursts of three spikes for the first 4 minutes of exploration in a familiar environment are shown as black bars and for the last 4 minutes are shown as gray bars. A significant (*$p < .05$, t test) reduction in amplitude attenuation was seen in all data sets ($n = 7$). Data and figure reproduced with permission from Quirk, Blum, and Wilson (12).

hippocampus is involved in perceiving and encoding temporal relationships, storing memory traces for brief periods of time in associative learning, and indeed that the hippocampus is involved in "episodic" perception in general. Simply stated, the hippocampus appears to be integral to forming a coherent representation of a temporal series of events, corresponding to what we would refer to as a single episode of personal experience.

Obviously if the hippocampus is ultimately involved in mediating the storage of a complex set of individual experiences, forming a representation with the appropriate temporal ordering is key. In Houston, a typical example would be: the cross-walk light changed, I entered the street, the car almost ran me over; this is quite a different experience from any other sequencing of those three items. Recent exciting work by the laboratories of Howard Eichenbaum, Matt Wilson, and John Disterhoft have begun to demonstrate nicely that order-dependent hippocampal information processing is indeed occurring; furthermore, recent elegant work from these labs has begun to explore the cellular and molecular basis for this role.

Early studies in this area asked a simple question: do hippocampal lesions have a greater effect on memory paradigms that involve a time lag during learning? The answer to this question is clearly yes. For example, in one pioneering study, Chiba, Kesner, and Reynolds investigated memories for temporal ordering in rats, who were learning the specific order of presentation of two spatial locations (13). They found that the greater the time-lag between visits to the first site and the second site, the more susceptible the memory formation was to hippocampal lesions. Thus, the hippocampus is involved selectively in forming a memory of event orders when there is a longer intervening time between the first event and the second event.

More recent work (14) has shown that hippocampal lesions disrupt the ability of rats to learn the ordering of olfactory cues. For example, a rat with a hippocampal lesion will have a deficit in remembering the specific order: orange, lemon, wintergreen. This is a very nice example of the role of the hippocampus in placing sensory stimuli in the appropriate temporal relationship with each other.

In additional recent studies from Howard Eichenbaum's group, recordings from the hippocampus in vivo in behaving animals has suggested that temporal factors can come into play in the firing of "place" cells. Howard's group has shown that place cells can fire selectively depending on the recent history of the animal (15). In this experiment, they trained rats to make alternating left-hand and right-hand turns as they repeatedly ran a T maze. An animal in the identical spot in a T maze can have a given place cell fire selectively depending on whether it is about to make a left-hand turn or a right-hand turn. These cells may be "intent" cells influencing what the animal will do next. Alternatively, they may be "recent history" cells because what the animal is *about* to do next depends on what it just finished doing. Regardless, this cell firing pattern clearly shows that "place" cells are not just place cells but something more complex, influenced by the animal's recent history.

In fact, it is intriguing to consider that a potential clue to this aspect of pyramidal neuron function was there in the very first description of place cells by O'Keefe and Dostrovsky. Place cells don't just fire depending on location, they also only fire when the animal is moving in a specific direction through the place field. Obviously an animal moving in one direction in a place field has had a different recent experience than when it crossed the same spot moving in the opposite direction. This is pure speculation, but interesting to consider as a possibility.

The most extensively studied example of hippocampal involvement in time-dependent information processing is trace associative conditioning. You will recall from the last chapter that in trace conditioning a time lag is introduced between the CS and the US, typically in the range of a few seconds to a few minutes. The most popular experimental model to study this is trace eye-blink conditioning, although trace cued fear conditioning has recently begun to be utilized as well. Hippocampal lesions of various sorts (anatomical, pharmacologic, molecular) lead to a loss of trace eye-blink or fear conditioning in animals up to and including the human (1, 16, 17). The time-dependent specificity of the involvement of the hippocampus is illustrated by the observation that delivery of the identical stimuli with no intervening time lag (unfortunately designated as "delay" conditioning, although there is no delay *between* CS and US) is perfectly normal in hippocampal lesioned animals. Thus, the hippocampus is selectively involved in memory formation that incorporates a time-dependent component.

What is happening in the hippocampus during trace associative conditioning? This fascinating question is being explored at present, and at least a few answers are available. Hippocampal pyramidal neurons in area CA1 show large increases in their firing rates during the learning period, especially early in training when pyramidal neurons show increased firing in response to both the CS and the US (see Figure 10 and references 18 and 19 for more details). Thus it is possible that pyramidal neurons maintain a representation of the CS over time so that it can be associated with the US. Howard Eichenbaum has proposed a more sophisticated model, which he refers to as the episodic encoding model (20, 21). In this model, the hippocampus forms a temporal representation of a single event based on the specific order of firing of individual (or groups of) CA1 pyramidal neurons. Thus, the firing of ensembles of cells in a particular order would represent a specific episode in the animal's life, preserving the temporal relationships with fidelity. This type of information could then be used in the storage of a learned relationship between two stimuli separated in time. Overall, while the circuit properties underlying the role of the hippocampus in temporal information processing are still unclear at this time, new insights have been gained, and much effort is being devoted to this problem.

If the circuitry is unclear, the cellular and molecular mechanisms are even more

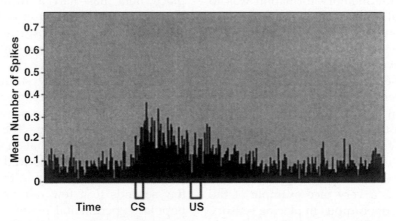

FIGURE 10 Increased hippocampal neuron firing during trace eye-blink conditioning. Average peri-event histograms (10 ms bins) for pyramidal cell response profile recorded from rabbits during trace conditioning. Action potentials (spikes) from each cell were summed across a single training session, then averaged across cells. The duration of the histogram is 3750 ms, and the duration of the baseline period prior to CS onset is 1000 ms. Of all tested pyramidal cells, 7.4% display this type of response profile. Data and figure reproduced with permission from McEchron, Weible, and Disterhoft (19).

It is worth noting that many neocortical neurons exhibit this same type of firing pattern, that is, a residual increase in firing after the presentation of an environmental stimulus. This has been most extensively documented in neurons in the visual system. This is important to keep in mind because clearly the hippocampus is not the only area of the brain encoding temporal information.

mysterious. Tantalizing clues have emerged, however. For example, trace fear conditioning is dependent on N-methyl-D-aspartate (NMDA) receptor function in CA1 pyramidal neurons, as was recently demonstrated in a very sophisticated study using genetically engineered mice (17). John Disterhoft's lab has also shown that trace eye-blink conditioning results in increases in CA1 pyramidal neuron membrane excitability and an increase in synaptic efficacy at the connections between neurons in area CA3 and area CA1 (see reference 22 and Figure 11). The contributions of these specific mechanisms to the role of the hippocampus in temporal information processing will hopefully become more clear as work in this area continues.

Overall, these studies directly demonstrating changes in hippocampal pyramidal neuron firing in time-dependent associative learning are a beautiful example of cognitive processing of real time. They suggest that hippocampal pyramidal neurons encode the maintenance of a representation of a sensory stimulus, in the absence of any continued presentation of the stimulus itself.[1] This representation functions to allow a subsequent association of that sensory input with a temporally removed, second sensory stimulus.

C. Multimodal Associations— The Hippocampus as a Generalized Association Machine and Multimodal Sensory Integrator

Even the earliest reports of place cells noted that they are multimodal sensory integrators. In an early study where O'Keefe began to investigate "why they fire where

they fire," he trained rats in a T maze using four different external visual cues as the spatial landmarks (6). He then proceeded to query the animal's hippocampus by recording how place cell firing patterns changed when one or several of the spatial cues were removed. He found that some place cells used one or two of the cues as the relevant landmarks while the remainder of the landmarks were immaterial to their firing—a fairly straightforward result. However, he also observed some place cells that were triggered by any combination of any two landmarks. As far as these cells were concerned, landmarks A + B was equivalent to landmarks C + D was equivalent to A + C, and so on. Thus, two environments that were different from each other visually (A + B versus C + D, for example) were treated as equivalent as long as the animal had had the opportunity to previously learn that A, B, C, and D were always present in a consistent spatial relationship to *each other*. The place cell firing apparently had come to represent an abstraction, an integration of four spatial cues. Apparently any two cues were sufficient to allow the place cell (or something upstream of it) to reconstruct a representation of the entirety of the space.

More recent work has made clear the role of the hippocampus in general, and "place" (i.e., pyramidal) cells in particular, in multimodal sensory integration. Howard Eichenbaum and his collaborators have been leaders in this pursuit, and they have made many seminal observations in this area. Their findings have completely changed the way we look at the function of the hippocampus. In this next section, I will highlight two of the studies from Howard Eichenbaum and his co-workers that I consider to be landmarks in the field.

Eichenbaum's lab has used the four-arm radial maze in many studies (see Figure 7). The set-up in the basic version of the experiment is quite simple—there are four arms to the plus-shaped maze, and the maze is in a room with one unique visual

---

[1]It is important to note that this may not take place entirely within the hippocampus. For example, a larger circuit of which the hippocampus is a part may carry out this function. Particularly appealing in this context is the possibility of reciprocal hippocampal-neocortical projections participating in a short-term memory store, given the variety of evidence demonstrating the maintained firing of cortical neurons in vivo after various sensory stimuli.

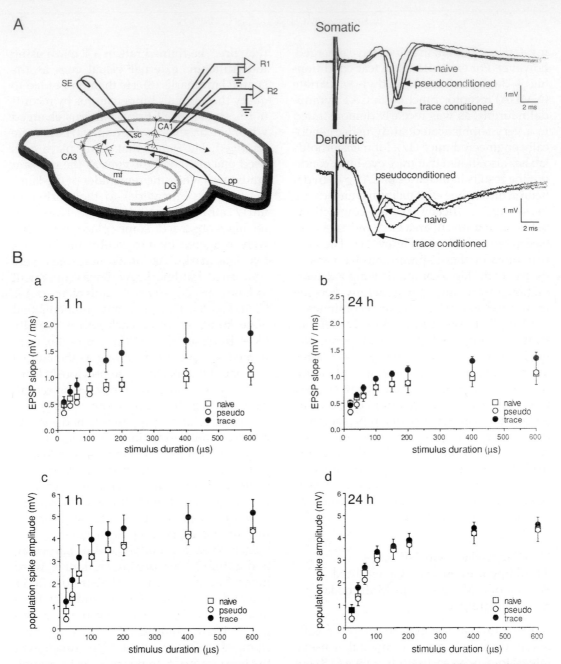

FIGURE 11 Increased connectivity in hippocampal pyramidal neurons with eye-blink conditioning. Hippocampal slices were prepared and physiologic responses monitored in vitro, using control animals and trace-conditioned animals. (A) Diagram showing rabbit hippocampal slices in vitro with placement of stimulating electrode (SE), and somatic (R1) and dendritic (R2) recording electrodes. To the right are representative field potentials (excitatory postsynaptic responses) from each type of recording one hour after conditioning. The following structures are also labeled: Schaffer collaterals (sc), perforant path (pp), dentate gyrus (DG), mossy fibers (mf), CA1 and CA3. (B) Effects of conditioning on Schaffer collateral evoked field potentials recorded in CA1. Means ± SE are given for trace-conditioned (1 hour, $n = 9$; 24 hour, $n = 13$), pseudoconditioned (1 hour, $n = 9$; 24 hour, $n = 8$), and naïve ($n = 7$) animals for each stimulus intensity value. (a) Excitatory Postsynaptic Potential (EPSP) slope recorded in dendrites was greater in slices prepared from conditioned animals 1 hour after conditioning. (b) No significant differences in initial EPSP slope were seen between conditioning groups 24 hours after conditioning. No conditioning effect was seen in population spike amplitude input-output function 1 hour (c) or 24 hours (d) after conditioning; population spikes indicate action potential firing in the post-synaptic CA1 pyramidal neurons. Diagram and data reproduced with permission from Power, Thompson, Moyer, and Disterhoft (22).

cue on each wall. The animal learns to use the spatial cues to navigate to food rewards in the maze. Firing patterns for hippocampal place cells recapitulate what we described previously—they fire dependent upon the animal's location in space relative to the distal visual cues. In addition, as expected, they are direction-dependent; that is, they fire selectively when the animal is moving either outward into an arm or inward back toward the center of the maze.

What happens when you have local cues within the arms of the maze? Eichenbaum's group addressed this question by preparing their four-arm maze with distinct visual, olfactory, and tactile cues in each of the four arms, in addition to the four distal visual cues on the wall (23, 24; see Figure 12). When they train their animals in this maze, they find cells that fire selectively dependent upon the texture of the floor and the olfactory cues that are present. If there are cells in the hippocampus that fire in response to distal visual cues and also cells that fire in response to local cues, are they

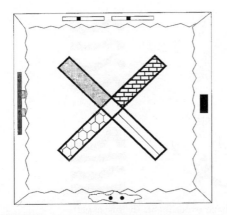

FIGURE 12   Four-arm radial maze with local and distal cues. The four-arm radial maze set-up used in the experiments such as those performed by Tanila et al. (7, 24; see text and Figure 13) is used to assess effects of manipulation of local and distal cues. Local cues are coverings of the arms that give a set of visual, tactile, and olfactory cues distinct form the other arms. The distal cues are objects on each wall surrounding the maze. Reproduced with permission from Tanila, Sipila, Shapiro, and Eichenbaum (7).

mutually exclusive? The answer is no—in fact, there are individual cells that fire in response to both local cues and distal cues when they are presented separately. Moreover, there are some cells that fire only when all the cues are presented together. Their firing depends on the simultaneous presence of all the various cues. This latter finding suggests that these cells are firing in response to (or in order to produce) an aggregate representation of all the cues!

Finally, we come to the *piece de resistance*— what happens to these multimodal cells, cells that respond to both local cues and distal cues, if you change the relationship of the local cues to the distal cues? Eichenbaum and his colleagues did a clever manipulation where they asked that question: the "double rotation" experiment (Figure 13). They trained animals in a multicue maze that contained both local cues and distal visual cues and then rotated the visual cues 90° counterclockwise and the local cues 90° clockwise. When the animal is placed back in the manipulated maze what happens to the firing of the cells? The firing of some cells tracks the visual cues, as expected of place cells. The firing of other cells tracks the local olfactory, tactile, and visual cues—sort of a variant of the classic place cell. However, there are some single cells that track both the local and distal cues. They continue to fire when the animal is in a particular arm of the maze with specific local cues, and fire in a *different* arm of the maze that is in the original orientation relative to the distal visual cues. Thus, hippocampal pyramidal neuron firing can track local cues, can track distal cues, or can track both independently. In the latter case the cell appears to encode an A + B + C + D representation as discussed earlier, where either A + B or C + D is sufficient to trigger firing. In this case, it is even more complex because the different cues are nonequivalent; that is, some are distal visual cues and some are local tactile and olfactory cues.

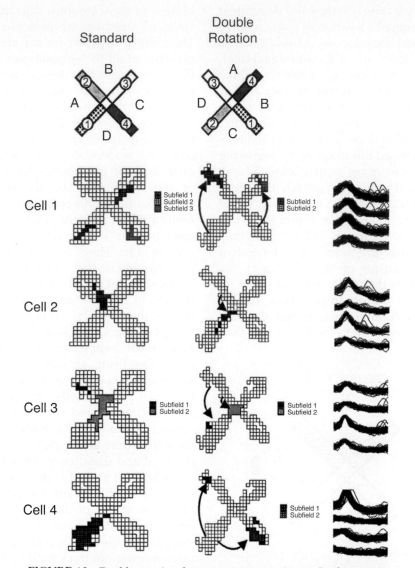

FIGURE 13   Double rotation four-arm maze experiment. In this experiment, the four local cues were rotated 90° to the left as the distal cues were rotated 90° to the right. The responses of four simultaneously recorded cells (cells 1–4) are shown here before and after the double rotation of the cues. Data and figure reproduced with permission from Tanila, Shapiro, and Eichenbaum (24). Copyright © 1997 John Wiley and Sons, Inc.

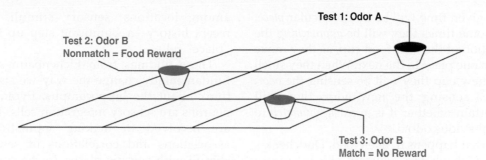

FIGURE 14   Continuous odor-guided non-matching to sample. This diagram outlines an experiment to assess the ability of the animal to distinguish a matching or non-matching stimulus. The animals must determine if the second smell that they experience is the same or different than the first, if the third is the same or different than the second and so on. In this example, Test 1 has Odor A; Test 2 has Odor B, a non-match. Test 3 also has Odor B so the third is a match to the second. Only non-matches contain a food reward.

Thus we have seen our first example of the fact that "place cell" is really a misnomer. Hippocampal pyramidal neurons are place cells, but they also can be texture cells and olfactory cells, and they also can be place + texture + olfactory cells. In the next experiment I will describe, Howard Eichenbaum's lab went on to show that the world of the hippocampal pyramidal neuron is even more complex than that. Hippocampal pyramidal neurons are multimodal association cells that are involved in encoding a wide variety of contingencies and relationships.

In preparing to do their experiment, Howard and his colleagues Emma Wood and Paul Dudchenko first trained rats in a contingency task—a task with the accurate but cumbersome descriptor "continuous odor-guided non-matching to sample" (25). One aspect of the task is that rats learn that small cups filled with sand sometimes have food rewards in them. Moreover, each sand cup has one of nine odor cues mixed in with it, spicy smells such as thyme and paprika. How does a rat know if a specific sand cup has food buried in it or not? The sand cups are presented sequentially, and if

the smell of the cup presented is different from the previous one, then the rat knows there is food buried in the new cup. Thus, continuous (presented sequentially) odor-guided (smell of the cup) non-matching (different) to sample (from the previous one). In presenting many odors in a row, the investigators were also careful to vary the order of presentation so that sequences of odors could not be used to predict the food—in other words, only the odor presented immediately before could be used to predict the food reward.

After rats learned this fundamental contingency, an additional layer of complexity was added that was irrelevant to the rats, but of fundamental import to the rat-testers (see Figure 14). The food cups were presented to the rats randomly at one of nine different locations in an open field surrounded by spatial cues (can you say place cell?). The positions of placement in the matrix were carefully controlled so that this variable did not allow prediction of the presence or absence of the food reward.

In considering the entirety of the task, then, a number of different individual components can be identified. The rats at any given time will be in a particular *place*. At some times they will be *approaching* the location of the new food cup, as they move from one place to the next. When they smell the new cup they will be sensing the *odor*. After sensing the new odor, they will ascertain whether it is a *match/nonmatch* to the previous odor.

What happens if, like Wood, Dudchenko, and Eichenbaum, you are able to record pyramidal neuron firing in the animals' hippocampi while they perform this task? If you were in this enviable position you would find that hippocampal pyramidal neurons exhibit an amazing array of sophisticated firing patterns (Figure 15). Some cells fire selectively only when the animal is approaching a food cup, regardless of where it is (Figure 15D). Perhaps they are encoding that the animal is about to have to make a decision about the content of the cup. Or perhaps they encode some abstract representation of the food cup itself. Some cells respond selectively to specific odors only (Figure 15A). Some cells fire selectively depending on whether the odor matches or doesn't match the previous odor, regardless of the odor being presented or where it is (Figure 15C). Perhaps they are reward/no reward cells, or perhaps they are contingency cells. Thus, specific hippocampal pyramidal neurons can be considered odor cells, or approach cells, or match/non-match cells—an amazing array of possibilities.

Not surprisingly, some cells are simply place cells (Figure 15B). However, some cells are specific place + odor cells, firing at only one place in the matrix and only upon the presentation of a specific odor. Some cells are place + match/nonmatch cells. Finally, a few cells were even so specialized as to be place + odor + match/nonmatch cells. Just think about it! These cells will fire only in a specific place in response to a specific odor and only if it does not match the previous odor. These cells appear to encode complex, multimodal associations

among locations, sensory stimuli, and recent history—a significant step up from "place" cells.

These findings from Eichenbaum's lab fundamentally change the way we should think about the hippocampus. Pyramidal neurons are sensory integration cells. They are involved in making sophisticated associations and correlations of sensory stimuli with specific places, in the context of the animal's prior history.

Overall, the wide variety of studies we discussed in this section, which used in vivo recording techniques in the behaving animal, suggest an amazingly complex involvement of the hippocampus in sensory processing—suggesting its involvement in cognitive processing of space, time, and relationships.

Finally, these experiments illustrate the power of, but also the important caveat for, the "measure" experiment when studying the behaving animal. Measuring things *in vivo* is quite powerful because you can ascertain that specific things are happening as the animal learns. However, there also is the limitation that the interpretation of the data may be limited by our own lack of discernment of what is going on in the animal's brain. Cells that in previous studies had been characterized as "place" cells likely were encoding information much more sophisticated than the experimenters realized. The interpretation of data in a behavioral "measure" experiment may fall short simply because the experimenter has not fully appreciated everything that is happening with the animal's cognitive processing.

Our interpretation is limited by what we think we are asking the animal to do, based on our own thinking about the task when we design the experiment. However, the animal may be learning many things about its environment, and about what is happening to it, that are not apparent to us. These learning events will result in real

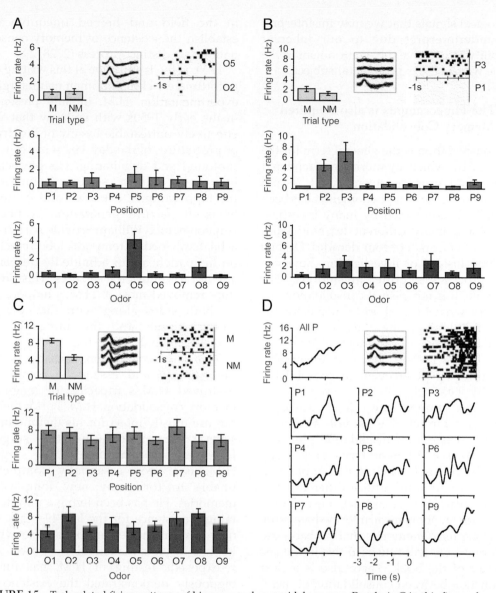

FIGURE 15 Task related firing patterns of hippocampal pyramidal neurons. Panels A–C in this figure show the firing rate in 1-second analysis period for each trial type (M = match; NM = non-match), cup location (P1–P9), and odor (O1–O9) for three different types of cells: (A) an odor cell (odor, $F_{(8,74)}$ = 8.59, P < .0001; trial type, $F_{(1,74)}$ = 0.04, not significant (NS); cup location $F_{(8,74)}$ = 1.03, NS; odor × trial type, $F_{(8,74)}$ = 1.74, NS); (B) a location cell (cup location, $F_{(8,74)}$ = 8.60; P <.0001; odor, $F_{(8,74)}$ = 0.84, NS; trial type $F_{(1,74)}$ = 2.76, NS; odor × trial type $F_{(8,74)}$ = 1.14, NS; cup × trial type, $F_{(8,74)}$ = 1.58, NS); (C) a match cell (trial type, $F_{(1,74)}$ = 22.95, P < .0001; odor, $F_{(8,74)}$ = 1.42, NS; location, $F_{(8,74)}$ = 1.17, NS; odor × trial type, $F_{(8,74)}$ = 0.68, NS; location × trial type, $F_{(8,74)}$ = 1.20, NS). Panel d shows firing rates (200 ms bins) for 3 second period when the rat approached each cup position (P1–P9), and averaged across all positions (all P) for an approach cell (trial period, t(1,107) = 10.77, P < .001; trial type, $F_{(1,74)}$ = 0.06, NS; odor $F_{(8,74)}$ = 0.47, NS; Location $F_{(8,74)}$ = 1.42, NS; Odor × trial type, $F_{(8,74)}$ = 0.96, NS; location × trial type, $F_{(8,74)}$ = 1.00, NS). Each panel also shows the waveform of the cell recorded on each tetrode channel and a raster display of firing patterns time-locked to the end of the odor sample period. Data, figure, and figure legend reproduced from Wood, Dudchenko, and Eichenbaum (25).

biological signals that we may misinterpret or underinterpret due to our inherent inability to perceive the environment in the same way as the experimental subject.

D. The Hippocampus is also Required for Memory Consolidation

Consolidation is the general term for the process by which memories are rendered stable and lasting (see references 21, 26, and 27). Its existence as a phenomenon has been reliably demonstrated by many investigators using many different learning paradigms over a span of four decades. Despite its long history of investigation, however, the process is quite mysterious. For example, it is not clear if consolidation is a process whereby a short-term memory is rendered long-lasting (i.e., a process of serial conversion of short-term to long-term memory), or if short-term and longer-term memories of a given event are consolidated entirely separately.

A few things are clear, however. Consolidation clearly is not a unitary process. There are consolidation processes that subserve different types of learning (explicit versus implicit, for example) and that, at a minimum, utilize different brain areas. There also are distinct consolidation processes for short-term, intermediate-term, and long-term memories that probably are different—we will return to this in the last chapter of the book. There also is a clear distinction between consolidation of memory versus storage of memory. Brain lesions to specific areas can lead to a selective disruption of consolidation of new memories without affecting storage and recall of old memories The classic studies illustrating this distinction involve patient "H.M." The story of H.M. has been told, retold, and analyzed repeatedly in the learning and memory literature, so I will only briefly review the case here. The first studies of H.M. and his memory deficits are landmarks

in the field and helped unequivocally establish the existence of memory consolidation as a distinct process (2, 28, 29).

H.M. is (he is still alive at this writing) an unfortunate victim of human neurosurgical experimentation. H.M. initially presented in the early 1950s with epilepsy that was effectively untreatable by any of the drugs or procedures of the day. His seizures were profound and debilitating. His physicians hypothesized that his seizures originated in the hippocampus, a known and common locus of seizure generation. A neurosurgeon named William Scoville performed a bilateral medial temporal lobe resection on his patient in an admittedly desperate attempt to control the seizures. This procedure removed most of H.M.'s hippocampi on both sides along with the adjacent cortical tissue, and the amygdala (see reference 29 and Figure 16).

This iatrogenic lesion partially treated the epilepsy and essentially completely destroyed H.M.'s capacity for long-term memory consolidation. H.M.'s prior memories are mostly intact for his lifetime up to several years predating the surgery. However, since the time of the surgery, H.M. has been essentially completely unable to form any new long-lasting memories. He has been living a minute-to-minute existence for the last 49 years. His only new memories are of facts to which he has been exhaustively exposed and re-exposed. Testing of H.M. has unambiguously demonstrated the existence of consolidation processes in human memory. He has preservation and stability of a large number of pre-existing memories and a clear capacity to recall them consistently. What he does not have is the capacity to make any new memories that last for more than a few seconds without continuous rehearsal.

There has been a general tendency to ascribe this deficit to loss of the hippocampus, which is consistent with a wide variety

BOX 3

RECONSOLIDATION OF MEMORIES

What if every time you recalled a memory you made that memory subject to erasure? A frightening thought, certainly. The idea also seems somewhat at odds with our perception of consistency in our own memories—recalling them seems to make them stronger, not weaker. Nevertheless, recent provocative studies have suggested that every time we recall a specific memory, we make it necessary for that memory to be reestablished. The word used to describe this attribute of memory is "reconsolidation" in reference to the well-known attribute that long-term memories, when initially formed, are labile and subject to disruption over a period of hours (see text). It appears that previously established long-term memories also are subject to disruption specifically during that period immediately after each time they are recollected.

The most definitive recent experiment concerning memory reconsolidation was performed by Karim Nader and Glenn Schafe in Joe LeDoux's lab (30), although important work in this area has also been performed by the laboratories of Susan Sara, Yadin Dudai, and Alcino Silva, among others. Nader et al. (30) studied memory reconsolidation using cued fear conditioning in rats, which as we discussed in Chapter 2 is an amygdala-dependent process. Basically, Nader et al. found that

when an animal is reexposed to a conditioned stimulus (an auditory cue in this case), which of course elicits recollection of a prior CS-US pairing, restorage of that memory can be disrupted by inhibiting protein synthesis in the amygdala. The same memory is impervious to an equivalent period of protein synthesis inhibition as long as the animal is not stimulated to recall the CS-US pairing during that time. The implication of these studies is that reactivated memories must be put back into long-term storage via a protein synthesis-dependent process similar to that used during the initial consolidation period. Hence the term "reconsolidation."

There are, of course, a great number of questions raised by these studies. Is the reconsolidation mechanism identical to the initial consolidation mechanism? Are all long-term memories subject to reconsolidation after each recollection, or is this mechanism restricted to particular brain areas or memory types? Might disruption of this process contribute to memory pathologies such as aging-related memory loss? Could pharmacologic means be used as a therapeutic intervention in "pathologic" memory such as post-traumatic stress disorder? Future studies will hopefully lead to new insights into these and other questions concerning this fascinating phenomenon.

of animal lesion studies and indeed with the memory consolidation deficits of other patients with more selective hippocampal lesions. However, it is important to remember that H.M. has lesions of the surrounding perihippocampal cortices and the

amygdala, which likely contribute to the particularly pronounced nature of his deficits (Figure 16).

Also, given what we discussed earlier in this chapter about the role of the hippocampus in multimodal cognitive processing,

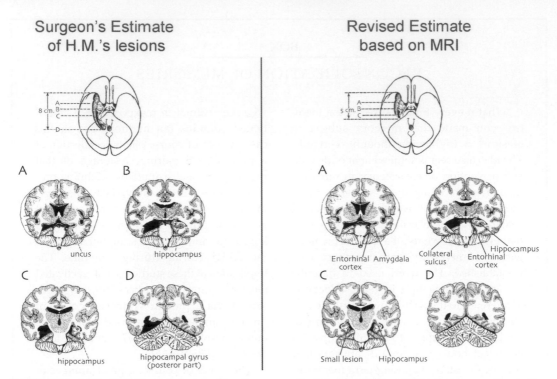

FIGURE 16 MRI of H.M.'s brain lesions. The diagram on the left shows Patient H.M.'s lesions as estimated by the surgeon who performed the original operation (2). The diagram on the right, shows Patient H.M.'s actual lesions as shown by magnetic resonance imaging (MRI). A through D in both diagrams are drawings of coronal sections from rostral (A) to caudal (D). In each cross-section (A–D), the right half of the brain is drawn as normal, for purposes of comparison. Figure and MRI data reproduced with permission from Corkin et al. (29).

one wonders about generalized cognitive deficits in H.M. as well. I am not referring to a loss of intelligence but rather to the possibility of a general inability to process information about his surroundings, correlations among items and events, and the like. These problems may contribute to his cognitive problems and his long-term memory deficits as well. I should make it clear that I don't believe these considerations negate the conclusion of a deficit in memory consolidation in H.M., but I am simply pointing out that interpreting the basis of H.M.'s cognitive deficits should take into consideration modern ideas about the important role of the hippocampus in

information processing as well as memory consolidation.

The role of the hippocampus in memory consolidation that was identified in the seminal studies of H.M. have been confirmed and extended in a wide variety of hippocampal lesion studies in experimental animals. Obviously animal experimentation allows a much more detailed and controlled experimental approach than human studies and a number of attributes of hippocampus-dependent memory consolidation have become clear. For example, inhibitors of protein synthesis block memory consolidation when they are applied after training. Consolidation is known to be a process that occurs over several hours after training. Hippocampus-dependent long-term memory consolidation is also dependent on altered gene expression. Activation of the N-methyl-D-aspartate subtype of glutamate receptor is involved, as are a number of signal transduction mechanisms and neuromodulatory neurotransmitter systems. Overall, a quite wide variety of studies using many different approaches have demonstrated that involvement in memory consolidation is a central attribute of hippocampal function. We will spend much of the rest of the book discussing the cellular and molecular particulars of this process. In brief, the hippocampus, in addition to its information processing role, serves as a short-term memory store that ultimately downloads information to the cortex for longer-term storage.

The basis for this process is mysterious, but one thing that is clear is that the hippocampus must be able to hold a memory trace for some appreciable period of time—hours to days or weeks at least.

In the next chapter, we will talk about a cellular mechanism likely to be critical to allowing the hippocampus to serve as this sort of memory buffer—long-term potentiation (LTP). Long-lasting synaptic potentiation of this sort *also* likely is involved in the precise formation and maintenance of hippocampal place cell firing patterns. We also will touch on shorter-lasting forms of synaptic plasticity that may be involved in short-term storage of information and information processing in the hippocampus as well as phenomena such as post-tetanic potentiation (PTP) and short-term potentiation (STP) that may be involved in the "time" aspect of hippocampal processing of CS-US contingencies over the period of a few seconds.

In Chapter 5, we will talk about complex mechanisms regulating the induction of LTP, specifically ending up with examples of how lasting plastic change in hippocampal neurons can be triggered dependent upon three-way or four-way contingencies. These latter examples are the types of cellular mechanisms that are likely to allow the multimodal sensory integration observed in the studies by Eichenbaum's group that we discussed in this chapter.

After we go through the physiology, we then will proceed to the molecules that allow these sophisticated cellular processes to occur. These will be the issues of Chapters 6, 7, and 8.

IV. SUMMARY

In this chapter, we explored hippocampal function in more detail, drawing specific examples from the literature for each of the four broad categories of cognition in which the hippocampus participates—space, time, multimodal associations, and memory consolidation. This outline of the complexities of hippocampal function prepares us for the next chapter, where we will begin to dissect the hippocampal synaptic circuit and its cellular physiology. This will allow us to begin to understand how the hippocampus achieves its various functions as a signal integrator and as a transient cellular memory store for subsequent downloading of information to the longer-term storage areas of the cortex.

References

1. Squire, L. R., and Zola-Morgan, S. (1991). "The medial temporal lobe memory system." *Science* 253:1380–1386.
2. Scoville, W. B., and Milner, B. (2000). "Loss of recent memory after bilateral hippocampal lesions. 1957." *J. Neuropsychiatry Clin. Neurosci.* 12:103–113.
3. Winson, J. (1978). "Loss of hippocampal theta rhythm results in spatial memory deficit in the rat." *Science* 201:160–163.
4. O'Keefe, J., and Dostrovsky, J. (1971). "The hippocampus as a spatial map. Preliminary

evidence from unit activity in the freely-moving rat." *Brain Res.* 34:171–175.

5. O'Keefe, J. (1976). "Place units in the hippocampus of the freely moving rat." *Exp. Neurol.* 51:78–109.

6. O'Keefe, J., and Conway, D. H. (1978). "Hippocampal place units in the freely moving rat: why they fire where they fire." *Exp. Brain Res.* 31:573–590.

7. Tanila, H., Sipila, P., Shapiro, M., and Eichenbaum, H. (1997). "Brain aging: impaired coding of novel environmental cues." *J. Neurosci.* 17:5167–5174.

8. Lever, C., Wills, T., Cacucci, F., Burgess, N., and O'Keefe, J. (2002). "Long-term plasticity in hippocampal place-cell representation of environmental geometry." *Nature* 416:90–94.

9. Muller, R. U., and Kubie, J. L. (1987). "The effects of changes in the environment on the spatial firing of hippocampal complex-spike cells." *J. Neurosci.* 7:1951–1968.

10. Muller, R. U., Kubie, J. L., and Ranck, J. B., Jr. (1987). "Spatial firing patterns of hippocampal complex-spike cells in a fixed environment." *J. Neurosci.* 7:1935–1950.

11. Mehta, M. R., Barnes, C. A., and McNaughton, B. L. (1997). "Experience-dependent, asymmetric expansion of hippocampal place fields." *Proc. Natl. Acad. Sci. USA* 94:8918–8921.

12. Quirk, M. C., Blum, K. I., and Wilson, M. A. (2001). "Experience-dependent changes in extracellular spike amplitude may reflect regulation of dendritic action potential back-propagation in rat hippocampal pyramidal cells." *J. Neurosci.* 21:240–248.

13. Chiba, A. A., Kesner, R. P., and Reynolds, A. M. (1994). "Memory for spatial location as a function of temporal lag in rats: role of hippocampus and medial prefrontal cortex." *Behav. Neural. Biol.* 61:123–131.

14. Fortin, N. J., Agster, K. L, and Eichenbaum, H. B. (2002). "Critical role of the hippocampus in memory for sequences of events." *Nat. Neurosci.* 5:458–462.

15. Wood, E. R., Dudchenko, P. A., Robitsek, R. J., and Eichenbaum, H. (2000). "Hippocampal neurons encode information about different types of memory episodes occurring in the same location." *Neuron* 27:623–633.

16. Clark, R. E., and Squire, L. R. (1998). "Classical conditioning and brain systems: the role of awareness." *Science* 280:77–81.

17. Huerta, P. T., Sun, L. D., Wilson, M. A., and Tonegawa, S. (2000). "Formation of temporal memory requires NMDA receptors within CA1 pyramidal neurons." *Neuron* 25:473–480.

18. McEchron, M. D., and Disterhoft, J. F. (1997). "Sequence of single neuron changes in CA1 hippocampus of rabbits during acquisition of trace eyeblink conditioned responses." *J. Neurophysiol.* 78:1030–1044.

19. McEchron, M. D., Weible, A. P., and Disterhoft, J. F. (2001). "Aging and learning-specific changes in single-neuron activity in CA1 hippocampus during rabbit trace eyeblink conditioning." *J. Neurophysiol.* 86:1839–1857.

20. Eichenbaum, H., Dudchenko, P., Wood, E., Shapiro, M., and Tanila, H. (1999). "The hippocampus, memory, and place cells: is it spatial memory or a memory space?" *Neuron* 23:209–226.

21. Eichenbaum, H. (2000). "A cortical-hippocampal system for declarative memory." *Nat. Rev. Neurosci.* 1:41–50.

22. Power, J. M., Thompson, L. T., Moyer, J. R., Jr., and Disterhoft, J. F. (1997). "Enhanced synaptic transmission in CA1 hippocampus after eyeblink conditioning." *J. Neurophysiol.* 78:1184–1187.

23. Shapiro, M. L., Tanila, H., and Eichenbaum, H. (1997). "Cues that hippocampal place cells encode: dynamic and hierarchical representation of local and distal stimuli." *Hippocampus* 7:624–642.

24. Tanila, H., Shapiro, M. L., and Eichenbaum, H. (1997). "Discordance of spatial representation in ensembles of hippocampal place cells." *Hippocampus* 7:613–623.

25. Wood, E. R., Dudchenko, P. A., and Eichenbaum, H. (1999). "The global record of memory in hippocampal neuronal activity." *Nature* 397:613–616.

26. Eichenbaum, H. (2001). "The long and winding road to memory consolidation." *Nat. Neurosci.* 4:1057–1058.

27. Schafe, G. E., Nader, K., Blair, H. T., and LeDoux, J. E. (2001). "Memory consolidation of Pavlovian fear conditioning: a cellular and molecular perspective." *Trends Neurosci.* 24:540–546.

28. Milner, B., Squire, L. R., and Kandel, E. R. (1998). "Cognitive neuroscience and the study of memory." *Neuron* 20:445–468.

29. Corkin, S., Amaral, D. G., Gonzalez, R. G., Johnson, K. A., and Hyman, B. T. (1997). "H. M.'s medial temporal lobe lesion: findings from magnetic resonance imaging." *J. Neurosci.* 17:3964–3979.

30. Nader, K., Schafe, G. E., and Le Doux, J. E. (2000). "Fear memories require protein synthesis in the amygdala for reconsolidation after retrieval." *Nature* 406:722–726.

31. Guzowski, J. F., McNaughton, B. L., Barnes, C. A., and Worley, P. F. (1999). "Environment-specific expression of the immediate-early gene Arc in hippocampal neuronal ensembles." *Nat. Neurosci.* 2:1120-1124.

32. Wilson, M. A., and McNaughton, B. L. (1994). "Reactivation of hippocampal ensemble memories during sleep." *Science* 265:676–679.

33. Graves, L., Pack, A., and Abel, T. (2001). "Sleep and memory: a molecular perspective." *Trends Neurosci.* 24:237–243.

34. Kudrimoti, H. S., Barnes, C. A., and McNaughton, B. L.

(1999). "Reactivation of hippocampal cell assemblies: effects of behavioral state, experience, and EEG dynamics." *J. Neurosci.* 19:4090–4101.

35. Louie, K., and Wilson, M. A. (2001). "Temporally structured replay of awake hippocampal ensemble activity during rapid eye movement sleep." *Neuron* 29:145–156.

36. Maquet, P. (2001). "The role of sleep in learning and memory." *Science* 294:1048–1052.

37. Lavie, P., Pratt, H., Scharf, B., Peled, R., and Brown, J.

(1984). "Localized pontine lesion: nearly total absence of REM sleep." *Neurology* 34:118–120.

38. McNaughton, B. L., Chen, L. L., and Markus, E. J. (1991). ""Dead reckoning," landmark learning, and the sense of direction: A neurophysiological and computational hypothesis." *J. Cognitive Neurosci.* 3:190–202.

39. Squire, L. R., and Lindenlaub, E. (Eds.). (1990). The Biology of Memory. F. K. Schattauer Verlag: Stuttgart.

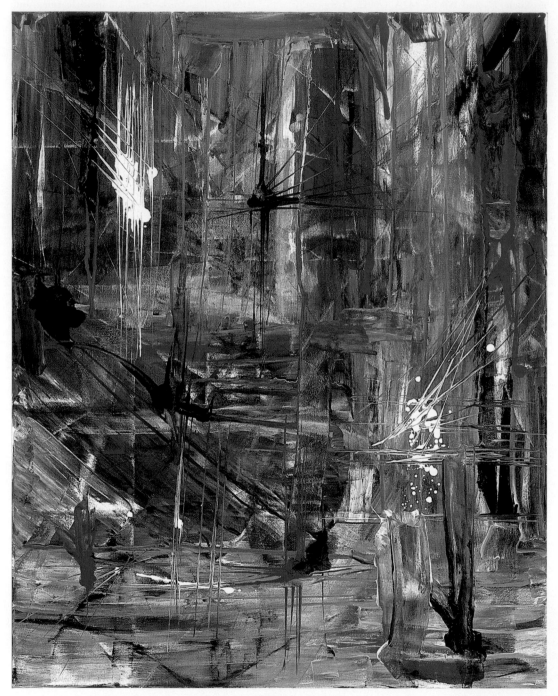

LTP Experiment
J. David Sweatt, Acrylic on canvas, 2002

Long-Term Potentiation as a Physiological Phenomenon

In the last two chapters we discussed a number of different hippocampus-dependent forms of learning and memory and the idea that in several instances the hippocampus serves as a short- and long-term "memory buffer." In this chapter, we will try to understand how it is that lasting changes in function are achieved in the hippocampus and elsewhere in the brain, focusing our attention at the cellular level. This represents a landmark step forward: our first attempt at formulating a hypothesis concerning the precise memory-related events occurring in the CNS that are *lasting* changes.

First off, I must note that there is a huge gap in our knowledge between the issues of Chapter 2 and 3, behavior, and the types of persistent neuronal modifications we will be focusing on for most of the rest of the book. The particular circuits and neuronal connections that underlie most forms of mammalian learning and memory are mysterious at present, particularly for hippocampus-dependent forms of learning. There really is very little understanding of the means by which complex memories are stored and recalled at the neural circuit level—this will be a very important avenue of future research.

All is not lost, however. Despite our limited understanding of the particulars of the circuitry involved, a general hypothesis of memory storage is available and broadly accepted. This hypothesis is that:

Memories are stored as alterations in the strength of synaptic connections between neurons in the CNS.

The significance of this general hypothesis should be emphasized—this is one of the few areas of contemporary cognitive research for which there is a unifying hypothesis. This makes many of us optimistic that memory will be the first high-order cognitive process to be understood at the cellular and molecular level.

This general hypothesis has a solid underlying rationale. As described in the first two chapters, learning and memory manifest themselves as a change in an animal's behavior, and scientists capitalize upon this in order to study these phenomena by observing and measuring changes in an animal's behavior in the wild or in experimental situations. However, all of the behavior exhibited by an animal is a result of activity in the animal's nervous system. The nervous system comprises many kinds of cells, but the primary functional units of the nervous system are neurons. Because neurons are cells, all of an animal's behavioral repertoire is a manifestation of an underlying cellular phenomenon. By extension, changes in an animal's behavior such as occurs with learning must also be subserved by an underlying cellular change.

By and large, the vast majority of the communication between neurons in the nervous system occurs at *synapses*, and a generic synapse can be thought of as consisting of a presynaptic component, a postsynaptic component, and a synaptic cleft. Communication between the presynaptic component and the postsynaptic component occurs across the synaptic cleft and is mediated by a chemical species, a *neurotransmitter*. Neurotransmitter is synthesized in the presynaptic cell and released in response to excitation of the presynaptic neuron. The neurotransmitter then diffuses across the synaptic cleft, where it binds to specific *receptors* on the postsynaptic cell.

As synapses mediate the neuron-neuron communication that underlies an animal's behavior, changes in behavior are ultimately subserved by alterations in the nature, strength, or number of interneuronal synaptic contacts in the animal's nervous system. The capacity for alterations of synaptic connections between neurons is referred to as *synaptic plasticity*, and as described earlier one of the great unifying theories to emerge out of neuroscience research in the last century was that synaptic plasticity subserves learning and memory.

One of the pioneers in advancing this line of thinking was the Canadian psychologist Donald Hebb, who published his seminal formulation as what is now generally known as Hebb's Postulate:

When an axon of cell A . . . excites cell B and repeatedly or persistently takes part in firing it, some growth process or metabolic change takes place in one or both cells so that A's efficiency as one of the cells firing B is increased.
D. O. Hebb, The Organization of Behavior, 1949 (28).

Note the important contrast between Hebb's Postulate and its popular contemporary formulation—one (Hebb's) specifies cell firing and the other (the modern formulation) specifies synaptic change. These two phenomena are clearly different, and the current, exclusively synaptic, variant is incomplete. Changes in synapses are certainly important in information storage in the CNS, but we need to consider that the postsynaptic receptors sit in a membrane whose biophysical properties are carefully controlled. Regulation of membrane sodium channels, chloride channels, and potassium channels also contribute significantly to the net effect in the cell that any neurotransmitter-operated process can achieve.

Thus, limitations arise from ignoring potential long-term regulation of membrane biophysical properties. We need to consider that local changes in dendritic membrane excitability may be involved in cellular information processing, and also that global changes in cellular excitability that alter the likelihood of the cell firing an action potential may be a mechanism for information storage.

This last point has been criticized as too limiting because with global changes in excitability one loses the computational power of selectively altering the response at a single synaptic input (i.e., synapse specificity). However, we don't know how the neuron or the CNS compute a memory output. The fundamental unit of information storage may not be the synapse but the neuron. Future experiments will be necessary to resolve this issue; nevertheless, it is worthwhile to keep in mind the possibility that regulation of excitability as well as alterations in synaptic connections may play a role in memory storage.

I. SYNAPSES IN THE HIPPOCAMPUS— THE HIPPOCAMPAL CIRCUIT

As Hebb had postulated, most contemporary theories regarding the cellular basis of learning suggest that information storage is subserved by activity-dependent alterations at the synapse. Because we are focusing on hippocampus-dependent forms of memory for the most part, we should therefore ask the question: what is the synaptic structure of the hippocampus?

The main excitatory (i.e., glutamatergic) synaptic circuitry in the hippocampus, in overview, consists of three modules (see Figure 1 and references 1, 2, and 3). As we

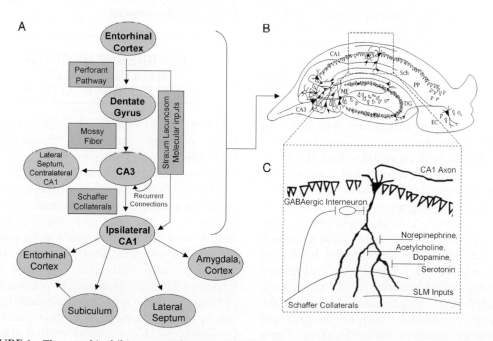

FIGURE 1   The entorhinal/hippocampal system. (A) This panel diagrams the principal inputs, outputs, and intrinsic connections. (B) In this panel, the central components of the circuit are delineated in a more anatomically correct fashion, illustrating the principal intrinsic connections of the dentate gyrus and hippocampus proper. (C) This is an expansion of area CA1 showing some of the synaptic inputs onto a single pyramidal neuron in area CA1. See text for additional details. Hippocampal diagram reproduced with permission from Johnston and Wu (25).

discussed in the last chapter, information enters the dentate gyrus of the hippocampal formation from cortical and subcortical structures via the perforant path inputs from the entorhinal cortex (Figure 1). These inputs make synaptic connections with the dentate granule cells of the dentate gyrus. After synapsing in the dentate gyrus, information is moved to area CA3 via the mossy fiber pathway, which consists of the axonal outputs of the dentate granule cells and their connections with pyramidal neurons in area CA3. After synapsing in area CA3, information is moved to area CA1 via the Schaffer-collateral path, which consists largely of the axons of area CA3 pyramidal neurons along with other projections from area CA3 of the contralateral hippocampus as well. After synapsing in CA1, information exits the hippocampus via projections from CA1 pyramidal neurons and returns to subcortical and cortical structures.

The connections in this synaptic circuit are retained in a fairly impressive manner if one makes transverse slices of the hippocampus, because the inputs, "trisynaptic circuit," and outputs are laid out in a generally laminar fashion along the long axis of the hippocampal formation. This is a great advantage for in vitro electrophysiological experiments, which I will return to shortly.

I also should emphasize that the trisynaptic circuit just outlined is a great oversimplification; there are a great many additional synaptic components of the hippocampus! I will highlight a few illustrative examples here, most of which we will return to later in the book (see also Figure 1). There are inhibitory gamma-amino-butyric acid containing (GABAergic) interneurons that make synaptic connections with all the principal excitatory neurons outlined earlier. These GABAergic inputs serve in both a feedforward and feedback fashion to control excitability. There are also many recurrent and collateral excitatory connections between the excitatory pyramidal neurons,

particularly in the area CA3 region. There is a direct projection from the entorhinal cortex to the distal regions of CA1 pyramidal neuron dendrites, a pathway known as the *stratum lacunosum moleculare.*

Finally, there are many modulatory projections into the hippocampus that make synaptic connections with the principal neurons (see Figure 1 and Box 1). These inputs are via long projection fibers from various anatomical nuclei in the brain stem region, and they are, by and large, not directly excitatory or inhibitory but rather serve to modulate synaptic connectivity in a fairly subtle way. There are four predominant extrinsic modulatory projections into the hippocampus. First, there are inputs of norepinephrine (NE)-containing fibers that project from the locus ceruleus. Second, there are dopamine (DA)-containing fibers that arise from the substantia nigra. There also are inputs using acetylcholine (ACh) from the medial septal nucleus and 5-hydroxytrypramine (5HT, serotonin) from the raphe nuclei.

II. A BREAKTHROUGH DISCOVERY—LTP IN THE HIPPOCAMPUS

To my great chagrin, I must note that there is very little understanding of how this complex hippocampal circuitry processes information and contributes to learning, memory, and ultimately the behavioral output of the animal. We are reduced to treating the hippocampus largely as a black box, known to be critical for cognition and memory formation, without really understanding how that happens. This will be a very important area of future research and many talented minds are applying themselves to this problem. Nevertheless, I am confident that understanding the basic mechanisms of synaptic alteration in the hippocampus, the topic we will cover for the next several chapters, will give us valuable insights into both general mechanisms of synaptic plasticity and CNS

BOX 1

TYPES OF RECEPTORS AND POTENTIAL SITES OF PLASTICITY

Neurotransmitters can be broadly categorized into two types, based on the types of receptors they bind to and their effects on the postsynaptic cell. Some neurotransmitters directly mediate neuron-neuron communication by binding to and opening *ligand (neurotransmitter)-gated ion channels*. A second major category generally serves a more subtle role—modulating neuronal function by eliciting intracellular *second-messenger generation*.

The first type of receptors form neurotransmitter-regulated pores that can open upon binding of neurotransmitter, allowing ions to flux across the cell membrane and resulting in an electrical change (generally *depolarizing* or *hyperpolarizing*) in the cellular membrane. Neurotransmission of this sort is typically how one neuron excites (or inhibits) another follower neuron within a neuronal circuit. The two predominant types of ligand-gated ion channels in the hippocampus and elsewhere in the CNS bind glutamate (excitatory) or gamma-amino-butyric acid (GABA, inhibitory). The major glutamate receptor subtype is named for a selective agonist at this receptor, alpha-amino-3-hydroxy-5-methyl-4-isoxazolepropionic acid (mercifully abbreviated AMPA). The AMPA subtype of receptors are glutamate-gated cation channels that when opened lead to membrane depolarization. Another subtype of glutamate receptor that is very similar is activated by kainic acid (KA, kainate), and this subtype is referred to as the kainate receptor. The typical EPSP in a hippocampal neuron is mediated by ion flux through the AMPA subtype of glutamate receptor. Inhibitory postsynaptic potentials (IPSPs) are mostly mediated by the GABA-A subtype of GABA receptors.

GABA-A receptors are GABA-gated chloride channels. Opening these channels moves the membrane potential in a negative direction, toward the hyperpolarized chloride ion equilibrium potential. This tends to hyperpolarize the membrane and clamp it there.

The second major category of neurotransmitter receptor doesn't directly produce electrical changes in the postsynaptic neuron but rather elicits biochemical changes within the postsynaptic neuron. Typically, these types of neurotransmitters couple to second-messenger-generating enzymes that can lead to alterations in a wide variety of cellular chemical processes. These types of neurotransmitters are referred to as *modulatory* because their effects typically (but by no means exclusively) sculpt and fine-tune the electrical and cellular responses to the neurotransmitters that open ligand-gated ion channels. Almost all neurotransmitters have specific subtypes of receptors that act in this fashion, including specific receptors for glutamate, GABA, norepinephrine, dopamine, serotonin, and acetylcholine, in addition to a large number of different neuropeptides.

The second-messenger-generating enzymes that these modulatory neurotransmitter receptors couple to are also quite diverse. A partial listing includes adenylyl cyclase, which makes cyclic AMP (cAMP) and activates the cAMP-dependent protein kinase (PKA); phospholipase C (PLC), which makes diacylglycerol (DAG) and activates protein kinase C (PKC); PLC also makes inositol *tris*-phosphate (IP3), which mobilizes intracellular calcium and can activate the calcium/calmodulin-dependent protein kinase type II (CaMKII);

Continued

BOX 1—cont'd

TYPES OF RECEPTORS AND POTENTIAL SITES OF PLASTICITY

and phospholipase A2 (PLA2), which liberates free arachidonic acid that can be converted into a wide variety of active metabolites. We will explore these systems and others in excruciating detail in Chapters 6–8.

Finally, it is important to note that the targets of these various signaling pathways are as diverse as the genome itself. In terms of neuronal function, particularly important targets are the presynaptic proteins associated with neurotransmitter release, membrane K^+ channels, Ca^{2+} channels and Na^+ channels, nuclear transcription factors regulating gene expression, the protein synthesis machinery, and the cytoskeleton.

function in a broad sense, and mechanisms of learning specifically.

When Tim Bliss was a young man, he likewise had (he still has) confidence that understanding long-term alterations in synaptic function in the hippocampus would yield valuable insights into the mechanisms of mammalian memory. He acted on this confidence by displacing himself as a postdoctoral researcher from England to Per Anderson's lab in Oslo, a focal point of physiologic studies of the hippocampus then and now. Tim set out to find a long-lasting form of synaptic plasticity in the hippocampus, and by teaming up with Terje Lomo he did just that. The seminal report by Bliss and Lomo in 1973, describing a phenomenon they termed "long-term potentiation" of synaptic transmission, set the stage for what is now three decades of progress in understanding the basics of long-term synaptic alteration in the CNS.

As a personal aside, I once asked Tim how LTP was discovered. His recollection was that, before he came to Anderson's lab, Terje Lomo had serendipitously discovered that brief periods of high-frequency synaptic stimulation could lead to an enhancement of synaptic transmission in hippocampal recordings from rabbits. The

physiologists there used this trick to prolong their experiments; when they started to lose their preparation they would give a quick "buzz" to the hippocampus to increase synaptic strength so that they could get some more data. I find this a fascinating example of chance favoring the prepared mind—Tim's insight was to appreciate the importance of the phenomenon.

In their experiments, Bliss and Lomo recorded synaptic responses in the dentate gyrus, stimulating the perforant path inputs from the entorhinal cortex (4). They used extracellular stimulating and recording electrodes that they implanted into the animal. The basic experiment was begun by recording baseline synaptic transmission in this pathway. Then they delivered a brief period of high-frequency (100 Hz "tetanic") stimulation, and after this brief period of stimulation they saw an increase in the strength of synaptic connections between the perforant path inputs from the entorhinal cortex onto the dentate granule neurons in the dentate gyrus (Figure 2). They also observed an increased likelihood of the cells firing action potentials in response to a constant synaptic input, a phenomenon they termed E-S (EPSP-to-Spike) potentiation. These two phenomena together were termed LTP. LTP lasted many, many hours

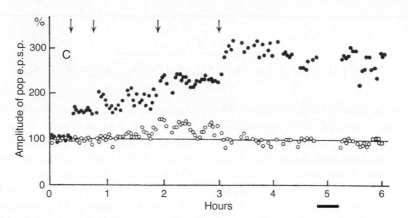

FIGURE 2   Bliss and Lomo's first published LTP experiment. As described in more detail in the text, in this pioneering work Tim Bliss and Terje Lomo demonstrated long-term potentiation of synaptic transmission. This specific experiment investigated synaptic transmission at perforant path inputs into the dentate gyrus (see Figure 1). Arrows indicate the delivery of high-frequency synaptic stimulation, resulting in LTP. Filled circles are responses from the tetanized pathways, open circles are a control pathway that did not receive tetanic stimulation. The bar, where no data points are available, indicates a period of time where Tim Bliss fell asleep. Data acquisition in this era involved the investigator directly measuring by hand synaptic responses from an oscilloscope screen. Moreover, it was not unusual for experiments to extend overnight owing to the long amount of time involved in preparing the rabbit for the experiment, implanting the electrodes into the brain, and establishing a stable recording configuration. Reproduced with permission from Bliss and Lomo (4).

in this intact rabbit preparation. The appeal of LTP as an analog of memory was immediately apparent – it is a long-lasting change in neuronal function that is produced by a brief period of unique stimulus, exactly the sort of mechanism that had long been postulated to be involved in memory formation. This pioneering work of Bliss and Lomo set in motion a several-decades-long pursuit by numerous investigators geared toward understanding the attributes and mechanisms of LTP.

A. The Hippocampal Slice Preparation

Bliss and Lomo did their experiment using the intact rabbit, stimulating and recording in the anesthetized animal using implanted electrodes. In recent times, this preparation has been largely supplanted by the use of recordings from hippocampal slices maintained in vitro. (See Figure 3.) Because most of the LTP experiments that I will be describing in the rest of the book come from this type of preparation, I will briefly describe one typical procedure for

preparation of hippocampal slices from rodents and then give an overview of extracellular recording in a typical LTP experiment (see Box 2).

To prepare the raw material for a hippocampal-slice experiment, brains of rats or mice are rapidly removed and

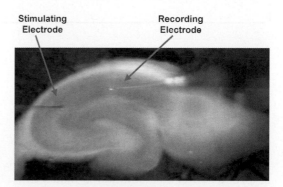

FIGURE 3   Electrodes in a living hippocampal slice. This photograph illustrates the appearance of a mouse hippocampal slice, maintained in a recording chamber. Responses in area CA1 are recorded using a saline-filled glass micropipette electrode (right) and a bipolar platinum stimulating electrode (left). See text and Figure 4 for additional details.

BOX 2

RECORDING FROM INDIVIDUAL NEURONS

Most of the data under discussion in this chapter were generated using extracellular recording techniques, but a number of much more sophisticated electrophysiologic techniques have been used to great effect in studies of LTP. These types of techniques fall into two broad categories generally referred to as *sharp electrode* recording and *patch clamp* recording. The basic difference in the two techniques is that sharp electrode recording impales the neuron with the recording electrode, while patch clamping involves forming a tight seal between the recording electrode and the cell membrane. In general, sharp electrode recording is used for *current clamp* experiments, or experiments where one monitors the membrane potential passively. Patch clamp experiments in general involve *voltage clamp* of the membrane potential. In these experiments, one can hold the membrane potential constant while measuring current flow through membrane channels. Alternatively, one can use the electrode to manipulate the membrane potential directly. This latter type of experiment was the sort used to

discover pairing LTP as described in the text, and it was also used in key experiments demonstrating that depolarization of the postsynaptic cell is required for LTP induction. More recent applications of patch-clamping approaches have allowed the direct recording of dendritic membrane potential (prior studies had all recorded from the much larger cell body region), and this *dendritic-patch-recording* technique allowed the seminal finding of back-propagating action potentials in dendrites.

One great strength that single-cell recording techniques have in common is that they allow access to the cytoplasm of a single postsynaptic neuron. This allows the introduction of pharmacologic agents, including large proteins, specifically into the single postsynaptic cell. Application of this approach has led to a number of landmark findings in investigations of LTP, including the discovery of a necessity for postsynaptic calcium for LTP induction, and the necessity of postsynaptic protein kinase activity for LTP induction.

---

briefly chilled in ice-cold "cutting" saline. For the sake of completeness, I will note that the cutting saline consists of 110 mM sucrose, 60 mM NaCl, 3 mM KCl, 1.25 mM NaH$_2$PO$_4$, 28 mM NaHCO$_3$, 500 µM CaC1$_2$, 5 mM D-glucose, 7 mM MgCl$_2$, and 600 µM ascorbate. After this solution is made, it is saturated with 95% O$_2$ and 5% CO$_2$ by bubbling this gas through the solution. A standard aquarium air stone serves quite nicely for this purpose. The high Mg^{2+} concentration in the cutting solution helps maintain the health of the tissue during

subsequent slicing, by decreasing neuronal excitability and lowering neurotransmitter release. As a practical matter, it is important to remove the brain from the animal and get it into the chilled cutting solution as quickly as possible in order to be able to get healthy slices. The current record in my lab is held by Coleen Atkins, who in her prime could get the brain out of a rat and into cutting solution in 15 seconds.

Once the brain is out and cold, one can be a little more deliberate but must still move expeditiously. Removing the hippocampus from the brain and making transverse slices, while still maintaining the tissue in a healthy state, generally involves idiosyncratic maneuvers, high anxiety, and no small amount of superstitious behavior. The principal component to success is clearly practice. Transverse slices approximately 400-µm thick are prepared with a MacIlwain tissue chopper or Vibratome (preferable but more expensive) and maintained at least 45 minutes in a holding chamber containing 50% artificial cerebrospinal fluid (ACSF) and 50% cutting saline. ACSF contains 125 mM NaCl, 2.5 mM KCl, 1.24 mM NaH$_2$PO$_4$, 25 mM NaHCO$_3$, 10 mM D-glucose, 2 mM CaCl$_2$, and 1 mM MgCl$_2$, saturated with 95% O$_2$ and 5% CO$_2$ as described previously and continuously bubbled throughout the experiment.

After slices and experimenter have recovered from the dissection, they are then transferred to an electrophysiology rig and slice recording chamber, respectively, and the slices are perfused with 100% ACSF. Slices are allowed to equilibrate for about 60–90 minutes before recording begins. This is generally the point at which the experimenter eats lunch, if he is a postdoc, or dinner, if he is a graduate student.

B. Measuring Synaptic Transmission in the Hippocampal Slice

As mentioned previously, the main information processing circuit in the hippocampus is the relatively simple trisynaptic pathway, and much of this basic circuit is preserved in transverse slices across the long axis of the hippocampus. Various types of long-term potentiation can be induced at all three of these synaptic sites, and we will discuss later some mechanistic differences among the various types of LTP that can be induced. Most experiments on the basic attributes and mechanisms of LTP have been studies of the synaptic connections between axons from area CA3 pyramidal neurons that extend into area CA1. These are the

synapses onto CA1 pyramidal neurons that are known as the Schaffer-collateral inputs.

In a popular variation of the basic LTP experiment, extracellular field potential recordings in the dendritic regions of area CA1 are utilized to monitor synaptic transmission at Schaffer-collateral synapses (see Figure 4). A bipolar stimulating electrode is placed in the stratum radiatum subfield of area CA1 and stimuli (typically constant current pulses ranging from 1–30 µA) are delivered. Stimuli delivered in this fashion stimulate the output axons of CA3 neurons that pass nearby, causing action potentials to propagate down these axons. Responses are typically recorded through an amplifier coupled to a personal computer, using any of a variety of data acquisition software. Recording electrodes typically are drawn from glass filament microcapillaries using an electrode puller and are filled with ACSF.

The typical waveform consists of a "fiber volley," which is an indication of the presynaptic action potential arriving at the recording site, and the excitatory postsynaptic potential (EPSP) itself. The EPSP responses are a manifestation of synaptic activation (depolarization) in the CA1 pyramidal neurons. For measuring "field" (i.e., extracellularly recorded) EPSPs, the parameter typically measured is the initial slope of the EPSP waveform (see Figure 4). Absolute peak amplitude of EPSPs can also be measured, but the initial slope is the preferred index. This is because the initial slope is less subject to contamination from other sources of current flow in the slice. For example, currents are generated by feed-forward inhibition due to GABAergic neuron activation. Also, if the cells fire action potentials, this also can contaminate later stages of the EPSP, even when one is recording from the dendritic region.

Extracellular field recordings measure responses from a population of neurons, so EPSPs recorded in this fashion are referred to as population EPSPs (pEPSPs). Note that pEPSPs are downward-deflecting for

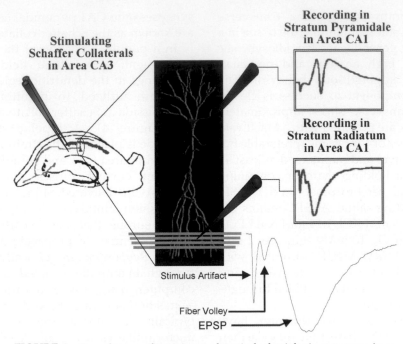

FIGURE 4 Recording configuration and typical physiologic responses in a hippocampal-slice recording experiment. Electrode placements and responses from stratum pyramidale (cell body layer) and stratum oriens (dendritic regions) are shown. In addition, the typical waveform of a population EPSP is illustrated, showing the stimulus artifact, fiber volley, and population EPSP. Figure and data by Joel Selcher.

stratum radiatum recordings (see Figure 4). If one is recording from the cell body layer (stratum pyramidale), the EPSP is an upward deflection; if the cells fire action potentials, the EPSP has superimposed upon it a downward deflecting "spike", the population spike. As mentioned earlier, for both stratum radiatum and stratum pyramidale recordings, the EPSP slope measurements are taken as early as possible after the fiber volley to eliminate contamination by population spikes.

Test stimuli are typically delivered and responses recorded at 0.05 Hz (once every 20 seconds); every six consecutive responses over a 2-minute period are pooled and averaged. As a prelude to starting an LTP experiment, input/output (I/O) functions for stimulus intensity versus EPSP magnitude are recorded in response to increasing intensities of stimulation (e.g.

from 2.5 to 45.0 µA, see Figure 5). For the remainder of the experiment, the test stimulus intensity is set to elicit an EPSP that is approximately 35–50% of the maximum response recorded during the I/O measurements. Baseline synaptic transmission at this constant test stimulus intensity is usually monitored for a period of 15–20 minutes to ensure a stable response.

Once the health of the hippocampal slice is confirmed as indicated by a stable baseline synaptic response, LTP can be induced using any one of a wide variety of different LTP induction protocols. Many popular variations include a single or repeated period of 1-second, 100 Hz stimulation (with delivery of the 100-Hz trains separated by 20 seconds or more) where stimulus intensity is at a level necessary for approximately half-maximal

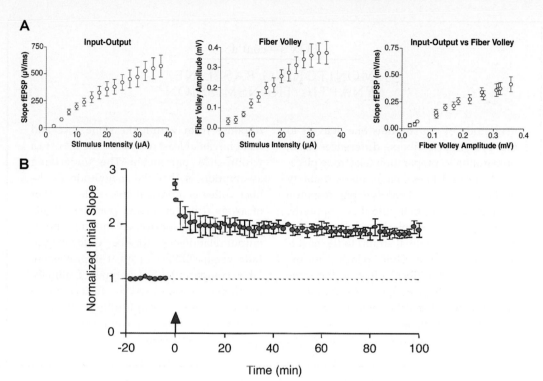

FIGURE 5 An input-output curve and typical LTP experiment. (A) This panel shows the relationship of EPSP magnitude versus stimulus intensity (in microamps) and the same data converted to an input-output relationship for EPSP versus fiber volley magnitude in order to allow an evaluation of postsynaptic response versus presynaptic response in the same hippocampal slice. (B) This panel illustrates a typical high-frequency stimulation-induced potentiation of synaptic transmission in area CA1 of a rat hippocampal slice in vitro. The arrow indicates the delivery of 100 Hz (100 pulses/second) synaptic stimulation. Data courtesy of Ed Weeber and Coleen Atkins.

BOX 3

MONITORING BASELINE SYNAPTIC TRANSMISSION

In most pharmacologic experiments using physiologic recordings in hippocampal slice preparations, the effects of drug application on baseline synaptic transmission can be evaluated by simply monitoring EPSPs before and after drug application, using a constant stimulus intensity. A more elaborate alternative is to produce input-output curves for EPSP initial slope (or magnitude) versus stimulus intensity for the presynaptic stimulus (see Figure 5).

These types of within-slice experiments are very straightforward; however, this type of within-preparation design is not possible in some experimental comparisons. For example, if one is comparing a wild-type with a knockout animal, there of necessity must be a comparison across preparations. How does one evaluate if there is a difference in basal synaptic transmission in this situation? The principal confound is that while one has control over the

Continued

BOX 3—cont'd

MONITORING BASELINE SYNAPTIC TRANSMISSION

magnitude of the stimulus one delivers to the presynaptic fibers, differences from preparation to preparation (electrode placement, slice thickness, etc.) cause variability in the magnitude of the synaptic response elicited by a constant stimulus amplitude. One approach commonly to compare one preparation (or animal strain) to the next is to quantitate the EPSP relative to the amplitude of the fiber volley in that same hippocampal slice (see figure 5A). The rationale is that the fiber volley, which represents the action potentials firing in the presynaptic fibers, is a presynaptic physiologic

response from within the same slice and that one can at least normalize the EPSP to a within-slice parameter. The underlying assumption is that the magnitude of the fiber volley is representative of the number of axons firing an action potential. While not a perfect control, evaluating input-output relationships for fiber volley magnitude versus EPSP is a great improvement when comparing different types of animals. If differences are observed, an increase in the fiber volley amplitude-EPSP slope relationship suggests an augmentation of synaptic transmission.

---

stimulation (see Figure 5). A variation is a "strong" induction protocol where LTP is induced with three pairs of 100 Hz, 1-second stimuli, where stimulus intensity is near that necessary for a maximal EPSP. This latter protocol gives robust LTP that lasts for essentially as long as one can keep the hippocampal slice alive.

III. NMDA RECEPTOR-DEPENDENCE OF LTP

Baseline excitatory synaptic transmission in the CNS, including at Schaffer-collateral synapses, depends on a glutamate-gated cation channel, the AMPA subtype of glutamate receptor (see Box 1). This is the basic housekeeping glutamate receptor that mediates most of excitatory synaptic transmission in the brain. In 1983 Graham Collingridge made the breakthrough discovery that induction of tetanus-induced

forms of LTP are blocked by blockade of a different subtype of glutamate receptor, the N-methyl-D-aspartate (NMDA) receptor (5). Collingridge's fascinating discovery was that the glutamate analog amino-phosphono-valeric acid (APV), an agent that selectively blocks the NMDA subtype of glutamate receptors, could block LTP induction while leaving baseline synaptic transmission entirely intact (Figure 6).

This was the first experiment to give a specific molecular insight into the mechanisms of LTP induction. The properties of the NMDA receptor that allow it to function in this unique role of triggering LTP are important, and we will return to a detailed analysis of regulation of the NMDA receptor several times in this book. For our purposes right now, suffice it to say that pharmacologic blockers of NMDA receptor function have allowed the definition of different types of LTP that can be selectively induced with various physiologic stimulation protocols. For example, subsequent

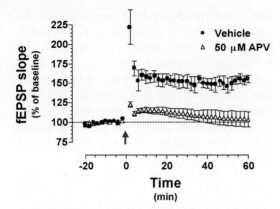

FIGURE 6   APV block of LTP. These data are from recordings in vitro from mouse hippocampal slices, demonstrating the NMDA receptor-dependence of tetanus-induced LTP. Identical high-frequency synaptic stimulation was delivered in control (filled circles) and NMDA receptor antagonist (APV, open triangles) treated slices. Data courtesy of Joel Selcher.

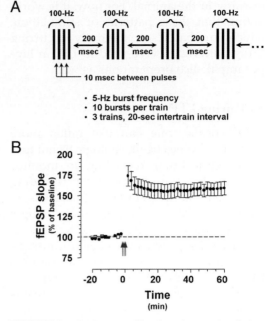

FIGURE 7   LTP Triggered by theta-burst stimulation in the mouse hippocampus. (A) This schematic depicts theta-burst stimulation. The LTP induction paradigm consists of three trains of 10 high-frequency bursts delivered at 5 Hz. (B), LTP induced with theta-burst stimulation (TBS-LTP) in hippocampal area CA1. The three red arrows represent the three TBS trains. Data courtesy of Joel Selcher.

work has shown that an NMDA receptor-independent type of LTP can be induced in area CA1, and elsewhere in the hippocampus (mossy fibers to be precise), as well as other parts of the CNS. We will return to a brief description of these types of LTP at the end of this chapter, but for now we will continue to focus on NMDA receptor-dependent types of LTP.

Early studies of LTP used mostly high-frequency (100-Hz) stimulation, in repeated 1-second-long trains, as the LTP-inducing stimulation protocol. Even though these protocols are still widely used to good effect, it is clear that such prolonged periods of high-frequency firing do not occur physiologically in the behaving animal. However, LTP can also be induced by stimulation protocols that are much more like naturally occurring neuronal firing patterns in the hippocampus. To date, the forms of LTP induced by these types of stimulation have all been found to be NMDA receptor-dependent in area CA1. Two popular variations of these protocols are based on the natural occurrence of an increased rate of hippocampal pyramidal neuron firing while a rat or mouse is

exploring and learning about a new environment. Under these circumstances hippocampal pyramidal neurons fire bursts of action potentials at about 5 bursts/sec (i.e., 5 Hz). This is the "theta" rhythm that was discussed in the last chapter. One variation of LTP-inducing stimulation that mimics this pattern of firing is referred to as theta-frequency stimulation (TFS), which consists of 30 seconds of single stimuli delivered at 5 Hz. Another variation, theta-burst stimulation (TBS) consists of three trains of stimuli delivered at 20-second intervals, each train is composed of ten stimulus bursts delivered at 5 Hz, with each burst consisting of four pulses at 100 Hz (see Figure 7). We will return to these types of LTP induction protocols in Chapters 5 and 9, where we will discuss modulation of LTP induction and the role of LTP in learning in the animal. For now, it is worth noting that these patterns of stimulation, which are based on naturally occurring firing patterns in vivo, lead to LTP in hippocampal slice preparations as well.

A. Pairing LTP

Of course, one can use much more sophisticated electrophysiologic techniques than extracellular recording to monitor synaptic function. Intracellular recording and patch clamp techniques that measure electrophysiologic responses in single neurons have also been used widely in studies of LTP, and as with field recordings, you can use these techniques and observe LTP (see Box 2). Of course, these types of recording techniques perturb the cell that is being recorded from and lead to "rundown" of the postsynaptic response in the cell impaled by the electrode. This limits the duration of the LTP experiment to however long the cell stays alive— somewhere in the range of 30 minutes to an hour for an accomplished physiologist. Regardless, in these recording configurations you can induce synaptic potentiation using tetanic stimulation or theta-pattern stimulation and measure LTP as an increase in post-synaptic currents through glutamate-gated ion channels, or as an increase in postsynaptic depolarization when monitoring the membrane potential.

Control of the postsynaptic neuron's membrane potential with cellular recording techniques also allows for some sophisticated variations of the LTP induction paradigm. In one particularly important series of experiments, it was discovered that LTP can be induced by pairing repeated single presynaptic stimuli with postsynaptic membrane depolarization, so-called "pairing" LTP (6). (See Figure 8.)

The basis for pairing LTP comes from one of the fundamental properties of the NMDA receptor (see Figure 9). The NMDA receptor is both a glutamate-gated channel and a voltage-dependent one. The simultaneous presence of glutamate and a depolarized membrane is necessary and sufficient (when the co-agonist glycine is present) to gate the channel. Pairing synaptic stimulation with membrane depolarization provided via the recording electrode (plus the low levels of glycine always normally present) opens the NMDA receptor channel and leads to the induction of LTP.

How is it that the NMDA receptor triggers LTP? The NMDA receptor is a calcium channel, and its gating leads to elevated intracellular calcium in the postsynaptic neuron. We will return to this calcium influx that triggers LTP in the next chapter, and indeed most of the rest of this book deals with the various processes this calcium influx triggers.[1]

These properties, glutamate dependence *and* voltage-dependence, of the NMDA receptor allow it to function as a coincidence detector. This is a critical aspect of NMDA receptor regulation and allows for a unique contribution of the NMDA receptor to information processing at the molecular level. Using the NMDA receptor, the neuron can trigger a unique event, calcium influx, specifically when a particular synapse is both active presynaptically (glutamate is present in the synapse) and postsynaptically (when the membrane is depolarized).

---

[1]It is important to remember that it is not necessarily the case that every calcium molecule involved in LTP induction actually comes through the NMDA receptor. Calcium influx through membrane calcium channels and calcium released from intracellular stores may also be involved. In fact, it is an interesting "thought experiment" to try to design a way to test this idea—as a practical matter it is much more difficult to determine than one might first think.) Mechanistically the gating of the NMDA receptor/channel involves a voltage-dependent Mg^{2+} block of the channel pore. Depolarization of the membrane in which the NMDA receptor resides is necessary to drive the divalent Mg cation out of the pore, which then allows calcium ions to flow through. Thus, the simultaneous occurrence of both glutamate in the synapse and a depolarized postsynaptic membrane is necessary to open the channel and allow LTP-triggering calcium into the postsynaptic cell.

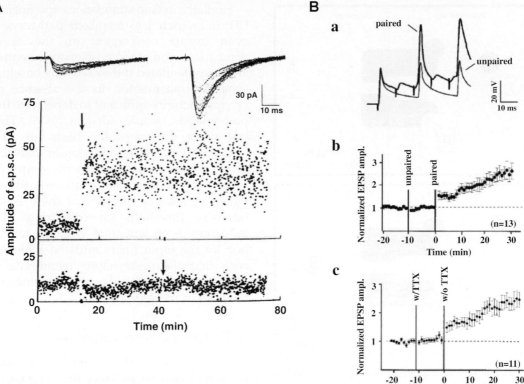

FIGURE 8   Pairing LTP. (A) LTP of synaptic transmission induced by pairing postsynaptic depolarization with synaptic activity. The upper panels illustrate postsynaptic currents recorded directly from the postsynaptic neuron using voltage clamp techniques (see Box 2). The lower panels are a pairing LTP experiment (upper), and control, nonpaired pathway (lower). In the pairing LTP experiment hippocampal CA1 pyramidal neurons were depolarized from –70 to 0 mV, while the paired pathway was stimulated at 2 Hz 40 times. Control received no stimulation during depolarization. From Malinow and Tsien (26). Reproduced with permission from Nature Publishing Group. (B) Pairing small EPSPs with back-propagating dendritic action potentials induces LTP. (a) Subthreshold EPSPs paired with back-propagating action potentials increase dendritic action potential amplitude. Voltage clamp recording at approximately 240 μm from soma, that is, in the dendritic tree of the neuron (see Figure 10). Action potentials were evoked by 2-ms current injections through a somatic whole-cell electrode at 20-ms intervals. Alone, action potential amplitude was small (unpaired). Paired with EPSPs (5 stimuli at 100 Hz), the action potential amplitude increased greatly (paired). (b) The grouped data show normalized EPSP amplitude after unpaired and paired stimulation. The pairing protocol shown in A was repeated five times at 5 Hz at 15-second intervals for a total of two times. (c) A similar pairing protocol was given with and without applying the sodium channel blocker tetrodotoxin (TTX, to block action potential propagation) to the proximal apical dendrites to prevent back-propagating action potentials from reaching the synaptic input sites. LTP was induced only when action potentials fully back-propagated into the dendrites. Reproduced with permission from Magee & Johnston (10). Copyright 1997 American Association for the Advancement of Science.

This confers a computational capacity at the molecular level. Using the NMDA receptor the neuron can confer a property of associativity on the synapse. This attribute is nicely illustrated by "pairing" LTP, as described previously, where low-frequency synaptic activity paired with postsynaptic depolarization can lead to LTP. The associative property of the NMDA receptor allows for many other types of sophisticated information processing as well, however. For example, activation of a weak

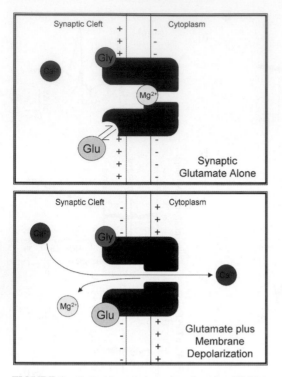

FIGURE 9 Coincidence detection by the NMDA receptor. The simultaneous presence of glutamate and membrane depolarization is necessary for relieving Mg^{2+} blockade and allowing calcium influx.

input to a neuron can induce potentiation, provided a strong input to the same neuron is activated at the same time (7). These particular features of LTP induction have stimulated a great deal of interest because they are reminiscent of classical conditioning, with depolarization and synaptic input roughly corresponding to unconditioned and conditioned stimuli, respectively.

The associative nature of NMDA receptor activation also allows for synapse specificity of LTP induction, which has been shown to occur experimentally. If you pair postsynaptic depolarization with activity at one set of synaptic inputs to a cell, while leaving a second input silent or active only during periods at which the postsynaptic membrane is near the resting potential, you get selective potentiation of the paired input pathway.

Similarly, in field stimulation experiments, LTP is restricted to tetanized pathways—even inputs convergent on the same dendritic region of the postsynaptic neuron are not potentiated if they see only baseline synaptic transmission in the absence of synaptic activity sufficient to depolarize the postsynaptic neuron adequately (8). This last point illustrates the basis for LTP "cooperativity." LTP induction in extracellular stimulation experiments requires cooperative interaction of afferent fibers, which in essence means that there is an intensity threshold for triggering LTP induction. Sufficient total synaptic activation by the input fibers must be achieved such that the postsynaptic membrane is adequately depolarized to allow opening of the NMDA receptor (9).

B. Dendritic Action Potentials

In the context of the functioning hippocampal neuron in vivo, the associative nature of NMDA receptor activation means that a given neuron must reach a critical level of depolarization in order for LTP to occur at any of its synapses. Specifically, in the physiologic context, the hippocampal pyramidal neuron generally must reach the threshold for firing an action potential, although there are some interesting alternatives to this that we will discuss later in this chapter and in Chapter 5. Even though action potentials are, of course, triggered in the active zone of the cell body, hippocampal pyramidal neurons along with many other types of CNS neurons can actively propagate action potentials into the dendritic regions: the so-called *back-propagating* action potential (10). (See Figure 10.) These dendritic action potentials are just like action potentials propagated down axons in that they are carried predominantly by voltage-dependent ion channels such as sodium channels. The penetration of the back-propagating action potential into the dendritic region provides a wave of membrane depolarization that allows for

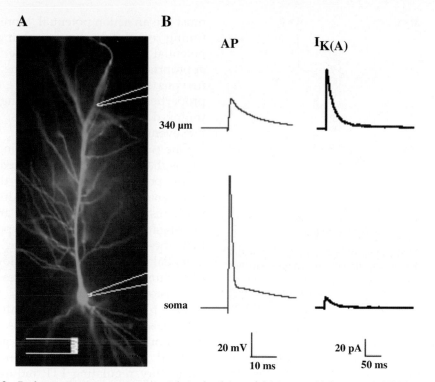

FIGURE 10   Back-propagating action potentials in dendrites of CA1 pyramidal neurons. (A) This panel shows the recording set-up, with a bipolar stimulating electrode used to trigger action potentials at the cell body region (lower left), a recording electrode in the cell soma to monitor firing of an action potential, and a recording electrode in the dendrites (upper right) to monitor propagation of the action potential into the distal dendritic region. (B) Traces here indicate the data recorded from the soma (lower) and dendritic (upper) electrodes. The left-hand traces (labeled AP) indicate the membrane depolarization achieved at the soma and dendrite when an action potential is triggered and propagates into the dendritic region. Note that the dendritic action potential is of lower magnitude and broader owing to the effects of dendritic membrane biophysical properties as the action potential propagates down the dendrite. The right-hand side shows current flow through "A-type" voltage-dependent potassium currents observed in the soma and dendrites. The density of A-type potassium currents increases dramatically as one progresses outward from the soma into the dendritic regions, as illustrated by the much larger potassium current observed in the distal dendritic electrode. These voltage-dependent potassium channels are key regulators of the likelihood of back-propagating action potentials reaching various parts of the dendritic tree. Data and figures reproduced with permission from Yuan *et al.* (27).

the opening of the voltage-dependent NMDA receptor/ion channels. *Active* propagation of the action potential is necessary because the biophysical properties of the dendritic membrane dampen the passive propagation of membrane depolarization; thus, an active process such as action potential propagation is required. As a generalization in many instances in the intact cell, back-propagating action potentials are what allow sufficient depolarization to reach hippocampal pyramidal

neuron synapses in order to open NMDA receptors. In an ironic twist, this has brought us back to a more literal reading of Hebb's Postulate, where as we discussed in the introduction to this Chapter, Hebb actually specified *firing* of the postsynaptic neuron as being necessary for the strengthening of its connections.

In fact, the timing of the arrival of a dendritic action potential with synaptic glutamate input appears to play an important part in precise, timing-dependent

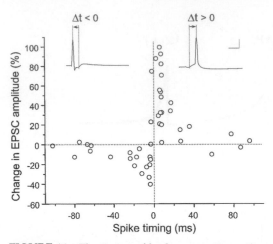

FIGURE 11 The timing of back-propagating action potentials with synaptic activity determines whether synaptic strength is altered, and in which direction. Precise timing of the arrival of a back-propagating action potential (a "spike") with synaptic glutamate determines the effect of paired depolarization and synaptic activity. A narrow window when the arrival of the synaptic EPSP immediately precedes or follows the arrival of the back-propagating action potential determines whether synaptic strength is increased, decreased, or remains the same. See text for additional discussion. Figure adapted with permission from Bi and Poo (12).

triggering of synaptic plasticity in the hippocampus (see reference 10 and Figures 8 and 11). It has been observed that a critical timing window is involved vis-à-vis back-propagating action potentials: glutamate arrival in the synaptic cleft must slightly precede the back-propagating action potential in order for the NMDA receptor to be effectively opened. This timing dependence arises in part due to the time required for glutamate to bind to and open the NMDA receptor. The duration of an action potential is, of course, quite short so in essence the glutamate must be there first and already bound to the receptor in order for full activation to occur. (Additional factors are also involved; see references 11, 12, and 13 for a discussion).

This order-of-paring specificity allows for a precision of information processing—not only must the membrane be depolarized, but also, as a practical matter, the cell

must fire an action potential. Moreover, the timing of the back-propagating action potential arriving at a synapse must be appropriate. It is easy to imagine how the nervous system could capitalize on these properties to allow for forming precise timing-dependent associations between two events.

One twist to the order-of-paring specificity is that if the order is reversed and the action potential arrives before the EPSP, then synaptic depression is produced. The mechanisms for this attribute are under investigation at present—one hypothesis is that the backward pairing by various potential mechanisms leads to a lower level of calcium influx, which produces synaptic depression (see chapter 5).

The role of back-propagating action potentials in regulating NMDA receptor activation raises the interesting possibility of local effects on dendritic membrane excitability regulating LTP induction in a dendritic branch-specific (or even branch subregion-specific) manner. Because dendrites are highly branched, nonuniform entities, regulating the ability of a back-propagating action potential to penetrate into a specific dendritic region could control the capacity of LTP induction for all the synapses in that branch. Although highly hypothetical at this point, such a mechanism could confer additional information processing capacity on hippocampal pyramidal neurons. Similarly, but even more speculatively, locally constrained action potential generation only within a dendritic subregion would allow for highly localized NMDA receptor activation as well.

Branch-specific regulation of LTP induction could occur through two easily conceived mechanisms. The first is through neuromodulation of local voltage-dependent Na^+ and K^+ channels, for example in the proximal region of a branch (11). Shutting down the capacity of an action potential to pass a branch point by down-regulating Na^+ channels or up-regulating K^+ channels is a possibility, based on the known capacity of neurotransmitter receptors and their attendant signal transduction mechanisms to regulate these channels (see Figures 10 and 12). The idea here is that local activation of NE, ACh, or serotonin receptors could increase (or decrease) the likelihood of LTP induction for an entire branch by controlling the likelihood of action potential propagation into that branch.

A second possible mechanism for regulating branch-specific action potential back-propagation is activity-dependent (10). The occurrence of EPSPs boosts action potential back-propagation in a given dendritic region through modulation of local voltage-dependent K^+ channels. In brief, membrane depolarization by an EPSP leads to a transient decrease in voltage-dependent K^+ channel function, by causing voltage-dependent inactivation of these channels. Thus, synaptic input into a particular branch point can increase the likelihood of action potential propagation into that region owing to increased membrane excitability because of diminution of active K^+ channels (see Figures 8 and 12). The duration of this effect is, of course, limited by the time-course of recovery of the K^+ channels, which is typically fairly quick. It is important to note that this mechanism and the one described in the previous paragraph are not mutually exclusive, but rather they might act in concert to confer additional information processing sophistication.

In later chapters, we will discuss additional implications of this type of information processing in more detail. Thus, we will discuss in more detail the molecular mechanisms by which these local effects regulating membrane depolarization within specific dendritic branches or dendritic subregions may be achieved. Moreover, we will discuss the signal transduction mechanisms by which modulatory neurotransmitter systems can regulate the likelihood of action potential back-propagation by controlling dendritic potassium channels, and we will discuss how this might allow

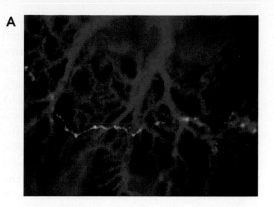

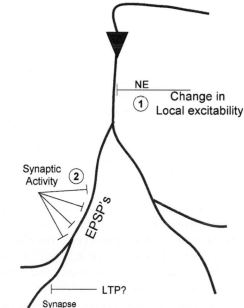

FIGURE 12 The dendritic tree and regulation of action potential propagation. (A) This photograph is of pyramidal neuron dendrites and a single axon fiber passing through them. Photo by Michael Hausser and Beverly Clark. (B) Two ways to regulate the likelihood of a back-propagating action potential reaching a given distal synapse are shown. One possibility is neurotransmitter (e.g., NE) regulation of local potassium channels determining the extent of action potential propagation (1). A second possibility is postsynaptic EPSPs, which inactivate potassium channels (see Figure 8B, part b), arriving in a dendritic region and allowing passage of an action potential through that region (2).

for sophisticated information processing through an interplay of action potential propagation, glutamate release, and neuro-modulation (see reference 10). All these things become possible because the dendritic membrane in which the NMDA receptors reside is not passive but contains voltage-dependent ion channels. This means that controlling the postsynaptic membrane biophysical properties can be a critical determinant for regulating the triggering of synaptic change; we will return to this issue in Chapter 6.

IV. NMDA RECEPTOR-INDEPENDENT LTP

Although the vast majority of studies of LTP and its molecular mechanisms have investigated NMDA receptor-dependent processes, as mentioned previously there also are several types of NMDA receptor-independent LTP. We will not discuss the mechanisms for these types of LTP very much in this book for two reasons. First, there have not been many studies investigating the molecular basis of NMDA receptor-independent LTP, at least relative to its NMDA receptor-dependent counterpart. Second, in those cases where mechanisms for this type of LTP have been investigated, there has been considerable controversy. I believe that it is wise to wait for the field to advance somewhat before attempting to integrate molecular mechanisms for NMDA receptor-independent LTP into the better-established models for NMDA receptor-dependent LTP. Nevertheless, it is clearly worthwhile to describe briefly a few different types of NMDA receptor-independent LTP as background material and to highlight them as important areas for future investigation.

A. 200-Hz LTP

NMDA receptor-independent LTP can be induced at the Schaffer-collateral synapses in area CA1, the same synapses we have been discussing thus far. This allows for somewhat of a compare-and-contrast of two different types of LTP at the same synapse. A protocol that elicits NMDA receptor-independent LTP in area CA1 is the use of four 0.5-second, 200-Hz stimuli separated by 5 seconds (14). LTP induced with this stimulation protocol is insensitive to NMDA receptor-selective antagonists such as APV (see Figure 13). It is interesting that simply doubling the rate of tetanic stimulation from 100 to 200 Hz appears to shift activity-dependent mechanisms for synaptic potentiation into NMDA receptor independence. At the simplest level of thinking, this indicates that there is some unique type of temporal integration going on at the higher-frequency stimulation that allows for superseding the necessity for NMDA receptor activation. What might the 200-Hz stimulation be uniquely stimulating? One appealing hypothesis arises from the observation that 200-Hz LTP is blocked by blockers of voltage-sensitive calcium channels. Thus, the current working model is that 200-Hz stimulation elicits sufficiently large and sufficiently prolonged membrane depolarization, resulting in the opening of voltage-dependent calcium channels, to trigger elevation of postsynaptic calcium sufficient to trigger synaptic potentiation. One observation consistent with this hypothesis is that injection of postsynaptic calcium chelators blocks 200-Hz stimulation-induced LTP.

B. TEA LTP

NMDA receptor-independent LTP in area CA1 can also be induced using tetraethylammonium (TEA$^+$) ion application, a form of LTP that is referred to as LTP$_K$ (15, 16). TEA$^+$ is a nonspecific potassium channel blocker, the application of which greatly increases membrane excitability. Like 200-Hz LTP, LTP$_K$ is insensitive to NMDA receptor antagonists and is blocked by blockade of voltage-sensitive calcium channels. Moreover, LTP$_K$ is blocked by postsynaptic calcium chelator

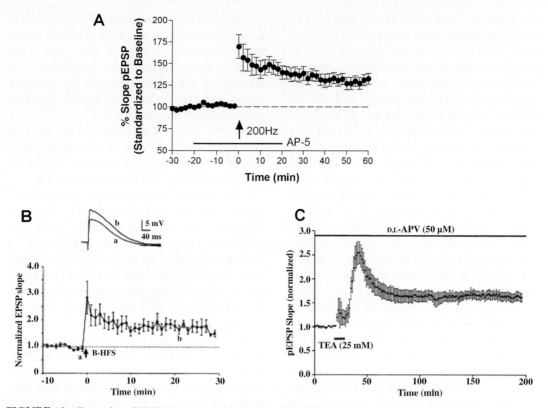

FIGURE 13   Examples of NMDA receptor-independent LTP. (A) 200-Hz stimulation in area CA1 elicits LTP even in the presence of the NMDA receptor antagonist APV. Data courtesy of Ed Weeber. (B) LTP at Mossy Fiber inputs into area CA3 is also NMDA receptor independent – the potentiation shown occurred in the presence of blockers of the NMDA receptor. Data courtesy of Rick Gray. Reproduced with permission from Kapur *et al.* (19). (C) Similarly, application of the K channel blocker Tetra-Ethyl Ammonium (TEA) also elicits NMDA receptor-independent LTP in area CA1. Data courtesy of Craig Powell (Ph.D. thesis pg 50; Powell *et al.* JBC 1994(16)).

injection as well. One twist is that the induction of LTP_K is dependent on synaptic activity, as its induction is blocked by AMPA receptor antagonists. Similar to 200-Hz LTP, the current model for TEA LTP is that synaptic depolarization via AMPA receptor activation, augmented by the hyperexcitable membrane owing to K^+ channel blockade, leads to a relatively large and prolonged membrane depolarization. This leads to the triggering of LTP through postsynaptic calcium influx.

C. Mossy Fiber LTP in Area CA3

The predominant model system for studying NMDA receptor-independent LTP is not the Schaffer-collateral synapses, but rather the mossy fiber inputs into area CA3 pyramidal neurons. Considerable excitement accompanied the discovery of NMDA receptor-independent LTP at these synapses by Harris and Cotman (17). The mossy fiber synapses are unique, large synapses with unusual presynaptic specializations, and there has been much interest in comparing the attributes and mechanisms of induction of mossy fiber LTP (MF-LTP) with those of NMDA receptor-dependent LTP in area CA1.

However, subsequent progress in investigating the mechanistic differences between these two types of LTP has been relatively slow for several reasons. First, the experiments are technically difficult physiologically—the CA3 region is "finicky," and typically area CA3 is the first part of the hippocampal slice preparation to die in vitro. The local circuitry in area CA3 is complex, with many recurrent excitatory connections between neurons there: synapses that also are plastic and exhibit NMDA receptor-dependent LTP. Most problematic has been that there has been an ongoing controversy about the necessity of postsynaptic events, especially elevations of postsynaptic calcium, for the induction of mossy fiber LTP. There basically are two schools of thought on mossy fiber LTP. One line of thinking is that MF-LTP is entirely presynaptic in its induction and expression (18). A second line of thinking is that MF-LTP has a requirement for postsynaptic signal transduction events for its induction (see for example references 19 and 20). The most prominent data supporting the second line of thinking comes from the laboratory of my colleague and collaborator, Dan Johnston. Thus, I cannot pretend to be unbiased in my thinking on this issue. For my purposes in this book, which focuses on NMDA receptor-dependent forms of LTP, I will simply note that this has been an area of controversy.

V. A ROLE FOR CALCIUM INFLUX IN NMDA RECEPTOR-DEPENDENT LTP

In contrast to the story with mossy fiber-LTP, NMDA receptor-dependent LTP at Schaffer-collateral synapses has achieved a broad consensus of a necessity for elevations of postsynaptic calcium for triggering LTP (21). In fact, this is one of the few areas of LTP research where there is almost universal agreement, and for that reason I am choosing this as the proper topic with which to end this chapter. In a very real sense, this topic is a break-point in the book, where we will transition from established thinking to more speculative areas. The elevation of postsynaptic calcium as a trigger for LTP is also appropriate as a

transitional topic because this is the point at which biochemically things become much more complex—most of the next four chapters will deal with the complexities of regulating the generation of the calcium signal and the plethora of events that this unique signal triggers.

But for one last section we can sit back and enjoy the harmony of consensus opinion, at least until I add in a few dissonant notes to spice up the composition a bit.

The case for a role for elevated postsynaptic calcium in triggering LTP is quite clear-cut and solid. It is well-established and has been reviewed adequately a sufficient number of times (22–25), so I will only overview the evidence here. Injection of calcium chelators postsynaptically blocks the induction of LTP. Inhibitors of a variety of calcium-activated enzymes also block LTP induction, as we will discuss extensively in chapters 6 and 7. Fluorescent imaging experiments using calcium-sensitive indicators have clearly demonstrated that postsynaptic calcium is elevated with LTP-inducing stimulation. Elevating postsynaptic calcium is sufficient to cause synaptic potentiation (although I must say there has been a little bit of controversy on this point). Thus, the hypothesis of a role for postsynaptic calcium elevation in triggering LTP has met the three classic criteria (block, measure, mimic) that we discussed in the last chapter and thus apparently is on solid ground.

I emphasize this, and the fact that there really is no disagreement about this conclusion, because something so well-established will serve nicely as a basis for a critique of the logic of this type of hypothesis testing. William of Ockham formulated *Occam's Razor* in the context of evaluating competing hypotheses. Basically, Occam's Razor states that when competing hypotheses are being evaluated, choose the one that is the simplest and still compatible with the available data. There is no doubt this is solid reasoning. The simplest hypothesis that is consistent with the available data described in the last paragraph is that elevations of postsynaptic calcium trigger LTP. However, consider the alternative interpretation of the block experiment, where the injection of calcium chelators postsynaptically blocks LTP induction. Say you hypothesize that what is really happening is that maintaining a tonic, low level of calcium is necessary to maintain the appropriate biochemical state of the cell. You think that chelating calcium disrupts this baseline process, which is not involved in LTP induction but is prerequisite for allowing LTP to happen. You say that the observed calcium elevation is an epiphenomenon not involved in LTP induction, and the sufficiency of postsynaptic calcium for triggering LTP is in question.

This is clearly not the most parsimonious interpretation of the data, à la Occams Razor. It requires much more mental gymnastics to justify. However, it is consistent with the available data and a perfectly tenable hypothesis. My point here is that the logic of hypothesis testing is not absolute, nor is it flawless. Testing the "big three" predictions experimentally is just about all you can do, and the more different ways you test them the better. However, we must always keep in mind that the underlying biology may not cooperate with us, and that things may be more complicated than we imagine. This of course becomes more and more of an issue the less data you have relevant to any hypothesis—in other words, for most of the rest of the topics we will be covering in this book. It also is important to keep in mind that, no matter what the area of investigation, the specific caveats for LTP experiments generalize to the rest of scientific investigation as well.

BOX 4

SHORT-TERM PLASTICITY: PPF AND PTP

There are two types of short-term plasticity exhibited at hippocampal Schaffer collateral synapses and elsewhere that are activity-dependent just as is LTP. These are paired-pulse facilitation (PPF) and post-tetanic potentiation (PTP). Paired-pulse facilitation is a form of short-term synaptic plasticity that is commonly held to be due to residual calcium augmenting neurotransmitter release presynaptically. When two single stimulus pulses are applied with interpulse intervals ranging from 20 to 300 msec, the second EPSP produced is larger than the first (see Panel A). This effect is referred to as PPF. The role of this type of synaptic plasticity in the behaving animal is unknown at this time; however, it clearly is a robust form of temporal integration of synaptic transmission and could be used in information processing behaviorally. The second form of short-term plasticity, PTP, is a large enhancement of synaptic efficacy observed after brief periods of high-frequency synaptic activity. For example, in experiments where LTP is induced with one or two 1-second, 100-Hz tetani, a large and transient increase in synaptic efficacy is produced immediately after high-frequency tetanus (see, for example, Figure 6 and Panel B). This is post-tetanic potentiation. The mechanisms for PTP are unknown, but both PTP and PPF are NMDA receptor-independent phenomena.

Continued

BOX 4—cont'd

SHORT-TERM PLASTICITY: PPF AND PTP

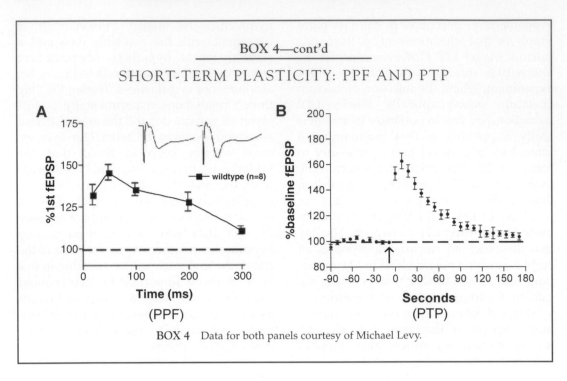

BOX 4   Data for both panels courtesy of Michael Levy.

VI. SUMMARY

Like learning, LTP can be defined as a long-lasting change in output in response to a transient input. The persistence of this effect has been demonstrated to extend many hours in vitro and several weeks in vivo. We do not know how LTP relates to memory and the entire ninth chapter of the book will be devoted to the evidence for and against the hypothesis that hippocampal LTP is involved in memory. Regardless, it is the best-understood example of long-lasting synaptic plasticity in the mammalian CNS, and it is a model for how long-lasting memory-associated changes are likely to occur in the CNS. One premise of this book is that understanding LTP will yield valid insights into the mechanisms of plasticity that underlie learning and memory in the brain. The bona fide changes in neuronal connections that occur in vivo may or may not be identical to LTP as it is presently studied in the laboratory, but this does not diminish its utility as a cellular model system for studying lasting neuronal change in the mammalian CNS.

References

1. Naber, P. A., and Witter, M. P. (1998). "Subicular efferents are organized mostly as parallel projections: a double-labeling, retrograde-tracing study in the rat." *J. Comp. Neurol.* 393:284–297.
2. van Groen, T., and Wyss, J. M. (1990). "Extrinsic projections from area CA1 of the rat hippocampus: olfactory, cortical, subcortical, and bilateral hippocampal formation projections." *J. Comp. Neurol.* 302:515–528.
3. Johnston, D., and Amaral, D. G. (1998). "Hippocampus." In: *The synaptic organization of the brain*, edited by Shepherd GM, 4th ed. New York: Oxford University Press; 417–458.
4. Bliss, T. V., and Lomo, T. (1973). "Long-lasting potentiation of synaptic transmission in the dentate area of the anaesthetized rabbit following stimulation of the perforant path." *J. Physiol.* 232:331–356.
5. Collingridge, G. L., Kehl, S. J., and McLennan, H. (1983). "Excitatory amino acids in synaptic transmission in the Schaffer collateral-commissural

pathway of the rat hippocampus." *J. Physiol.* 334:33–46.

6. Wigstrom, H., and Gustafsson, B. (1986). "Postsynaptic control of hippocampal long-term potentiation." *J. Physiol. (Paris)* 81:228–236.

7. Barrionuevo, G., and Brown, T. H. (1983). "Associative long-term potentiation in hippocampal slices." *Proc. Natl. Acad. Sci. USA* 80:7347–7351.

8. Andersen, P., Sundberg, S. H., Sveen, O., and Wigstrom, H. (1977). "Specific long-lasting potentiation of synaptic transmission in hippocampal slices." *Nature* 266:736–737.

9. McNaughton, B. L., Douglas, R. M., and Goddard, G. V. (1978). "Synaptic enhancement in fascia dentata: cooperativity among coactive afferents." *Brain Res.* 157:277–293.

10. Magee, J. C., and Johnston, D. (1997). "A synaptically controlled, associative signal for Hebbian plasticity in hippocampal neurons." *Science* 275:209–213.

11. Johnston, D., Hoffman, D. A., Magee, J. C., Poolos, N. P., Watanabe, S., Colbert, C. M., and Migliore, M. (2000). "Dendritic potassium channels in hippocampal pyramidal neurons." *J. Physiol.* 525 (1):75–81.

12. Bi, G. Q., and Poo, M. M. (1998). "Synaptic modifications in cultured hippocampal neurons: dependence on spike timing, synaptic strength, and postsynaptic cell type." *J. Neurosci.* 18:10464–10472.

13. Linden, D. J. (1999). "The return of the spike: postsynaptic action potentials and the induction of LTP and LTD." *Neuron* 22:661–666.

14. Grover, L. M., and Teyler, T. J. (1990). "Two components of long-term potentiation induced by different patterns of afferent activation." *Nature* 347:477–479.

15. Aniksztejn, L., and Ben-Ari, Y. (1991). "Novel form of long-term potentiation produced by a K+ channel blocker in the hippocampus." *Nature* 349:67–69.

16. Powell, C. M., Johnston, D., and Sweatt, J. D. (1994). "Autonomously active protein kinase C in the maintenance phase of N-methyl-D-aspartate receptor-independent long term potentiation." *J. Biol. Chem.* 269:27958–27963.

17. Harris, E. W., and Cotman, C. W. (1986). "Long-term potentiation of guinea pig mossy fiber responses is not blocked by N-methyl D-aspartate antagonists." *Neurosci. Lett.* 70:132–137.

18. Zalutsky, R. A., and Nicoll, R. A. (1990). "Comparison of two forms of long-term potentiation in single hippocampal neurons." *Science* 248:1619–1624.

19. Kapur, A., Yeckel, M. F., Gray, R., and Johnston, D. (1998). "L-Type calcium channels are required for one form of hippocampal mossy fiber LTP." *J. Neurophysiol.* 79:2181–2190.

20. Yeckel, M. F., Kapur, A., and Johnston, D. (1999). "Multiple forms of LTP in hippocampal CA3 neurons use a common postsynaptic mechanism." *Nat. Neurosci.* 2:625–633.

21. Lynch, G., Larson, J., Kelso, S., Barrionuevo, G., and Schottler, F. (1983). "Intracellular injections of EGTA block induction of hippocampal long-term potentiation." *Nature* 305:719–721.

22. Nicoll, R. A., and Malenka, R. C. (1995). "Contrasting properties of two forms of long-term potentiation in the hippocampus." *Nature* 377:115–118.

23. Chittajallu, R., Alford, S., and Collingridge, G. L. (1998). "Ca^{2+} and synaptic plasticity." *Cell. Calcium* 24:377–385.

24. Johnston, D., Williams, S., Jaffe, D., and Gray, R. (1992). "NMDA-receptor-independent long-term potentiation." *Annu. Rev. Physiol.* 54:489–505.

25. Johnston, D., and Wu, S. M-s. (1995). *Foundations of cellular neurophysiology.* Cambridge, MA: MIT Press.

26. Malinow, R., and Tsien, R. W. (1990). "Presynaptic enhancement shown by whole-cell recordings of long-term potentiation in hippocampal slices." *Nature* 346:177–180.

27. Yuan, L. L., Adams, J. P., Swank, M., Sweatt, J. D., and Johnston, D. (2002). "Protein kinase modulation of dendritic K+ channels in hippocampus involves a mitogen-activated protein kinase pathway." *J. Neurosci.* 22:4860–4868.

28. Hebb, D. O. (1949). The Organization of Behavior; a neuropsychological theory. New York, Wiley Press: p862.

Complexities of LTP
J. David Sweatt, Acrylic on canvas, 2002

5

Complexities of Long-Term Potentiation

I. INTRODUCTION

The problem with LTP is that it is deceptively simple-looking. Buzz a slice and get a lasting change, what could be simpler? It looks for all the world like you had simply flipped a biochemical "light switch" and turned on LTP. We now know the error of this mindset: we now know that LTP is immensely complex as both a physiologic and biochemical phenomenon. In this chapter, we continue our discussion of LTP physiology, highlighting a few of the complexities that LTP exhibits at the physiologic level. This will help us transition to our discussion of LTP biochemistry in the next section, where things are going to start to get really hairy.

I find it ironic that there was an influx of stellar scientists into the LTP field in the late

1980s and early 1990s, when there was a general sense that LTP would be solved in 5 years or so and that everybody had better hurry in order to be the first. Although nobody ever came right out and said it, I'm sure that more than a few people thought there was a Nobel Prize ripe for the taking. It turned out that LTP was more complicated than most of us imagined, and it seemed like the more we learned, the worse it got. The quick answer was not there to be had, and these days the general mindset in some quarters is to question if the molecular complexity of LTP might not in fact be overwhelming.

From one perspective, this complexity in itself suggests the physiologic relevance of LTP—such an immensely complicated biochemical process is very unlikely to pop up as an experimental artifact. One imagines that a great deal of selection pressure over time is necessary for the evolution of the subtleties and complexities manifest in the biochemistry of LTP. By inference, this also suggests that LTP is doing something very important but also complicated in the behaving animal, such as subserving learning and memory. Thus, one can make the argument that the molecular complexity of LTP is inferential evidence of its involvement in memory in the animal, or at least some evolutionarily important process that has been rigorously selected for over great distances of evolutionary time.

We might call this the "blind watchmaker" argument for a role for LTP in memory formation. Dr. Richard Dawkins has written a book entitled *The Blind Watchmaker*— one theme of which is that the presence of biological complexity implies functional importance from an evolutionary perspective (1). While Dr. Dawkins was discussing this concept in the context of creationism versus Darwinism, the argument might also, in my opinion, be applied to LTP and memory formation.

In this chapter I will highlight a few of the interesting complexities of LTP. We will expand upon the basics of LTP presented in the last chapter by discussing in more detail some specific attributes of LTP induction and expression that go beyond the fundamental activity-dependence of LTP that we have already covered. In this chapter, we also will touch on many areas that are current topics of investigation, some of which are unresolved, controversial, or speculative. For our purposes here, I will for the most part limit the discussion to complexities that can be observed or demonstrated using physiologic techniques.

II. PRESYNAPTIC VERSUS POSTSYNAPTIC MECHANISMS

One of the most intensely studied and least satisfactorily resolved aspects of LTP concerns the locus of LTP maintenance and expression. One component of LTP is an increase in the EPSP, which could arise from somehow increasing glutamate concentrations in the synapse or by increasing the responsiveness to glutamate by the postsynaptic cell (see Figure 1). In short, the "pre"-versus-"post" debate is whether the relevant changes reside presynaptically, manifest as an increase in neurotransmitter release or similar phenomenon, or postsynaptically, as a change in glutamate receptor responsiveness, etc. Over the last

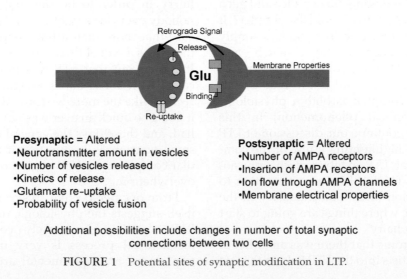

Presynaptic = Altered
•Neurotransmitter amount in vesicles
•Number of vesicles released
•Kinetics of release
•Glutamate re-uptake
•Probability of vesicle fusion

Postsynaptic = Altered
•Number of AMPA receptors
•Insertion of AMPA receptors
•Ion flow through AMPA channels
•Membrane electrical properties

Additional possibilities include changes in number of total synaptic connections between two cells

FIGURE 1   Potential sites of synaptic modification in LTP.

15 years or so, *numerous* experiments were performed to try to address this question, and as of yet there is no clear consensus answer. Popularity of the "Pre" hypothesis versus the "Post" hypothesis has waxed and waned, and this oscillation may continue for some time yet. In the next few paragraphs, I will summarize a few representative findings to give a little background on the issues. Those readers looking for an interesting "homework" assignment would find the following exercise edifying: in one sitting read the recent papers by Choi, Klinguaf, and Tsein (2); Bolshakov, Golan, Kandel, and Siegelbaum (3); and Nicoll and Malenka (4). This will give you a feel for the nature of the ongoing debate, and also illustrate that a lot of really smart people have been working on the problem and have yet to reach a consensus.

In some of the earliest studies that began to get at LTP mechanistically, it became clear that infusing compounds into the postsynaptic cell led to a block of LTP. A few of these studies involving calcium chelators were described in the last chapter, and some studies investigating protein kinases are described in Box 1 in this chapter. If compounds that are limited in their distribution to the postsynaptic compartment block LTP, the most parsimonious hypothesis is that LTP resides postsynaptically.

BOX 1

A NEED FOR POSTSYNAPTIC PROTEIN KINASE ACTIVITY IN LTP INDUCTION

Experiments using intracellular electrodes to perfuse membrane-impermeant peptides directly and selectively into the postsynaptic cell have been instrumental in clarifying a necessity for postsynaptic events in LTP induction. Based on many studies of this sort, it is clear that LTP induction is blocked by infusion of compounds whose permeation is restricted to the intracellular compartment of the postsynaptic cell. Some of the pioneering studies of this sort utilized injection of protein kinase inhibitors postsynaptically, which not only illustrated a need for postsynaptic events generally but also clarified a need for postsynaptic signal transduction events specifically for the induction of LTP.

In some of the earliest studies, involvement of Ca^{2+}-dependent protein kinases was tested by intracellular injection of peptides that inhibited either PKC or CaMKII (26). As we will discuss later, many second messenger-regulated protein kinases have within their amino acid sequence autoinhibitory domains. Synthetic peptides that inhibit these domains are some of the most selective pharmacologic tools available anywhere. In one early experiment peptides corresponding to the protein kinase C autoinhibitory domain were infused postsynaptically and found to block LTP induction (see, for example, reference 26). (See figure.) While a variety of other earlier studies had shown that less-selective kinase inhibitors could block LTP induction, these early studies were landmark findings because of the specificity of the experimental manipulation.

In other early studies, a role for postsynaptic CaMKII was also investigated using a similar approach. Two different

Continued

BOX 1—cont'd

A NEED FOR POSTSYNAPTIC PROTEIN KINASE ACTIVITY IN LTP INDUCTION

types of peptides were used to inhibit CaMKII activation in these studies. In one series of studies the investigators used the pseudosubstrate peptide CaMKII(273–302), which inhibits CaMKII by mimicking the autoinhibitory domain (26). In a separate series of experiments, a different type of approach was used—the infusion of calmodulin-binding peptides (27). These peptides bind to the calcium signal-transducing protein calmodulin and inhibit its activation of downstream targets including CaMKII. The results from both experiments are consistent with a role for postsynaptic signal transduction events in LTP induction in general and suggest a role for CaMKII specifically. It turns out that subsequent work has shown that both manipulations are doing more than just blocking CaMKII activation because both types of peptides can affect other relevant signal transduction cascades. Nevertheless, these were key findings at the time, motivating pursuit of the CaMKII system as

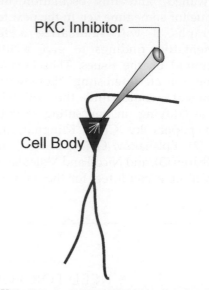

BOX 1   Injection of PKC inhibition directly into the cell body of a pyramidal neuron via an intra-cellular recording electrode.

a player in LTP induction, and a wide variety of subsequent work has supported a role for CaMKII activation in LTP.

Not too long afterward, however, evidence began to accumulate suggesting that there were presynaptic changes involved in LTP expression as well. For example, various types of "quantal" analysis that had been successfully applied at the neuromuscular junction to dissect presynaptic changes from postsynaptic changes suggested that LTP is associated with changes presynaptically. In a series of investigations, several laboratories used whole-cell recordings of synaptic trans-mission in hippocampal slices and found an increase in the probability of release, a strong indicator of presynaptic changes in

classic quantal analysis (5–8). These findings fit nicely with earlier studies from Tim Bliss's laboratory suggesting an increase in glutamate release in LTP as well (8). OK, so why not just say that there are changes both presynaptically and postsynaptically? The rub came in that some of the quantal analysis results seemed to exclude the occurrence of post-synaptic changes.

These findings in the early 1990s ushered in an exciting phase of LTP research that was important independent of the pre-versus-post debate per se. If there are changes presynaptically but these changes are triggered by events originating in the postsynaptic cell, as the earlier inhibitor-perfusion experiments had indicated, then the existence of a *retrograde messenger* is implied. A retrograde messenger is a compound generated in the postsynaptic compartment that diffuses back to and signals changes in the presynaptic compartment—the opposite (retrograde) direction from normal synaptic transmission. Moreover, if the compound is generated intracellularly in the postsynaptic

neuron, then the compound must be able to traverse the postsynaptic membrane somehow. The data supporting presynaptic changes in LTP implied the existence of such a signaling system, and this hypothesis launched a number of interesting and important experiments to determine what types of molecules might serve such a role— some of these are highlighted in Box 2.

However, in the mid-1990s the pre/post pendulum began to swing back in the opposite direction, toward the postsynaptic

---

BOX 2

CANDIDATE RETROGRADE SIGNALING MOLECULES

As described in the text, biochemical evidence makes it clear that molecular changes occur in both the presynaptic and postsynaptic compartments. While the existence of changes in both compartments does not resolve the important issue of the precise locus of increased synaptic strength, the existence of presynaptic biochemical changes that depend on postsynaptic events for their induction makes clear the necessity of a retrograde signaling mechanism of some sort. How does the postsynaptic cell communicate with the presynaptic terminal? The principal requirement is that the retrograde messenger must be able to traverse the synapse, and this could happen through either diffusion of a molecule or a direct physical coupling of molecules across the synapse (see figure). These are, of course, not mutually exclusive possibilities.

There is considerable evidence available supporting the existence of diffusible messengers that can serve as retrograde signaling molecules. Popular candidates include nitric oxide free radical ($NO^{\cdot}$), superoxide anion (O_2^-), and arachidonic acid (AA). These

molecules have in common that they are able to cross cell membranes, and thus can be generated in the postsynaptic cell and diffuse across to local presynaptic compartments to effect changes. Their diffusion is, of course, not limited to the presynaptic terminal they are directly activated by, but rather they may also diffuse to other local synapses. We will return to the mechanisms for generating these compounds and their likely targets in the next two chapters.

A different concept for signaling is to have a protein complex that physically links the postsynaptic compartment with the presynaptic compartment. A requirement for this type of signaling is that a post-translational modification of a postsynaptic cytoplasmic domain of the complex must be able to transduce, presumably through a conformational change, a signal to the presynaptic compartment. This type of mechanism is much more speculative at present. However, cell adhesion molecules such as integrins have the necessary signal-transducing capacity. These proteins traverse the membrane and

Continued

BOX 2—cont'd

CANDIDATE RETROGRADE SIGNALING MOLECULES

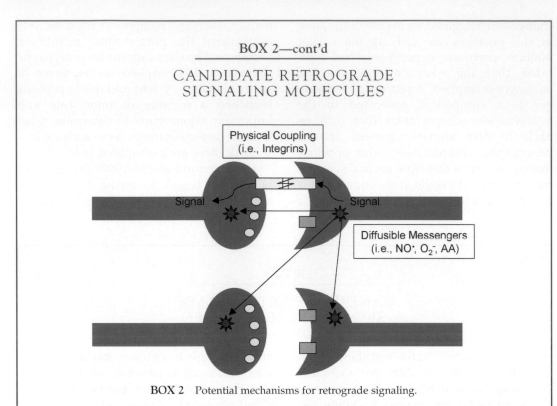

BOX 2   Potential mechanisms for retrograde signaling.

connect with a partner molecule on an adjacent cell, which also crosses its cell membrane. Thus, they connect the cytoplasmic compartments of two cells. In addition, signal transduction by these molecules is a two-way street—cytoplasmic domain conformational changes can be transferred to the extracellular domain of the same molecule, which is linked to its partner in the adjacent cell. We will return to some specific candidates in this category for retrograde signaling in Chapter 6.

side. Several groups found evidence for postsynaptic changes that could account for the apparently presynaptic changes identified by quantal analysis studies. Specifically, evidence was generated for what are termed *silent synapses* (see Box 3). These are synapses that contain NMDA receptors but no AMPA receptors— they are capable of synaptic plasticity mediated by NMDA receptor activation but are physiologically silent in terms of baseline synaptic transmission. Silent synapses are rendered active by NMDA receptor-triggered activation of latent AMPA receptors postsynaptically. Such an uncovering of silent AMPA receptors could involve membrane insertion or post-translational activation of already-inserted receptors. Activation of silent synapses is a postsynaptic mechanism that could explain the effects (decreased failure rate, for example) in quantal analysis experiments that implied presynaptic changes. Thus, there is now an argument that all of LTP physiology and biochemistry could be postsynaptic.

BOX 3

SILENT SYNAPSES, WHISPERING SYNAPSES

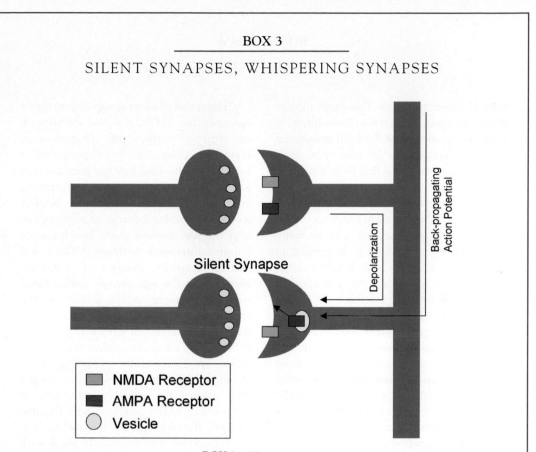

BOX 3   Silent synapses.

Silent synapses are all-or-none. The popular model for silent synapses is insertion of postsynaptic AMPA receptors into a synapse that previously had only NMDA receptors, activating the synapse (see figure). The prior existence in the synapse of the NMDA receptor is, of course, necessary for the synapse to be capable of sensing the simultaneous presence of synaptic glutamate and membrane depolarization and to trigger the AMPA receptor insertion. The NMDA receptor is normally silent for baseline synaptic transmission because the voltage-dependence keeps the ion channel blocked by Mg^{2+}; thus, at the outset, the entire synapse is "silent." The AMPA receptor insertion renders the synapse active at baseline synaptic transmission levels, and this is hypothesized to happen in an all-or-none fashion.

Because the postsynaptic membrane of a silent synapse is devoid of AMPA receptors, the membrane depolarization necessary to allow unblocking of the NMDA channel must be provided from some distal source. Any membrane depolarization reaching a silent synapse must be propagated from a site of depolarization elsewhere in the cell—either another synapse that has AMPA receptors or a back-propagating action

Continued

BOX 3—cont'd

SILENT SYNAPSES, WHISPERING SYNAPSES

potential from the soma. Thus, activation of silent synapses is likely to be exquisitely sensitive to control of the local membrane electrical properties. In this light, it is interesting to consider that local control of membrane excitability may serve as a particularly important component in controlling the activation of silent synapses.

Given this consideration, and for many other reasons as well, it is interesting to contemplate a role for local dendritic action potentials in regulating the activation of NMDA receptors (see reference 25). Gyorgi Buzsaki's lab has found that local dendritic spikes can be generated in the dendrites of CA1 pyramidal neurons, especially during periods of rhythmic activity such as those associated with learning. These local spikes are action potentials generated in the dendrite itself, that propagate within a restricted dendritic subregion, independent of an action potential firing in the cell body. The existence of these local spikes has important implications for dendritic subregion-specific information processing in a general sense, and it is also interesting to consider a potential role for these local actions in activating silent synapses.

Conversion of silent synapses into active synapses by AMPA receptor insertion is an entirely postsynaptic phenomenon. However, there has been proposed a variation of this idea that has been referred to as a "whispering" synapse. A whispering synapse has both AMPA and NMDA receptors in it, but because of a number of hypothetical factors such as glutamate affinity differences between NMDA and AMPA receptors, kinetics of glutamate elevation in the synapse, or spatial localization of the receptors, the AMPA receptors are silent (see also Box 4). A *presynaptic* mechanism converts a whispering synapse to being fully active. An increase in glutamate release presynaptically, resulting in an elevation of glutamate levels in the synapse then allows the effective activation of pre-existing AMPA receptors with baseline synaptic transmission. By this mechanism, a synapse that was previously silent with respect to baseline synaptic transmission is rendered detectably active. However, this alternative mechanism requires no change in the postsynaptic compartment whatsoever.

Like the retrograde messenger hypothesis, the silent synapses hypothesis has also led to a number of important and interesting experiments that warrant attention aside from the pre-versus-post debate. Specifically, these experiments have focused new attention on the importance of considering the postsynaptic compartment in a cell-biological context. Mechanisms of receptor insertion, trafficking, and turnover that had been studied in non-neuronal cells are now beginning to get the attention they

deserve in neurons as well. Like retrograde signaling, experiments arising from investigating mechanisms for activation of silent synapses have led to important "spin-off" studies that are important independent of the precipitating issue of pre-versus-post. Retrograde signaling and silent synapses represent to me excellent examples of the robustness of hypothesis testing in science— regardless of the final answer on pre-versus-post, tangible benefits have already arisen out of testing the attendant hypotheses.

So what is the bottom line? Pre or Post? My reading of the literature leads me to conclude that changes are occurring in both the presynaptic and postsynaptic compartments. Even though the wide variety of physiologic studies have been inconclusive, even to those expert in the techniques and approaches, which I am not, a variety of other kinds of experiments suggest that changes are occurring in both compartments. I will highlight two different types of approaches. First, a number of experiments using sophisticated imaging techniques have found LTP to be associated with increased vesicle recycling and increased presynaptic membrane turnover (9, 10). Also, direct biochemical measurements of the phosphorylation of proteins selectively localized to the presynaptic compartment have shown LTP-associated changes. Conceptually similar experiments looking at phosphorylation of postsynaptic proteins have found the same thing. (We will return to these experiments in chapters 6 and 7.) Thus, in my mind, the imaging and biochemistry studies have fairly clearly illustrated that sustained biochemical changes are happening in both the presynaptic and postsynaptic cell.

This conclusion and indeed all of the pre-versus-post experiments have a very important caveat to keep in mind. In trying to reach a consensus conclusion one is making a comparison across a wide spectrum of different types of experiments and different preparations. For example, one is comparing results with cultured cells versus hippocampal slices. One is trying to compare results for different types of LTP, LTP induced using pairing versus tetanic stimulation protocols. One likely is looking at different stages of LTP in comparing results from different experimental time points. Finally, in these experiments the various investigators are using material from different developmental stages in the animal, where the neurons under study are in different stages of their differentiation pathway. These considerations are a good reason to exercise caution in interpreting the experiments at this point; indeed, these issues may be contributing greatly to the apparent incompatibility of the results obtained in different labs.

BOX 4

ALTERNATIVE MECHANISMS FOR LTP

It seems obvious that if there is an increase in synaptic strength, it must be the result of either an increase in neurotransmitter release or an increase in postsynaptic responsiveness. However, what if it's neither of these? Are there alternative models that can explain synaptic potentiation that involve neither mechanism? Two alternate possibilities have received some attention. They are the possibilities of diminished re-uptake of glutamate, leading to increased synaptic glutamate levels; and altered kinetics of glutamate release, where the same number of glutamate molecules are released but at a faster rate, such that the peak synaptic glutamate concentration is higher.

Does decreased glutamate re-uptake account for LTP? Jonathan Levenson and his collaborators recently directly tested this hypothesis, and the answer was a resounding no. In fact, LTP-inducing stimulation at Schaffer-collateral synapses leads to an *increase* in glutamate re-uptake through neuronal membrane glutamate

Continued

BOX 4—cont'd

ALTERNATIVE MECHANISMS FOR LTP

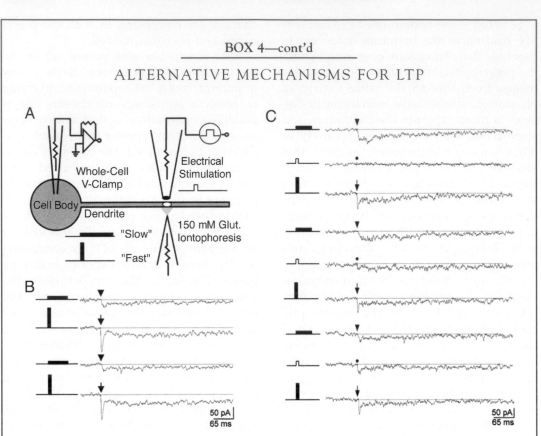

BOX 4 Concentration profile of neurotransmitter delivery determines AMPA receptor activation. (A) Representation of the experimental design for concurrently stimulating presynaptic release and iontophoretically examining the postsynaptic receptors. Iontophoresis and stimulating electrodes are brought to within 1 mm of an isolated synapse. Filled vertical and horizontal bars, used throughout the figures, represent the fast (1 ms, 100 nA) and slow (10 ms, 10 nA) iontophoretic application parameters. (B) AMPA receptors are not activated by a slow flux of glutamate. Slow pulses elicited NMDA receptor-only responses, while fast pulses elicited AMPA and NMDA receptor responses from the same site. (AMPA receptor responses are the fast peaks at the beginning of the responses, NMDA receptor responses are the slower, more sustained response.) Because AMPA receptor activation was sensitive to the instantaneous changes in the concentration of neurotransmitter, AMPA-quiet responses could be generated at synapses with functional AMPA Receptors. (C) Silent synapses contain functional AMPA receptors. Excitatory Post-Synaptic Current (EPSC) AMPA-quiet responses, resulting from endogenous transmitter release, were evoked by presynaptic electrical stimulation at a synapse in a cultured hippocampal neuron (open vertical bars). Evoked synaptic events were interleaved with alternating iontophoretic applications of neurotransmitter. Although EPSCs AMPA-quiet were evoked presynaptically, AMPA receptor responses were clearly visible at this synapse during fast iontophoretic pulses, indicating that endogenous AMPA-quiet synaptic events occurred at synapses containing functional AMPARs ($n = 4$). Figure and figure legend from Renger, Egles, and Liu (29).

transporters (28). This counterintuitive effect may be involved in limiting glutamate spillover from potentiated synapses. An alternative possibility is that increased re-uptake might protect potentiated synapses from desensitization, if there would otherwise be a too-prolonged elevation of glutamate at the synapse.

Certain aspects of the second alternative, the "altered kinetics of release"

BOX 4—cont'd

ALTERNATIVE MECHANISMS FOR LTP

hypothesis, have also been evaluated experimentally. Renger, Egles, and Liu (29) found that rapid elevations of glutamate at the synapse are more effective at activating synaptic AMPA receptors than are slower elevations. There are several reasons why rapid elevations of glutamate might be particularly efficacious. For any given number of glutamate molecules, more rapid release of glutamate will give a higher peak glutamate level. This factor is compounded by the kinetics of glutamate binding to AMPA receptors and receptor desensitization—AMPA receptors have a fast on-rate of glutamate binding and also rapidly desensitize. Thus, a slow elevation of glutamate concentration in the synapse can lead to desensitization of a fraction of the AMPA receptors before the peak

glutamate concentration is reached. Overall, the model is that rapid, transient elevations of synaptic glutamate cause greater AMPA receptor responses so that simply changing the kinetics of glutamate release, without changing the total number of glutamate molecules released, leads to a net synaptic potentiation (see figure). Thus, all of LTP might be accounted for by speeding up the presynaptic release process itself. While this hypothesis is at a very early stage of testing, it is an intriguing idea. I also find it interesting that the increased rate of glutamate re-uptake observed by Levenson et al. (28) is also consistent with this idea—increased re-uptake may serve to sharpen the peak of glutamate at the synapse and diminish AMPA receptor desensitization.

III. LTP CAN INCLUDE AN INCREASED AP FIRING COMPONENT

Another caveat to keep in mind is that the preceding discussion deals only with mechanisms contributing to increases in synaptic strength. The increased EPSP is typically measured in field recording experiments as an increase in the initial slope of the EPSP (or EPSP magnitude), as was discussed in the previous chapter. A second component of LTP is referred to as EPSP-spike (E-S) potentiation. E-S potentiation was identified by Bliss and Lomo in the first published report of LTP (11) and is defined as an increase in population spike amplitude that cannot be attributed to an increase in synaptic transmission (i.e., initial EPSP slope in field recordings). Thus, E-S potentiation is a term used to refer to

the postsynaptic cell having an increased probability of firing an action potential at a constant strength of synaptic input.

E-S potentiation at Schaffer-collateral synapses can be observed using recordings in stratum pyramidale, as illustrated in Figure 2. In this example Eric Roberson in my lab generated input-output curves for the initial slope of the EPSP and the population spike amplitude, using various stimulus intensities, before and after LTP induction. E-S potentiation is manifest as an increase in population spike amplitude even when responses are normalized to EPSP slope. I should note that we have found that the probability of induction and magnitude of E-S potentiation in area CA1 is more variable than LTP of synaptic transmission. A similar greater variability in E-S potentiation was also observed by Bliss and Lomo in their original report.

A

B

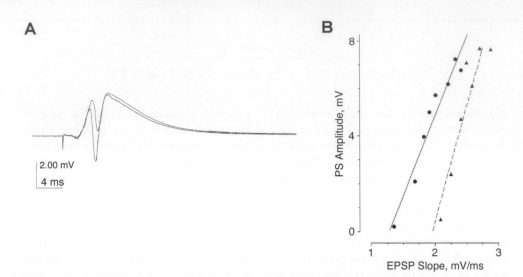

FIGURE 2   E-S potentiation in area CA1. Extracellular recordings were made in the cell body layer of area CA1 (using stimulation of the Schaffer-collateral inputs), and input-output curves were performed using a range of 5–45 μA constant current stimulation. Initial slopes of the EPSP and population spike (PS) amplitude were then determined from the tracings, and the data were plotted as population spike amplitude versus EPSP slope. (A) Superimposed representative tracings for before and 75 minutes after tetanic stimulation, show the increased population spike amplitude after tetanic stimulation. (B) Plots are shown for pre-tetanus (triangles) and 75 minutes post-tetanus (circles). In this experiment, five 100-Hz tetani were delivered. E-S coupling was assayed in hippocampal slices by taking a second set of input-output measurements after the induction of LTP. The baseline I/O curve and the post-stimulation I/O curve were then compared to assess whether a change in excitability had occurred over the course of the experiment. Although we measured both EPSP slope and population spike amplitude from the same waveform recorded from the cell body layer, the preferred approach is to record EPSPs in the dendritic region and simultaneously record spikes independently from the cell body layer. This approach minimizes cross-contamination of the pop spike in the EPSP measurements, and vice versa. Data and figure courtesy of Erik Roberson.

What is the mechanism for this long-term increase in the likelihood of firing an action potential? One possibility that comes to mind is that there could be changes in the intrinsic excitability of the postsynaptic neuron. Particularly appealing is the idea that long-term down-regulation of dendritic potassium channel function could cause a persisting increase in cellular excitability and action potential firing. While investigations of this hypothesis are still at an early stage, some recent work has suggested that E-S potentiation has a component that is the result of intrinsic changes in the postsynaptic neuron.

Progress in testing this hypothesis has been slow owing to the technically difficult nature of the experiments. Most patch-clamp physiologic studies of LTP have utilized recordings from the cell body, which are not capable of detecting changes in channels localized to the dendrites due to technical limitations. Thus, testing the idea of changes in dendritic excitability as a mechanism contributing to E-S potentiation requires dendritic patch-clamp recording, which at present only a few laboratories do routinely.

However, a more thoroughly investigated mechanism for E-S potentiation is based on alterations in feed-forward inhibitory connections onto pyramidal neurons in area CA1 (see Figure 3). A number of different types of neurons in the hippocampus are called interneurons (or intrinsic neurons) because their inputs and outputs are restricted to local areas of the hippocampus

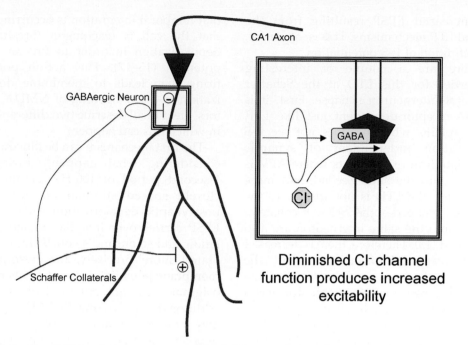

Diminished Cl⁻ channel function produces increased excitability

FIGURE 3 The GABAergic interneuron model of E-S potentiation. One potential mechanism for E-S potentiation is diminution of inhibitory feed-forward inhibition through GABA-ergic interneurons in area CA1. Specific possible sites for this effect include LTD of the Schaffer-collateral inputs onto GABAergic neurons or synaptic depression of the interneuron-CA1 pyramidal neuron synapse.

itself (see reference 12). In other words, they only communicate with other neurons nearby in the hippocampus. Most of these neurons in area CA1 use the inhibitory neurotransmitter GABA, and their actions are to inhibit firing of CA1 pyramidal neurons. Different GABAergic interneurons make connections in all the dendritic regions of CA1 pyramidal neurons as well as the initial segment of the axon where the action potential originates. A single GABAergic interneuron may contact a thousand pyramidal neurons; thus, the effects of altered interneuron function are not generally limited to a single follower cell.

Interneurons in area CA1 receive glutamatergic Schaffer-collateral projections just as the pyramidal neurons do; in fact, the inputs to the interneurons are branches of the same axons impinging the pyramidal neurons. Glutamate release at these interneuron synapses activates the interneurons

and causes downstream release of GABA onto the pyramidal neurons. This inhibitory action is, of course, slightly delayed at the level of the single cell that receives input from the same Schaffer-collateral axon that is activating the GABAergic interneuron because there is an extra synaptic connection involved.

How does this local circuit contribute to E-S potentiation? Two different groups have shown that the same stimulation that produces LTP at the Schaffer collateral–pyramidal neuron synapses simultaneously produces a decreased efficacy of coupling (long-term depression, LTD) of the Schaffer collateral–interneuron synapses (13, 14). Thus, while the excitatory input to the pyramidal neuron is being enhanced, the feed-forward inhibitory GABA input is diminished. This causes a net increase in excitability and increased likelihood of firing an action potential, added on top of the increased EPSP resulting from the normal LTP mechanisms. This is, of course, the definition of E-S potentiation.

There are a couple of interesting properties for this LTD at the Schaffer collateral–interneuron synapse. First, it is NMDA-receptor-dependent just like LTP. This explains why one does not see E-S potentiation independent of synaptic potentiation in experiments where APV is infused onto the slice. Second, and more interesting, the LTD is not specific to the activated synapse—other Schaffer-collateral inputs onto the same interneuron are also depressed (13). Therefore, there is decreased feed-forward inhibition across all the inputs (and outputs of course) for the whole interneuron. The interneuron has a diminished response to all its inputs, and therefore decreased feed-forward inhibition to all its outputs. Thus, the interneuron LTD appears to be serving to modulate the behavior of an entire small local circuit of neuronal connections. The precise role this interesting attribute plays in hippocampal information processing is unclear at present, but it is under study.

IV. TEMPORAL INTEGRATION IN LTP INDUCTION

At one level, it is a statement of the obvious to say that LTP induction depends on temporal integration. After all, the only thing that distinguishes the LTP induction protocols from baseline stimulation is that, during the LTP induction protocol, stimulation is delivered at a higher rate. It obviously is the case that if the only thing that is different is that the synapse is seeing activity at 100 pulses per second rather than once every 20 seconds, then LTP is being triggered by unique timing-dependent processes, which is simply a restatement of one definition of temporal integration. But what unique events are happening physiologically with high-frequency stimulation? Stated briefly, the answer to this question is

that temporal integration is occurring such that the cell is reaching a threshold of depolarization in order to fire an action potential (15–17). This action potential firing then leads to membrane depolarization to allow opening of NMDA receptors. Next I will describe two different ways in which this can happen.

The first mechanism can be illustrated by considering what happens during the 1-second period of 100-Hz tetanus. Such closely spaced stimulation means that postsynaptic depolarization from the first EPSP carries over into the second stimulation, and so on, and so on, 96 more times. Stated more precisely, the postsynaptic membrane potential does not recover to the original resting potential before an additional depolarizing EPSP is triggered, and temporal summation of postsynaptic depolarization occurs. The summed depolarization eventually reaches threshold for the cell to fire an action potential (see Figure 4). This is one of the classic examples of neuronal temporal integration, and, of course, such a process is not limited to hippocampal pyramidal neurons. One unique aspect of this in hippocampal neurons, and

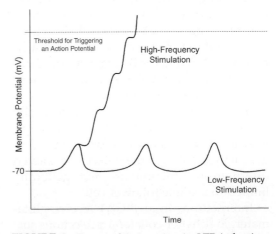

FIGURE 4 Temporal integration in LTP induction. Temporal summation of EPSPs is one mechanism contributing to bringing the postsynaptic neuron to threshold for firing an action potential, one contribution to the selective ability of high-frequency stimulation to produce LTP.

probably other cortical neurons as well, is that triggering of the action potential is used to generate a back-propagating action potential into the dendrites, which is involved in depolarizing the NMDA receptor and triggering synaptic plasticity.

A second example comes from considering LTP induced by theta-pattern stimulation. With this type of LTP induction protocol, delivered at the slower 5-Hz (once every 200 ms) rate, temporal integration is similarly involved but occurs via a different route. After all, 200 ms is long enough for the postsynaptic membrane potential to recover completely before the next wave of depolarization, so temporal integration of the sort described here is inadequate as an explanation. Joel Selcher in my laboratory investigated this question by examining the physiologic events occurring during the period of theta-frequency stimulation. For illustrative purposes, I will discuss Joel's results with theta-frequency stimulation, although he and others observed similar effects with theta-burst stimulation as well.

For these experiments, Joel used theta-frequency stimulation (TFS) consisting of 30 seconds of 5-Hz stimulation. This stimulation paradigm evokes stable LTP as described earlier and as illustrated in Figure 5. Joel then assessed population spikes during the theta-frequency stimulation period, utilizing a dual-recording electrode technique. The stimulating electrode remained in hippocampal area CA3 and activated Schaffer-collateral fibers innervating area CA1. One recording electrode was positioned in stratum radiatum of area CA1 in order to record synaptic responses, field EPSPs (Figure 5B). Joel placed another electrode in stratum pyramidale, the cell body layer, in order to record action potential firing in response to the same input. For each single stimulus, the initial slope of the EPSP recorded in stratum radiatum and the amplitude of the population spike recorded in stratum pyramidale were measured throughout the period of 5-Hz stimulation.

Theta-frequency stimulation resulted in a short-lived increase in action potential firing during the 30 seconds of 5-Hz stimulation (see Figure 5C, D). For roughly the first 20 seconds of the stimulation, the amplitude of the population spike increased dramatically. Meanwhile, over this same time period, the EPSP slope recorded in stratum radiatum gradually declined. Therefore, the ratio of the population spike amplitude to the EPSP slope increased over time, indicating an increased likelihood of action potential firing over the short time course of the TFS (Figure 5D). Once again, for TFS as for 100-Hz tetanic stimulation, some temporal integration process is taking place to cause action potential firing during the period of LTP-inducing stimulation.

The mechanism for this temporal integration is not clear at present: clearly temporal summation of the sort operating in 100-Hz stimulation is not sufficient to explain it. However, a variety of previous studies have suggested that for LTP induced by TFS there is an important role for attenuation of feed-forward GABAergic inhibition onto pyramidal neurons (see references 18, 19, and 20 and Figure 6). One current hypothesis is that short-term synaptic depression in the GABAergic local circuit during theta-frequency stimulation, which is a result of stimulation of presynaptic GABA-B autoreceptors, leads to a loss of GABA-mediated inhibition, increased excitability, and increased firing of action potentials during the period of theta-frequency stimulation.

V. LTP CAN BE DIVIDED INTO PHASES

Contemporary models divide very long-lasting LTP (i.e., LTP lasting in the range of 5 to 6 hours) into at least three phases. LTP comprising all three phases can be induced with repeated trains of high-frequency stimulation in area CA1 (see Figure 7), and the phases are expressed

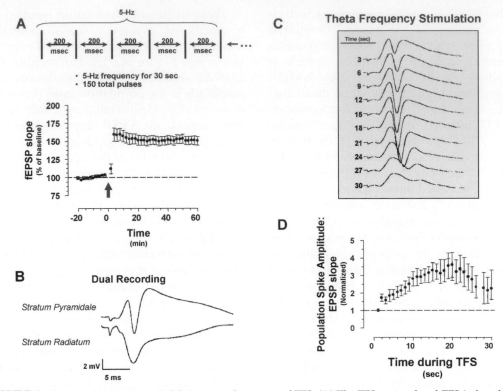

FIGURE 5 Increased action potential firing over the course of TFS. (A) The TFS protocol and TFS-induced LTP in mouse hippocampal slices. (B) Electrode placement configuration for recording EPSP and population spikes simultaneously during TFS. (C) Representative traces in response to TFS from a hippocampal slice. Note the difference in the population spike between the first and 18th stimulation of the stimulation paradigm. (D) Quantitation of increased spike amplitude during TFS. Population spike amplitudes recorded in stratum pyramidale of hippocampal area CA1 during theta-frequency stimulation are plotted normalized to EPSP slope. Slices showed a progressive increase in spike generation during the first two-thirds of TFS. Data and figures courtesy of Joel Selcher.

sequentially over time to constitute what we call LTP. Late LTP (L-LTP) is hypothesized to be dependent for its induction on changes in gene expression, and this phase of LTP lasts many hours. Early LTP (E-LTP) is likely subserved by persistently activated protein kinases, as we will discuss in Chapter 7, and starts at around 20 minutes or less post-tetanus and is over in about 2–3 hours. The first stage of LTP, generally referred to as short-term potentiation, is independent of protein kinase activity for its induction and lasts about 30 minutes. I prefer to refer to the first stage of LTP as Initial LTP (I-LTP) to emphasize that it is a persistent form of NMDA receptor-dependent synaptic plasticity that

is induced by LTP-inducing tetanic stimulation and is a prelude to E-LTP and L-LTP (see reference 21). We will not really discuss I-LTP (aka STP) much more in this book because the mechanisms for its induction are essentially a complete mystery at present.

Two different groups have proposed an additional phase of LTP, intermediate LTP (22, 23). Unfortunately these two groups are not referring to the same thing, in all likelihood. At this time, I am not incorporating an intermediate phase of LTP into our discussion because intermediate-LTP might be explained as a prolonged form of E-LTP. Also, even though there is generally a consensus about different mechanisms for

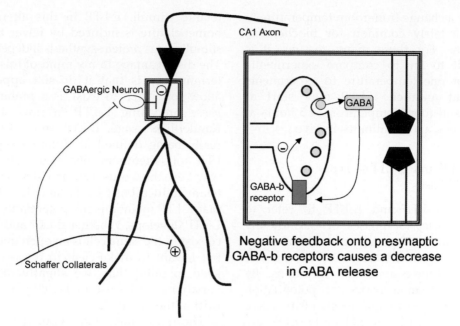

FIGURE 6   GABA-B receptors in temporal integration with TBS. This figure presents one model for the increased excitability that occurs during TBS, based on autoinhibition at GABAergic inputs onto CA1 pyramidal neurons during the period of stimulation.

E-LTP and L-LTP, it is unclear where intermediate LTP might fit into this scheme.

Readers may note some degree of ambiguity in the times specified for each phase of LTP. This is in part because the phases are very descriptive and different labs often use slightly different conditions for their LTP experiments. For example, for technical reasons, most L-LTP experiments are performed at room temperature or 27–28°C because it is much easier to maintain a healthy slice for many hours at these lower temperatures. Many E-LTP experiments, especially those involving direct biochemical measurements, are performed at 32–35°C. Comparing studies done at different temperatures is complicated by the pronounced temperature-dependence of essentially all chemical reactions—any physical chemist far afield enough to be reading this book will remember that this is described by the Arrhenius Equation. Plugging some back-of-the-envelope numbers into this equation shows that a doubling of reaction

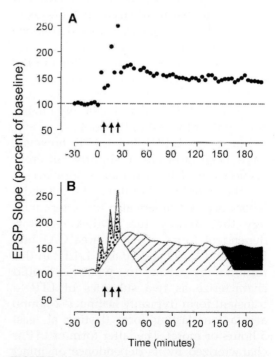

FIGURE 7   Immediate, early, and late LTP. (A) Real data from a late-phase LTP experiment. Courtesy of Eric Roberson. (B) A cartoon adaptation of the same data approximating the Initial, Early, and Late stages of LTP. Adapted from Roberson, English, and Sweatt (21).

rate for a change from room temperature to 32°C is fairly common for biochemical reactions. For these many reasons, it is difficult to try to compare experiments done at one temperature to experiments done at another. L-LTP may start at 3 hours at room temperature, 1.5 hours at 32 degrees, and 45 minutes in vivo.

A. E-LTP and L-LTP—Types Versus Phases

I use E-LTP and L-LTP to refer to different *temporal* phases of LTP. By my definition, these phases are subserved by different *maintenance* mechanisms of different time-courses and durations. By phase, I mean a period of potentiation subserved by a unique mechanism. These two phases of LTP—E-LTP and L-LTP—are not exclusive of each other. In fact, my model is that E-LTP is ongoing while L-LTP is developing, and that one supplants the other over time. This has certain theoretical implications that are discussed in more detail in reference 21. I emphasize these definitions here because they are very important as we transition to molecular mechanisms in the next chapters. These definitions contain an underlying assumption about the biochemistry of LTP that is an organizing principle for the rest of the book.

The terms E-LTP and L-LTP, however, have been used in a slightly different fashion as well, in particular as popularized by the Kandel laboratory. The Kandel laboratory and others also use a terminology that divides the NMDA receptor-dependent form of LTP in area CA1 into E-LTP and L-LTP. E-LTP and L-LTP in this terminology refer to what I would characterize as two subtypes of LTP—a transient form (typically lasting 1–2 hours) and a long-lasting form (lasting at least 5 hours or more). The latter form of LTP is characterized by its dependence on intact protein synthesis, and the induction of this form of LTP requires delivery of multiple tetanic stimuli. E-LTP in this alternative nomenclature is induced by fewer tetanic stimuli and is protein-synthesis-independent. The disadvantage in my mind of this latter terminology is that it doesn't appear to allow for E-LTP to exist as a preliminary *phase* preceding L-LTP in time. In the Kandel-like usage, E-LTP and L-LTP are really being defined as different types of LTP, not as temporal phases of LTP. In the way I use the words, I assume that multiple tetani induce both E-LTP and L-LTP, and that E-LTP maintains the potentiation until L-LTP develops. Whether E-LTP and L-LTP coexist in the same cell is an open question, but I want to make clear to the reader to keep in mind that two slightly different variations in the use of E-LTP and L-LTP exist in the literature.

The thing that I like about the Kandel laboratory's use of the terms E-LTP and L-LTP is that their usage emphasizes that different and unique things happen with multiple tetani. Multiple, spaced tetani elicit very long-lasting LTP and appear to recruit a unique protein synthesis-dependent mechanism for L-LTP. This is a great example of temporal integration—tetani delivered in close temporal sequence with other tetani appear to be able to trigger a uniquely long-lasting event: L-LTP. This is a cellular analog to the graded acquisition of memory—as we discussed in the first two chapters multiple training trials elicit more robust and long-lasting memory. The E-LTP/L-LTP dichotomy drawn by the Kandel lab highlights this attribute, and that is, I believe, the rationale behind their use of the terms. Again, I point this out to help avoid confusion because of the different applications of the terms E-LTP and L-LTP. This is particularly important because later on in this section and in Chapter 12 I will discuss some theoretical implications of LTP having different phases. In these sections, I will be referring to E-LTP and L-LTP as being at different points on a temporal continuum, not as different types of LTP.

Before turning to a discussion of some implications of LTP having phases, I must introduce one final set of three terms— three terms widely used and abused in the LTP literature. These terms arose from pharmacological inhibitor studies of LTP, and I will go through these types of studies in a moment. However, for now I will simply introduce the terms.

Induction refers to the transient events serving to trigger the formation of LTP. *Maintenance*, or more specifically a maintenance mechanism, refers to the persisting biochemical signal that lasts in the cell. This persisting biochemical signal acts upon an effector, for example a glutamate receptor or the presynaptic release machinery, resulting in the *expression* of LTP.

It is important to keep in mind that, depending on the design of the experiment, induction, maintenance, and expression could be differentially inhibited (see Figure 8). The simplest type of experiment doesn't do this—imagine, for example, that you apply an enzyme inhibitor (or knockout a gene) before, during, and after the period of LTP-inducing high-frequency stimulation and find that your manipulation blocks LTP. You cannot distinguish whether the missing activity is required for the induction, the expression, or the maintenance of LTP. To distinguish among these possibilities, imagine instead applying the inhibitor selectively at different time points during the experiment. If you apply the inhibitor only during the tetanus and then wash it out, but it blocks the generation of LTP, you can conclude that the enzyme is necessary for LTP induction. If you apply the inhibitor after the tetanus, and it reverses the potentiation, it may be blocking either the maintenance or expression of LTP, as was nicely illustrated in an early experiment by Malinow, Madison, and Tsien (24) where they applied a protein kinase inhibitor after LTP induction. In this experiment, transient application of a kinase inhibitor after tetanus blocked synaptic potentiation, but the potentiation recovered after removal of the inhibitor. This is a blockade of LTP *expression*. However, if the kinase inhibitor had caused the potentiation to be lost irreversibly, the inhibitor would then by definition have blocked the *maintenance* of LTP.

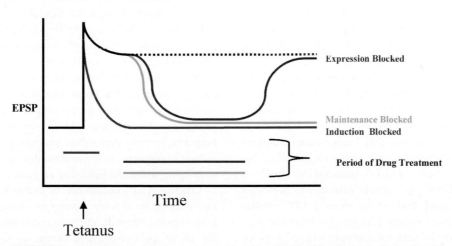

FIGURE 8   Induction, maintenance, and expression of LTP. This schematic illustrates the different experimental approaches to dissecting effects on the biochemical mechanisms subserving LTP induction, maintenance, or expression. See text for additional details.

BOX 5

MODULATION OF LTP INDUCTION

In one sense, the hippocampal slice is a denervated preparation. In the intact animal, the hippocampus receives numerous input fibers that provide modulatory inputs of the neurotransmitters dopamine (DA), norepinephrine (NE), serotonin (5HT), and acetylcholine (ACh). Functionally these inputs are largely lost as a necessity of physically preparing the hippocampal slice for the experiment. However, these lost modulatory inputs can be partially reconstituted by directly applying the neurotransmitters (or more commonly pharmacologic substitutes) to the slice preparation in vitro. This approach has been used quite successfully to gain insights into the physiologic mechanisms and functional roles of these inputs in the intact brain.

NE-, DA-, and ACh-mimicking compounds can all modulate the induction of LTP at Schaffer-collateral synapses. Specifically, agents acting at various subtypes of receptors for these compounds can increase the likelihood of LTP happening and the magnitude of LTP that is induced. Several examples of this type of modulation experiment are shown in the figure. In one example, 5-Hz stimulation of Schaffer-collateral synapses, for 3 minutes, gives essentially no potentiation. Coapplication of isoproterenol, a beta-adrenergic receptor agonist that mimics endogenous NE, converts a nonpotentiating signal into a potentiating one (33). Under other conditions beta-adrenergic agonists can augment the *magnitude* of LTP induced as well, if different physiologic stimulation protocols are used that evoke modest LTP. Similar types of effects can be observed for activation of various subtypes of receptors for ACh and DA (see reference 15). The basis for this modulation is complex, and

we will discuss some of the many sites at which these agents might act in the next chapter.

One known site of action of neuromodulators is regulation of back-propagating action potentials in pyramidal neuron dendrites. All these agents, which modulate LTP induction, can modulate the magnitude of back-propagating action potentials (see Panel B). The augmentation of back-propagating action potentials is a means by which these neurotransmitters can enhance membrane depolarization and thereby enhance NMDA receptor opening. We will discuss how this happens at the molecular level in the next chapter.

The growth factor BDNF (brain-derived neurotrophic factor) can also modulate the induction of LTP by a number of mechanisms, at least one of which is presynaptic (see references 34, 35, and 36 and Panel C). BDNF, acting through its cell-surface receptor TrkB, acts on presynaptic terminals to facilitate neurotransmitter release selectively during high-frequency stimulation. This is an interesting example of modulation of LTP induction that is activity-dependent but localized to the presynaptic compartment. The mechanisms controlling the levels of BDNF in the adult hippocampus are not entirely clear at this point, but it is fairly well established that hippocampal BDNF levels can be regulated by a variety of neuronal activity-dependent processes and indeed in response to environmental signals impinging upon the behaving animal.

Overall LTP induction is subject to modulation by a wide variety of extracellular signals. We will return to mechanisms for these processes, and some of their implications for memory formation in the animal, in later chapters.

BOX 5—cont'd

MODULATION OF LTP INDUCTION

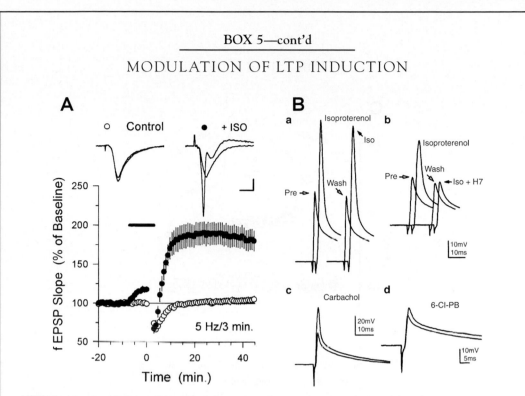

BOX 5   Neuromodulation of LTP induction. (A) Modulation of LTP induction by the beta-adrenergic agonist Isoproterenol (ISO). Activity-dependent β-adrenergic modulation of low-frequency stimulation-induced LTP in the hippocampus CA1 region. (A) In control experiments (no ISO), 3 minutes of 5-Hz stimulation (delivered at time = 0, open symbols, n = 26) had no lasting effect on synaptic transmission (45 minutes after 5-Hz stimulation, fEPSPs were not significantly different from pre–5-Hz baseline, t(25) = 1.01). However, 3 minutes of 5-Hz stimulation delivered at the end of a 10-minute application of 1.0 mM ISO (indicated by the bar) induced LTP (closed symbols, $p < .01$ compared with baseline). The traces are fEPSPs recorded during baseline and 45 minutes after 5-Hz stimulation in the presence and absence (control) of ISO. Calibration bars are 2.0 mV and 5.0 ms. Reproduced from Thomas, Moody, Makhinson, and O'Dell (33).

   (B) One potential mechanism for neuromodulation is regulation of back-propagating action potentials in CA1 dendrites. The data shown illustrate amplification of dendritic action potentials by isoproterenol (a) and its susceptibility to inhibition by the protein kinase inhibitor H7 (b). The traces shown are from dendritic patch-clamp recordings from hippocampal pyramidal neurons. Muscarinic agonist (carbachol, c) and the dopamine receptor agonist 8-Cl-PB also can give various degrees of action-potentail modulation as well. (a) Bath application of 1 μM isoproterenol resulted in a 104% increase in amplitude, from 41 mV(Pre) to 84 mV, of an antidromically initiated action potential recorded 220 μm from the soma. (Wash-out of isoproterenol is indicated by wash). With a second application of isoproterenol (dark arrow labeled 'Iso'), the amplitude again increased twofold to 80 mV. (b) In a different recording (300 μM H-7), a generic kinase inhibitor was included in the control saline during the wash-out of isoproterenol. The subsequent second application of isoproterenol failed to lead to a second increase in amplitude (dark arrow labeled 'Iso + H7'). (c) In a similar recording, 1 μM carbachol increased the action potential amplitude by 81%, from 27 to 60 mV. In the carbachol experiments, cells were held hyperpolarized to –80 mV to remove Na$^+$ channel inactivation. (d) One of the 6 out of 10 recordings where 6-Cl-PB led to an increase in amplitude. In a recording 220 μm from the soma, 10 μM 6-Cl-PB increased dendritic action potential amplitude by 26%, from 21 to 26.5 mV. The cells were held at –70 mV in all 6-Cl-PB experiments. Adapted from Johnston, Hoffman, Colbert, and Magee (15).

Continued

Continued

BOX 5—cont'd

MODULATION OF LTP INDUCTION

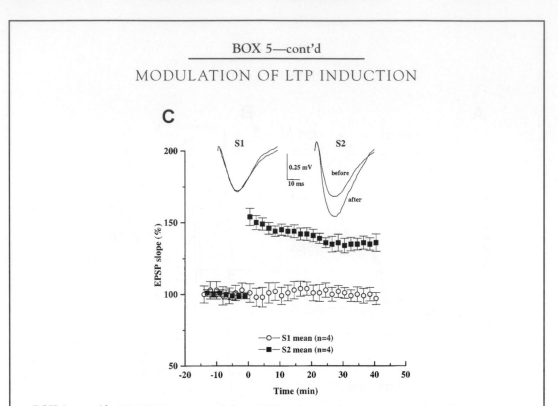

BOX 5, cont'd (C) BDNF also modulates LTP induction in response to theta-frequency-type stimulation. Two stimulating electrodes were positioned on either side of a single recording electrode to stimulate two different groups of afferents converging in the same dendritic field in CA1. Stimulation was applied to Schaffer collaterals alternately at low frequency (one per minute). After a period of baseline recording, LTP was induced with a theta-burst stimulation applied at time 0 only to one pathway (S2, filled squares). Simultaneous recording of an independent pathway (S1, open circles) showed no change in its synaptic strength after the theta burst was delivered to S1. BDNF (closed squares) selectively facilitates the induction of LTP in the tetanized pathway without affecting the synaptic efficacy of the untetanized pathway. EPSPs were recorded in the CA1 area of BDNF-treated slices. Synaptic efficacy (initial slope of field EPSPs) is expressed as a percentage of baseline value recorded during the 20 minutes before the tetanus. Representative traces of field EPSPs from S1 and S2 pathways were taken 10 minutes before and 40 minutes after the theta-burst stimulation. Adapted from Gottschalk, Pozzo-Miller, and Figurov (35).

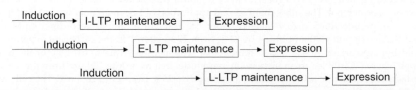

FIGURE 9   Mechanisms of induction, maintenance, and expression. This diagram highlights the importance of considering that each different phase of LTP may have separate and parallel induction, maintenance, and expression mechanisms.

Finally, it is important for the reader to synthesize the concepts of induction, maintenance, and expression with the concept of phases. Simply stated, three phases of LTP (I-, E-, and L-LTP) times three distinct underlying mechanisms for each phase (induction, maintenance, and expression) gives nine separate categories into which any particular molecular mechanism contributing to LTP may fit (see Figure 9). Added to this is the complexity that one phase could be largely presynaptic and another largely postsynaptic. Interesting implications begin to arise from thinking about LTP this way. How is it that the different mechanisms for the different phases interact with each other? Is the maintenance mechanism for one phase the induction mechanism for the next, or do the mechanisms for the phases operate independently? If the maintenance and expression mechanisms for the phases are independent, how does the magnitude of LTP stay constant as the shorter-lasting phase decays? How does the mechanism for L-LTP know where to stop, so that the magnitude of L-LTP is the same as the magnitude that E-LTP had attained? In reference 21, Joey English, Eric Roberson, and I discussed some hypothetical answers to these questions. While in this earlier publication we discussed them in the context of LTP specifically, it also is important to keep in mind that in many ways the same considerations apply to memory itself. If memory is encoded as some complex set of molecular changes, how is it that fidelity of memory is maintained as short-term memory transitions into long-term memory, for example. Although we won't arrive at an answer to these many questions, I believe that it is instructive to begin to formulate a hypothetical framework for their discussion. We will return to these hypothetical issues in the last chapter of the book.

In some cases for these questions, we can begin to formulate specific answers in molecular terms. Those cases where a molecular mechanism can be hypothesized constitute the issues that are addressed in the next three chapters. In Chapter 6, I will discuss mechanisms contributing to the induction of E-LTP, although, of course, many of those same molecular events are prerequisites for L-LTP as well. In Chapter 7, I will discuss mechanisms contributing to the maintenance and expression of E-LTP. In Chapter 8, I will discuss mechanisms that appear to be unique to the induction and expression of L-LTP.

BOX 6

DEPOTENTIATION AND LTD

When scientists began to think seriously about the possible involvement of LTP in memory in the animal, a theoretical conundrum arose. If synapses can be potentiated and this potentiation is very long-lasting, over time the synapses will be driven to their maximum synaptic strength. In this condition, there is no longer synaptic plasticity and no further capacity for that synapse to participate in synaptic-plasticity-dependent processes. Worse yet, over the lifetime of an animal, synapses will by random chance experience LTP-inducing conditions (presynaptic activity coincident with a postsynaptic action potential, for example) numerous times. If LTP is irreversible, ultimately every synapse will be maximally potentiated—obviously not a desirable condition vis-à-vis memory storage.

Consideration of this conundrum raises two implications. First, synapses that are involved in lifelong memory storage must

Continued

BOX 6—cont'd

DEPOTENTIATION AND LTD

be rendered essentially aplastic. In order to have good fidelity of memory storage over the lifetime of an animal, a synapse involved in permanent memory storage must be rendered immutable to a change in synaptic strength resulting from the random occurrence of what would normally be LTP-inducing stimulation. We will return to this issue in the last chapter of the book.

But what about synapses like those in the hippocampus that are not sites of memory storage, but rather whose plasticity is part of the active processing of forming new long-term memories? In order to retain their plasticity and hence their capacity to contribute to memory formation, their potentiation must be reversible. Schaffer-collateral synapses can undergo activity-dependent reversal of LTP; a phenomenon termed depotentiation (see figure). Another activity-dependent way to decrease synaptic strength is Long-term Depression, the mirror image of LTP. LTD is a long-lasting decrease of synaptic strength below baseline. Using a logic similar to that of the first paragraph, the phenomenon of dedepression of synaptic transmission is implied, although this has not been widely studied at this point.

As a practical matter, it is often difficult to separate depotentiation from LTD experimentally. For example, a "baseline" response in hippocampal slices or in vivo likely is a mixture of basal synaptic activity and activity at previously potentiated synapses. Moreover, for the most part, the stimulation protocols used to induce depotentiation are variations of the protocols used to induce LTD. Nevertheless, mechanistic investigations have made clear that depotentiation and LTD use different mechanisms (see references 30 and 31), and

thus must be considered as distinct processes.

Physiologic LTD (and depotentiation) induction protocols generally involve variations of repetitive 1-Hz stimulation (see references 30 and 32). A common protocol is to deliver 900 stimuli at 1 Hz, but there also are LTD protocols that use random small variations in frequency in the 1-Hz region, and variations that use paired-pulse stimuli delivered at 1 Hz. Synaptic depression appears to be fairly robust in vivo but is quite difficult to get in hippocampal slices from adult animals. LTD in vitro is almost always studied using slices from immature animals, or cultured immature neurons, and it is possible that LTD as it is currently studied in vitro is largely a manifestation of what is normally a developmental mechanism.

One ironic aspect of the LTP/LTD story is that both phenomena at Schaffer-collateral synapses can be blocked by NMDA receptor antagonists. This suggests that calcium influx triggers both processes, and indeed current models of LTD induction hypothesize that LTD is caused by an influx of calcium that achieves a lower level than that needed for LTP induction. This lower level of calcium is hypothesized to activate protein phosphatases selectively, and by this mechanism lower synaptic efficacy (see Box 1).

Another very different type of LTD is cerebellar LTD. Cerebellar LTD occurs at synapses onto Purkinje neurons in the cerebellar cortex. Cerebellar LTD is a very interesting phenomenon because its behavioral role is much better understood than the hippocampal plasticity phenomena we are discussing throughout this book. Among other things, cerebellar LTD is

BOX 6—cont'd

DEPOTENTIATION AND LTD

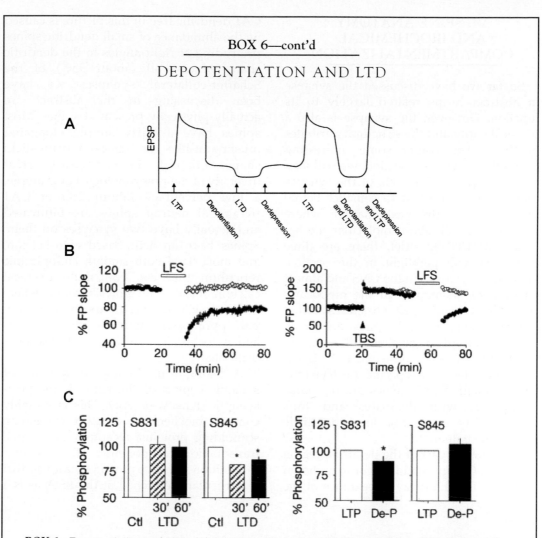

BOX 6   Depotentiation and LTD. (A) Schematic illustrating LTP, Depotentiation, LTD, dedepression, and combinations of them. (B) This figure shows LTD and depotentiation in hippocampal neurons where slices receiving baseline stimulation (control, open circles) and 1-Hz stimulation (closed circles) were recorded simultaneously. FP indicates field potential. (C) These data show regulation of distinct AMPA receptor phosphorylation sites during bidirectional synaptic plasticity. Homosynaptic LTD in CA1 is associated with dephosphorylation of GluR1 at a PKA site (ser845). Depotentiation gives dephosphorylation at a CaMKII/PKC site (ser 831). Adapted from Lee et al. (31).

involved in associative eye-blink conditioning, a cerebellum-dependent classical conditioning paradigm. Considerable progress has been made in investigating the roles and mechanisms of cerebellar LTD, and prominent investigators in this field are Masao Ito, Richard Thompson, Mike Mauk, and David Linden. Literature searches for the work of these investigators would be a good place to start for those interested in this area, but we will return briefly to cerebellar LTD in Chapter 9.

VI. SPINE ANATOMY AND BIOCHEMICAL COMPARTMENTALIZATION

So far we have discussed the synapse in abstract terms related largely to its function. However, the synapse is also a physical entity and the structural attributes of this entity confer some interesting properties. In this last section, we will look at certain physical aspects of the synapse that will be important to consider before moving on to the next chapter, where we begin to talk about molecular mechanisms for LTP. In brief, there are three points we will highlight in this section. First, most synapses in the CNS and almost all excitatory synapses in the hippocampus are at specialized structures called *dendritic spines*. Second, spines are small, well-circumscribed biochemical compartments that localize proteins and signaling molecules to a specific postsynaptic compartment. Third, spines are of course contiguous with dendrites and thus continuously sense the local dendritic membrane potential.

A picture of part of the dendritic region of an area CA1 pyramidal neuron is shown in Figure 10. The fuzzy appearance of the CA1 dendritic tree in this picture is caused by the abundance of small dendritic spines protruding at right angles to the dendritic shaft. Almost all (about 95%) of the Schaffer-collateral synapses we have been discussing in the abstract are actually physically present at spines. Most spines have a fairly simple elongated mushroom-like (i.e., chicken drumstick) shape, although there is clearly great diversity of their morphology. For example, a low percentage (about 2%) of CA1 pyramidal neuron spines are bifurcated and actually have two synapses on them. Spines have an actin-based cytoskeleton, and most have both smooth endoplasmic reticulum that can contribute to local calcium release and polyribosomes where local protein synthesis occurs. In hippocampal pyramidal neurons microtubules and mitochondria are limited to the dendritic shaft.

A distinguishing feature of the area of synaptic contact at the spine is the postsynaptic density, or PSD. This is a highly compact biochemical structure containing scaffolding proteins, receptors, and signal transduction components. The calcium/calmodulin sensitive protein kinase CaMKII is particularly enriched at the PSD, as is a

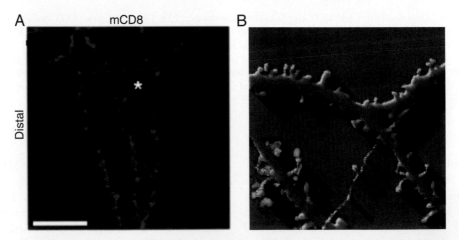

FIGURE 10 Dendrites with spines in a hippocampal pyramidal neuron. This figure illustrates the presence and shapes of dendritic spines on pyramidal neurons in the hippocampus. The spines are the small mushroom-shaped lateral projections containing synaptic contacts. (A) Courtesy of Liqun Lou, Stanford University. (B) Courtesy of E. Korkotian, The Weizmann Institute.

structural protein called PSD-95, a name based on its molecular weight. We will return to these molecules in much more detail in Chapters 6 and 7.

The dendritic spine membrane surrounds the PSD and the area immediately below it and thus circumscribes a discrete biochemical compartment. The spine neck, however, is open to the dendritic shaft so there is still considerable diffusion of soluble spine contents (such as calcium and second messengers) into the local dendritic

---

BOX 7

LTP OUTSIDE OF THE HIPPOCAMPUS

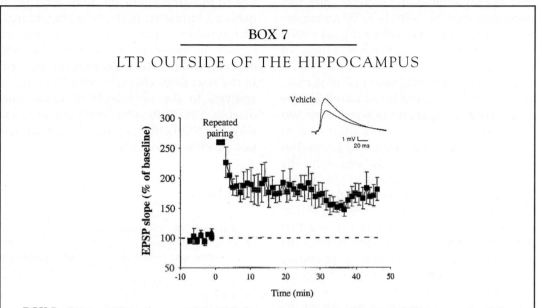

BOX 7 Pairing LTP in the amygdala. This figure shows "pairing"-induced LTP in neurons of the basolateral nucleus of the amygdala. The plot shows mean ± SE percent EPSP slope (relative to baseline) in cells treated with 0.1% DMSO vehicle (black squares) before and after LTP induction. Traces from an individual experiment before and 40 minutes after induction are shown in the inset. Traces are averages of five responses. Adapted from Schafe et al. (37).

The abundance of literature dedicated to studying LTP in the hippocampus might lead a newcomer to the field to suppose that LTP is somehow restricted to these synapses. However, plasticity of synaptic function, including phenomena such as LTP and LTD, is the rule rather than the exception for most forebrain synapses. LTP outside the hippocampus has been mostly studied in the cerebral cortex and the amygdala (see figure). The likely functional roles for LTP at these other sites are quite diverse, but two specific examples are worth highlighting. LTP-like processes in the cerebral cortex play a role in activity-dependent development of the visual system and other sensory systems. LTP in the amygdala has received prominent attention as a mechanism contributing to cued fear conditioning. The role of LTP in amygdala-dependent fear conditioning in fact is the area for which the strongest case can be made for a direct demonstration of a behavioral role for LTP. It is important to bear in mind through the rest of the book, the next three chapters in particular, that cortical LTP and amygdalar LTP probably exhibit some mechanistic differences from the NMDA receptor-dependent LTP that we will be focusing on. However, in my opinion, the molecular similarities are likely to greatly outweigh the differences.

region. Nevertheless, on short time scales, the spine compartment may serve to localize signaling molecules effectively to a specific synapse. Moreover, molecules tethered to the PSD by scaffolding proteins and the like probably have fairly limited diffusion because the spine compartment will make them tend to rebind at the same PSD as they unbind and rebind. Thus, this spine morphology is likely to be an important component for achieving synaptic specificity in LTP and other forms of synaptic plasticity.

The compartmentalization of molecules by the dendritic spine is not paralleled by an electrical compartmentalization, by and large. At one point, a popular line of thinking was that the shape and properties of the spine neck might regulate the capacity of electrical signals to get to and from the spine head compartment. This idea is no longer considered tenable, and as a first approximation we can assume that the spine membrane potential reflects the local dendritic shaft membrane potential. However, it is likely that electrical compartmentalization does occur in dendrites, but this is at the level of the various dendritic branches as well as a component contributed by their overall distance from the soma (see reference 25). This introduces the fascinating possibility that local generation and restricted propagation of action potentials within a specific dendritic subregion might be used as a mechanism for generating dendritic branch-specific plasticity.

VII. SUMMARY

In this chapter, we transitioned from thinking about LTP as a straightforward activity-dependent form of synaptic plasticity. We saw, for example, that LTP induction is subject to a great number of modulatory influences. Also, temporal integration mechanisms are key to regulating LTP induction. In addition to these issues, we discussed the fact that regulating membrane excitability, directly by modulating membrane ion channels and indirectly through local GABAergic circuits, can play a pronounced role in regulating LTP induction. Finally, we noted the existence of altered probability of action potential firing as a persisting effect superimposed upon synaptic potentiation. All these issues are key to thinking about the roles for LTP in memory formation in the behaving animal. The synapse integrates a wide variety of signals in order to make a biochemical decision whether to trigger lasting change. In the next three chapters we will take our analysis to the next level of detail and discuss the molecular mechanisms that allow for this complex physiologic information processing to occur.

References

1. Dawkins, R. (1986). *The blind watchmaker*, 1st American edn. New York: Norton.
2. Choi, S., Klingauf, J., and Tsien, R. W. (2000). "Postfusional regulation of cleft glutamate concentration during LTP at 'silent synapses'." *Nat. Neurosci.* 3:330–336.
3. Bolshakov, V. Y., Golan, H., Kandel, E. R., and Siegelbaum, S. A. (1997). "Recruitment of new sites of synaptic transmission during the cAMP-dependent late phase of LTP at CA3-CA1 synapses in the hippocampus." *Neuron* 19:635–651.
4. Nicoll, R. A., and Malenka, R. C. (1999). "Expression mechanisms underlying NMDA receptor-dependent long-term potentiation." *Ann. NY Acad. Sci.* 868:515–525.
5. Malinow, R., and Tsien, R. W. (1990). "Presynaptic enhancement shown by whole-cell recordings of long-term potentiation in hippocampal slices." *Nature* 346:177–180.
6. Bekkers, J. M., and Stevens, C. F. (1990). "Presynaptic mechanism for long-term potentiation in the hippocampus." *Nature* 346:724–729.
7. Malinow, R. (1991). "Transmission between pairs of hippocampal slice neurons: quantal levels, oscillations, and LTP." *Science* 252:722–724.
8. Dolphin, A. C., Errington, M. L., and Bliss, T. V. (1982). "Long-term potentiation of the perforant path in vivo is associated with increased glutamate release." *Nature* 297:496–498.
9. Zakharenko, S. S., Zablow, L., and Siegelbaum, S. A. (2001). "Visualization of changes in presynaptic function during long-term synaptic plasticity." *Nat. Neurosci.* 4:711–717.

10. Malgaroli, A., Ting, A. E., Wendland, B., Bergamaschi, A., Villa, A., Tsien, R. W., and Scheller, R. H. (1995). "Presynaptic component of long-term potentiation visualized at individual hippocampal synapses." *Science* 268:1624–1628.

11. Bliss, T. V., and Lomo, T. (1973). "Long-lasting potentiation of synaptic transmission in the dentate area of the anaesthetized rabbit following stimulation of the perforant path." *J. Physiol.* 232:331–356.

12. Johnston, D., and Amaral, D. G. (1998). "Hippocampus." In: *The synaptic organization of the brain* edited by Shepherd GM, 4th ed. New York: Oxford University Press; 417–458.

13. McMahon, L. L., and Kauer, J. A. (1997). "Hippocampal interneurons express a novel form of synaptic plasticity." *Neuron* 18:295–305.

14. Lu, Y. M., Mansuy, I. M., Kandel, E. R., and Roder, J. (2000). "Calcineurin-mediated LTD of GABAergic inhibition underlies the increased excitability of CA1 neurons associated with LTP." *Neuron* 26:197–205.

15. Johnston, D., Hoffman, D. A., Colbert, C. M., and Magee, J. C. (1999). "Regulation of back-propagating action potentials in hippocampal neurons." *Curr. Opin. Neurobiol.* 9:288–292.

16. Scharfman, H. E., and Sarvey, J. M. (1985). "Postsynaptic firing during repetitive stimulation is required for long-term potentiation in hippocampus." *Brain Res.* 331:267–274.

17. Linden, D. J. (1999). "The return of the spike: post synaptic action potentials and the induction of LTP and LTD." *Neuron* 22:661–666.

18. Mott, D. D., and Lewis, D. V. (1991). "Facilitation of the induction of long-term potentiation by GABAB receptors." *Science* 252:1718–1720.

19. Chapman, C. A., Perez, Y., and Lacaille, J. C. (1998). "Effects of GABA(A) inhibition on the expression of long-term potentiation in CA1 pyramidal cells are dependent on tetanization parameters." *Hippocampus* 8:289–298.

20. Davies, C. H., Starkey, S. J., Pozza, M. F., and Collingridge, G. L. (1991). "GABA autoreceptors regulate the induction of LTP." *Nature* 349:609–611.

21. Roberson, E. D., English, J. D., and Sweatt, J. D. (1996). "A biochemist's view of long-term potentiation." *Learn. Mem.* 3:1–24.

22. Winder, D. G., Mansuy, I. M., Osman, M., Moallem, T. M., and Kandel, E. R. (1998). "Genetic and pharmacological evidence for a novel, intermediate phase of long-term potentiation suppressed by calcineurin." *Cell.* 92:25–37.

23. Shulz, P: Personal communication.

24. Malinow, R., Madison, D. V., and Tsien, R. W. (1988). "Persistent protein kinase activity underlying long-term potentiation." *Nature* 335:820–824.

25. Kamondi, A., Acsady, L., and Buzsaki, G. (1998). "Dendritic spikes are enhanced by cooperative network activity in the intact hippocampus." *J. Neurosci.* 18:3919–3928.

26. Malinow, R., Schulman, H., and Tsien, R. W. (1989) "Inhibition of postsynaptic PKC or CaMKII blocks induction but not expression of LTP." *Science* 245:862–866.

27. Malenka, R. C., Kauer, J. A., Perkel, D. J., Mauk, M. D., Kelly, P. T., Nicoll, R. A., and Waxham, M. N. (1989). "An essential role for postsynaptic calmodulin and protein kinase activity in long-term potentiation." *Nature* 340:554–557.

28. Levenson, J., Weeber, E., Selcher, J. C., Kategaya, L. S., Sweatt, J. D., and Eskin A. (2002). "Long-term potentiation and contextual fear conditioning increase neuronal glutamate uptake." *Nat. Neurosci.* 5:155–161.

29. Renger, J. J., Egles, C., and Liu, G. (2001). "A developmental switch in neurotransmitter flux enhances synaptic efficacy by affecting AMPA receptor activation." *Neuron* 29:469–484.

30. Lee, H. K., Kameyama, K., Huganir, R. L., and Bear, M. F. (1998). "NMDA induces long-term synaptic depression and dephosphorylation of the GluR1 subunit of AMPA receptors in hippocampus." *Neuron* 21:1151–1162.

31. Lee, H. K., Barbarosie, M., Kameyama, K., Bear, M. F., and Huganir, R. L. (2000). "Regulation of distinct AMPA receptor phosphorylation sites during bidirectional synaptic plasticity." *Nature* 405:955–959.

32. Kemp, N., McQueen, J., Faulkes, S., and Bashir, Z. I. (2000). "Different forms of LTD in the CA1 region of the hippocampus: role of age and stimulus protocol." *Eur. J. Neurosci.* 12:360–366.

33. Thomas, M. J., Moody, T. D., Makhinson, M., and O'Dell, T. J. (1996). "Activity-dependent beta-adrenergic modulation of low frequency stimulation induced LTP in the hippocampal CA1 region." *Neuron* 17:475–482.

34. Lu, B., and Chow, A. (1999). "Neurotrophins and hippocampal synaptic transmission and plasticity." *J. Neurosci. Res.* 58:76–87.

35. Gottschalk, W., Pozzo-Miller, L. D., Figurov, A., and Lu, B. (1998). "Presynaptic modulation of synaptic transmission and plasticity by brain-derived neurotrophic factor in the developing hippocampus." *J. Neurosci.* 18:6830–6839.

36. Xu, B., Gottschalk, W., Chow, A., Wilson, R. I., Schnell, E., Zang, K., Wang, D., Nicoll, R. A., Lu, B., and Reichardt, L. F. (2000). "The role of brain-derived neurotrophic factor receptors in the mature hippocampus: modulation of long-term potentiation through a presynaptic mechanism involving TrkB." *J. Neurosci.* 20:6888–6897.

37. Schafe, G. E., Atkins, C. M., Swank, M. W., Bauer, E. P., Sweatt, J. D., and LeDoux, J. E. (2000). "Activation of ERK/MAP kinase in the amygdala is required for memory consolidation of pavlovian fear conditioning." *J. Neurosci.* 20:8177–8187.

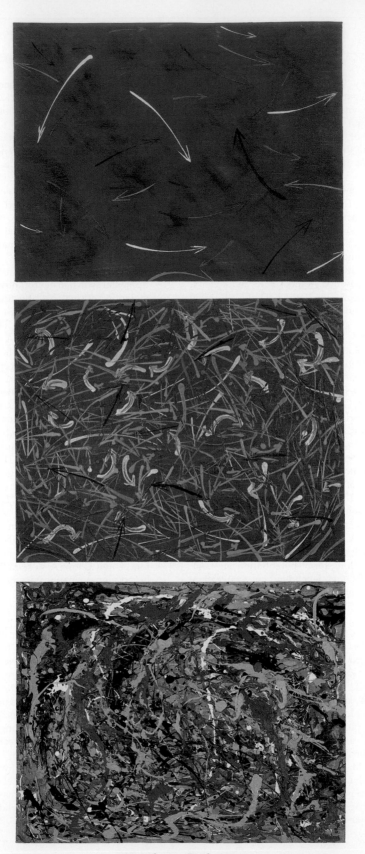

LTP Induction Biochemistry

J. David Sweatt, Acrylic on canvas, 2002

6

The Biochemistry of LTP Induction

I. INTRODUCTION

As we discussed in the last chapter, one problem with LTP is that it *looks* simple. You give a hippocampal slice a brief period of high-frequency stimulation, and for all the world it looks like you flipped a light switch and put the synapses in a potentiated state. In Chapter 4, we talked about the consensus that elevation of postsynaptic calcium is what triggers LTP. In this chapter, we will talk about the complex biochemical mechanisms involved in this process.

The typical discussion of LTP induction starts out with something like: "NMDA receptors open, a triggering burst of calcium comes in, and then many complicated LTP induction processes are started." To my embarrassment, I have promulgated that idea many times, but now I realize that it is exactly the wrong way to look at the LTP induction process. Most people, including myself, have historically thought of the LTP induction process as *starting* with calcium elevation postsynaptically. It is more appropriate to think of the LTP induction process as *ending* with postsynaptic calcium being elevated. This is because many important biochemical components of the LTP induction machinery are upstream of the NMDA receptor. There probably also are postsynaptic biochemical events triggered by the initial stages of calcium influx that feed back and regulate later stages of calcium influx.

One point here is that once postsynaptic calcium gets to a sufficient concentration, it will trigger LTP. However, many important mechanisms upstream of reaching the triggering level of calcium determine whether that threshold level of calcium gets reached. These upstream mechanisms are extremely important as well—they are the biochemical computation that the synapse performs in deciding if LTP should be triggered.

A second point is that these processes are mechanisms for sophisticated signal integration at the molecular level, and many of these mechanisms are themselves *associative* in nature. In this chapter, we will see several examples where the simultaneous presence of two signals leads to a unique event—biochemical coincidence detection. The neuron capitalizes on these biochemical simultaneity detectors, where they are necessary for LTP induction to be triggered, in order to be able to achieve the sort of sophisticated logical operations necessary for the hippocampus to serve as a multimodal signal integrator as we discussed in Chapter 3.

Given the hundreds of individual molecular events that have been reported as being involved in LTP induction in the literature, how can one begin to organize this immense molecular system into a coherent picture? In order to help myself think about this complicated, interactive molecular system, I have begun to think about the biochemistry of LTP induction as comprising several basic systems. Specifically, I have found it useful to think about LTP induction as involving the following components:

1. Mechanisms upstream of the NMDA receptor that directly regulate NMDA receptor function.
2. Mechanisms upstream of the NMDA receptor that control membrane depolarization.
3. The components of the synaptic infrastructure that are necessary for the NMDA receptor and the synaptic signal transduction machinery to function normally.
4. Feed-forward and feedback mechanisms that regulate the level of calcium attained.
5. Extrinsic signals that regulate the response to the calcium influx.
6. The mechanisms for the generation of the actual persisting biochemical signals.

These various stages and components of the LTP induction machinery are schematized in Figure 1. Essentially in this chapter we will be filling in the molecular details necessary to flesh out this general model.

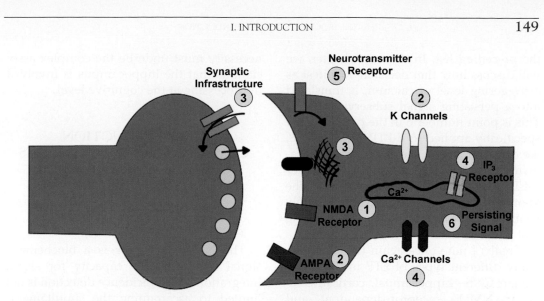

FIGURE 1 LTP induction machinery. This schematic diagram summarizes examples of the six different components of LTP induction discussed in this chapter. See text for explanations.

As an editorial aside, I believe that the general lack of appreciation of the role of all these mechanisms, which are upstream of calcium reaching a level sufficient to trigger LTP, is a big part of why there has been so much confusion about LTP induction mechanisms. Perturbing the system at any point can lead to a block of LTP. The typical block-mimic-measure hypothesis testing approach is not sufficiently robust to parse out such a complicated mechanism when the read-out (LTP measured physiologically) is (1) so far downstream and (2) triggered largely in an all-or-none fashion.

Note that we will be discussing mechanisms for the induction of E-LTP by and large, although, of course, the same sophisticated control mechanisms could also participate in regulating the triggering of L-LTP. However, it's not clear to what extent the induction mechanisms for E-LTP and L-LTP are sequential versus parallel in the context of the intact cell. For example, the same signal transduction enzymes that contribute to E-LTP induction locally at a postsynaptic spine compartment likely also contribute to altered gene expression in the nuclear compartment. However, these two processes may be completely sequestered

from each other in the cell (or not). The answer to this specific question will, of course, require a great deal of detailed information at the cytoarchitectural level that we simply don't have at this point.

Nevertheless, in some instances it is known, by definition, that there are unique mechanisms contributing to L-LTP induction. We will talk about mechanisms that uniquely contribute to L-LTP induction and expression in Chapter 8, and focus on the complexities of the very earliest steps in the induction of E-LTP and L-LTP in this chapter. In the next chapter (Chapter 7), we will discuss the mechanisms for generating persisting signals that contribute to E-LTP maintenance and expression. Lest you become complacent with how clearly delineated this is starting to sound, keep in mind that some of the persisting signals in E-LTP maintenance (Chapter 7) may well contribute to L-LTP induction as well (Chapter 8), although this is quite speculative at this point.

To re-cap: in this chapter, we will talk about the complex biochemical mechanisms that compute whether the right signals have arrived at a synapse so that LTP should be induced. This is numbers 1–5 in the preceding list. In the next chapter, we will discuss how that decision, manifest as a triggering level of calcium, is translated into a persisting signal subserving E-LTP. This is point number 6 in the preceding list specifically applied to E-LTP. In Chapter 8, we will talk about the additional mechanisms involved in computing whether L-LTP should also be triggered, and the known biochemical mechanisms uniquely contributing to inducing and maintaining that phase of LTP.

Finally, I note once again that there are many different types of LTP in the mammalian CNS—hippocampal, cortical, cerebellar, NMDA receptor-dependent, and -independent, just to name a few prominent categories. I therefore need to specify to the best extent possible exactly which LTP I am discussing. In the next three chapters, I will be discussing NMDA receptor-dependent LTP at Schaffer-collateral/commissural synapses in area CA1 of rat or mouse hippocampus. In most cases, I will be discussing LTP induced using multiple, spaced trains of 1 second, 100-Hz stimuli. I chose this subtype of LTP because it has available the widest variety of direct biochemical data, and this type of protocol induces both E-LTP and L-LTP.

Several sections later in this chapter, I also will discuss LTP induced with theta-frequency stimulation or theta-burst stimulation. This type of LTP induction protocol is most interesting in the context of the signal integration aspects of LTP induction (1–3). LTP induction using these types of protocols is subject to modulation by a wide variety of external signals and regulation of membrane properties. Theta-type LTP provides the richest examples of how the biochemical machinery of LTP induction might be involved in the complex multimodal information processing that the hippocampus performs. Specifically, for this form of LTP, we can see examples of how the synapse has the capacity at the molecular level to ascertain if three, four, five, or more signals are simultaneously present. These are the types of mechanisms that of

necessity must underlie the complex associations that the hippocampus is involved in processing at the cognitive level.

II. LTP INDUCTION COMPONENT 1—MECHANISMS UPSTREAM OF THE NMDA RECEPTOR THAT DIRECTLY REGULATE NMDA RECEPTOR FUNCTION

The NMDA receptor is a biochemical signal integrator. It's capacity for signal integration and coincidence detection is not limited to ascertaining the simultaneous presence of glutamate and depolarization. It also senses biochemical signals used in computing the degree of calcium influx that it will allow. In this section, we will discuss the biochemical mechanisms known to regulate the NMDA receptor directly, which have been implicated in LTP induction, memory formation, or both. These biochemical processes, as far as I know at present, are not all-or-none like the glutamate/depolarization mechanism but rather serve to modulate the magnitude of postsynaptic calcium influx. (In the section after this one, we will talk about biochemical processes that are used to control the NMDA receptor in an all-or-none fashion, indirectly through controlling the membrane potential.)

The NMDA receptor is also a temporal integrator, and these mechanisms are limited to biochemical processes, as opposed to biophysical processes. The time frame in which the NMDA receptor can detect the simultaneous presence of depolarization and glutamate is, of course, quite limited because the membrane depolarization is so brief. In contrast, a biochemical signal such as elevation of a second messenger or increased protein kinase activity has a much longer half-life. Thus if the synapse wants to set up a temporal integration mechanism on the seconds (or longer) time-scale, it must use these types of processes. The capacity of the NMDA receptor to be modulated by protein kinases and other messenger molecules allows for this sort of temporal integration as well.

A. The Structure of the NMDA Receptor

The NMDA receptor is a glutamate-gated cation channel and as such is a multisubunit transmembrane protein. Current models hypothesize that it is a tetrameric hetero-oligomeric protein with more than one glutamate binding site. It is, of course, voltage-dependent, and this arises from the voltage-dependent Mg block of the pore that we discussed in Chapter 4. The protein has binding sites for zinc, polyamines, and glycine (a co-agonist necessary for activity).

Abundantly expressed individual subunits of the receptor are named NR1, NR2A, NR2B, NR2C, and NR2D—the somewhat complex nomenclature arose for historical reasons related to different groups that cloned the first NMDA receptor subunits. One functional NMDA receptor is comprised of one or more NR1 subunits plus one or more NR2-type subunits. The NR2 subunits determine the calcium permeability of the channel and can influence the voltage-dependence of its activation,

kinetics of opening, and other biophysical properties. NR1 and NR2A and 2B are phosphorylated at a number of different sites—NR1 by PKC and the cyclic AMP dependent protein kinase (PKA), NR2A by cyclin-dependent kinase 5, and NR2A and NR2B by various tyrosine kinases such as src and fyn.

The NMDA receptor is subject to a wide variety of direct modulatory influences, some of which are listed in Table 1. Please keep in mind that not every single biochemical factor known to man to influence the NMDA receptor is listed in Table 1. The table is limited to the intersection of those things that (1) I know about and (2) have been experimentally implicated as being involved in LTP per se. The same general rule applies to all the tables included in this chapter, and I welcome feedback on any missing items.

B. Kinase Regulation of the NMDA Receptor

One of the oncogene products produced by the Rous sarcoma virus, which also has a homologue in the mammalian genome, is the tyrosine kinase src. Src family tyrosine kinases like src and fyn directly

Table 1   Direct Modulators of the NMDA Receptor

Modulator	Mechanism	Effect
Src family tyrosine kinases (src, fyn)	Tyrosine phosphorylation Loss of Zn inhibition	Enhancement
Scaffolding proteins		
RACK1	Binding	Inhibitory
PSD-95	Scaffolding	Modulatory
PKC	Ser/thr phosphoryation (direct) Src activation (indirect)	Enhancement Enhancement
PKA/PP1/Yotiao	Phosphorylation Dephosphorylation	Enhancement Inhibition
Cyclin-dependent kinase 5	Ser/thr phosphorylation	Enhancement
Nitric oxide/reactive oxygen species	Sulfhydryl nitrosylation or oxidation	Inhibition
Polyamines (e.g., spermine, spermidine)	Direct binding to a modulatory site	Augmentation
Caseine kinase II	Ser/thr phosphorylation modulation of polyamine effects	Enhancement

phosphorylate the NMDA receptor (4, 5), increasing calcium flux through the receptor. Tyrosine phosphorylation of the NMDA receptor increases current flow[1] through the ion channel by reducing a tonic, Zinc-dependent inhibition (6).

Protein tyrosine kinase phosphorylation of the NMDA receptor may be required for LTP induction and at a minimum serves an important modulatory role controlling the likelihood of LTP induction (7). The activities of src and fyn in Area CA1 are controlled by a number of upstream signal transduction cascades. One important regulator of src is the focal adhesion kinase (FAK) CAKbeta, also known as pyk2, and this cascade has been shown to be involved, through src, in regulating LTP induction (8). In addition, the Extracellular Signal Regulated Kinase (ERK) MAP kinase cascade and the PKC cascades, which we will return to later, also can activate src-family kinases, and these pathways may also modulate NMDA receptor function and LTP induction via Src (9). Dephosphorylation of the src/fyn sites on NMDA receptors likely occurs through the action of the tyrosine phosphatase STEP.

A number of interesting cell surface receptors modulate NMDA receptor function, and thus potentially LTP induction, acting through the src cascade (see Figure 2).

---

[1]There are a number of different mechanisms that can cause "increased current flow" through a ligand-gated ion channel: (1) The probability that the channel will open can be increased, which is referred to as increased *"channel open probability"*. (2) The *conductance*, that is, the rate at which ions flow through the channel, can be increased. (3) The *number* of channels in the membrane can increase. (4) The *affinity* of the channel for its ligand can increase—a mechanism that, of course, can only operate at subsaturating ligand concentrations. By and large, throughout the book, I will not go into detail on which of these mechanisms is involved in channel modulation, except where the mechanism is directly relevant to the molecular mechanisms that are involved (e.g., increased membrane insertion of a channel implies the involvement of specific molecular processes). In addition, in many cases, the specifics are not known or the channel modulation involves multiple mechanisms. For your reference, src modulation of the NMDA receptor at a minimum involves increased channel open probability.

The Ephrins, which have been mostly studied in the context of nervous system development, modulate NMDA receptors in cultured neurons (10). EphrinB2, acting through its receptor EphB2, activates src and modulates NMDA receptors via this mechanism. Genetic deletion of EphB2 leads to an attenuation of LTP in area CA1 (11, 12). Recent data from Ed Weeber in my laboratory has implicated the Apolipoprotein E receptors in hippocampus as modulating LTP induction via a src/NMDA receptor pathway—we will return to this system in Chapter 11 on mechanisms contributing to Alzheimer's disease. Finally, the *obese* gene product leptin acts through its cell surface receptor and a PI3-Kinase/MAPK/src pathway to modulate NMDA receptors and LTP induction in the hippocampus (13). Thus, the src/fyn pathways serve an important role in funneling cell surface signals to the NMDA receptor itself, modulating its activity and regulating LTP induction.

Src tyrosine kinase potentiation of NMDA receptors is also subject to a variety of other influences. RACK1 (Receptor for Activated C Kinase 1) promotes formation of a fyn/RACK1/NR2B complex that actually inhibits fyn phosphorylation of the NMDA receptor and diminishes current through the receptor (14). Also, the Postsynaptic Density core protein PDS-95 modulates src phosphorylation of NMDARs, and src potentiation of NMDAR currents appears to require the presence of PSD-95 (15).

Protein kinase C not only can act indirectly through src to modulate the NMDAR but also can directly phosphorylate the receptor on serine/threonine residues and affect its function (16, 17). Phosphorylation of the NMDAR by PKC causes increased calcium flow through the receptor (18). The potential import of this is quite straightforward—any cell surface receptor coupled to a phospholipase C cascade can modulate the likelihood of LTP induction through direct regulation of the NMDA receptor complex (see Figure 2).

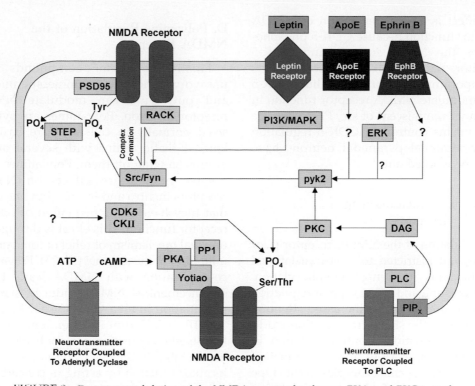

FIGURE 2 Receptor modulation of the NMDA receptor by the src, PKA, and PKC cascade. These kinase cascades are represented here in relation to modulation of NMDA receptors, which could potentially lead to regulating LTP induction. See text for discussion and definitions.

The cAMP-dependent protein kinase (PKA) also can augment NMDA receptor function, although the mechanism is complex and not entirely worked out (19). PKA binds to the NMDA receptor via an associated protein, Yotiao (Yotiao is a specific isoform of A Kinase Anchoring Protein, which we will discuss again in a later section of this chapter). Yotiao binds both PKA and Protein Phosphatase 1 (PP1) to the NMDA receptor, and when all three are bound together the PP1 activity predominates and keeps the NMDA receptor phosphorylation (and activation) low. PKA activation by cAMP leads to enhancement of NMDA currents, although it is not entirely clear whether this is the result of PKA phosphorylation of the NMDA receptor, loss of tonic dephosphorylation by PP1, or both. Again, in the context of the hippocampal pyramidal neuron, this mecha-

nism represents a basis for any neurotransmitter receptor coupled to adenylyl cyclase to be able to modulate NMDA receptor function and the induction of LTP.

The cyclin-dependent kinases (CDKs) are key regulators of cell division, controlling progression through the cell cycle. However, this role is, of course, not germane to understanding the function of nondividing neurons in the adult CNS. However, one CDK isoform, CDK-5, is selectively expressed in postmitotic neurons and functions in regulating neuronal migration and neurite outgrowth in development. Moreover, recent work has shown that this kinase is involved in synaptic plasticity and learning in adult animals (20). Specifically, inhibition of CDK-5 blocks NMDA receptor-dependent LTP in area CA1 and blocks contextual fear conditioning. One possible mechanism for this effect is CDK-5 regulation of NMDA receptor function because CDK-5 phosphorylates the NR2A subunit and CDK-5 inhibitors reduce NMDA-induced currents in hippocampal neurons (21). Thus, CDK-5 may modulate NMDA receptor function in a manner reminiscent of src, PKC, etc. The mechanisms controlling CDK-5 regulation in hippocampal pyramidal neurons have yet to be worked out.

C. Redox Regulation of the NMDA Receptor

Modulation of the NMDA receptor is, of course, not restricted to post-translational modifications involving phosphorylation. An interesting and novel type of regulation that is starting to gather increased attention in general in the signal transduction world is redox modulation of protein function. In the context of NMDA receptor function there are two specific examples of this type of regulation, both of which elicit inhibition of NMDA receptor function. The reactive nitrogen species nitric oxide (NO), a free radical, can react with sulfhydryl moieties in cysteine side chains, a reaction leading to S-nitrosylation of the side chain. This reaction occurs in NR2A subunits at reasonably low levels of free NO and leads to decreased channel opening (22). A second example of redox regulation of NMDA receptors involves reactive oxygen species (ROS) such as superoxide and peroxynitrite, the product of the reaction of superoxide plus NO (23). ROS inhibition of the NMDA receptor likely occurs via cysteine oxidation in a fashion reminiscent of the effects of NO, although the mechanisms of this effect are not clear at present. Likewise, the physiologic role of NO and ROS inhibition of NMDA receptor function is also not clear. One interesting speculation is that oxidative inhibition of NMDA receptors might serve to "lock" the synapse in a particular state after plasticity had been triggered, or the mechanism might serve as a basis for inhibitory cross-talk limiting the capacity of a synapse to undergo LTP.

D. Polyamine Regulation of the NMDA Receptor

Finally, polyamine compounds with unsavory names like spermine, spermidine, and putrescine can modulate NMDA receptor function. Polyamines are synthesized normally in cells and are basically long aliphatic chains with several amino groups hanging off them. Polyamines have diverse modulatory effects on NMDA receptors in vitro and in vivo, but one effect that they have is augmentation of NMDA receptor function. This effect is through the unusual mechanism of relief of tonic proton inhibition of the channel (24, 25). Polyamine co-application with NMDA leads to an enhancement of NMDA-induced synaptic potentiation in area CA1. Casein Kinase II (CKII), a calcium-independent protein kinase whose function has not been widely investigated in the CNS, augments NMDA receptor function by acting in concert with polyamine binding to the receptor intracellular domain (26). The role of this mechanism in LTP induction in the intact cell is unknown. However, CKII is activated by LTP-inducing stimulation (27) and evidence exists suggesting activity-dependent increased polyamine synthesis in the hippocampus (28). These mechanisms might serve a role in temporal integration with repeated stimulation or in setting a baseline likelihood of LTP induction.

III. LTP INDUCTION COMPONENT 2—MECHANISMS UPSTREAM OF THE NMDA RECEPTOR THAT CONTROL MEMBRANE DEPOLARIZATION

As we discussed in the last chapter, recent discoveries have highlighted the importance of mechanisms for controlling membrane depolarization in LTP induction, membrane depolarization necessary for NMDA receptor activation. One important factor is the discovery of back-propagating action potentials and of their involvement in providing the depolarization of the synaptic membrane necessary for LTP induction (29–31). A second relevant consideration is the "silent synapse" model of LTP induction, wherein there are synapses that contain NMDA receptors but no AMPA receptors. Obviously, in the second scenario, the membrane depolarization necessary for NMDA receptor activation cannot come from local AMPA receptors but must be propagated via the membrane from a distal site. Taken together, these two considerations bring into focus the necessity of understanding the mechanisms that control the electrical properties of the dendrite and dendritic spines.

Table 2 lists a number of the important molecules contributing to regulation of membrane depolarization in pyramidal neuron dendrites. Progress in this area has been greatly facilitated by relatively recent technical advances that allow direct cell-attached-patch recording from the distal dendritic regions of CA1 pyramidal neurons. These studies have identified a number of relevant membrane currents that control dendritic membrane depolarization and excitability, and in most cases there are reasonable hypotheses about the molecules underlying these currents. However, keep

in mind that as is the case in most of neurobiology right now, linking a specific molecule with a specific ionic current involves some degree of speculation.

In the next section, wherever possible I will use the term "current" to refer to an entity identified in physiology experiments, and use the term "channel" to refer to specific molecules. Also, in some cases the molecules can be referred to by their own names (e.g., Kv4.2).

A. Dendritic Potassium Channels

A-Type Currents

"A-type", or voltage-dependent, rapidly inactivating K^+ channels localized to the dendrites of hippocampal pyramidal neurons play a critical role in shaping the local electrical responses of the dendritic membrane and dendritic tree. The functions of A-type channels in general are to repolarize the membrane after an action potential, contribute to the resting membrane potential (modestly), and regulate firing frequency. My colleague Dan Johnston and his co-workers have proposed a model in which A-type channels in distal dendrites of the hippocampus are critical

Table 2   Mechanisms Upstream of the NMDA Receptor Involved in Membrane Depolarization

Ionic Current	Molecules Involved	Role	Mechanisms of Modulation
K currents			
Voltage-dependent	Kv4.2 (and Kv4.3)	Limit bpAPs	ERK, PKA, CaMKII
"A" currents		Limit EPSP magnitude	
"H" currents	NCN channels (HCN)	Regulate excitability	Cyclic nucleotides (direct)
Na currents			
AMPA receptors	GluR1, GluR2 aka GluR-A,B	Depolarize membrane	PKA, CaMKII, PKC
Voltage-dependent Na$^+$ currents	Na(v)1.6, 1.1,1.2	AP propagation	PKC (decreased inactivation)
Ca currents	?—likely many	AP propagation (hypothetical)	PKA
Cl currents			
GABA receptors	All GABA-A receptor subunits	AP firing, excitability	Numerous

regulators of back-propagating action potentials, regulating LTP induction by controlling voltage-dependent NMDA receptor activation.

Moreover, this type of regulatory mechanism is subject to modulation by cellular signal transduction cascades. Dax Hoffman and Jeff Magee, working in Dan Johnston's laboratory, found that activation of PKA or PKC shifts the activation curve of A-type K^+ currents recorded in hippocampal area CA1 dendrites (32). The voltage-dependence of their activation is shifted in the depolarizing direction, leading to increases in dendritic excitability and increased back-propagating action potentials in dendrites. More recent work by Dan's group, some of it in collaboration with Paige Adams in my lab, has shown that the alterations in A-current voltage-dependence caused by application of PKA, PKC, or β-adrenergic receptor activators is secondary to activation of ERK MAP kinase (33, 34). Overall, these observations indicate that K channel regulation of dendritic membrane properties is regulated by cell surface neurotransmitter receptors coupled to ERK activation. The implication of this, as will be discussed in more detail later, is that neuromodulation of K channel function could serve a critical role in controlling action potential back-propagation and local membrane electrical properties. This mechanism would then allow indirect but critical control over the membrane depolarization necessary for NMDA receptor activation.

What is the molecular basis for this regulation of voltage-dependent K channel function? The A-type potassium channel pore-forming subunit Kv4.2 is localized to subsynaptic compartments of dendrites in CA1 pyramidal neurons and is likely the pore-forming subunit of dendritic A-type channels in these regions.

Morover, Paige Adams in my laboratory tested the idea that Kv4.2 might be a target for ERK, and found that Kv4.2 is a substrate for ERK in hippocampal pyramidal neurons

(35). In additional recent studies in collaboration with Lilian Yuan in Dan Johnston's lab, we found that activation of PKA and PKC, as well as stimulation of β-adrenergic receptors, leads to ERK activation and Kv4.2 phosphorylation by ERK in hippocampal area CA1 (33). Furthermore, in these studies, we found that modulation of A currents by PKA, PKC, and beta-adrenergic receptors are secondary to ERK activation, and that this mechanism is a basis for controlling back-propagating action potentials in pyramidal neuron dendrites.

Our working hypothesis is that ERK phosphorylation of Kv4.2, the K^+ channel pore-forming subunits likely to mediate A currents in hippocampal dendrites, decreases the probability of channel opening or the number of channels in the membrane. Once these channels in a particular region of a dendrite are rendered nonfunctional as a result of phosphorylation, the ability of a back-propagating action potential to invade that particular dendrite increases. This will allow, or increase the likelihood of, NMDA receptor activation and Ca^{2+} influx locally, and thus control the induction of LTP at that synapse.

Available data suggest the particular importance of this mechanism in theta-type LTP induction protocols (2, 3). Theta-frequency stimulation causes complex spike bursting in area CA1 cells, which can back-propagate into the dendrites and depolarize synapses. Several groups, including the laboratories of Eric Kandel, Danny Winder, and Tom O'Dell have shown that blocking ERK activation in mouse area CA1 blocks not only the complex spike bursting seen with the theta-frequency stimulation protocol, but also the LTP that is so induced (2, 3). It seems likely that blocking ERK in these experiments decreases the phosphorylation of Kv4.2, leading to an increase in the probability of current flux through these channels. Moreover, Danny Winder's group has found that beta-adrenergic receptor-mediated modulation of LTP induced with theta-frequency stimulation is blocked by inhibitors of ERK activation. Again, these findings are consistent with a model wherein ERK regulation of membrane electrical properties, via control of Kv4.2 channels, regulates back-propagating action potentials and controls NMDA receptor activation.

KV4.2 as a Signal Integrator

Finally, I should note that Anne Anderson, Laura Schrader, and their colleagues in my lab have found evidence that Kv4.2 is a substrate for three different kinases known to be involved in LTP induction: PKC, PKA, and ERK (33, 35). Thus, Kv4.2 may serve as a functional integrator of the actions of these protein kinases by serving as a convergence point for their actions. PKA, PKC, and ERK all lead to a diminution of Kv4.2 function, actions that will tend to promote LTP induction through the mechanisms outlined previously.

The "H" Current

My long-time colleague Dan Johnston told me recently that even hard-core cellular physiologists have a hard time understanding "H" currents, so the odds of a biochemist like me understanding them were slim. He was right. I do know that the

---

BOX 1

MAPK AS A SIGNAL INTEGRATOR CONTROLLING Kv4.2

While regulation of cell proliferation is the best-studied function of the ERK mitogen Activated Protein Kinase (MAPK) cascade, it is now known that hippocampal ERK activation is necessary for LTP and a wide variety of forms of hippocampus-dependent memory formation (see reference 92). It is interesting to consider that this cascade so critical for normal development is utilized for memory formation in the adult, suggesting a generalized mechanistic conservation between development and adult learning (see reference 52).

Regulation of the ERK cascade is complex, but this complexity allows for some interesting possibilities in terms of hippocampal information processing and neuronal coincidence detection. The ERK cascade, like MAPK cascades in general, is distinguished by a characteristic core cascade of three kinases (see figure). The first kinase in the sequence is Raf-1 (or B-Raf), which activates the second kinase,

MEK, by serine/threonine phosphorylation. MEKs are "dual-specificity" kinases, which means they phosphorylate both a threonine and tyrosine side chain in their substrates. Via this dual phosphorylation, they activate a downstream MAP kinase (p44 MAPK = ERK1, p42 MAPK = ERK2). One important feature of the cascade is that ERK (both ERK1 and ERK2) activity is exclusively regulated by MEK. Dual phosphorylation by MEK both necessary and sufficient for ERK activation. This allows the use of MEK inhibitors to selectively block activation of the ERKs.

Several second-messenger-regulated kinases have been shown to activate the ERK/MAPK cascade in the hippocampus. Stimulation of protein kinase C produces a robust activation of ERK2 in acute hippocampal slices, and activation of the cAMP cascade also leads to secondary activation of MAPK in hippocampal area CA1 (see figure). In addition, activation of β-adrenergic receptors (βARs) using

Continued

BOX 1—cont'd

MAPK AS A SIGNAL INTEGRATOR CONTROLLING Kv4.2

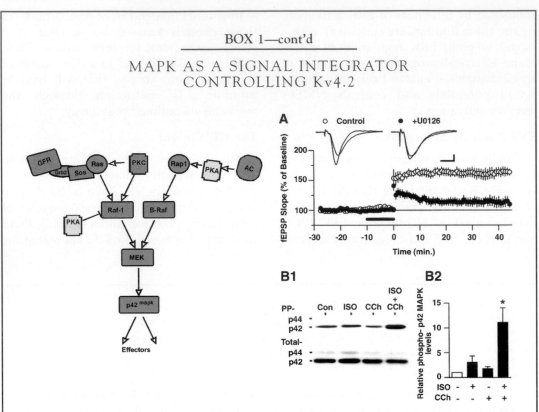

BOX 1   MAPK Activation may underlie the effects of Isoproterenol (ISO) plus carbachol on 5-Hz stimulation-induced LTP. The digram to the left illustrates the basic components of the ERK MAP kinase cascade in the hippocampus. (A) The MEK inhibitor U0126 inhibits the induction of LTP by 5 seconds of 5-Hz stimulation delivered during the coapplication of ISO and carbachol. A 5-second train of 5-Hz stimulation delivered at the end of a 10-minute bath application of ISO plus carbachol (200 nM each; the presence of agonists in the bath indicated by the bar) induced robust LTP in vehicle (0.2% DMSO) control experiments (open symbols; fEPSPs were potentiated to 163.9 ± 6.8% of baseline; n = 5) but had little effect on synaptic strength in slices continuously bathed in 20 μM U0126 (filled symbols; fEPSPs were 112.8 ± 7.3% of baseline; n = 5). The traces show superimposed fEPSPs recorded during baseline and 45 minutes post-5-Hz stimulation in a control experiment (left) and in a slice bathed in U0126 (right). Calibration: 1 mV, 5 msec. (B) Synergistic activation of MAPK by coactivation of β-adrenergic and cholinergic receptor agonists. (B1) Representative Western immunoblots showing protein bands visualized with antibodies to dually phosphorylated p42/44 MAPK (PP) and total p42/44 MAPK (Total) in control, untreated slices (Con), and slices bathed for 10 minutes in a CSF containing 200 nM ISO, 200 nM carbachol (CCh), or ISO plus carbachol (ISO 1 CCh). (B2) Average results ± SEM from seven separate experiments like that shown in B1. Only coapplication of ISO plus carbachol induced a statistically significant (*p < .05) increase in phospho-p42 MAPK levels. Reproduced from Watabe, Zaki, and O'Dell (2).

isoproterenol application leads to MAPK activation in area CA1, an effect attenuated by PKA inhibition. Metabotropic glutamate receptors, muscarinic acetylcholine receptors, DA receptors, alpha7 nicotinic acetylcholine receptors, and serotonin receptors all also lead to ERK activation in the hippocampus. Moreover, regulation of ERK activation in the hippocampus is not limited to neurotransmitter receptors. One of the most widely studied activators of hippocampal ERKs is BDNF; BDNF receptors couple to

---

BOX 1—cont'd

MAPK AS A SIGNAL INTEGRATOR CONTROLLING Kv4.2

ERK activation in hippocampal neurons, and the ERK activation contributes to BDNF-induced synaptic plasticity in area CA1. Other intriguing possible regulators of ERK in the hippocampus include a novel GTPase activating protein, SynGAP, that potentially links Ca^{2+}/calmodulin activation to ERK stimulation and reactive oxygen species, including superoxide, that can lead to ERK activation in the hippocampus.

This wide variety of upstream regulators of ERK suggests that this signal transduction cascade may serve to integrate diverse cell-surface signals into a coherent intracellular response. Especially intriguing is the possibility that this signal integration may not simply serve to sum up signals but rather, in some cases, serve to allow synergistic effects or coincidence detection. Recent important results from Tom O'Dell's laboratory suggest that this type of

information processing is indeed occurring. For example, Watabe, Zaki, and O'Dell (see figure) found synergistic activation of hippocampal ERKs by convergent sub-threshold activation of β-adrenergic receptors and muscarinic acetylcholine receptors. These data suggest that the ERK cascade can serve as a coincidence detector in its own right.

In considering a role for the ras/raf/MEK/ERK pathway in learning and memory, it certainly warrants emphasis that this pathway has been implicated in learning and memory in a wide variety of species. Published and unpublished studies in Aplysia, Lymnaea, Hermissenda, C. elegans, crayfish, Zebra Finch, Drosophila, mice, and rats have all directly or indirectly implicated a role for this cascade in learning and memory. Studies that we will discuss in Chapter 10 also suggest that it is appropriate to add the human to this list.

H stands for *hyperpolarization*—these are cation (sodium + potassium) channels that are partially active at the resting membrane potential and that open more with membrane hyperpolarization. Thus, they are voltage-dependent, hyperpolarization-activated channels. They also are directly gated by cyclic nucleotides (cAMP and cyclic Guanosine Mono Phosphate cGMP), which open the channels, but there also is good evidence that some of the enhancing effects of cAMP on Ih are mediated by PKA-dependent phosphorylation. The net effect of H channel function in dendrites is to dampen membrane excitability as other potassium channels do, at least in CA1 pyramidal neurons. However, they dampen membrane excitability without significantly attenuating the peak depolarization

of back-propagating action potentials (hyperpolarization activated therefore shut down when the membrane is strongly depolarized, get it?).

What does augmentation of H channels do, then? As a first approximation, you can think of enhancing H channel function as sharpening a back-propagating action potential, narrowing the window of membrane depolarization (36). They are open and counteracting membrane depolarization when the membrane is modestly depolarized, but inactive when the membrane is at the peak of the action potential. This effect might play an important role in timing-dependent plasticity mechanisms, restricting the time-frame over which associative actions like NMDA receptor activation might occur. A second, more tonic effect of augmenting H channels is to limit the ability of modest depolarization to penetrate a dendritic region. Overall, one can think of H channels as a cyclic nucleotide/PKA-dependent filtering mechanism for limiting membrane depolarization—in other words, a mechanism for enhancing the signal-to-noise ratio for depolarization-dependent associative events. cAMP/PKA, acting through H channels, might serve to ensure that associative events occur only when sufficiently robust electrical signals are seen.

B. Voltage-Dependent Sodium Channels (and Calcium Channels?)

Just like in axons, propagation of action potentials along dendrites depends on voltage-gated sodium channels. In situations where back-propagating action potentials provide the depolarization necessary for NMDA receptor activation, this effect is of course dependent on the function of these channels. Work from Costa Colbert and his colleagues has demonstrated that this is a potential site of plasticity for the regulation of LTP induction (37). Specifically, Costa has shown that PKC can regulate the rate of inactivation of sodium channels in pyramidal neuron dendrites, a mechanism allowing PKC control of the extent of action potential back-propagation. Specifically, PKC decreases the extent of sodium channel inactivation, allowing for repetitive action potentials (where Na channel inactivation is relevant) to penetrate the dendrites more effectively (30, 38). By this mechanism, PKC activation could promote the induction of LTP.

Back-propagating action potentials also activate voltage-dependent calcium channels in the dendritic membrane (30, 39). This is a critical source of dendritic calcium influx, but under certain conditions voltage-gated calcium channels (VGCCs) can contribute to the action-potential associated membrane depolarization as well. In various experimental circumstances, VGCCs can even propagate a dendritic "calcium spike," a regenerative action potential mediated by calcium flux across the membrane. Thus, modulation of calcium channels, aside from being a mechanism for regulating calcium influx, also can theoretically contribute to controlling local membrane depolarization.

C. AMPA Receptor Function

In the next chapter we will cover in detail a variety of mechanisms by which protein kinases augment AMPA receptor function. This is one of the principal mechanisms by which synaptic strength is enhanced during the *expression* of E-LTP. However, it should not escape our attention that these mechanisms could play a critical role in the *induction* of LTP as well. In this context it is important to note that CaMKII, PKC, and PKA all enhance AMPA receptor function—any cell surface receptor or calcium influx process that leads to activation of these kinases could influence the likelihood of LTP induction by augmenting AMPA receptor membrane depolarization.

This amplification of AMPA receptor function could be important in several contexts. First, AMPA receptors provide the initial depolarization of the membrane that brings the cell to threshold for firing an action potential. An augmentation of AMPA receptor function means that, for any given level of glutamate at the synapse, there is greater depolarization, at least until the concentration of glutamate reaches a saturating level. Thus, the cell is more likely to reach threshold for firing an action potential, and thus be more likely to trigger NMDA receptor activation. In "non-silent" synapses where AMPA receptors and NMDA receptors are both present, AMPA receptor augmentation will directly lead to greater local membrane depolarization and enhanced NMDA receptor function. This is an appealing model in the context of second-messenger-coupled neurotransmitter receptors modulating LTP induction.

Second, enhanced AMPA receptor function can serve as a temporal integration mechanism. Protein kinase activation and substrate phosphorylation typically are much longer lasting (relatively) than glutamate elevation at the synapse. Depolarization-associated calcium influx or second messenger elevation can set in motion a positive feedback mechanism over time, such that subsequent stimulation of AMPA receptors is enhanced relative to an initial response. This could occur via calcium-activated kinases phosphorylating AMPA receptors, or even through AMPA receptor insertion into the membrane. Although this idea is quite speculative at this time, these mechanisms nicely fit the classical definition of a temporal integration system.

D. GABA Receptors

As described in the last chapter, GABA-gated chloride ion channels (GABA-A receptors) control numerous processes relevant to the triggering of LTP. Because these processes were described in the last chapter in the context of hippocampal circuit information processing mechanisms, I won't cover them further here. Moreover, at present the role of GABA-A receptors has largely been studied in the context of controlling the likelihood of action potential firing and membrane depolarization in the cell-body region, as opposed to local control of the membrane electrical properties in the distal dendritic regions. While it is clear that dendritic GABA-A receptor activation could play a powerful role in controlling

---

BOX 2

COUPLING OF RECEPTORS TO INTRACELLULAR MESSENGERS

Neurotransmitters that act by binding to receptors on the cell surface can elicit a wide variety of biochemical effects inside a neuron. How does a signal at the cell's surface manage to alter the activities of enzymatic processes intracellularly? In many cases, this is achieved by virtue of the neurotransmitter receptor coupling to and altering the catalytic activity of second-messenger-generating enzymes on the inner leaflet of the cell membrane. The second messengers thus produced typically activate downstream *protein kinases*, which are enzymes that regulate the activity of a wide variety of intracellular proteins by attaching phosphate groups to (*phosphorylating*) specific amino acids in the protein's sequence.

Typically, coupling of the receptor to the effector enzyme is mediated by *G proteins*, or *guanine nucleotide binding proteins*. G proteins are themselves enzymes that bind Guanosine triphosphate (GTP) and hydrolyze it to Guanosine diphosphate (GDP). Receptors activate G proteins by causing an allosteric change in the protein that causes an exchange of GTP onto the protein, replacing the GDP that is there in the inactive state. The GTP-bound version of the G protein is active and interacts with second-messenger-generating enzymes (or ion channels in some cases), greatly increasing their catalytic rate and producing elevations of the intracellular levels of the second messengers. After the G protein has hydrolyzed GTP to GDP, the G protein relaxes back to its inactive state, where it can remain unstimulated or once again be activated by the neurotransmitter/receptor complex (see figure).

Continued

BOX 2—cont'd

COUPLING OF RECEPTORS
TO INTRACELLULAR MESSENGERS

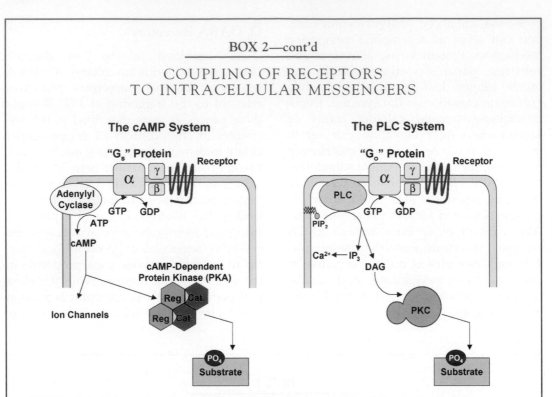

BOX 2 Coupling of cell surface receptors to PKA and PKC. This illustration indicates the connecting pathway between the receptor and the downstream effects of the protein kinases. In both pathways the receptor is linked though G protein interactions with the second messenger producing enzymes that modulate PKA and PKC, which in turn effects phosphorylation of a variety of substrates. See text for full explanation.

Why does this elaborate machinery exist? Why not have the receptor directly interact with the second-messenger-generating enzyme? One answer to this question lies in the *kinetics* of the GTP hydrolysis reaction. On the kinetic scale at which enzymes typically operate, G proteins are notably slow. This means that once the receptor stimulates the exchange of GTP onto the G protein, the G protein will stay in the GTP-bound, active conformation for a relatively extended period of time, on the order of a few minutes. However, after GTP is bound, the G protein quickly dissociates from the ligand/receptor complex. The ligand-occupied receptor can then proceed to activate additional G protein molecules. The net effect of the G protein involvement,

then, is both an amplification and a prolongation of the neurotransmitter-stimulated event. Overall, the cell trades energy (in the form of GTP hydrolysis) for the benefit of augmented signal transduction across the membrane.

Two well-characterized second-messenger-generating enzymes are activated by G proteins: *adenylyl cyclase* and *phospholipase C*. Adenylyl cyclase converts ATP to adenosine 3′, 5′-cyclic monophosphate, using magnesium as a cofactor. cAMP is known to activate two downstream effectors: the *cAMP-dependent protein kinase (PKA)* and certain types of *cyclic nucleotide-gated ion channels*. The activity of phospholipase C results in the production of two different second messengers. Phospholipase C

BOX 2—cont'd

COUPLING OF RECEPTORS
TO INTRACELLULAR MESSENGERS

hydrolyzes the membrane phospholipid *phosphatidylinositol 4,5-bis phosphate* at the linkage between the glycerol backbone and the phospho-head group, liberating *diacylglycerol (DAG)* and *inositol 1,4,5-tris phosphate*. Both of these compounds serve as second messengers. DAG binds to and activates the downstream effector *protein kinase C (PKC)*. IP_3 binds to an intracellular receptor in the endoplasmic reticulum that is a calcium channel, leading to calcium mobilization from intracellular stores. Calcium of course is a pluripotent messenger in its own right and can activate a side variety of intracellular proteins and enzymes, including CaMKII.

Because second messengers are such powerful agents, regulation of their levels is carefully controlled. In cells specific enzymes for the breakdown of each of these messengers keep the levels of the compounds low in the resting cell. *Phosphodiesterase* is an enzyme that hydrolyzes cAMP into the inactive product 5'-AMP. Similarly, *DAG lipase* hydrolyzes DAG into its component parts, a glycerol molecule and two free fatty acids. DAG can also be inactivated by phosphorylation to phosphatidic acid, via the actions of *DAG kinase*. IP_3 is further metabolized by a very elaborate enzymatic system. IP_3 can be both broken down by phosphatases, leading ultimately to production of free inositol, or phosphorylated at additional sites by various kinases, leading eventually to the production of additional signaling molecules.

NMDA receptor activation locally, at present the specific molecular mechanisms that might operate in plasticity of this system have not been well defined.

IV. LTP INDUCTION COMPONENT 3—THE COMPONENTS OF THE SYNAPTIC INFRASTRUCTURE THAT ARE NECESSARY FOR THE NMDA RECEPTOR AND THE SYNAPTIC SIGNAL TRANSDUCTION MACHINERY TO FUNCTION NORMALLY

Don't be misled by my use of the term "infrastructure." The term sounds very static and boring. In fact, the synaptic infrastructure that I am referring to is quite a dynamic place. The components of the synaptic infrastructure such as scaffolding proteins, cytoskeletal proteins, and cell surface adhesion molecules are now coming to be appreciated as important signaling components in the cell that respond rapidly and with great variety to extracellular and intracellular signals. I use the term "infrastructure" to describe these cellular components not because they are boring or immutable but rather because they have in common that they provide the underpinnings of the physical structure of the synaptic and dendritic regions.

However, there's a problem with studying these molecules. Most enzymes catalyze the conversion of one chemical species into another, Adenosine triphosphate (ATP) to cAMP, for example, and catalysis of this sort is fairly straightforward to identify, characterize, and study in detail. The molecules of the "synaptic infrastructure" that we will be discussing in this section by and large do not catalyze reactions of this sort. Many of them are not enzymes at all. Even where they are enzymes, the functional consequence of their catalysis is to cause a conformational change in another protein—they are allosteric modulators that achieve their effects by causing another protein to assume an altered shape in three-dimensional space. It is much more difficult to characterize these types of molecules because their effects do not lend themselves to easy quantification in vitro.

Futhermore, the tools necessary to do the block, mimic, and measure experiments that we have been discussing throughout the book are largely unavailable for these types of proteins at present. As an additional complication, think about what it means to do a "mimic" experiment on a protein whose functional role is to change from one conformation to another. An agent that locks the protein in *any* particular conformation disrupts the capacity of the protein to change conformation and thus to transduce a signal. An "agonist" can block function just as effectively as an antagonist.

The upshot of all this is that we are at a very early stage in studying these types of mechanisms—this is likely to be a rich area of future discovery. However, for right now, I am left mostly with the option of listing molecules that fit into this category, that have been implicated in LTP based on knockout or inhibitor studies. Placing them into a scheme for LTP induction is fairly speculative at this point, and in some cases the most that can be said is that they are known to interact with other proteins known to be involved in LTP. With these caveats in mind, I proceed with a brief listing of the more notable components of the synaptic infrastructure that have been implicated as contributing to LTP induction.

A. Cell Adhesion Molecules and the Actin Matrix

A prominent category of synaptic "adhesion" molecules are the integrins (40).

Integrins are cell surface molecules that transduce signals from the extracellular matrix to the inside of the cell. They are single-transmembrane-domain   proteins that usually function as heterodimers of alpha and beta subunits. Knockout mice deficient in alpha5 and beta3 integrin exhibit hippocampus-dependent learning deficits and deficits in NMDA receptor-dependent LTP in area CA1 (41).

Integrins interact with a wide variety of intracellular effectors, three categories of which are clearly important to keep in mind in terms of LTP induction in general and regulating NMDA receptor function specifically (see Figure 3). First, integrins couple to src activation in many cells, and as we discussed in the first section of this chapter this is a mechanism for directly augmenting NMDA receptor function. Second, integrins couple to ras and via this mechanism can lead to ERK activation— this might play a role in K channel regulation (and regulating other effectors) as we discussed in the second section of this chapter. Finally, the prototype function of integrins is in regulating the actin cytoskeleton. This potential role of integrins has taken on special significance given recent findings by a number of laboratories, principally among them John Lisman's, that normal dynamic regulation of the actin cytoskeleton is necessary for LTP induction. Exactly how the actin cytoskeleton regulates LTP induction is unclear at present, but there will be many examples of candidate mechanisms that we will discuss in the rest of this section.

Integrin regulation of the actin cytoskeletal matrix is complex. One principal role is linking the extracellular matrix to sites of actin matrix adhesion on the cytoplasmic side of the membrane. Integrin cytoplasmic tails bind to alpha-actinin and talin, which in turn recruit actin binding proteins such as vinculin to the complex. This complex serves to anchor the cytoskeleton to the perisynaptic plasma membrane and synaptic zone.

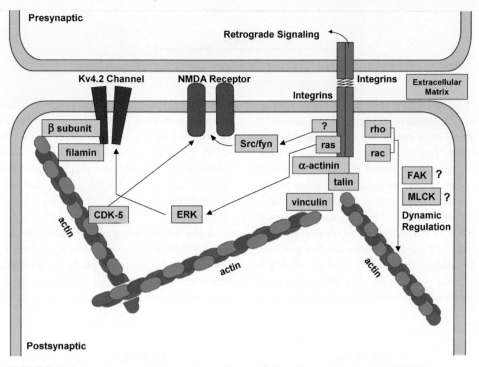

FIGURE 3 Interactions among integrins and intracellular effectors that regulate NMDA receptor function. See text for discussion and definitions.

Integrins also regulate the small G proteins rho (*ras ho*mologue, first identified in *Aplysia*) and rac (which regulate actin dynamics)—this dynamic regulation of the actin matrix is especially appealing to consider in the context of activity-dependent changes in spine morphology. These types of rapid morphological changes in spine morphology have been studied quite elegantly by the laboratories of Gang-yi Wu, Richard Tsien, and Tobias Bonhoffer, to whose publications I refer you for further details. Consideration of integrin regulation of rho activity is especially appealing in this context because the classic role of rho is in regulating actin-myosin-based movement by activating myosin light-chain kinase. Another potential integrin effector in this context is the Focal Adhesion Kinase (FAK), which also serves to control cell morphology via the actin cytoskeletal matrix in many cells.

The actin cytoskeletal matrix may also contribute to NMDA receptor regulation in fairly direct ways. For example, actin microfilaments can serve as anchors for signaling components that affect the NMDA receptor directly. One example of this is actin filaments serving as the anchor for CDK-5, which as we discussed earlier can phosphorylate and activate the NMDA receptor. Also, A-potassium channels interact with the actin-binding protein filamin via their cytoplasmic C-terminal domain, and potassium channel beta subunits couple these channels to the actin cytoskeleton as well. These interactions certainly help localize A-channels appropriately in the dendritic spine. Perhaps more importantly, disruption of these interactions can cause attenuation of potassium channel function, and, as we discussed earlier, A-channel inhibition promotes increased membrane excitability and enhanced NMDA receptor function.

An additional interesting aspect of integrin function, one that is perhaps key in

BOX 3

REGULATION OF RAS BY GAPS AND GEFS

Ras is a low-molecular-weight GTP-binding protein (G protein) classically studied as a target for particular receptor tyrosine kinases. Ras acts as a critical relay in signal transduction by cycling between an active conformational state when bound to GTP, and an inactive state when bound to GDP (see figure). The GTPase, or turn-off activity of ras is dependent on the opposing effects of two distinct classes of regulatory ras-binding molecules; GAPs and GEFs (guanine nucleotide exchange factors). GAPs promote formation of the GDP-ras complex through increasing ras GTPase activity, and thus inactivate ras. GEFs act by catalyzing the exchange of GTP for GDP, causing ras activation. The best-known GEFs fall into two major classes; the son of sevenless (SOS) class and the ras-guanine-nucleotide releasing factor (ras-GRF) class.

It also is important to note that there are three different isoforms of ras: H, N, and K. These different ras types likely have similar functions but they exhibit distinct tissue distributions—all are found in the brain.

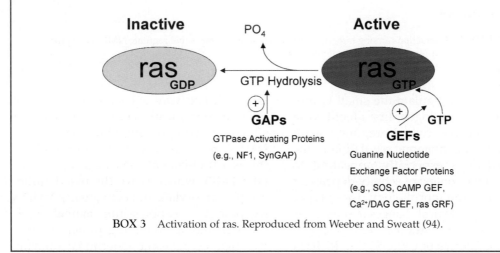

BOX 3   Activation of ras. Reproduced from Weeber and Sweatt (94).

the context of retrograde signaling in synaptic plasticity, is that integrins can transduce a signal from inside the cell back out to the extracellular domain. Specifically, phosphorylation of integrins on their cytoplasmic domain can cause a conformational change in their extracellular domain. Because a postsynaptic integrin molecule can directly bind to another presynaptic integrin molecule, this is a potential mechanism for sending a signal from the postsynaptic compartment back to the presynaptic compartment (i.e., retrograde signaling). Although this idea is still speculative at present, this type of direct conformational signal transduction from post- to presynaptic cells is an appealing idea for allowing coordinated, simultaneous functional changes in both compartments. Although this is not hypothesized to regulate NMDA receptor function specifically, I would be remiss if I did not mention this potentially quite important role for integrins as one potential component of LTP induction.

An additional transmembrane, extracellular-matrix-binding protein that has been directly implicated in LTP induction is Syndecan-3. Inhibition of this molecule using various approaches leads to deficits in LTP (42). Syndecan-3 binds heparan sulfates in the extracellular space, which are components of the glycosamino-glycan family of molecules present there. Syndecan-3 associates with the tyrosine kinase fyn, which might regulate NMDA receptor activity through direct tyrosine phosphorylation. The cell adhesion molecules L1 and Neural Cell Adhesion Molecule (N-CAM) have also been implicated in the expression of LTP in some studies, however, recent results from knockout mice have suggested that loss of these molecules does not lead to LTP deficits (43–45). Finally, the N-cadherin subtype of cell adhesion molecule has been implicated in LTP induction and maintenance (see reference 46 for a review). A likely role for the cadherins is in stabilizing strong connections between the presynaptic and postsynaptic membranes, although like other cell adhesion molecules the cadherins also interact with and can regulate the actin cytoskeleton.

B. Presynaptic Processes

It is a statement of the obvious that any presynaptic process that regulates gluta-mate release can impinge upon the likeli-hood of LTP induction by controlling the level of synaptic glutamate that is attained. We discussed a number of specific examples of this type of mechanism in the last chapter—for example, BDNF receptor regu-lation of LTP induction and the potential role for alterations in glutamate re-uptake as a mechanism for controlling NMDA receptor desensitization. I will not reiterate the details here, but simply note that they fit equally well into a discussion of regu-lating NMDA receptor function as they did in the prior context of "complexities of LTP."

Of course, many other specific molecular processes are involved in mediating and modulating the likelihood of vesicle fusion presynaptically, and thus modulating the likelihood of NMDA receptor activation postsynaptically. A complete treatment of this area of plasticity would require an entire monograph in its own right; more-over, many of the molecular details of these processing are still being worked out. For the present purposes, I will limit myself to pointing out that knockouts and inhibitors that affect the presynaptic infrastructure are quite likely to disrupt indirectly the proper function of the NMDA receptor as well.

C. Anchoring and Interacting Proteins of the Postsynaptic Compartment

Postsynaptic Density Proteins

The postsynaptic density warrants dis-cussion as a cellular organelle in its own right. It is a multiprotein assembly that is the organizing center for many receptors and effectors, and the cytoskeleton, in the postsynaptic compartment (47, 48).

PSD-95 is a protein enriched in the postsynaptic density and a prominent player in this context (49). Identification of this protein by Mary Kennedy helped launch a great increase in our under-standing of the molecular basis for the organization of the complex postsynaptic infrastructure. What follows is a brief overview summarizing many years of work by many laboratories, including those of Mary Kennedy, Morgan Sheng, and Rick Huganir.

PSD-95 binds to NMDA receptors (specifically the NR2 subunit) postsynap-tically and serves as a multidomain anchor-ing protein for a large number of scaffold-ing and structural proteins postsynaptically (see Figure 4). PSD-95 helps anchor nitric oxide synthase (NOS), localizing this source of the reactive nitrogen species NO. PSD-95

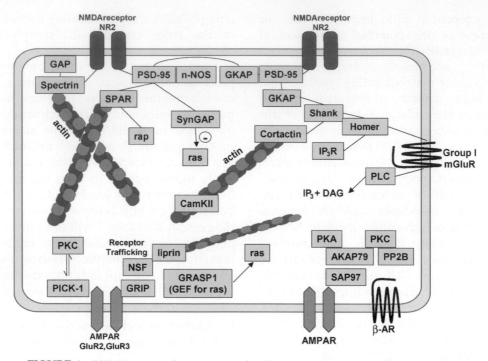

FIGURE 4   PSD-95 as an anchoring protein for NMDA receptors. See text for explanation.

also binds the ras Guanosine triphos-phatase Activating Protein synGAP, whose function is still under investigation but which may regulate the ras/ERK cascade locally at the synapse (see Box 3). PSD-95 also anchors the cytoskeleton through its interations with a protein termed SPAR, which is a Guanosine triphos-phatase Activating Protein (GAP) for rap and also an actin-interacting protein in its own right. Rap helps control the cytoskele-ton indirectly through its target signal transduction processes such as the MAP kinase cascades.

PSD-95 also binds to proteins that seem to be more explicitly structural, such as the scaffolding protein Shank. Shank is another multidomain molecule that links the PSD-95 binding protein Guanylate Kinase-Associated Protein (GKAP) to the actin skeleton through cortactin. Shank also binds to Homer, a metabotropic receptor binding protein. Thus, via Shank and Homer, group I metabotropic receptors

coupled to PLC can be localized near the NMDA receptor. Homer also binds the IP3 receptor, which may help localize the ER close to the NMDA receptor, allowing for proximity of intracellular calcium release mechanisms to the principal pathway for extracellular calcium influx, the NMDA receptor.

Genetic deletion of PSD-95 leads to striking alterations in LTP in area CA1—LTP is enhanced (49). This is associated with learning deficits. It is unclear how the loss of PSD-95 leads to the augmentation of LTP—obviously interpretation of the result is difficult because of the many complex roles of PSD-95 at the synapse, as outlined earlier. Overall, the data suggest that PSD-95 is somehow altering the threshold for LTP induction, a result consistent with the idea that PSD-95 and its associated proteins serve as dynamic modulators of NMDA receptor function.

The preceding discussion makes clear that the NMDA receptor does not reside in isolation in the membrane. In fact, Seth Grant's laboratory has clearly established that the NMDA receptor is the anchor for a large multiprotein complex of structural proteins and signal transduction components, as discussed in Box 4. This consideration leads to the inclusion of the NMDA receptor in the list of proteins necessary for proper NMDA receptor function (see Table 3). What is meant by this apparent statement of the obvious is that it is important to remember that the NMDA receptor is functioning as much more than a ligand-and-voltage-gated calcium channel. It also is a critical component of the synaptic infrastructure in a physical sense— serving as a membrane anchor for a wide variety of important postsynaptic proteins.

BOX 4

THE NMDA RECEPTOR SUPRAMOLECULAR COMPLEX

Probably the most-studied molecule in the short history of molecular studies of learning and memory is the NMDA subtype of glutamate receptor. As described in the Chapter 4, the breakthrough discovery in this area was made by Graham Collingridge and his colleagues, who found a necessity for the NMDA receptor for LTP induction at Schaffer-collateral synapses in hippocampal area CA1. Many studies subsequent to this work have brought into sharp relief the importance of the NMDA receptor in synaptic plasticity and memory formation. Recent work by Seth Grant and his colleagues has shown that the "NMDA receptor" is in fact a large multiprotein complex (90, 91). This complex includes a striking representation of many different types of scaffolding proteins and signal transduction molecules (see table). In fact, the NMDA receptor supramolecular complex includes a number of proteins whose function has been directly implicated in human learning, including NF1, PKA, raf-1, MEK, ERK, and RSK-2. These gene products have all directly or indirectly been implicated in human learning because they are associated with various types of human mental retardation syndromes (see Chapter 10). As Grant and his colleagues mentioned in their report (90), the presence of gene products linked to human mental retardation within the NMDA receptor complex was intriguing and consistent with a role for this complex in human cognition.

The NMDA receptor supramolecular complex has been referred to as the Hebbosome. I am not particularly fond of this nomenclature because Hebbian plasticity involves much more than just the NMDA receptor in my opinion. One of the major themes of this book is that we need to begin to think of Hebbian plasticity as not sufficiently described by just considering the function of the NMDA receptor and its associated proteins in isolation. In particular, regulation of membrane excitability properties are being emphasized here, so I don't want to do myself a disservice by adapting the Hebbosome nomenclature.

Of course, the Hebbosome terminology also makes a variation of this point as well. The Hebbosome nomenclature emphasizes the enormously complex molecular machine that is involved in NMDA receptor-dependent processes. I do not wish to take away from the importance of this concept. It just seems to me that what we might call the

Continued

BOX 4—cont'd

THE NMDA RECEPTOR
SUPRAMOLECULAR COMPLEX

Molecule	Mr (kD)
Glutamate Receptors	
NR1	120
NR2A	180
NR2B	180
GluR6 + 7	117
mGluR1a	200
Scaffolding and adaptors	
PSD-95	95
ChapSyn110/PSD-93	110
Sap102	115
GKAP/SAPAP	95-140
Shank	200
Homer	28/45
Yotiao	200
AKAP150	150
NSF	83
PKA	
PKA catalytic subunit	40
PKA-R2β	53
PKC	
PKCβ	80
PKCγ	80
PKCε	90
CaM Kinase	
CaM Kinase II β	60
phospho-CaM Kinase	60

Molecule	Mr (kD)
Phosphatases	
PP1	36
PP2A	36
PP2B(calcineurin)	61
PPs	50
PTPID/SHP2	72
Tyrosine Kinases	
Src	60
PYK2	116
MAP Kinase pathway	
ERK (pan ERK)	42/44
ERK1	44
ERK2	42
MEK1	45
MEK2	46
MKP2	43
Rsk	90
Rsk-2	90
c-Raf1	74
Small G-proteins and modulators	
Rac1	21
Rap2	21
SynGAP	10,12,35,60
NF1	60,101

Molecule	Mr (kD)
Other signaling molecules	
Calmodulin	15
nNOS	155
PI3 Kinase	85
PLCγ	130
cPLA2	110
Citron	183
Arg3.1	55
Cell adhesion and cytoskeletal proteins	
N-Cadherin	150
Desmoglein	165
β-Caternin	92
LI	200
pp120cas	120
MAP2B	280
Actin	45
α-actinin 2	110
Spectrin	240/280
Myosin (brain)	205
Tubulin	50
Cortactin	80/85
CortBP-1	180/200
Clathryn heavy chain	180
Dynamin	100
Hsp-70	70

TABLE BOX 4   Summary of molecular composition of the NMDAR supramolecular complex. The component molecule and its molecular weight are list. Adapted from Husi et al. (90).

Hebbosome is even bigger than the huge molecular complex already described. In fact, the Hebbosome may be the entire postsynaptic spine compartment. Even this idea leaves out presynaptic factors.

Consideration of the NMDA receptor supramolecular complex raises an additional important point to bear in mind. Briefly stated, Figures 2–4 are inadequate in a structural sense. As illustrated in these figures, signaling by the various protein kinase cascades is greatly influenced by

scaffolding proteins that serve to localize the signal transduction machinery to appropriate subcellular compartments. However, it is useful to also think of "signaling compartments" within neurons. A given molecular cascade in some locales within the cell will be constricted in its range of effects and effectors, achieving effects locally. The NMDA receptor supramolecular complex including NF1, ras/ERK, and the like is likely to function in this manner. The NMDA receptor complex also serves

---

BOX 4—cont'd

THE NMDA RECEPTOR
SUPRAMOLECULAR COMPLEX

to localize protein kinases such as CaMKII postsynaptically.

However, the ERK, PKA, and src cascades in other cellular domains may achieve effects more broadly, and indeed be subject to additional mechanisms of regulation. This has been demonstrated in studies investigating ERK signaling to the nucleus. At a minimum, it appears that there are at least two (likely more) functional pools of ERK and PKA in neurons—one involved in local regulation of the dendritic spine compartment and a second involved in regulating gene expression.

Table 3   Components of the Synaptic Infrastructure Necessary for NMDA Receptor Function

Component	Targets	Role
Cell adhesion molecules		
Integrins	Src, rho, rac, ras/MAPKs	Transmembrane signaling, interactions with extracellular matrix, NMDAR regulation
Syndecan-3	MLCK, FAK? fyn, NMDAR	Spine morphology? Signaling from matrix heparan sulfates to the NMDA receptor
N-Cadherin	Other cadherins, cytoskeleton	spine morphology? Pre-post adhesion?
Actin cytoskeleton/associated proteins		
Rho	Membrane/cytoskeleton interactions	Regulate synaptic structure
CDK-5	NMDA receptor	Increase NMDA receptor function
Filamin	K channels	K channel localization
Presynaptic processes		
Glutamate release	Synaptic glutamate	NMDA receptor activation
Glutamate re-uptake	Synaptic glutamate	Limiting NMDA receptor desensitization
Anchoring/interacting proteins		
PSD-95	Receptors, signal transduction nNOS, SynGAP, GKAP	Postsynaptic organization
NMDA receptor	Multiple proteins	Effector localization, structural organization
Rack1/fyn	NMDA receptor	Direct regulation of NMDA receptor
Shank/HOMER	Metabotropic receptors	Effector localization, cytoskeleton
GRIP	AMPA receptors, PICK-1/PKC	Postsynaptic organization
AKAP	PKA, PP2B	Kinase and phosphatase localization
CaMKII	Signal transduction	Regulate likelihood of LTP induction

This consideration also serves as an important caveat for interpreting results from NMDA receptor knockout mice. This apparently "clean" experimental manipulation, wherein the NMDA receptor is entirely lost, likely results in a large number of secondary effects on molecules normally associated with the NMDA receptor postsynaptically. In fact, experiments using various deletion mutants missing the cytoplasmic anchoring domains of the NMDA receptor have allowed dissection of the role of the NMDA receptor as a scaffolding protein versus its role as a ligand-gated ion channel (50). Deletion of the intracellular domain of the NMDA receptor appears to be sufficient to account for essentially all the physiologic and behavioral deficits observed in NMDA receptor knockout mice—the upshot is that the role of the NMDA receptor as a component of the PSD infrastructure is just as important as its role as a ligand-gated ion channel.

Additional Direct Interactions with the NMDA Receptor

The NMDA receptor NR1 and NR2 subunits also bind spectrin, the actin-binding protein. This may serve as an additional cytoskeleton anchoring site postsynaptically. Moreover, this interaction is subject to regulation by phosphorylation—tyrosine phosphorylation of NR2B leads to decreased interactions of spectrin with the receptor, and NR1 interaction with spectrin is modulated by serine/threonine phosphorylation. However, the role of these effects in synaptic plasticity is not clear at this point.

Finally, as described earlier in the section on direct modulation of NMDA receptors, the scaffolding protein RACK1 promotes formation of a fyn/RACK1/NR2B complex that actually inhibits fyn phosphorylation of the NMDA receptor and diminishes current through the receptor (see Figure 2). Also, PDS-95 modulates src phosphorylation of NMDARs, and src potentiation of

NMDAR currents appears to require the presence of PSD-95.

Consideration of the complicated structure and regulation of the postsynaptic density complex highlights the importance of thinking of the entire postsynaptic domain as a large functional unit. The NMDA receptor is embedded in a dynamic multiprotein complex that it regulates and in turn that regulates it. While many details of the structural components of the PSD complex are still being worked out and their roles in LTP induction are being actively investigated, it is clear that disrupting one or more of the cogs in this machine can lead to disruption of the proper function of the NMDA receptor.

AMPA Receptors

AMPA receptors, of course, provide the initial depolarization, either locally or distally in the neuron, that ultimately results in NMDA receptor activation. As such, alterations in the AMPA receptor protein or its associated interacting proteins can lead to loss of proper regulation of NMDA receptor activation. However, in this section we will focus on the AMPA receptor as a *structural* component of the synapse.

AMPA receptors, like NMDA receptor, also reside postsynaptically but are in much more of a state of flux than NMDA receptors. In fact, the average half-life for an AMPA receptor in the postsynaptic membrane is 15 minutes. We will return to some implications of this in the next chapter. Also, as we have discussed in previous chapters, AMPA receptor membrane insertion can be activity-dependent. Thus, the AMPA receptor should probably not be thought of like the NMDA receptor—the NMDA receptor likely serves a frankly structural role in addition to its function as a ligand-gated ion channel while the AMPA receptor is more peripherally associated with the PSD (see reference 51).

The AMPA receptor binds at least two "structural" proteins—Protein Interacting with C Kinase-1 (PICK-1), which binds PKC, and Glutamate Receptor Interacting Protein (GRIP) (see reference 47). GRIP is a multidomain scaffolding protein that likely functions in AMPA receptor trafficking. GRIP also binds to GRIP Associated Protein-1 (GRASP1), a Guanine nucleotide Exchange Factor (GEF) for ras (see references 52 and 53)—the functional role of GRASP1 at the synapse is unclear at present. AMPA receptors can also bind N-Ethyl maleimide Sensitive Factor (NSF), a vesicle-associated protein that may also be involved in receptor membrane insertion is in a fashion reminiscent of its role presynaptically in neurotransmitter vesicle fusion.

AMPA receptors also bind the A kinase anchoring protein AKAP79, an interaction that appears to be mediated by the PSD-95 homologue SAP-97 (54–56). As the name implies, AKAPs bind and localize PKA by interacting with the regulatory subunits of the kinase. The general role of AKAPs is to help localize PKA near relevant targets such as the AMPA receptor postsynaptically. The story is actually more complicated than that, because AKAP79 in the hippocampus also binds and localizes a protein phosphatase, PP2B (aka Calcineurin). As a first approximation, it is useful to think of proteins such as AKAPs as serving a role to increase the signal-to-noise ratio for signal transduction—localizing kinases close to their substrates to increase the efficacy of phosphorylation, but also localizing phosphatases to those same substrates in order to keep their basal phosphorylation low and to allow for rapid reversal of phosphorylation events once the kinase activation is over (56). AKAP79 may also serve specifically to localize the calcium-sensitive phosphatase PP2B to the AMPA receptor in order to facilitate calcium-dependent AMPA receptor dephosphorylation and down-regulation in LTD (57).

AKAP79 also serves an additional scaffolding protein function. It binds to cyclase-coupled receptors such as the beta-adrenergic receptor, localizing receptor, effector, kinase, substrate, and phosphatase all together in a supramolecular complex. In the context of the hippocampal pyramidal neuron synapse, this might allow for enhanced beta adrenergic receptor modulation of AMPA receptor function, enhancing AMPA receptor function via PKA-dependent phosphorylation. This might serve in the induction of LTP as a mechanism whereby cyclase-coupled receptors can augment AMPA receptor-mediated membrane depolarization and indirectly augment NMDA receptor activation.

AKAP79 also binds to PKC, again localizing this kinase near its substrate, the AMPA receptor. By analogy to the scenario outlined earlier for AKAP/PKA, this scaffolding activity might facilitate PKC-coupled receptor augmentation of AMPA receptor function during the induction of LTP as well. As we will discuss in the next chapter, PKC phosphorylation of AMPA receptors also contributes to E-LTP expression, and of course AKAP79 localization of PKC near AMPA receptors would help facilitate this mechanism as well.

CaMKII

CaMKII is highly enriched at the postsynaptic density complex. This enrichment in part occurs through CaMKII binding to the actin cytoskeleton, and the anchor for the cytoskeleton is the NMDA receptor as we have discussed extensively. Thus, one purpose of the NMDA receptor/PSD-95/cytoskeleton complex is to help localize CaMKII to the PSD domain. This keeps a critical effector of the NMDA receptor, CaMKII, tightly bound and localized for effective responsiveness to NMDA receptor activation. Interaction of CaMKII with the PSD also can be regulated by CaMKII autophosphorylation—John Lisman has proposed this as a mechanism contributing to the maintenance of E-LTP, a model that we will return to in the next chapter.

While the various scaffolding proteins—PSD-95 and the like—that we discussed ealier are involved upstream of the NMDA receptor, regulating its function, CaMKII is downstream of the NMDA receptor. However, I list it as a component of the synaptic infrastructure necessary for proper NMDA receptor function because it is such an important and direct target of the NMDA receptor—in essence loss of CaMKII function may functionally translate as equivalent to loss of NMDA receptor function. In addition, CaMKII binding to the PSD complex may play a structural role in concert with the actin cytoskeleton to serve as part of the infrastructure necessary for the NMDA receptor to function appropriately.

V. LTP INDUCTION COMPONENT 4—FEED-FORWARD AND FEEDBACK MECHANISMS THAT REGULATE THE LEVEL OF CALCIUM ATTAINED

There is a clear consensus that elevation of postsynaptic calcium is necessary for LTP induction, so clearly any process that modulates the postsynaptic calcium level has the capacity to affect LTP induction. Unfortunately that's about where the clarity ends. In this section, we will deal with some of the known processes whereby calcium levels in the postsynaptic spine are regulated. (See table for summary.)

In one sense, dendritic spines are specialized calcium-handling compartments (see Sabatini, Oertner, and Svoboda

(58) for a very nice treatment of this idea). They contain many molecules dedicated to calcium handling that affect the kinetics of calcium elevation, kinetics which are a critical determinant for (a) whether synaptic strength is changed and (b) whether LTP or LTD is induced. A few generalizations can be made in this context based on published work in this area. One, calcium elevation in a spine is largely compartmentalized to that spine—the narrow spine neck greatly limits calcium diffusion out of the spine in response to NMDA receptor activation, for example. Two, the level of calcium attained determines whether synaptic strength goes up or down—modest levels yield synaptic depression (LTD or depotentiation) and higher levels yield LTP. Three, the kinetics of calcium entry secondary to NMDA receptor activation versus back-propagating action potential/VDCC-dependent calcium influx are different—NMDA receptor activation gives a much longer-lasting elevation of spine calcium than does activation of VDCCs. Four, a seminal finding from Rob Malenka's lab made clear that a relatively prolonged (> 2 seconds) elevation of postsynaptic calcium is necessary for LTP induction in CA1 pyramidal neurons. The basic idea is that this prolonged calcium elevation is necessary to trigger the biochemical processes subserving LTP maintenance (which we will discuss in the next chapter). With these four principles in mind it becomes quite clear that regulating the kinetics of calcium handling and the steady-state level of

Table 4   Calcium Feedback and Feed-Forward Mechanisms

Molecule/Organelle	Role	Modulator/Regulator
VDCCs	Augment NMDA receptor-dependent Ca influx Ca influx due to bpAPs Regulate ERK activation	PKA
Endoplasmic reticulum (Ca-ATPase/IP3R/RyR)	Ca efflux from ER, limit LTP?	PLC-coupled receptors
Presynaptic mitochondria	Regulate presynaptic Ca levels	Unknown

calcium achieved locally in the dendritic spine is going to be a critical component of LTP induction. What is not clear are the exact molecular processes that impinge upon these variables.

In this section, I will briefly overview two postsynaptic processes and one presynaptic process that are involved in synaptic calcium handling and describe some of the available literature investigating the role of these processes in LTP induction. The specific systems I will describe are postsynaptic Voltage-dependent Calcium Channels (VDCCs), the postsynaptic endoplasmic reticulum (ER), and presynaptic mitochondria. The precise roles of these three systems/processes in LTP induction are quite murky at present, and many more years of work are likely to be necessary before a clear picture emerges concerning exactly what is happening with these molecules and organelles during LTP induction. However, a number of studies using inhibitors and knockouts of various components of these systems have been published, and a brief review of these studies is appropriate in order to set the stage for thinking about this category of molecular mechanisms.

A. VDCCs

The role of VDCCs in LTP induction is difficult to study because VDCCs are necessary for the synapse to function at all—presynaptic VDCCs are what allow the calcium influx necessary for neurotransmitter release. However, the presynaptic channels involved in release are largely "N" and "P"-type VDCCs (59), and "L"-type (aka high-voltage activated) VDCCs appear to be the principal dendritic VDCCs, at least as far as LTP induction is concerned. Thus, one can use L-type VDCC antagonists such as nifedipine and nitrendipine to try to dissect out the contributions of VDCCs versus NMDA receptors in triggering LTP induction.

A wide variety of studies have made it clear that L-type VDCCs are necessary for NMDA receptor-*independent* LTP at CA1

synapses—LTP induced, for example, by 200-Hz stimulation or K channel blockade. This necessity for VDCC function for these forms of LTP helped establish that this type of LTP is indeed distinct from NMDA receptor-dependent LTP (60, 61). Also, based on these studies, it is clear that calcium influx through VDCCs is sufficient to cause synaptic potentiation. However, are VDCCs necessary for NMDA receptor-dependent LTP as well? Might calcium influx through VDCCs augment the calcium influx that occurs via NMDA receptors? This is clearly a possibility given that Ito et al. (62) have found that theta-stimulation-induced LTP is significantly attenuated by blockade of VDCCs. (100 Hz HFS-induced LTP is generally held to be independent of VDCCs.) In addition, Dudek and Fields (63) also found that VDCC activation occurs with theta-type stimulation, and that downstream activation of the ERK cascade is dependent upon calcium influx through VDCCs.

One potential mechanism for this effect is activation of VDCCs by back-propagating action potentials (63, 64). Thus, calcium influx due to back-propagating action potentials might sum with calcium coming in via NMDA receptors, augmenting the postsynaptic calcium signal. Additional considerations involving K channel inactivation also apply in this scenario (see reference 64), which also serves to augment membrane depolarization and calcium influx.

This process might also be subject to neuromodulation as well. An early collaborative study by Chetkovich, Gray, Johnston, and Sweatt (65) showed that postsynaptic VDCCs are directly up-regulated by the cAMP/PKA cascade. This would allow the opportunity for adenylyl cyclase-coupled receptors, such as beta-adrenergic receptors, to modulate VDCCs by this mechanism as well. As we discussed in the last chapter, coincidence detection mechanisms such as this appear to be particularly important for theta-type LTP induction in area CA1.

B. The Spine Apparatus

The postsynaptic spine has a specialized form of endoplasmic reticulum referred to as the spine apparatus. The spine apparatus performs like the ER in other parts of the cell, as an intracellular calcium store. The spine apparatus has at least three types of calcium channels in it. The first is the Ca ATPase that pumps calcium out of the cytoplasm and into the spine apparatus. The second is the ryanodine receptor (RyR), which is a calcium-gated calcium channel that allows calcium out of the ER. The RyR functions in calcium-induced calcium release (CICR). The third channel is the inositol tris-phosphate (IP$_3$)-gated calcium channel that responds to the second messenger IP$_3$ to cause calcium efflux. IP$_3$ receptors and RyR generally act in concert—IP$_3$ triggers local calcium release, which activates RyR (66). You also may recall that we have seen the IP$_3$ receptor already in this chapter—it is one of the proteins that interacts with the mGluR anchoring protein HOMER, localizing these receptors near the ER and vice versa. It also is clear that calcium influx through NMDA receptors can trigger secondary CICR from the spine apparatus (67).

The literature on the role of the spine apparatus in LTP could at best be considered "messy." Depletion of spine apparatus calcium with the Ca ATPase inhibitor thapsigargin blocks the induction of LTP, although this effect may be limited to modest tetanic stimulation protocols (68, 69). This suggests that mobilization of intracellular calcium from the spine apparatus is necessary for LTP induction under some conditions. However, additional studies with inhibitors/knockouts of the RyR and the IP$_3$ receptor have yielded ambiguous results. Various groups have reported that loss of RyR3 receptor function leads to an attenuation of LTP (70, 71), no effect on LTP (72), or an augmentation of LTP (73). Genetic deletion of IP$_3$ receptors leads to a complex phenotype—generally not affecting LTP induced with HFS, but augmenting lower-frequency stimulation such that stimuli normally causing LTD now elicit LTP (72, 74). In general, it is difficult to come up with a model for the role of the spine apparatus in LTP induction at this point. It seems as if the spine apparatus may somehow serve to limit LTP induction, perhaps by biasing the synapse toward depotentiating mechanisms. However, investigations of these mechanisms is clearly at a very early stage, and the studies are made more difficult by the complex interacting machinery of the spine apparatus.

C. Mitochondrial Calcium-Handling

Mitochondria are generally not found in the postsynaptic spine but rather are restricted in distribution to the presynaptic terminal and postsynaptic dendritic shaft. One of the many roles of mitochondria is in presynaptic calcium handling—they can serve as calcium buffers by taking up cytoplasmic calcium. Michael Levy in my laboratory, in collaboration with Bill Craigen, has been investigating the potential role of mitochondria in regulating calcium handling, and thus synaptic plasticity at Schaffer-collateral synapses (75). While these studies are at an early stage, Michael would kill me if I didn't take the opportunity in this section of the book to present a synopsis of his interesting findings in this area (76).

The mitochondrial outer membrane has within it one of three isoforms of a family of porin proteins, known as the voltage-dependent anion channels (VDACs). Mitochondrial porins conduct small molecules and constitute one component of the permeability transition pore that opens in response to mitochondrial membrane depolarization, such as occurs with cytoplasmic calcium elevation. Because mitochondrial porins have significant roles in diverse cellular processes including regulation of mitochondrial ATP and calcium flux, my colleagues Michael Levy, Bill Craigen, and Ed Weeber sought to determine their importance in learning and synaptic plasticity using knockout mice. They found that fear conditioning and Morris water maze spatial learning are disrupted in VDAC1- and VDAC3-deficient mice. They also found that LTP induction was similarly blocked in these mice, and moreover that acute inhibition of the mitochondrial permeability transition pore by cyclosporin A in wild-type hippocampal slices reproduces the electrophysiological phenotype of VDAC-deficient mice. All these effects occurred in the absence of gross disruptions of baseline synaptic transmission. These results demonstrate a dynamic functional role for mitochondrial porins and the permeability transition pore in learning and synaptic plasticity. Our current working hypothesis is that presynaptic mitochondria contribute to regulating acute and baseline presynaptic calcium levels, selectively affecting calcium handling and presynaptic neurotransmitter release during periods of high-frequency synaptic activity.

VI. LTP INDUCTION COMPONENT 5—EXTRINSIC SIGNALS THAT REGULATE THE RESPONSE TO THE CALCIUM INFLUX

This is one of the most fascinating areas of investigation into the biochemistry of LTP induction. Rich in associative mechanisms, this category is more widely studied than some of the other areas we have been discussing. We will be discussing two signal transduction cassettes that can serve to "gate" LTP induction. The first example will draw from PKA regulation of protein phosphatase activity—a system referred to as the "cAMP Gate" for LTP induction. Strong evidence exists in the literature that this is an important mechanism for regulating the likelihood of LTP induction at Schaffer collateral synapses. The second example is the PKC/Neurogranin system—a postsynaptic system for regulating the level of free calmodulin, and, hence, for regulating calmodulin-responsive enzymes. The role for this system in regulating the likelihood of LTP induction is slightly more speculative than the cAMP gate, but it still is based on a substantial body of literature.

A. The cAMP Gate for LTP Induction

Bob Blitzer, Ravi Iyengar, and Manny Landau were among the first scientists to truly appreciate the biochemical complexity of LTP induction. They have proposed and investigated a model for regulating the likelihood of LTP induction that they have termed the cAMP gate (77). I find this neologism very appealing—it succinctly captures the essential function of a somewhat complex mechanism for augmenting protein kinase activation in response to the initial elevations of calcium with LTP-inducing stimulation.

When considering protein phosphorylation, most neuroscientists think first of protein kinases, the "on" switches, relegating protein phosphatases to the subordinate role of turning enzymes back "off"

Table 5   Extrinsic Signals Modulating the Calcium Response

Regulatory System	Molecules Involved	Role
The cAMP gate	PKA/PP1/I1/PP2B	Phosphatase inhibition Augmented kinase signaling
The PKC/neurogranin system	PLC/PKC/neurogranin/CaM	Augmenting CaMKII activation Augmenting Ca-sensitive cyclase

after their job is completed. However, protein phosphatases play a dynamic and important role in regulating synaptic plasticity and triggering memory formation (see reference 78). A new understanding is emerging of how protein phosphatases are quite active participants in regulating neuronal function, and that a dynamic interplay occurs between phosphatases and kinases in order to set thresholds determining whether a given neuronal input will be able to trigger a long-lasting neuronal change. In the next two paragraphs, I will illustrate this concept with a brief description of the components of the cAMP gate—it likely will be helpful to refer to Figure 5 in envisioning how the cAMP gate works.

As has been described in more detail by Blitzer et al. (77), there is an interesting interplay of the calcium-sensitive phosphatase, calcineurin, and PKA in controlling the activity of another protein phosphatase, PP1 (protein phosphatase 1). The activity of PP1 is regulated by an inhibitory protein, inhibitor 1 (I1); and only the phosphorylated version of I1 is effective at inhibiting PP1. Thus, the capacity of I1 to block PP1 activity is regulated by PKA-dependent phosphorylation of I1–PKA through phosphorylation of I1 leads to PP1 inhibition. Calcineurin-dependent dephosphorylation of I1 leads to increased PP1 activity by relieving the I1-dependent inhibition. Thus, calcineurin counteracts the effects of PKA, indirectly activating PP1 through I1 dephosphorylation. The net result is that elevation of cAMP levels and activation of PKA leads to phosphatase inhibition—a mechanism for the PKA

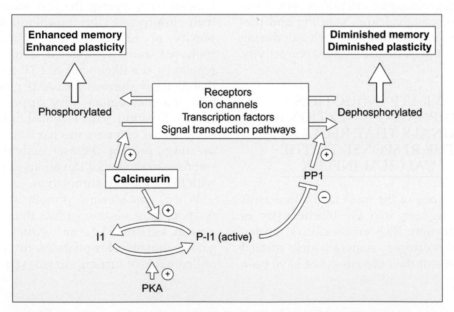

FIGURE 5   Model for the cAMP gate. The model illustrates an interaction of calcineurin and the cAMP-dependent protein kinase (PKA) in regulating the phosphorylation of proteins important for setting a threshold for triggering long-lasting synaptic effects. Blocking calcineurin leads to protein phosphatase 1 (PP1) inhibition indirectly through increasing inhibitor 1 (I1) phosphorylation. Loss of calcineurin and PP1 activity leads to a shift in the balance of substrate protein phosphorylation (receptors, channels, etc.). Increased phosphorylation of these effectors changes synaptic function in such a way that there is an increased likelihood of reaching a threshold for triggering lasting effects. Reproduced from Sweatt (93).

cascade to amplify the activity of any protein kinase that is activated with LTP-inducing stimulation.

These known regulatory mechanisms lead to a model for how PKA controls protein dephosphorylation and the triggering of synaptic plasticity (see Figure 5). PKA, in part, regulates the induction of long-lasting changes by inhibiting activity, enhancing the phosphorylation of key enzymes whose activity is necessary for triggering and maintaining synaptic potentiation. In essence, in this model calcineurin and PP1 act like a brake on the formation of synaptic potentiation, and PKA relieves this breaking mechanism. Moreover, the mechanism can serve as the basis for a biochemical coincidence detector—simultaneous activation of the PKA cascade with other protein kinases can lead to signal amplification and the triggering of unique phosphorylation-dependent events.

Bob Blitzer and his colleagues have tested key aspects of this model for regulating LTP induction and have developed a substantial body of evidence in accordance with their hypothesis (see 1, 77, 79). Isabel Mansuy, Danny Winder, and Eric Kandel have also studied certain aspects of the role or protein phosphate regulation in synaptic plasticity in vivo and in learned behavior in the intact animal (80, 81). These latter investigators have found that genetically engineered, calcineurin-inhibited animals exhibit an increased likelihood of triggering robust long-term potentiation in several hippocampal subregions including area CA1—a test of a key prediction of the cAMP gate model. In an interesting additional experiment, Malleret et al. (81) showed that calcineurin blockade-dependent augmentation of long-term potentiation in hippocampal slices was blocked by blocking the cAMP-dependent protein kinase, again in concordance with the cAMP gate model.

They also found that calcineurin inhibition enhanced the duration of object recognition in learning tasks in vivo—in effect calcineurin inhibition led to memory improvement. They found significant effects for tasks involving memories of minutes-to-hours duration, and also effects in a variation of the procedure that measures longer-term memory that lasts for one week. These data extend the relevance of the cAMP gate into the behaving animal.

Of course, a key question concerns the identity of the substrate proteins whose phosphorylation is augmented by the cAMP gate. Blitzer et al. (77), have focused on CaMKII as a target of the gate, and this certainly is an important target as we will discuss at the end of this chapter and in the next chapter. Additional candidates at this point include protein kinase C, voltage-dependent potassium channels, glutamate receptors and their associated proteins, and any of a number of components of the ERK MAP kinase cascade as we discussed in earlier sections of this chapter. In short, any phosphorylation event involved in LTP induction is subject to regulation by this mechanism, making it a pluripotent system for controlling synaptic plasticity.

B. The PLC/PKC/Neurogranin System

The capacity of extrinsic synaptic signals to enhance Ca-triggered events postsynaptically is not limited to the PKA system. PKC, acting through the calmodulin (CaM)-binding protein neurogranin (NG), can also lead to enhancement of the activation of Ca/CaM responsive enzymes. (Neurogranin was originally identified by subtractive cloning and termed RC3, and it is also referred to as P17. I use "neurogranin" because that is the name used most frequently in the literature; (see reference 82). Relevant targets of this system include both CaMKII and the Ca/CaM sensitive forms of adenylyl cyclase that are known to be important for LTP induction. The concept is the same as the cAMP gate—amplification of calcium signals through regulation of its target effectors. However, the PKC/Neurogranin system resides upstream of Ca/CaM-sensitive enzymes, increasing their activation by increasing the level of postsynaptic free CaM. This is in contrast to the cAMP gate, which amplifies downstream effects by enhancing substrate phosphorylation.

How does the neurogranin gate work? Neurogranin is a low-molecular-weight member of the calpacitin family of proteins. NG is localized to the postsynaptic cell and in fact is one of those proteins, like CaMKII, whose mRNA is selectively targeted to the dendritic region. NG functions as a calmodulin-binding protein and binds calmodulin in the *absence* of calcium (see Figure 6). The notable attribute of NG is that it is a PKC substrate, and when phosphorylated by PKC, it is unable to bind CaM. Thus, PKC phosphorylation of NG regulates the postsynaptic level of free calmodulin. PKC activation leads to inhibition of CaM binding to its NG localization scaffold, increasing the concentration of free CaM postsynaptically. This free CaM is then able to respond to calcium signals— PKC acting via NG can amplify Ca/CaM signaling postsynaptically.

Principal workers in figuring all this out have been Dan Gerendasy and Gregor Sutcliffe, Pierre DeGraan, Freesia and Kuo-Ping Huang, Dan Storm, and Eric Klann and Shu-Jen Chen from my lab. Various experiments by these investigators and others have demonstrated that PKC phosphorylation of NG occurs with LTP-inducing stimulation (83, 84), that PKC phosphorylates NG and regulates CaM binding and CaM level (85), that inhibition of NG function affects LTP induction (81, 86, 87), and that PKC/CaMKII crosstalk occurs in LTP induction (88). I refer the reader to an excellent comprehensive review by Dan Gerendasy and Gregor Sutcliffe for further details and references (82).

The upshot of all this is that the PKC/NG system can serve as a modulator of LTP induction. Moreover, the system in concert with a calcium signal can serve as a coincidence detector—a modest calcium signal coupled with PKC activation and

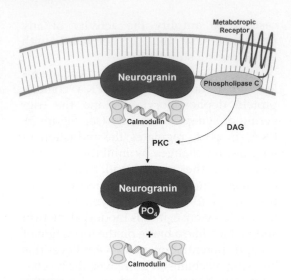

FIGURE 6 PKC phosphorylation of neurogranin regulates the level of free calmodulin. Neurogranin binds calmodulin in the absence of calcium. However, when PKC phosphorylates neurogranin, it is unable to bind calmodulin, freeing it to respond to calcium signals. See further explanation in text.

enhanced levels of free CaM will elicit a response not attainable by either signal in isolation.

Finally, it is very important to note that the cAMP gate and the PKC/neurogranin system do not necessarily operate in isolation. As shown in Figure 7, it is quite straightforward to interdigitate these two systems in a mutually reinforcing cascade (86). The figure shows that an initial calcium signal through the NMDA receptor can be reinforced by a PKC signal (the PKC neurogranin gate) and a cAMP signal (the cAMP gate) to give an augmented CaMKII stimulation. In essence, the CaMKII activation is amplified on the front end by the PKC/NG gate and on the output side by the cAMP gate. The cAMP Gate and the PKC/NG gate also can interact with each other in a mutually reinforcing fashion.

Cooperative, amplified systems such as this are the hallmark of biochemical cascades set up to serve as step-functions—allowing for an essentially all-or-none response after the appropriate preconditions

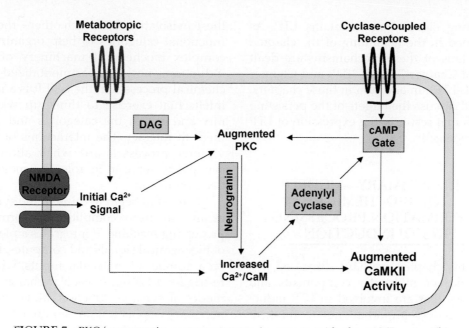

FIGURE 7   PKC/neurogranin system operates in concert with the cAMP gate. This diagram presents a schematic of the effects of the PKC/neurogranin system and the cAMP gate when considered together. CamKII activity is robustly activated by the simultaneous action of a cAMP coupled neurotransmitter, a DAG coupled neurotransmitter and an active NMDA receptor. See further discussion in text.

are met. In the case of the example shown in Figure 7, the simultaneous presence of a cAMP-coupled neurotransmitter, a DAG-coupled neurotransmitter, and an active NMDA receptor (depolarization plus glutamate) would give a robust output in terms of CaMKII activation. This, of course, is four-way coincidence detection—precisely the type of biochemical information processing capacity that is necessary for CA1 pyramidal neurons to trigger long-lasting changes in synaptic strength in response to multimodal sensory inputs as we discussed in Chapters 3 and 5. We will proceed to other examples of this type of multiple-input coincidence detection later.

With respect to Figure 7, keep in mind that while it is a static figure, the system may operate as a temporal integrator as well. An initial calcium signal may activate the cAMP gate and the PKC/NG system, allowing for enhanced responsiveness to a subsequent calcium signal when it arrives.

In fact, data from the Huang's laboratories investigating neurogranin knockout mice suggest directly that this is a role for this system—the augmentation of potentiating responses with repetitive stimulation (87, 89).

VII. LTP INDUCTION COMPONENT 6—THE MECHANISMS FOR THE GENERATION OF THE ACTUAL PERSISTING BIOCHEMICAL SIGNALS

Point number 6 begins a transition. Thus far, we have been discussing the mechanisms for regulating postsynaptic calcium and its immediate effectors, mechanism that determine if an LTP-inducing level of calcium is reached. Point 6 transitions us into the mechanisms whereby this triggering level of calcium is converted into a persisting signal that maintains LTP. As described in the beginning of the chapter, the details of these mechanisms are dealt with in Chapter 7 (for E-LTP) and Chapter 8 (for L-LTP). In addition in those chapters, we will discuss the targets of the persisting signals that result in the expression of LTP physiologically.

VIII. SUMMARY—MODELS FOR BIOCHEMICAL INFORMATION PROCESSING IN LTP INDUCTION

In this chapter, we have discussed five categories of molecular components and processes that are involved in LTP induction. It is *very* important not to think of

these in isolation from each other—they are functional categories to help organize the complex biochemical machinery of LTP induction, not compartmentalized biochemical processes in the cell! It is a useful intellectual exercise to think up ways to mix and match the categories and allow them to interact. The interactions of these various processes are what allow the synapse to serve in its role as a molecular decision maker.

We need to begin to think of the synapse as an immensely complicated information processing machine. It integrates a plethora of biochemical signals and computes, based on a number of molecular inputs, whether to trigger a lasting molecular change. This model of synaptic function allows for the necessary sophistication required for triggering memory formation in the animal in vivo. By way of providing a summary and overview for this chapter, I will finish up with a specific example of how these processes might interact. Please keep in mind that this example is illustrative and somewhat speculative.

A. Four-Way Coincidence Detection

This example is a combination of the NMDA receptor in its classical role, the cAMP gate, PKC activation of ERK, and potassium channel regulation by ERK. CaMKII activation is taken for our purposes as necessary for LTP induction, as we will discuss in the next chapter. The model is actually not even a far-fetched idea; it draws directly from data published by Manny Landau and colleagues (1, 79), Danny Winder and his collaborators (3), Tom O'Dell's group (2), and several of my colleagues (32–35). The model is schematized in Figure 8.

Imagine that LTP is going to be triggered by a back-propagating action potential (bpAP), caused in response to strong firing at a distal synapse, coupled with local synaptic glutamate. As we have discussed,

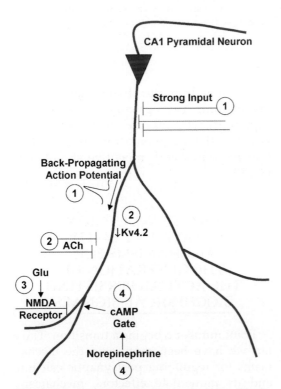

FIGURE 8 Four-way coincidence detection. This is an illustration of a model of one possible interaction of the NMDA receptor's activity, the cAMP gate, PKC activation of ERK, and K channel regulation by ERK. See summary in text for explanation

this is because NMDA receptor activation is going to require bpAP-associated membrane depolarization coupled with synaptic glutamate at the synapse of interest. In addition, imagine that Kv4.2 channels would limit the capacity of the bpAP to reach the synapse and thus depolarize the NMDA receptor, except that a PLC/PKC-coupled muscarinic ACh receptor has activated ERK and down-regulated these channels. Thus, the muscarinic receptor has gated the bpAP and allowed it to enter the relevant dendritic region. Let's say there's modest NMDA receptor activation and the calcium influx through the NMDA receptor would be insufficient to cause robust CaMKII activation (and hence LTP), except that the cAMP gate has been opened in the vicinity due to local beta-adrenergic receptor activation by NE. This amplification allows robust CaMKII activation and LTP induction.

In this example, a strong synaptic input, plus a weak synaptic input and two neuromodulatory inputs, has uniquely triggered lasting synaptic plasticity: four-way coincidence detection. It is a molecular analogue of a common behavioral situation: an aroused animal (NE) receiving a salient environmental cue (strong synaptic input) at the peak of the theta rhythm (ACh) coupled with a second sensory signal (weak synaptic input). The resulting increase in synaptic strength might contribute to the animal forming an associative memory for the event.

It's also completely straightforward to construct a five-way coincidence detection system. All that you have to do is add one more of the components described in this chapter—synergistic activation of ERK by two receptors, BDNF modulation of presynaptic glutamate release, or Ephrin modulation of NMDA receptor function via src. With longer-lasting extracellular signals like the Ephrins or reelin or BDNF, it is easy to construct a temporal component to the model so that the synapse can determine its set-point for LTP based on its recent history, or the recent history of other nearby neurons.

The point of these examples is to illustrate how the molecular complexity of LTP induction can require that a precise and multifactorial set of conditions be met in order to trigger plasticity. This allows for sophisticated information processing at the synaptic level. It allows for complex decision making at the molecular and cellular level. The complex biochemical machinery of the synapse allows for a complicated logic to operate in determining whether a persisting effect is triggered in the CNS. Moreover, while we have focused on hippocampal LTP specifically, these issues and mechanisms are almost certainly involved in hippocampus-dependent learning in the intact animal and at a variety of sites outside the hippocampus, for example the cortex and amygdala. We will return to this issue in Chapter 9.

As a final parting comment, I will note that in my estimation the Hebb model concerning activity-dependent synaptic plasticity in the CNS is inadequate. Strengthening of synaptic connections simply based upon repetitive firing is insufficient to account for memory formation in my opinion. This line of thought comes out of considering all the many processes we have discussed in this chapter. The molecular complexity of LTP induction has implications for thinking about memory formation in general terms. The synapse is a complex signal integration machine. To integrate information and decide whether to change its state, it responds to multiple signals, and its recent history. It's not just static and it's not just Hebbian. I posit that, in the functioning hippocampus, one presynaptic terminal merely consistently or repeatedly participating in the firing of a postsynaptic neuron typically is not enough to trigger plasticity—many more factors come into play, factors that are critical in allowing the synapse sufficient computational power to perform sophisticated information processing.

References

1. Brown, G. P., Blitzer, R. D., Connor, J. H., Wong, T., Shenolikar, S., Iyengar, R., and Landau, E. M. (2000). "Long-term potentiation induced by theta frequency stimulation is regulated by a protein phosphatase-1-operated gate." *J. Neurosci.* 20:7880–7887.

2. Watabe, A. M., Zaki, P. A., and O'Dell, T. J. (2000). "Coactivation of beta-adrenergic and cholinergic receptors enhances the induction of long-term potentiation and synergistically activates mitogen-activated protein kinase in the hippocampal CA1 region." *J. Neurosci.* 20:5924–5931.

3. Winder, D. G., Martin, K. C., Muzzio, I. A., Rohrer, D., Chruscinski, A., Kobilka, B., and Kandel, E. R. (1999). "ERK plays a regulatory role in induction of LTP by theta frequency stimulation and its modulation by beta-adrenergic receptors." *Neuron* 24:715–726.

4. Raymond, L. A., Tingley, W. G., Blackstone, C. D., Roche, K. W., and Huganir, R. L. (1994). "Glutamate receptor modulation by protein phosphorylation." *J. Physiol. Paris* 88:181–192.

5. Suzuki, T., and Okumura-Noji, K. (1995). "NMDA receptor subunits epsilon 1 (NR2A) and epsilon 2 (NR2B) are substrates for Fyn in the postsynaptic density fraction isolated from the rat brain." *Biochem. Biophys. Res. Commun.* 216:582–588.

6. Zheng, F., Gingrich, M. B., Traynelis, S. F., and Conn, P. J. (1998). "Tyrosine kinase potentiates NMDA receptor currents by reducing tonic zinc inhibition." *Nat. Neurosci.* 1:185–191.

7. Lu, Y. M., Roder, J. C., Davidow, J., and Salter, M. W. (1998). "Src activation in the induction of long-term potentiation in CA1 hippocampal neurons." *Science* 279:1363–1367.

8. Huang, Y., Lu, W., Ali, D. W., Pelkey, K. A., Pitcher, G. M., Lu, Y. M., Aoto, H., Roder, J. C., Sasaki, T., Salter, M. W., and MacDonald, J. F. (2001). "CAKbeta/Pyk2 kinase is a signaling link for induction of long-term potentiation in CA1 hippocampus." *Neuron* 29:485–496.

9. Grosshans, D. R., and Browning, M. D. (2001). "Protein kinase C activation induces tyrosine phosphorylation of the NR2A and NR2B subunits of the NMDA receptor." *J. Neurochem.* 76:737–744.

10. Takasu, M. A., Dalva, M. B., Zigmond, R. E., and Greenberg, M. E. (2002). "Modulation of NMDA receptor-dependent calcium influx and gene expression through EphB receptors." *Science* 295:491–495.

11. Grunwald, I. C., Korte, M., Wolfer, D., Wilkinson, G. A., Unsicker, K., Lipp, H. P., Bonhoeffer, T., and Klein, R. (2001). "Kinase-Independent Requirement of EphB2 Receptors in Hippocampal Synaptic Plasticity." *Neuron* 32:1027–1040.

12. Henderson, J. T., Georgiou, J., Jia, Z., Robertson, J., Elowe, S., Roder, J. C., and Pawson, T. (2001). "The Receptor Tyrosine Kinase EphB2 Regulates NMDA-Dependent Synaptic Function." *Neuron* 32:1041–1056.

13. Shanley, L. J., Irving, A. J., and Harvey, J. (2001). "Leptin enhances NMDA receptor function and modulates hippocampal synaptic plasticity." *J. Neurosci.* 21:RC186.

14. Yaka, R., Thornton, C., Vagts, A. J., Phamluong, K., Bonci, A., and Ron, D. (2002). "NMDA receptor function is regulated by the inhibitory scaffolding protein, RACK1." *Proc. Natl. Acad. Sci. USA* 99:5710–5715.

15. Liao, G. Y., Kreitzer, M. A., Sweetman, B. J., and Leonard, J. P. (2000). "The postsynaptic density protein PSD-95 differentially regulates insulin- and Src-mediated current modulation of mouse NMDA receptors expressed in Xenopus oocytes." *J. Neurochem.* 75:282–287.

16. Logan, S. M., Rivera, F. E., and Leonard, J. P. (1999). "Protein kinase C modulation of recombinant NMDA receptor currents: roles for the C-terminal C1 exon and calcium ions." *J. Neurosci.* 19:974–986.

17. Liao, G. Y., Wagner, D. A., Hsu, M. H., and Leonard, J. P. (2001). "Evidence for direct protein kinase-C mediated modulation of N-methyl-D-aspartate receptor current." *Mol. Pharmacol.* 59:960–964.

18. Ben-Ari, Y., Aniksztejn, L., and Bregestovski, P. (1992). "Protein kinase C modulation of NMDA currents: an important link for LTP induction." *Trends Neurosci.* 15:333–339.

19. Westphal, R. S., Tavalin, S. J., Lin, J. W., Alto, N. M., Fraser, I. D., Langeberg, L. K., Sheng, M., and Scott, J. D. (1999). "Regulation of NMDA receptors by an associated phosphatase-kinase signaling complex." *Science* 285:93–96.

20. Fischer, A., Sananbenesi, F., Schrick, C., Spiess, J., and Radulovic, J. (2002). "Cyclin-dependent kinase 5 is required for associative learning." *J. Neurosci.* 22:3700–3707.

21. Li, B. S., Sun, M. K., Zhang, L., Takahashi, S., Ma, W., Vinade, L., Kulkarni, A. B., Brady, R. O., and Pant, H. C. (2001). "Regulation of NMDA receptors by cyclin-dependent kinase-5." *Proc. Natl. Acad. Sci. USA* 98:12742–12747.

22. Choi, Y. B., Tenneti, L., Le, D. A., Ortiz, J., Bai, G., Chen, H. S., and Lipton, S. A. (2000). "Molecular basis of NMDA receptor-coupled ion channel modulation by S-nitrosylation." *Nat. Neurosci.* 3:15–21.

23. Choi, Y. B., and Lipton, S. A. (2000). "Redox modulation of the NMDA receptor." *Cell. Mol. Life Sci.* 57:1535–1541.

24. Traynelis, S. F., Hartley, M., and Heinemann, S. F. (1995). "Control of proton sensitivity of the NMDA receptor by RNA splicing and polyamines." *Science* 268:873–876.

25. Gallagher, M. J., Huang, H., Grant, E. R., and Lynch, D. R. (1997). "The NR2B-specific interactions of polyamines and protons with the N-methyl-D-aspartate receptor." *J. Biol. Chem.* 272:24971–24979.

26. Lieberman, D. N., and Mody, I. (1999). "Casein kinase-II regulates NMDA channel function in hippocampal neurons." *Nat. Neurosci.* 2:125–132.

27. Charriaut-Marlangue, C., Otani, S., Creuzet, C., Ben-Ari, Y., Loeb, J. (1991). "Rapid activation of hippocampal casein kinase II during long-term potentiation." *Proc. Natl. Acad. Sci. USA* 88:10232–10236.

28. Ingi, T., Worley, P. F., and Lanahan, A. A. (2001) "Regulation of SSAT expression by synaptic activity." *Eur. J. Neurosci.* 13:1459–1463.

29. Stuart, G. J., and Sakmann, B. (1994). "Active propagation of somatic action potentials into neocortical pyramidal cell dendrites." *Nature* 367:69–72.

30. Spruston, N., Schiller, Y., Stuart, G., and Sakmann, B. (1995). "Activity-dependent action potential invasion and calcium influx into hippocampal CA1 dendrites." *Science* 268:297–300.

31. Magee, J. C., and Johnston, D. (1995). "Synaptic activation of voltage-gated channels in the dendrites of hippocampal pyramidal neurons." *Science* 268:301–304.

32. Hoffman, D. A., Magee, J. C., Colbert, C. M., and Johnston, D. (1997). "K^+ channel regulation of signal propagation in dendrites of hippocampal pyramidal neurons." *Nature* 387:869–875.

33. Yuan, L. L., Adams, J. P., Swank, M., Sweatt, J. D., and Johnston, D. (2002). "Protein kinase modulation of dendritic K^+ channels in hippocampus involves a mitogen-activated protein kinase pathway." *J. Neurosci.* 22:4860–4868.

34. Watanabe, S., Hoffman, D. A., Migliore, M., and Johnston, D. (2002). "Dendritic K^+ channels contribute to spike-timing dependent long-term potentiation in hippocampal pyramidal neurons." *Proc. Natl. Acad. Sci. USA* 99:8366–8371.

35. Adams, J. P., Anderson, A. E., Varga, A. W., Dineley, K. T., Cook, R. G., Pfaffinger, P. J., and Sweatt, J. D. (2000). "The A-type potassium channel Kv4.2 is a substrate for the mitogen-activated protein kinase ERK." *J. Neurochem.* 2000, 75:2277–2287.

36. Magee, J. C. (1998). "Dendritic hyperpolarization-activated currents modify the integrative properties of hippocampal CA1 pyramidal neurons." *J. Neurosci.* 18:7613–7624.

37. Colbert, C. M., and Johnston, D. (1998). "Protein kinase C activation decreases activity-dependent attenuation of dendritic Na^+ current in hippocampal CA1 pyramidal neurons." *J. Neurophysiol.* 79:491–495.

38. Tsubokawa, H. (2000). "Control of Na^+ spike backpropagation by intracellular signaling in the pyramidal neuron dendrites." *Mol. Neurobiol.* 22:129–141.

39. Andreasen, M., and Nedergaard, S. (1996). "Dendritic electrogenesis in rat hippocampal CA1 pyramidal neurons: functional aspects of Na^+ and Ca^{2+} currents in apical dendrites." *Hippocampus* 6:79–95.

40. Martin, K. H., Slack, J. K., Boerner, S. A., Martin, C. C., and Parsons, J. T. (2002). "Integrin connections map: to infinity and beyond." *Science* 296:1652–1653.

41. Davis, R., and Weeber, E. J. (2001): Personal Communication.

42. Lauri, S. E., Kaukinen, S., Kinnunen, T., Ylinen, A., Imai, S., Kaila, K., Taira, T., and Rauvala, H. (1999). "Regulatory role and molecular interactions of a cell-surface heparan sulfate proteoglycan (N-syndecan) in hippocampal long-term potentiation." *J. Neurosci.* 19:1226–1235.

43. Bliss, T., Errington, M., Fransen, E., Godfraind, J. M., Kauer, J. A., Kooy, R. F., Maness, P. F., and Furley, A. J. (2000). "Long-term potentiation in mice lacking the neural cell adhesion molecule L1." *Curr. Biol.* 10:1607–1610.

44. Holst BD, Vanderklish PW, Krushel LA, Zhou W, Langdon RB, McWhirter JR, Edelman GM, Crossin KL: "Allosteric modulation of AMPA-type glutamate receptors increases activity of the promoter for the neural cell adhesion molecule, N-CAM." *Proc. Natl. Acad. Sci. USA* 1998, 95:2597–2602.

45. Luthl, A., Laurent, J. P., Figurov, A., Muller, D., and Schachner, M. (1994). "Hippocampal long term potentiation and neural cell adhesion molecules L1 and NCAM." *Nature* 372:777–779.

46. Huntley, G. W., Gil, O., and Bozdagi, O. (2002). "The cadherin family of cell adhesion molecules: multiple roles in synaptic plasticity." *Neuroscientist* 8:221–233.

47. Sheng, M., and Pak, D. T. (2000). "Ligand-gated ion channel interactions with cytoskeletal and signaling proteins." *Annu. Rev. Physiol.* 62:755–778.

48. Sheng, M. (2001). "Molecular organization of the postsynaptic specialization." *Proc. Natl. Acad. Sci. USA* 98:7058–7061.

49. Migaud, M., Charlesworth, P., Dempster, M., Webster, L. C., Watabe, A. M., Makhinson, M., He, Y., Ramsay, M. F., Morris, R. G., Morrison, J. H., O'Dell, T. J., and Grant, S. G. (1998). "Enhanced long-term potentiation and impaired learning in mice with mutant postsynaptic density-95 protein." *Nature* 396:433–439.

50. Sprengel, R., Suchanek, B., Amico, C., Brusa, R., Burnashev, N., Rozov, A., Hvalby, O., Jensen, V., Paulsen, O., Andersen, P., Kim, J. J., Thompson, R. F., Sun, W., Webster, L. C., Grant, S. G., Eilers, J., Konnerth, A., Li, J., McNamara, J. O., and Seeburg, P. H. (1998). "Importance of the intracellular domain of NR2 subunits for NMDA receptor function in vivo." *Cell.* 92:279–289.

51. Passafaro, M., Piech, V., and Sheng, M. (2001). "Subunit-specific temporal and spatial patterns of AMPA receptor exocytosis in hippocampal neurons." *Nat. Neurosci.* 4:917–926.

52. Sweatt, J. D. (2001). "Protooncogenes subserve memory formation in the adult CNS." *Neuron* 31:671–674.

53. Vetter, I. R., and Wittinghofer, A. (2001). "The guanine nucleotide-binding switch in three dimensions." *Science* 294:1299–1304.

54. Colledge, M., Dean, R. A., Scott, G. K., Langeberg, L. K., Huganir, R. L., and Scott, J. D. (2000). "Targeting of PKA to glutamate receptors through a MAGUK-AKAP complex." *Neuron* 27:107–119.

55. Coghlan, V. M., Perrino, B. A., Howard, M., Langeberg, L. K., Hicks, J. B., Gallatin, W. M., and Scott, J. D. (1995). "Association of protein kinase A and protein phosphatase 2B with a common anchoring protein." *Science* 267:108–111.

56. Dodge, K., and Scott, J. D. (2000). "AKAP79 and the evolution of the AKAP model." *FEBS Lett.* 476:58–61.

57. Tavalin, S. J., Colledge, M., Hell, J. W., Langeberg, L. K., Huganir, R. L., and Scott, J. D. (2002). "Regulation of GluR1 by the A-kinase anchoring protein 79 (AKAP79) signaling complex shares properties with long-term depression." *J. Neurosci.* 22:3044–3051.

58. Sabatini, B. L., Oertner, T. G., and Svoboda, K. (2002). "The life cycle of Ca$^{(2+)}$ ions in dendritic spines." *Neuron* 33:439–452.

59. Wheeler, D. B., Randall, A., and Tsien, R. W. (1994). "Roles of N-type and Q-type Ca^{2+} channels in supporting hippocampal synaptic transmission." *Science* 264:107–111.

60. Huang, Y. Y., and Malenka, R. C. (1993). "Examination of TEA-induced synaptic enhancement in area CA1 of the hippocampus: the role of voltage-dependent Ca^{2+} channels in the induction of LTP." *J. Neurosci.* 13:568–576.

61. Morgan, S. L., and Teyler, T. J. (1999). "VDCCs and NMDARs underlie two forms of LTP in CA1 hippocampus in vivo." *J. Neurophysiol.* 82:736–740.

62. Ito, K., Miura, M., Furuse, H., Zhixiong, C., Kato, H., Yasutomi, D., Inoue, T., Mikoshiba, K., Kimura, T., Sakakibara, S., and Miyakawa, H. (1995). "Voltage-gated Ca^{2+} channel blockers, omega-AgaIVA and Ni^{2+}, suppress the induction of theta-burst induced long-term potentiation in guinea-pig hippocampal CA1 neurons." *Neurosci. Lett.* 183:112–115.

63. Dudek, S. M., and Fields, R. D. (2001). "Mitogen-activated protein kinase/extracellular signal-regulated kinase activation in somatodendritic compartments: roles of action potentials, frequency, and mode of calcium entry." *J. Neurosci.* 21:RC122.

64. Magee, J. C., and Johnston, D. (1997). "A synaptically controlled, associative signal for Hebbian plasticity in hippocampal neurons." *Science* 275:209–213.

65. Chetkovich, D. M., Gray, R., Johnston, D., and Sweatt, J. D. (1991). "N-methyl-D-aspartate receptor activation increases cAMP levels and voltage-gated Ca^{2+} channel activity in area CA1 of hippocampus." *Proc. Natl. Acad. Sci. USA* 88:6467–6471.

66. Johenning, F. W., and Ehrlich, B. E. (2002). "Signaling microdomains: InsP(3) receptor localization takes on new meaning." *Neuron* 34:173–175.

67. Emptage, N., Bliss, T. V., and Fine, A. (1999). "Single synaptic events evoke NMDA receptor-mediated release of calcium from internal stores in hippocampal dendritic spines." *Neuron* 22:115–124.

68. Behnisch, T., and Reymann, K. G. (1995). "Thapsigargin blocks long-term potentiation induced by weak, but not strong tetanisation in rat hippocampal CA1 neurons." *Neurosci. Lett.* 192:185–188.

69. Harvey, J., and Collingridge, G. L. (1992). "Thapsigargin blocks the induction of long-term potentiation in rat hippocampal slices." *Neurosci. Lett.* 139:197–200.

70. Balschun, D., Wolfer, D. P., Bertocchini, F., Barone, V., Conti, A., Zuschratter, W., Missiaen, L., Lipp, H. P., Frey, J. U., and Sorrentino, V. (1999). "Deletion of the ryanodine receptor type 3 (RyR3) impairs forms of synaptic plasticity and spatial learning." *Embo. J.* 18:5264–5273.

71. Shimuta, M., Yoshikawa, M., Fukaya, M., Watanabe, M., Takeshima, H., and Manabe, T. (2001). "Postsynaptic modulation of AMPA receptor-mediated synaptic responses and LTP by the type 3 ryanodine receptor." *Mol. Cell. Neurosci.* 17:921–930.

72. Nishiyama, M., Hong, K., Mikoshiba, K., Poo, M. M., and Kato, K. (2000). "Calcium stores regulate the polarity and input specificity of synaptic modification." *Nature* 408:584–588.

73. Futatsugi, A., Kato, K., Ogura, H., Li, S. T., Nagata, E., Kuwajima, G., Tanaka, K., Itohara, S., and Mikoshiba, K. (1999). "Facilitation of NMDAR-independent LTP and spatial learning in mutant mice lacking ryanodine receptor type 3." *Neuron* 24:701–713.

74. Fujii, S., Matsumoto, M., Igarashi, K., Kato, H., and Mikoshiba, K. (2000). "Synaptic plasticity in hippocampal CA1 neurons of mice lacking type 1 inositol-1,4,5-trisphosphate receptors." *Learn. Mem.* 7:312–320.

75. Weeber, E. J., Levy, M., Sampson, M. J., Anflous, K., Armstrong, D. L., Brown, S. E., Sweatt, J. D., and Craigen, W. J. (2002). "The role of mitochondrial porins and the permeability transition pore in learning and synaptic plasticity." *J. Biol. Chem.* 277:18891–18897.

76. Levy, M. (2002). Personal Communication.

77. Blitzer, R. D., Connor, J. H., Brown, G. P., Wong, T., Shenolikar, S., Iyengar, R., and Landau, E. M. (1998). "Gating of CaMKII by cAMP-regulated protein phosphatase activity during LTP." *Science* 280:1940–1942.

78. Winder, D. G., and Sweatt, J. D. (2001). "Roles of serine/threonine phosphatases in hippocampal synaptic plasticity." *Nat. Rev. Neurosci.* 2:461–474.

79. Giovannini, M. G., Blitzer, R. D., Wong, T., Asoma, K., Tsokas, P., Morrison, J. H., Iyengar, R., and Landau, E. M. (2001). "Mitogen-activated protein kinase regulates early phosphorylation and delayed expression of Ca^{2+}/calmodulin-dependent protein kinase II in long-term potentiation." *J. Neurosci.* 21:7053–7062.

80. Winder, D. G., Mansuy, I. M., Osman, M., Moallem, T. M., and Kandel, E. R. (1998). "Genetic and pharmacological evidence for a novel, intermediate phase of long-term potentiation suppressed by calcineurin." *Cell.* 92:25–37.

81. Malleret, G., Haditsch, U., Genoux, D., Jones, M. W., Bliss, T. V., Vanhoose, A. M., Weitlauf, C., Kandel, E. R., Winder, D. G., and Mansuy, I. M. (2001). "Inducible and reversible enhancement of learning, memory, and long-term potentiation by genetic inhibition of calcineurin." *Cell.* 104:675–686.

82. Gerendasy, D. D., and Sutcliffe, J. G. (1997). "RC3/ neurogranin, a postsynaptic calpacitin for setting the response threshold to calcium influxes." *Mol. Neurobiol.* 15:131–163.

83. Ramakers, G. M., Pasinelli, P., van Beest, M., van der Slot, A., Gispen, W. H., and De Graan, P. N. (2000). "Activation of pre- and postsynaptic protein kinase C during tetraethylammonium-induced long-term potentiation in the CA1 field of the hippocampus." *Neurosci. Lett.* 286:53–56.

84. Chen, S. J., Sweatt, J. D., and Klann, E. (1997). "Enhanced phosphorylation of the postsynaptic protein kinase C substrate RC3/neurogranin during long-term potentiation." *Brain Res.* 749:181–187.

85. Ramakers, G. M., Gerendasy, D. D., and de Graan, P. N. (1999). "Substrate phosphorylation in the protein kinase Cgamma knockout mouse." *J. Biol. Chem.* 274:1873–1874.

86. Krucker, T., Siggins, G. R., McNamara, R. K., Lindsley, K. A., Dao, A., Allison, D. W., De Lecea, L., Lovenberg, T. W., Sutcliffe, J. G., and Gerendasy, D. D. (2002). "Targeted disruption of RC3 reveals a calmodulin-based mechanism for regulating metaplasticity in the hippocampus." *J. Neurosci.* 22:5525–5535.

87. Wu, J., Li, J., Huang, K. P., and Huang, F. L. (2002). "Attenuation of protein kinase C and cAMP-dependent protein kinase signal transduction in the neurogranin knockout mouse." *J. Biol. Chem.* 277:19498–19505.

88. Wang, J. H., and Kelly, P. T. (1995). "Postsynaptic injection of CA^{2+}/CaM induces synaptic potentiation requiring CaMKII and PKC activity." *Neuron* 15:443–452.

89. Pak, J. H., Huang, F. L., Li, J., Balschun, D., Reymann, K. G., Chiang, C., Westphal, H., and Huang, K. P. (2000). "Involvement of neurogranin in the modulation of calcium/calmodulin-dependent protein kinase II, synaptic plasticity, and spatial learning: a study with knockout mice." *Proc. Natl. Acad. Sci. USA* 97:11232–11237.

90. Husi, H., Ward, M. A., Choudhary, J. S., Blackstock, W. P., and Grant, S. G. (2000). "Proteomic analysis of NMDA receptor-adhesion protein signaling complexes." *Nat. Neurosci.* 3:661–669.

91. Husi, H., and Grant, S. G. (2001). "Proteomics of the nervous system." *Trends Neurosci.* 2001, 24:259–266.

92. Adams, J. P., and Sweatt, J. D. (2002). "Molecular psychology: roles for the ERK MAP kinase cascade in memory." *Annu. Rev. Pharmacol. Toxicol.* 42:135–163.

93. Sweatt, J. D. (2001). "Memory mechanisms: the yin and yang of protein phosphorylation." *Curr. Biol.* 11:R391–394.

94. Weeber, E. J., and Sweatt, J. D. (2002). "Molecular neurobiology of human cognition." *Neuron* 33:845–848.

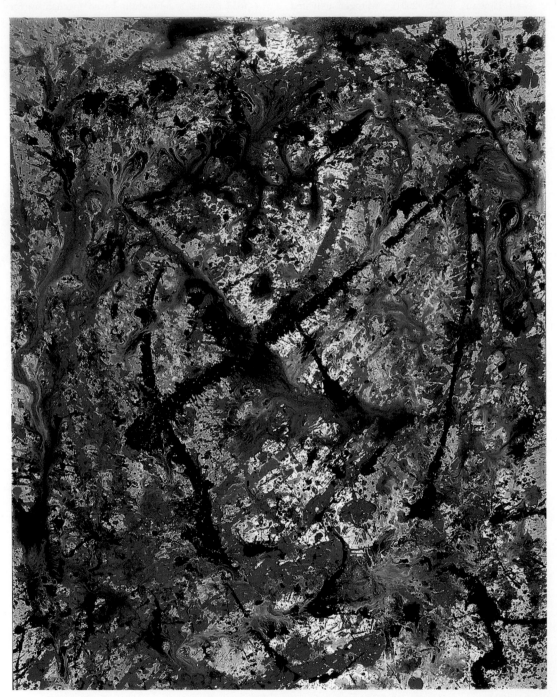

Autonomous Kinases in the PSD

J. David Sweatt, Acrylic on canvas, 2002

Biochemical Mechanisms for Short-Term Information Storage at the Cellular Level

Chapter Overview

In the last chapter, we discussed the complex mechanisms and biochemical "computations" involved in deciding whether an LTP-inducing level of calcium will be reached postsynaptically. In this chapter, we will deal with the first stages of those processes that are actually triggered by that calcium signal when it is attained. In essence, this chapter deals with the transition of LTP *induction* mechanisms into the *maintenance and expression* of LTP. For this chapter, we will deal specifically with the early stage of LTP, E-LTP. In the next chapter we will move on to later stages of LTP and the unique biochemical processes involved in L-LTP.

In this chapter, we begin to deal with the fundamental biochemical problem that has to be solved in order for memory to exist— the generation of a persisting biochemical signal by a transient inducing stimulus. In many ways, this is the heart of the matter for memory at the molecular level, the reduction of the problem to its smallest finite components. We will deal specifically in this chapter with the issue of how a transient calcium signal gets converted to a persisting biochemical trace in a CA1 pyramidal neuron. Almost all the mechanisms we will discuss have been studied in the context of NMDA receptor-dependent LTP, predominantly that form induced with 100-Hz tetanic stimulation. Of course, we also will draw extensively from in vitro biochemical studies of relevant molecular processes to round out our understanding of the biochemistry relevant to LTP.

A second issue we will deal with in this chapter is how the biochemical traces involved in maintaining E-LTP get converted into potentiation of synaptic transmission. These are the mechanisms of E-LTP expression. For the most part, this means discussing mechanisms of augmenting AMPA receptor function, although we also will touch on facilitation of presynaptic glutamate release and potential alterations in postsynaptic excitability.

The standard demarcation for distinguishing E-LTP from L-LTP is dependency upon new protein synthesis and altered gene expression, and I will use this criterion for defining the scope of this chapter. E-LTP is typically defined as being independent of new protein synthesis (1, 2). You should realize, however, that this is by no means a universally accepted idea. Various opinions run the gamut. At one end of the spectrum is the idea that some mechanisms for E-LTP are also dependent upon new protein synthesis. A specific example of this is Todd Sacktor's data indicating that de novo synthesis of an active fragment of PKC-zeta is involved in E-LTP maintenance, and I will cover this topic in this chapter. At the other end of the spectrum is the idea that no alterations in gene expression or protein synthesis are necessary for any phase of LTP. I also will discuss this idea briefly in this chapter, and we will return to a more theoretical treatment of the idea in the last chapter of the book. Please note that no one believes that E-LTP maintenance is independent of protein *synthesis*—at a minimum replenishment of proteins as

they are degraded is necessary for maintaining any cellular function. What is at issue is whether alterations from baseline protein synthesis (or gene expression) are necessary—hence the use of the terms "*new* protein synthesis" and "*altered* gene expression."

By and large, however, we will be limiting our discussion to mechanisms operating in E-LTP that are independent of altered protein synthesis. This interpretation is implicit to the oft-replicated observation that E-LTP can be maintained in the face of effective concentrations of protein synthesis inhibitors. This means that we will by definition be limiting our discussion in this chapter to persisting post-translational modifications of proteins. This biochemical reality helps keep the list of possible relevant mechanisms more manageable. After all, there are a finite number of possible chemical reactions in which the twenty amino acids of a protein can participate. A brief listing of known post-translational modifications of proteins[1] likely will be helpful at this point:

- Phosphorylation and dephosphorylation of serine, threonine, and tyrosine side chains
- Proteolysis—breaking the peptide amide bond of the backbone
- Oxidation and reduction of cysteine side chains (includes S-S bond formation)
- Nitrosylation of tyrosine and cysteine side chains
- ADP-ribosylation of arginine side chains
- Ubiquitination of lysine side chains
- Acetylation of lysine side chains
- Prolyl cis-trans isomerization

This is the list of candidates that we get to choose from in thinking about mechanisms for generating persisting, post-translational

---

[1] I am leaving out several of the more exotic and esoteric examples, including N-terminal acylation reactions of a variety of sorts (e.g., myristoylation), C-terminal farnesylation, cysteine palmitoylation, lysine methylation, and proline hydroxylation, plus the entire category of glycosylation reactions.

biochemical signals in cells. Of course, phosphorylation has been studied the most extensively, and we'll spend most of our time talking about phosphorylation-related mechanisms. However, any and all of these are possible mechanisms for making a persisting signal in a neuron, and the resourcefulness of evolution in capitalizing on all the tools available in the toolbox is legendary. In fact, there is direct or indirect evidence for all the mechanisms listed here as being involved in synaptic plasticity in the adult CNS (references 3, 4, and 5, and the rest of this chapter), and all but the last two have been directly implicated in NMDA receptor-dependent LTP in area CA1 (so far). It will be interesting to see what the future has in store for us as our understanding increases concerning the roles of these various processes in memory storage.

CHAPTER OVERVIEW

The chapter will be broken down into three broad sections (see Figure 1). The first section will deal with two well-established targets of the triggering calcium for LTP—CaMKII and PKC. In this section, I will focus principally on the known mechanisms for generation of persistently activated forms of these kinases, forms of the molecules that are capable of serving as molecular memory traces in LTP and memory in

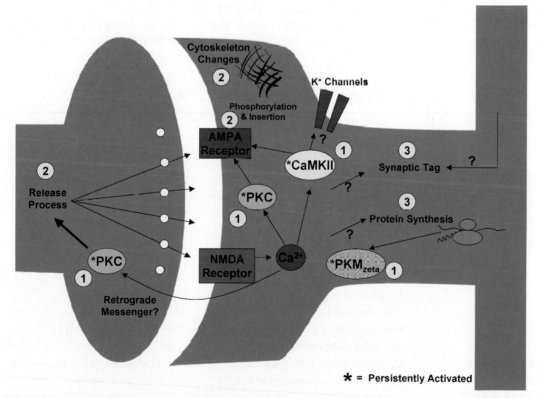

FIGURE 1 Chapter summary. This chapter deals with three primary issues related to mechanisms for E-LTP. First, describing mechanisms for generating and maintaining persisting signals at the synapse (1). Second, discussing molecular sites of action of these persisting signals that operate in the expression of E-LTP (2). Third, reviewing some of the mechanisms involved in the regulation of local dendritic protein synthesis and synaptic tagging, mechanisms involved in the E-LTP to L-LTP transition (3).

general. This, then, deals with E-LTP main-tenance. The second section of the chapter will deal with potential effectors of the persistently activated kinases: postsynaptic glutamate receptors, the presynaptic release mechanism, and the cytoskeleton. This section deals with mechanisms of E-LTP expression. The final section deals with dendritic protein synthesis plus the idea that synaptic "tags" are generated in response to LTP-inducing stimulation. This is not a component of E-LTP per se, but rather is a mechanism likely to contribute to the E-LTP-to-L-LTP transition. It may be helpful to think of the generation of synaptic tags and the regulation of local protein synthesis as a parallel mechanism triggered by some of the events associated with E-LTP induction (or maintenance). These parallel mechanisms also entail an early and persisting signal but are basi-cally a complex part of the initial stage of L-LTP induction.

I. TARGETS OF THE CALCIUM TRIGGER

We discussed in the last chapter the elaborate mechanisms involved in gener-ating a level of postsynaptic calcium suf-ficient to trigger LTP. What is it that this calcium signal does? The potential direct targets of the calcium signal are listed in Table 1. Obviously any direct target of the calcium signal has to be a calcium-binding protein. While there are a number of calcium-binding proteins in cells, based on the known functional categories of calcium-binding proteins and those that have been implicated in LTP, there are four proteins we need to pay particular attention to: calmodulin, PKC(s), calpain, and phospholipases. In this section of the chapter, we will discuss these four proteins and their targets, focusing mostly on CaM-regulated kinases and PKC because

TABLE 1   Potential Targets of the Ca^{2+} Signal

	Effect	Role
Calmodulin		
CaMKII α and β	Kinase activation	LTP induction/maintenance
CaMKIV	Kinase activation	Possibly L-LTP induction
ACI & VIII	cAMP production	Induction
NOS	NO, O_2^- production	Retrograde signals? Ras?
PKC and its targets		
α	Kinase activation	?
βI	Kinase activation	Not 100 Hz LTP
βII	Kinase activation	Not 100 Hz LTP
γ	Kinase activation	Induction
ζ	Kinase activation (not direct Ca^{2+} target)	Induction & maintenance
PHOX Proteins	O_2^- production (not direct Ca^{2+} target)	Phosphatase inhibitor/PKC activator
Calpain	Proteolysis of the cytoskeleton? GRIP?	Structural rearrangement
Phospholipases		
PLA$_2$	AA release	Retrograde signals
PLC	DAG release	PKC activation, pre and post

"Induction" mechanisms refer to the many processes reviewed in Chapter 6.

these have by far been the most extensively studied in the context of E-LTP.

Interestingly, CaM and the calcium-binding isoforms of PKC are the prototype molecules for the two major categories of calcium-binding proteins (see Figure 2). Each of these molecules has calcium-binding domains in their structure that define whole families of calcium-binding proteins. CaM is the prototype molecule for the "E-F hand" family of calcium-binding proteins. The E-F hand terminology derives

from esoteric naming of the calcium-binding domain based on a lettered alpha-helix nomenclature (the E-F part), coupled with the fact that the domain could be modeled to look like a human hand in a specific configuration. (OK, since you asked, the hand configuration is the classic "six-shooter" configuration that boys use when they want to pretend to shoot each other). As a first approximation, you can think of the E-F hand structure as the generic calcium binding domain in proteins. A wide variety

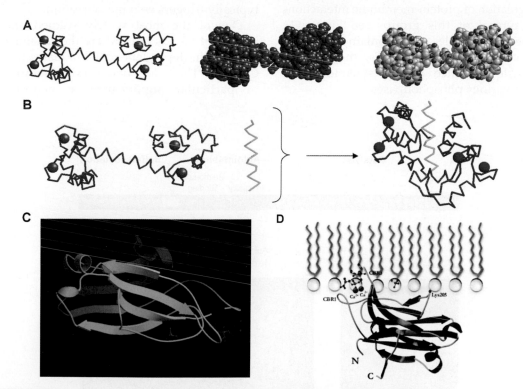

FIGURE 2 Structures of calcium-binding proteins. (A) This panel gives three views of calcium (red spheres) bound to calmodulin, illustrating the structure of the E-F-hand subtype of calcium-binding protein. The first rendering shows the peptide backbone of calmodulin in dark blue. The second rendering is identical to the first except that the calmodulin structure is illustrated in space-filling spheres. The third rendering is identical to the second except that amino acids are rendered in the CPK convention (red = oxygen, blue = nitrogen, gray = carbon, yellow = sulfur). (B) This panel illustrates the interaction of Ca/calmodulin with a target effector. An alpha-helical domain of CaMKII is illustrated in light green to the right of the calmodulin molecule. As part of achieving its effects on target effectors calmodulin changes the structure of its own interdomain alpha helix, wrapping itself around the target. (C and D) Illustrations of the "C2 domain" subtype of calcium binding domain. These figures illustrate two different conformations of this type of calcium-binding domain, typified by the C2 domain of PKC alpha. (D) Structural changes induced by calcium (shown as red spheres) binding to the calcium-binding domain and adjacent regions of the molecule typically cause allosteric changes, promoting binding to phospholipid membranes. Structures based on data in Verdaguer et al. (124).

of proteins, including CaM, troponin C, the S100s, and the calcium-binding subunits of the protease calpain and protein phosphatase 2B all contain E-F hand calcium-binding domains.

PKC is the prototype for the "C2 domain" family of calcium-binding proteins. As we will discuss later, the PKC superfamily is a heterogeneous group of proteins with variable (V) and conserved (C) domains. The second conserved domain (C2) is a calcium-binding domain. The C2 domain family of calcium-binding proteins typically bind both calcium and phospholipids, and calcium regulation of protein-membrane interactions is typical of this group (see Figure 2). Specific examples of C2 domain-containing proteins include the PKCs, the synaptic vesicle-associated protein synaptotagmin, and various phospholipases.

A. CaMKII in E-LTP

Calmodulin-Sensitive Enzymes

Calmodulin in the absence of calcium (apo-calmodulin) has a dumbbell-shaped structure with four E-F-hand calcium-binding domains (see Figure 2). Upon binding of calcium, which is a cooperative interaction, CaM undergoes an extensive conformational change in which the "handle" part of the dumbbell twists itself around a target molecule alpha helix (see Figure 2). This calcium-dependent interaction leads to a conformational change in the target and typically triggers enzyme activation.

One of the most widely studied and important targets of CaM are the calcium/calmodulin-dependent protein kinases (the CaMKs). There are two CaMK isoforms of particular significance in neurons:

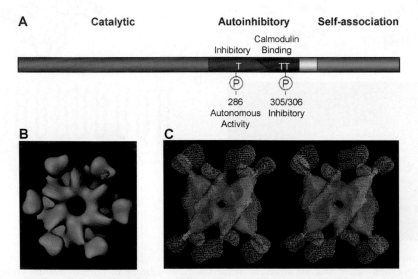

FIGURE 3   Structure of CaMKII. (A) Line diagram illustrating the catalytic, autoinhibitory, and association domains of CaMKII, as well as two sites of autophosphorylation. Reproduced from Lisman, Schulman, and Cline (6). Panels B and C illustrate a detailed and realistic model of CaMKII based on sophisticated high-resolution electron microscopy and X-ray diffraction techniques. (B) A top-down view of CaMKII showing 6 of the 12 individual subunits comprising the holoenzyme. Adapted from Lisman, Schulman, and Cline (6). (C) A stereo rendering of a side view of the same structure. This model shows that the core comprises an aggregate of 12 association domains (residues 315-478) and that the 12 "foot" regions extending from the core are the functional domains (residues 1-314). The ATP- and calmodulin-binding sites are near the middle of the foot (as indicated by the shaded region on one foot in Panel B). Reproduced from Kolodziej, Hudmon, Waxham, and Stoops (125).

CaMKII and CaMKIV. CaMKIV is most likely involved in regulating neuronal gene expression, and we will return to this molecule in the next chapter. CaMKII has achieved especial notoriety for its importance in the induction, maintenance, and expression of LTP, as we will discuss in the next section. Before proceeding, I point out that a particularly outstanding review of the role of CaMKII in LTP has been published recently by John Lisman, Howard Schulman, and Holly Cline (6). I refer you to this review for additional details and insightful analysis.

The Ca^{2+}/calmodulin-dependent protein kinase II (CaMKII) is enriched in the brain and exhibits multifunctional roles in calcium-mediated signal transduction processes. CaMKII is composed of homologous alpha and beta subunits with a size of 52 and 60 kDa, respectively. The CaMKII holoenzyme (i.e., the functional structure)

is a dodecamer (12 subunits) and is a mixture of both alpha and beta subunits. The individual subunit structure and the structure of the holoenzyme are given in Figure 3. Each subunit comprises three domains: an interaction domain that allows formation of the holoenzyme complex, a regulatory domain that binds calmodulin and regulates the enzyme's activity, and a catalytic domain that executes the phosphotransfer reaction from Mg^{2+}/ATP to the substrate protein.

The activity of CaMKII is highly sensitive to calcium influx, and the calcium-dependency of activation has an absolute requirement for calmodulin. In the simplest mode of regulation of CaMKII activity, calcium binds to calmodulin, the complex activates CaMKII, and enzymatic activity returns to baseline after calcium levels diminish (see Figure 4). This obviously can be relevant to LTP induction but is not a

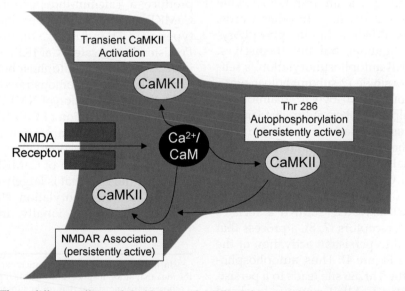

FIGURE 4 Three different effects of Ca/CaM on CaMKII. Calcium and calmodulin can produce CaMKII activation by various mechanisms, with the duration of the activation differing among the mechanisms. CaMKII can be transiently activated by direct binding of Ca/CaM—the activation terminates when calcium levels return to baseline. CaMKII can also be translocated to the NMDA receptor, independent of autophosphorylation, which leads to a calcium-independent activation lasting seconds to minutes. CaMKII which undergoes autophosphorylation at Thr286 can be rendered active independent of Ca/CaM, which is a mechanism for persistent activation. This persistently activated, autophosphosphorylated CaMKII can also associate with the NMDA receptor as well. See text for additional discussion.

mechanism for generating a persistently activated enzyme that can serve as an LTP maintenance molecule.

However, the activity of the enzyme and its sensitivity to successive increases in calcium concentrations are altered following CaMKII *autophosphorylation*. Autophosphorylation, the act of a kinase phosphorylating itself, occurs in CaMKII in response to calcium/calmodulin stimulation. Changes in the phosphorylation state of the alpha or beta subunits of CaMKII alter the kinetic properties of the holoenzyme—the enzyme becomes active independent of any need for calcium/calmodulin. Thus, autophosphorylation of CaMKII can generate a persistently active (aka autonomously active) enzyme—a persisting biochemical signal in response to a transient intitiating event!

The principal autophosphorylation site, and the site that renders the enzyme autonomously active, is Thr286 in CaMKII alpha (and the homologous Thr 287 site in the beta subunit). Autophosphorylation at this site occurs via an intraholoenzyme but intersubunit reaction. In other words, individual CaMKII subunits phosphorylate their neighbors, but not themselves. Thus, CaMKII autophosphorylation is self-delimited to a single 12-subunit holoenzyme. Activation of CaMKII by Ca^{2+}/calmodulin causes the alpha and beta subunits to undergo autophosphorylation at Thr286/287, rendering the enzyme autonomously active and partially insensitive to further increases in Ca^{2+}/CaM concentrations. An additional consequence of autophosphorylation is that activated CaMKII associates with NMDA receptors (7, 8), a process that also can lead to persistent activation of the enzyme (see Figure 4). Thus, autophosphorylation at the Thr286 site leads to a persistently activated CaMKII enzyme, localized postsynaptically at its site of activation—an ideal molecular memory trace.

How is it that the autophosphorylation of CaMKII is maintained in the face of protein phosphatases that can reverse the

autophosphorylation? Current models[2] (9) capitalize on data indicating that protein phosphatase activity is low in the PSD, where the autophosphorylated CaMKII is located. Thus, all that needs occur is that the rate of intersubunit autophosphorylation be greater than the net rate of CaMKII dephosphorylation in order for the phosphorylation to persist for the life of the enzyme. Thus, the capacity for intersubunit trans-phosphorylation synergizes with a low level of phosphatase activity to give a persisting signal in the cell.

The necessity of CaMKII autophosphorylation in LTP is reasonably well established. The induction of NMDA receptor-dependent LTP requires CaMKII activation in the postsynaptic neuron (10, 11), and mice deficient for alpha CaMKII show deficits in hippocampal LTP (12, 13). The sites of CaMKII autophosphorylation are also important in LTP induction. Mutations of the Thr286 site to prevent autophosphorylation or, conversely to produce a calcium-independent form of CaMKII, result in LTP deficits for some types of LTP-inducing stimulation (14). Persistently activated CaMKII, and indeed increased CaMKII autophosphorylation at Thr286, have been demonstrated in LTP.

Moreover, activation of NMDA receptors results in translocation of CaMKII from the cytosol to the postsynaptic density regions, and LTP-inducing stimulation triggers a transient translocation of CaMKII from the cytosol to the PSD that is largely dependent on the autophosphorylation state of the CaMKII at Thr286. Finally, injection or

---

[2]In the mid-1980s there was much excitement about the idea that autophosphorylated CaMKII might serve as a self-perpetuating signal that could subserve permanent memory storage. We will return to this idea in more detail in Chapter 12. The bottom line, however, is that a variety of experimental results suggest that perpetual activation of CaMKII does not occur with LTP-inducing stimulation. Direct assays for autonomously activated CaMKII indicate that the autophosphorylated enzyme only persists for 1 to 2 hours in the cell.

transfection of autonomously active CaMKII into neurons likewise leads to enhancement of synaptic strength and an occlusion of LTP induced by tetanic stimulation, further data consistent with a role of autonomously active CaMKII in E-LTP maintenance.

There is, however, one fly in the ointment concerning the present model for a role for CaMKII as an LTP maintenance molecule—CaMKII inhibitors applied after LTP-inducing stimulation may not reverse LTP (15). How can one rationalize that a compound that blocks CaMKII phosphotransferase activity does not lead to a reversal of LTP? One possibility is that CaMKII is playing a structural role in LTP that does not necessitate phosphorylation of substrates per se. Another possibility is that simultaneous CaMKII and PKC activity are triggered in LTP, and either is sufficient for E-LTP expression. Finally, it is possible that phosphatase inhibition synergizes with CaMKII autophosphorylation in LTP maintenance and expression, so that even if CaMKII phosphotransferase activity is blocked, the synapse can still stay potentiated for some period of time before substrate dephosphorylation occurs. (None of these possibilities excludes any of the others.) Thus, some mechanistic details still need to be worked out regarding the role of CaMKII as a persisting signal in E-LTP. Regardless, autonomously active, autophosphorylated CaMKII still serves as the prototype molecular information storage device at present.

Inhibitory Autophosphorylation of CaMKII

Additional in vitro experiments indicate that autophosphorylation of CaMKII at additional sites can also occur. Specifically, autophosphorylation of Thr 305/306 sites on alpha and beta CaMKII occurs following Thr286 autophosphorylation under circumstances of prolonged or robust stimulation. This can inhibit both the calcium/CaM-independent activity and the calcium/CaM-dependent activity. Thr305/ 306 autophosphorylation also leads to dissociation of the enzyme from the PSD. We will return to a possible role for this event in a human mental retardation syndrome, Angelman Syndrome, in Chapter 10.

CaMKII as a Temporal Integrator

Finally, it is important to note that while CaMKII can serve as an information storage molecule in E-LTP maintenance, a role for this mechanism is not limited to longer-term information storage. CaMKII can by similar mechanisms serve to allow temporal integration between spaced periods of NMDA receptor activation. That CaMKII can by itself serve as a temporal integrator was elegantly demonstrated in a series of studies by DeKoninck and Schulman (16). When CaMKII sees repeated, spaced pulses of calcium and calmodulin, it integrates these signals and gives a readout of calcium spike frequency in terms of autonomous CaMKII activity (see Figure 5). Thus, increasing frequencies and levels of calcium give increased autonomous

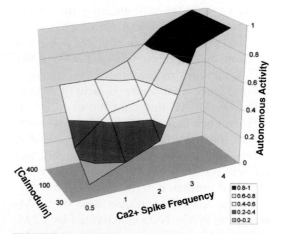

FIGURE 5 Temporal integration of a Ca signal by CaMKII, as a function of availability of calmodulin. Graphical representation of autonomous CaMKII activity illustrating dependence on the frequency of calcium concentration spikes and the concentration of calmodulin. Adapted from data in De Koninck and Schulman (16). Reproduced with permission from Dineley et al. (126).

CaMKII activity. In this amazing example, all that is needed for temporal integration is a single molecular complex sensing the ambient level of free calcium. This is likely a means by which multiple, spaced tetanic stimuli are able to selectively produce unique long-lasting effects on CaMKII activity postsynaptically. The generation of autonomous activity is also dependent on the level of free calmodulin, recalling the possible role of the PKC/neurogranin gate in regulating CaMKII, which we discussed at the end of the last chapter.

Two Additional Targets of CaM: Adenylyl Cyclase and NOS

Adenylyl cyclase (AC), the enzyme that converts ATP to the second messenger cAMP, is also a target of CaM in neurons. The CaM-sensitive AC isoforms are AC1 and AC8, and work from Dan Storm and his colleagues has demonstrated that simultaneous knockout of these two genes gives a pronounced LTP phenotype (see Figure 6, reviewed in 17). Both E-LTP and L-LTP are affected in the double knockouts. Calcium/calmodulin stimulation of AC likely contributes to regulating the cAMP gate in a temporal integration fashion (see the last chapter), and this may be the mechanism of attenuation of E-LTP in the AC knockout mice. However, there is no evidence that there is any *persisting* activation of AC that contributes to E-LTP maintenance (18) so AC likely serves only in the induction phase of E-LTP. L-LTP is completely lost in AC knockout mice, and we will return to the important role of AC in L-LTP induction in the next chapter.

Nitric Oxide Synthase also is CaM-sensitive. When NOS is activated by CaM, it converts arginine to citrulline plus the free radical species NO (nitric oxide). It is clear that generation of NO through NOS activation modulates LTP induction, but the precise mechanisms by which this happens are still being worked out (19). As we discussed in the last chapter, NMDA receptors are modulated by NO, and

NO-sensitive guanylyl cyclase has also been implicated as a target of NO in LTP induction, although there has been substantial argument over the role of this mechanism in LTP (see references 20, 21, and 22). The ras/ERK cascade is also a potential target of NO. These are all relevant mechanisms for NO in modulating LTP induction, but as with AC it seems unlikely that there is any role for ongoing NOS activation in E-LTP maintenance.

One of the most interesting potential roles for NO derives from its capacity to cross cell membranes directly. Thus, NO like other membrane-permeant species could be a "retrograde messenger" that carries a signal from the postsynaptic compartment to the presynaptic compartment (23). One specific retrograde messenger role that has been proposed for NO is activation of presynaptic guanylyl cyclase and the cyclic GMP-dependent protein kinase (PKG; 24). This proposed role also is limited to LTP induction as well and has not been proposed to serve an LTP maintenance function. However, presynaptic NO and NO-derived reactive species might also be particularly important in generating persisting signals presynaptically. We will return to this idea later when we talk about the possible role of oxidatively modified PKC in E-LTP maintenance.

In summary, then, both AC and NOS are additional targets of CaM in E-LTP induction. They serve as important triggering mechanisms, involved in generating persisting signals. They are not, however, persistently activated and do not directly participate in E-LTP maintenance.

B. A Second Target of Calcium: PKC

The calcium/phospholipid-dependent protein kinases (PKCs) are pluripotent regulators of synaptic transmission and neuronal function. PKC has not been as extensively studied as its cousin CaMKII in the context of LTP; nevertheless, there is a fairly broad literature implicating PKC as a

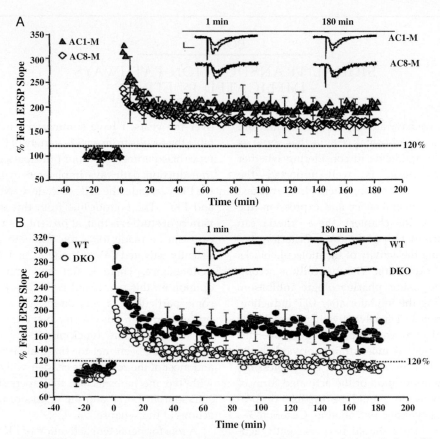

FIGURE 6   LTP in adenylyl cyclase-deficient mice. DKO mice lacking both the AC1 and AC8 calmodulin-sensitive isoforms of adenylyl cyclase have a defect in LTP. (A) LTP was induced in AC1 mutant (AC1-M, shaded triangles; n = 9 mice, 17 slices) and AC8 mutant mice (AC8-M, open diamonds; n = 13 mice, 25 slices) slices by four tetanic trains of 100-Hz (200 ms, 6 seconds apart) stimulus. There was no statistically significant difference between the mean fEPSP of AC1-M and AC8-M mutant mice 180 minutes after tetanization (p = .28). Representative fEPSP traces taken from area CA1 in AC1-M and AC8-M slices at 1 minute and 180 minutes after tetani are shown in the insets. Each trace is superimposed over a baseline trace taken 2 minutes before tetani for ease of comparison. Scale bar, 1 mV, 10 ms. (B) LTP was diminished in DKO mice. Wild-type mice (closed circles; n = 13 mice, 26 slices) preparations gave an L- LTP lasting up to 180 minutes, whereas potentiation in the DKO (open circles; n = 8 mice, 19 slices) preparations declined to near baseline values within 80 minutes. Representative fEPSP traces taken from area CA1 in wild-type and DKO brain slices at 1 minute and 180 minutes after tetani are shown in insets. The dashed lines represent an arbitrary cutoff (120%), below which potentiation was considered to be near baseline. Scale bar, 1 mV, 10 ms. Figure and legend reproduced from Wong et al. (127).

molecule contributing to the maintenance of E-LTP. PKC inhibitors can block the expression of E-LTP (25–28), PKC is persistently activated in E-LTP (29–36), and activation of PKC or injection of the enzyme into the postsynaptic cell elicits synaptic potentiation (37–40; reviewed in Weeber et al. (42); see Box 1). Thus, the molecule meets the three principal criteria establishing it as a candidate E-LTP maintenance molecule.

In mammals the PKC enzyme family is quite heterogeneous and comprises 11

BOX 1

SIGNAL TRANSDUCTION PATHWAYS IMPLICATED IN LTP

As we have already discussed, there are several experimental criteria that serve as a useful guideline in considering whether a hypothesis is well-supported—the block-mimic-measure criteria. In the context of E-LTP maintenance and expression (the topic of this chapter), these criteria can be formulated as follows. Criterion 1—Blocking the activity of the molecule blocks E-LTP expression. This typically is accomplished using pharmacologic inhibition, applying the inhibitor after LTP induction. Criterion 2—Directly activating the molecule should produce synaptic potentiation. This experiment is most straightforward in the context of mechanisms for LTP expression, where application of the activated form of the molecule should be capable of producing synaptic potentiation. Criterion 3—The molecule should be persistently activated (or elevated) with LTP-inducing stimulation.

Without going into a detailed review of the literature, because numerous writers including myself have reviewed these data over the years, I have summarized in the table the results from a wide variety of these types of experiments for four principal signal transduction pathways implicated in LTP: the PKA cascade, the ERK cascade, CaMKII, and PKC. The bottom line from this wide variety of studies is that, at present, a strong case can be made for a role for both persistently activated CaMKII and PKC in E-LTP maintenance. There is not unanimity of opinion on this point, and we will address some particulars of this discussion as we proceed through this chapter. Nevertheless, by and large, the block-mimic-measure criteria have been met for these molecules, and most of the rest of this chapter will deal with the mechanisms for their persistent activation in E-LTP and the targets of their actions at the synapse.

A role for persistent activation of PKA or ERK has been ruled out for E-LTP maintenance, although prolonged activation of these molecules may be involved in L-LTP induction. We will return to this discussion in the next chapter.

---

known isozymes that have been divided into three major subsets: conventional (α, βI, βII, and γ), novel (δ, ϵ, η, θ, and μ), and atypical (λ and ζ) (See Figure 7). Each isoform is encoded by a separate gene with the exception of the βI and βII isoforms, which are splice variants from a single gene. Each subfamily of PKC isoforms is subject to distinct control mechanisms. The conventional isoforms are regulated by calcium in concert with diacylglycerol and membrane phospholipid. The novel and atypical classes are structurally homologous but can be regulated independent of calcium. Brain subregion-and neuronal

subtype-specific expression is the rule rather than the exception for the various isoforms. Almost all the various subtypes are expressed to varying degrees in the hippocampus.

Good evidence exists from Todd Sacktor's lab that a wide variety of PKC isoforms are activated in response to LTP-inducing stimulation (34). For the present purposes, we will focus on the calcium-responsive isoforms: alpha, beta, and gamma. In a later section of the chapter, we will cover PKC zeta.

One would like to begin to dissect the contributions of the various isoforms of PKC

BOX 1—cont'd

SIGNAL TRANSDUCTION PATHWAYS IMPLICATED IN LTP

Cascade	Phase	Induction or Maintenance/ Expression	Inhibitors Block?	Activators Mimic?	Demonstrated to Occur?
CaMKII	E-LTP	Induction	Yes (62, 100)	Yes (101)	Yes (62, 102)
		Maint/Expr	Yes (when PKC inhib, (28, 103))	Yes (104)	Yes (62, 102, 105)
	L-LTP	Induction	?	?	Yes (62, 102, 105)
		Maint/Expr	?	?	No (105)
PKC	E-LTP	Induction	Yes (10, 25, 26, 103)	Yes? (37–40, 101)	Yes (29, 30, 34, 39)
		Maint/Expr	Yes, when CaMKII inhib, (26, 28)	Yes (37–40)	Yes (29, 30, 34, 39)
	L-LTP	Induction	Partially (106–109)	?	Yes (29, 30, 34, 39)
		Maint/Expr	?	?	No (29, 30, 34, 39)
PKA	E-LTP	Induction	Partially (110–112)	No (113)	Yes (18, 114, 115)
		Maint/Expr	No (18)	Yes (116, 117)	No (18)
	L-LTP	Induction	Yes (110, 113)	Yes (113)	Yes (18, 114, 115)
		Maint/Expr	No (117, 118)	?	No (18)
MAPK	E-LTP	Induction	Partially (119–121)	?	Yes (119, 122)
		Maint/Expr	No (119)	?	No (119)
	L-LTP	Induction	Yes (119–121)	Yes (113, 121, 123)	Yes (119, 122)
		Maint/Expr	No (119, 121)	?	No (119)

in synaptic plasticity. However, those PKC inhibitors reported to be isoform-selective do not generally differ greatly in their potency for inhibiting the various isoforms of PKC, limiting their effectiveness for hippocampal slice physiology studies. Obviously, transgenic mouse knockout technologies have been used to good effect to selectively eliminate specific protein kinase isoforms. Thus, at the present time, utilization of knockout technology to evaluate the roles of PKC isoforms in LTP and learning is a very appealing prospect.

The first isoform-specific investigation of a role for PKC in LTP involved characterization of a knockout of the brain-specific gamma isoform of PKC (41). Indeed, this was one of the very first knockout animal studies ever published. In these studies, very modest effects on hippocampus-dependent memory were observed with the loss of PKCγ. However, the PKCγ knockout animal has a very pronounced but idiosyncratic LTP deficit. Tetanus-induced LTP in area CA1 is completely lost in gamma knockout animals (see Figure 8). However, LTP can be recovered in PKCγ-deficient mice by delivery of an LTD-inducing stimulus prior to LTP-inducing tetanic stimulation (41).

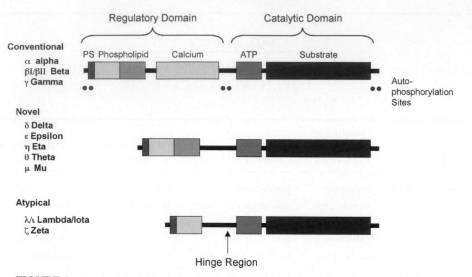

FIGURE 7   Domain structures of isoforms of PKC. The regulatory and catalytic domains of various PKC isoforms illustrated regions of structural conservation. Autophosphorylation sites in the conventional isoforms are indicated by red dots. Figure courtesy of Coleen Atkins.

These data suggest that the role of PKCγ is limited to the induction of LTP and that the gamma isoform of PKC is not necessary for LTP maintenance. (One alternative possibility is that LTD-inducing stimulation recruits the capacity of another PKC isoform to compensate for the lack of PKCγ.) The intriguing model has been proposed that a loss of phosphorylation of the postsynaptic PKC substrate neurogranin contributes to this phenotype, via the neurogranin gate mechanism that we discussed in the last chapter. Overall, these studies suggest the hypothesis that while PKCγ is involved in regulating LTP induction, other isoforms of PKC are involved in LTP maintenance.

Along these lines, Ed Weeber in my lab, in collaboration with Michael Leitges and others, evaluated a PKCβ knockout mouse model (42). The PKCβ knockout phenotype was in some ways the mirror image of the PKCγ knockout. Deletion of the PKCβ gene resulted in pronounced memory defects: strong attenuation of cued and contextual fear conditioning. However, the beta knockout animal had no discernable LTP phenotype in area CA1 of hippocampus[3] (see Figure 8). Based on these studies it

seems clear that the beta isoforms of PKC are not necessary for tetanus-induced, NMDA receptor-dependent LTP induction or early maintenance in area CA1 of hippocampus.

These observations do not, of course, preclude the involvement of PKCβ in other forms of LTP in area CA1 and in synaptic plasticity in other brain regions. The data specifically suggest an important role for the beta isoforms of PKC in the synaptic plasticity underlying amygdala-dependent associative learning because of the loss of amygdala-dependent fear conditioning in these animals. There is, moreover, a potential role for PKCβ in synaptic plasticity in area CA1, as we observed an attenuation of phorbol ester-induced potentiation of synaptic transmission in area CA1. Interestingly, this finding contrasts with mice deficient in the gamma isoform of PKC, which have no loss of phorbol ester-induced synaptic facilitation (43). These several observations, when taken

---

[3]This also is an example of a result that dissociates hippocampal LTP from learning behavior. We will return to this issue in detail in Chapter 9.

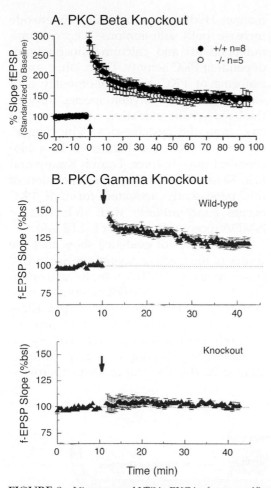

A. PKC Beta Knockout

B. PKC Gamma Knockout

FIGURE 8 Hippocampal LTP in PKC isoform-specific knockout mice. Hippocampal slices obtained from PKC beta (upper)-, and gamma (middle)-, (lower)-deficient mice or wild-type mice (+/+ in upper panel) were given an LTP-inducing stimulus (arrows) delivered after stable baseline responses were recorded for 20 minutes. Each set of tetani consisted of a single train of 100-Hz stimulation for 1 second, while maintaining slices at 25°C. Reproduced with permission from Weeber et al. (42) and Abeliovich, et al. (41).

altogether, suggest the possible specific involvement of the beta isoforms of PKC in neuromodulation in area CA1.

The PKC beta knockout studies indicate that, in and of itself, loss of the function of the PKCβ isoforms does not lead to a loss of E-LTP maintenance. Similarly, loss of PKCγ also does not lead to an inability to maintain E-LTP. That leaves us with the final calcium-sensitive isoform of PKC,

PKCα. Recent studies from my lab, again by Ed Weeber in collaboration with Michael Leitges and others, support the hypothesis that the alpha isoform of PKC is involved in E-LTP maintenance. Knockout of PKCα leads to a loss of tetanus-induced LTP in area CA1 in the absence of effects on baseline synaptic transmission or hippocampal morphology. While these studies are at a very early stage, hopefully future work will clarify the mechanisms involved in the regulation of PKCα activity in E-LTP, and the role of this PKC isoform in E-LTP maintenance.

Persistent Activation of PKC in E-LTP

How is it that PKC is utilized in generating a persisting signal in E-LTP? In 1991 Eric Klann and his colleagues published the first direct demonstration of persistent protein kinase activation in LTP, and they specifically identified PKC as one of the kinases involved in this process (29). Since that time Eric, and independently Todd Sacktor, have done an extensive series of studies to define the mechanisms for persistent activation of PKC in E-LTP. No aspect of this work has been straightforward. It is safe to say that none of the mechanisms that we all initially thought were the most likely to be involved in persistent PKC activation in LTP have subsequently turned out to be involved. Specifically, the two main hypotheses in the early days were membrane insertion and calpain-mediated proteolysis. Neither of these turned out to be involved in maintaining NMDA receptor-dependent LTP in area CA1, although they likely are involved in other forms of LTP (36).

In the next sections, I will describe some of the mechanisms that *have* turned out to be involved in persistent PKC activation in E-LTP in area CA1: oxidation, autophosphorylation, and increased synthesis. These all serve as unique and interesting examples of now neurons can solve the biochemical problem of generating a lasting signal capable of affecting synaptic function.

Oxidation of PKC

Eric Klann and his colleagues have discovered a quite novel route for persistent PKC activation in LTP, and indeed a novel signal transduction mechanism in its own right. In oxidative activation of PKC (and other proteins regulated by oxidation), a reactive oxygen species directly reacts chemically with its target. Thus, instead of binding reversibly to an allosteric site, the second messenger, in this case, causes a direct and persistent modification of an amino acid side chain of its effector enzyme. This reaction is probably not readily reversible—thus, the modification has a built-in persistence, lasting until the PKC molecule is broken down completely.

In the case of oxidative PKC activation in LTP, the reactive species is superoxide or a superoxide-derived reactive oxygen species such as peroxynitrite or hydrogen peroxide (see Figure 9 and and 44). PKC is activated by reactive oxygen species in a complex manner. Hydrogen peroxide and superoxide increase both autonomous (i.e., calcium-independent) and calcium/phospholipid-dependent PKC activity. The α, βII, ε, and ζ isoforms of PKC are autonomously activated by reactive oxygen species through thiol side-chain oxidation and release of zinc from the cysteine-rich "zinc finger" regions of PKC (see Figure 9). In a biochemical tour de force, Lauren Knapp and Eric Klann showed that the generation of this persistently activated form of PKC occurs concomitantly with induction of NMDA receptor-dependent E-LTP (45).

Several lines of evidence show that the source of the reactive oxygen species in LTP is secondary to NMDA receptor activation (44). For example, NMDA receptor activation in area CA1 of hippocampal slices results in superoxide free-radical production, providing a source of reactive oxygen species. This finding is nicely complemented by the observation that superoxide

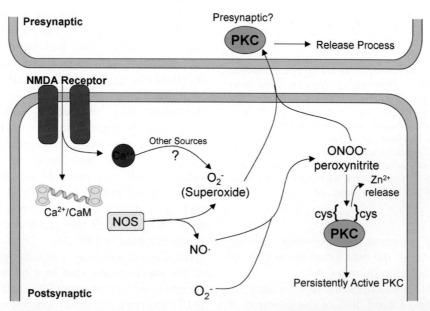

FIGURE 9 A model for oxidative activation of PKC in LTP. Calcium influx through the NMDA receptor triggers production of reactive oxygen species (NO, superoxide, and peroxynitrite), which directly act on cysteine side-chains in PKC. This oxidation results in Zn release and autonomously active PKC. Reactive oxygen species can also cross the synapse as retrograde messengers to activate PKC presynaptically.

scavengers inhibit E-LTP induction in area CA1. Finally, NMDA receptor blockade blocks the generation of the persistently activated oxidized form of PKC in E-LTP. However, the precise source of the superoxide-derived messenger is not known at this time, and this is an area of active investigation. Possibilities include NOS (which can produce superoxide as well as nitric oxide), NADPH oxidases, mitochondrial electron transport, and lipid peroxidases.

One additional interesting aspect of this model is that superoxide and other reactive oxygen species, like NO, can cross cell membranes by mechanisms that are still under investigation. Thus, oxidative activation of PKC may not be limited to the postsynaptic compartment (see Figure 9). This mechanism presents an intriguing possibility for a retrograde signaling mechanism in E-LTP, especially given that presynaptic PKC activation apparently is sufficient to give increased neuro-transmitter release.

Finally, I should note that not just PKC but several protein kinases and phosphatases are regulated by reactive oxygen species, as are a variety of transcription factors. Typically, protein kinases are activated by reactive oxygen species, whereas protein phosphatases are inhibited, potentially enabling a concerted modulation of protein phosphorylation levels within the cell similar to what we have already talked about with the cAMP gate. Persistent phosphatase inhibition in E-LTP is also a potential mechanism contributing to E-LTP maintenance (see reference 6; reviewed in reference 44).

PKC Autophosphorylation in LTP

PKC autophosphorylation is also a mechanism for generating a persisting signal in E-LTP. As part of his early studies into the mechanisms of persistent PKC activation in LTP, Eric Klann also observed that E-LTP is associated with a phosphatase-reversible alteration in PKC

immunoreactivity (30). This finding suggested that increased phosphorylation of PKC might contribute to its autonomous activation in LTP. In a follow-up series of studies, we tested the hypothesis that PKC phosphorylation is increased during E-LTP expression, utilizing an antibody we generated that is selective for autophosphorylated PKC (46).

PKC is known to autophosphorylate at sites in three domains in vitro: an amino-terminal pair of sites near the autoinhibitory domain, a pair of sites in the hinge region, and a carboxy-terminal pair of sites (47; see Figure 7). Additional studies have revealed that the enzyme is phosphorylated at two other sites; a transphosphorylation on the activation loop (T500 in PKC βII) and an autophosphorylation at an additional C-terminal site (S660 in PKC βII) (48). Three of the known phosphorylation sites (T500, T641, and S660) are likely to be phosphorylations occurring concomitant with maturation of the kinase (49, 50).

We studied autophosphorylation at the carboxy-terminal pair of autophosphorylation sites (S634/T641) for several reasons. First, there is a high degree of sequence conservation among the classical PKC isoforms in this domain (see Figure 7). Second, site-directed mutagenesis studies demonstrated that autophosphorylation in this domain has important functional consequences (51, 52), including protection of the enzyme from down-regulation and causing the enzyme to associate with the actin cytoskeleton, a potential localization mechanism.

In our studies of PKC autophosphorylation in LTP, we found that PKC has its C-terminal autophosphorylation persistently increased in LTP (46; see Figure 10). Thus, one persisting signal in E-LTP is an elevated level of autophosphorylated PKC. While this may sound reminiscent of the preceeding story with CaMKII autophosphorylation, it is known that PKC autophosphorylation occurs by an *intramolecular* reaction (49, 53). This means that,

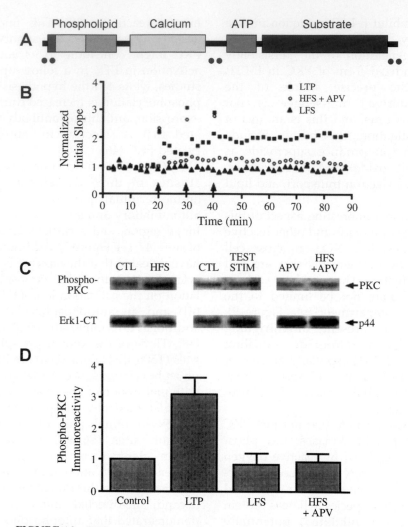

FIGURE 10   PKC autophosphorylation in LTP. (A) The three pairs of PKC autophosphorylation sites in the classical isoforms of PKC (red dots). Panels B through D show increased PKC phosphorylation in LTP. (B) Representative physiologic recording data for the three conditions used to investigate PKC phosphorylation in LTP. The Y-axis is the normalized initial slope of the field EPSP. Note that the high-frequency stimulation (HFS) and HFS + APV (50 μM D, L-APV) samples each received three pairs of tetanic stimulation trains (marked with *arrows*). All HFS and HFS + APV samples were taken 45 minutes to1 hour after delivery of the third period of tetanic stimulation. (C) Representative Western blots of individual area CA1 subregions for each of the 3 conditions employed in these studies. Each is paired with an appropriate control slice (CTL) from the same hippocampus. In the upper panels, blotting is with antiserum 96160 (phospho-PKC). In the lower panels, anti-p44 MAP kinase blot is used to control for protein loading (Erk1-CT). (D) Mean normalized phospho-PKC immunoreactivity. Error bars are SEM: for LTP $n = 9$, for test stim (LFS) $n = 3$, for HFS + APV, $n = 4$. HFS is significantly different from control, LFS, and HFS + APV ($p < .05$, one-way ANOVA). Adapted from Sweatt et al. (46).

unlike CaMKII, which can self-perpetuate its autophosphorylation by transphosphorylation of adjacent subunits, PKC autophosphorylation at these sites cannot be self-perpetuating by having one PKC molecule phosphorylate another.

This led us to wonder how the increased autophosphorylation of PKC was preserved in the presence of ongoing phosphatase activity in the neuron. To explain our observation, we developed the "protected site" model for PKC phosphorylation in LTP. In this model, PKC phosphorylation occurs at sites protected sterically by adjacent portions of the PKC molecule, limiting accessibility of phosphatase and preserving the enzyme in a phosphorylated state. Atomic resolution modeling and in vitro experiments supported key predictions of this model (see Box 2).

BOX 2

PROTECTED-SITE PHOSPHORYLATION IN PKC

Dephosphorylation of PKC, either in vitro or in LTP samples, requires the presence of cofactors normally serving to activate PKC (i.e., Ca^{+2}/PS/DAG). These observations lead to the hypothesis that phosphatase accessibility of phosphorylation sites on PKC is conformation-dependent. Sweatt et al. (46) tested this hypothesis by examining the phosphatase sensitivity of PKC, autophosphorylated with ^{32}P-ATP in vitro, in the presence and absence of its activators, PS/DAG, and Ca^{+2}. The presence of activators dramatically increased the rate of dephosphorylation of autophosphorylated PKC (see Panels A and B). In the presence of activators PKC was 83% dephosphorylated after incubation with protein phosphatase for 2 minutes, whereas in controls PKC was only 21% dephosphorylated after the 2-minute phosphatase treatment. Likewise, after a 30-minute incubation with phosphatase, PKC incubated in the presence of activators was completely dephosphorylated while control incubations exhibited notable phosphatase resistance. Western blot analysis with a C-terminal domain autophosphorylation-sensitive antiserum revealed that the rate of ^{32}P release parallels the rate at which immunoreactivity decreased. Thus, dephosphorylation of PKC is markedly stimulated in the membrane-bound "activated" conformation of PKC.

MODELING THE C-TERMINAL AUTOPHOSPHORYLATION SITES ON PKC

How are the sites of phosphorylation on PKC rendered inaccessible to phosphatases? We proposed a "protected site" model, whereby the conformation of PKC regulates accessibility of the phosphates to phosphatase. In this model, in the unstimulated conformation, sites of PKC phosphorylation are protected through steric hindrance by the surrounding areas of the protein. Upon binding of activating ligands, a conformational change occurs, making the phosphorylation sites accessible at the surface of the molecule. This model has the interesting implication that the dephosphorylation of PKC is regulatable. Only when PKC is in the appropriate conformation (e.g., in the presence of activating factors), will the protein be susceptible to dephosphorylation.

In order to gain preliminary insights into the structural correlates of protected sites of PKC phosphorylation, we undertook computer modeling studies of the catalytic core and carboxy-terminal autophosphorylation domain of PKC, based upon the known crystal structure of the catalytic subunit of PKA. The lower right-hand panel of the

Continued

BOX 2—cont'd

PROTECTED-SITE PHOSPHORYLATION IN PKC

figure shows several renderings of our model of the PKC catalytic core and C-terminal phosphorylation sites.

Our modeling suggests two potential types of protected phosphorylation sites in the C-terminal autophosphorylation domain of PKC. The first type is exemplified by the T641 phosphorylation site. The phosphate at T641 is immersed in a cleft in the upper lobe of the catalytic core, pointed inward toward the center of the molecule (right-hand panels, white arrows). In addition, T641 sits on the interior of a pronounced angle in the peptide backbone of the adjacent residues, limiting accessibility of the phosphate from the exterior of the molecule. This conformation suggests that the phosphate at T641 is normally well-protected

by the catalytic core on one face and also by the adjacent peptide backbone.

Interestingly, the other autophophorylation site, T634, presents another type of configuration. In our model of the catalytic core of PKC, the phosphate at T634 appears to point outward and be at the surface of the catalytic core. Thus, protection of this type of site would necessitate that other regions of PKC beyond the catalytic core extend over or near the site to limit phosphatase accessibility. Although at present no direct structural information is available, domains potentially involved include both the Ca^{+2} and lipid-binding domains of PKC (see Figures 2 and 7). In the future, it will be interesting to determine the configuration of these domains relative to the PKC catalytic core.

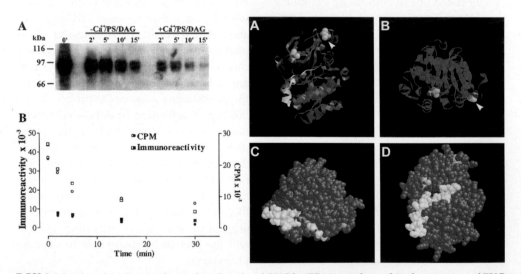

BOX 2 Dephosphorylation of autophosphorylated PKC by PP1 is accelerated in the presence of PKC activators. (Left-hand panel A) Purified PKC βII (100 ng per lane) was autophosphorylated in vitro, then dephosphorylated with PP1 for the indicated time in the presence of either 210 μM/6 μM PS/DAG (97 mol% and 3 mol%, respectively) and 400 μM Ca^{+2} (activating conditions, right half), or Triton X-100 (2 mM) mixed micelles containing 35 μM/1 μM PS/DAG (2 mol% and 0.05 mol%, respectively) with 100 μM Ca^{+2} (nonactivating conditions, left half). (Left-hand panel B) Quantitation of the data. Immunoreactivity refers to binding of antibody 96160 (see Figure 10) to these samples (blots not shown). Aliquots were removed into SDS-PAGE sample buffer and electrophoresed using 7% SDS-PAGE, transferred to nitrocellulose, and ^{32}P quantitated by phosphoimaging. The right-hand panels are space-filling models of the PKC catalytic domain and associated autophosphorylation sites. Reproduced from Sweatt et al. (46).

Our data suggest that the protection from phosphatase activity is conformation-dependent. For example, in the presence of its normal activators PKC is readily dephosphorylated (see Box 2 and references 30 and 48). This observation suggests that PKC phosphorylation is reversible under specific conditions, such as might occur when the cell receives a depotentiating signal. Specifically, in thinking about regulation of PKC autophosphorylation in depotentiation, we proposed that upon entry of low levels of Ca^{2+}, protein phosphatase 2B is activated, leading to dephosphorylation of protein phosphatase inhibitor 1, thereby causing activation of protein phosphatase 1. The depotentiation-associated Ca^{2+} signal (in conjunction with other activators, for example transient DAG production) also changes the conformation of PKC, exposing the phosphate at the "protected" site. Protein phosphatase 1 can then dephosphorylate PKC, returning the enzyme to its original state. Alternatively, protein phosphatase 2B could directly dephosphorylate PKC.

Finally, although we have proposed the "protected site" model based on our studies of PKC autophosphorylation in LTP, phosphorylation of protected sites might be a general biochemical mechanism for the generation of stable, long-lasting physiologic changes. This idea is appealing because such a mechanism confers three attributes upon a change in an enzymatic system: stability, constancy, and regulated reversibility. The change is stable in the sense that it is long-lasting in the cell. The magnitude of the change is constant because a constant fraction of the enzyme stays phosphorylated, unless additional stimulation occurs. Finally, although the change can be long-lasting, upon receiving a specific signal the change can be readily reversed, restoring the system to its original state. It will be interesting in the future to determine if protected site phosphorylation is used in other enzyme systems in the generation of persisting cellular signals.

Calpain and PKMζ

PKC was originally discovered not as second-messenger-regulated enzyme, but rather as a kinase activated secondary to proteolytic cleavage. Various proteases like trypsin and the calcium-activated protease calpain can clip PKC in its central "hinge" region (see Figure 7), releasing the N-terminal inhibitory domain and liberating the free, active C-terminal catalytic domain. This active fragment of PKC is referred to as PKM.

Of course, this mechanism of proteolytic activation of PKC has great appeal as a potential mechanism for generating a long-lasting signal in LTP. Making a long story short, it turns out that this acute proteolysis of PKC is not a dominant mechanism in NMDA receptor-dependent LTP in area CA1, although it does appear to be involved in NMDA receptor-independent LTP in this same region (34, 36). (We will return to an additional potential target of calpain proteolysis, the cytoskeleton, in the next section.)

However, there is a role for a constitutively active PKM as a persisting signal in E-LTP, it is just that the mechanism of its generation is not proteolysis. Todd Sacktor's research group has spent many years tracking down the basis for generation of this persistent signal in LTP, and I will briefly summarize their findings.

Todd's group has shown that a constitutively active PKC isoform, the PKM zeta (PKMζ) isoform, is synthesized de novo after LTP induction (see reference 54 and Figure 1). PKMζ is a second-messenger-independent, constitutively active fragment of PKCζ that lacks the regulatory domain. This fragment is synthesized from a unique mRNA that codes for the truncated form of the enzyme. An LTP-associated increase in the amount of PKMζ protein lasts at least 2 hours after LTP-inducing tetanus, an effect that is NMDA receptor-dependent (34, 54). Also, inhibitors of PKMζ applied after LTP-inducing stimulation reverse the expression of LTP (55). Interestingly, a decrease of PKMζ is seen after LTD induction in area CA1, which suggests that bi-directional regulation of PKMζ may contribute to potentiation and depression of synaptic transmission in area CA1 (56).

Thus, increased synthesis of a constitutively active PKC fragment represents a fourth category of persisting signal in LTP. It is interesting that the seemingly more straightforward mechanism of direct proteolysis of pre-existing PKCζ is not used—perhaps this mechanism has been reserved by evolution for use in other forms of synaptic plasticity (36). Finally, I note that because the formation of PKMζ in LTP is protein-synthesis-dependent, this is not strictly speaking a mechanism for E-LTP as I have defined it. However, I included the

example in this section because it is an example of a mechanism for generating an autonomously active kinase, like the other examples presented, and the time course of PKMζ formation is compatible with a role in early stages of LTP.

C. A Final Potential Target of Calcium—Phospholipases

There are a number of calcium-activated phospholipases in neurons that are potential targets of the LTP-inducing calcium signal. These include phospholipases C, D, and A2, which cleave off various parts of membrane phospholipids (summarized in Figure 11). We have already talked about PLC in the context of PKC activation in LTP

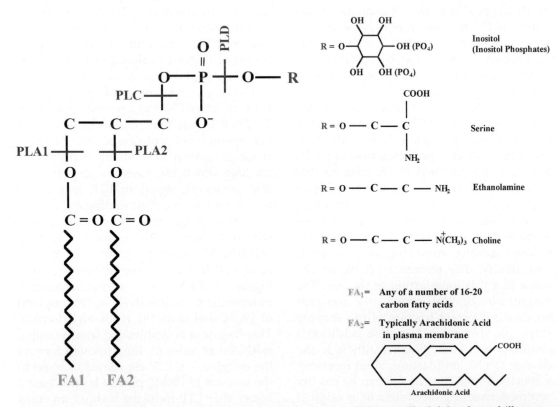

FIGURE 11 Sites of cleavage of membrane phospholipids by phospholipases. The left-hand panel illustrates bonds that are hydrolyzed by phospholipases A1, A2, C, and D. Note that each cleavage is a hydrolysis reaction, leaving free hydroxyl (OH) groups at the cleavage site for each of the two products. PLA1 and PLA2 liberate a free fatty acid (FA, see lower right panel) and a lyso-phospholipid. PLC liberates diacyl glycerol (DAG) and a phosphorylated head group (see upper right panel). PLD liberates phosphatidic acid (PA) and the free, hydroxylated head group.

induction, but what about phospholipases in LTP maintenance? Phospholipases are noteworthy in this context because they can generate membrane-permeant compounds like arachidonic acid (AA) and DAG, which if persistently produced could serve as retrograde signaling compounds in order to maintain changes in the presynaptic compartment.

One specific mechanism that has been proposed in this context is the persistent generation of AA by postsynaptic PLA2 (57). Tim Bliss's group has published evidence that there is a persisting increase in AA after LTP-inducing stimulation in vivo and proposed that this might serve as a persisting potentiating signal in E-LTP. Potential targets of AA are numerous. For example, AA can activate PKC, and this could serve as a presynaptic facilitation mechanism. However, AA can also be converted to a wide variety of active metabolic products by the cyclo-oxygenase pathway (which produces prostaglandins and associated compounds) and the lipoxygenase pathway (which produces active *hydroxy peroxy eicosa tetraenoic* acid (HPETE) metabolites). Any of a number of these compounds could serve as potentiating signals by binding to cell surface receptors pre- or postsynaptically.

The potential mechanisms for generating a persistent increase in AA or other phospholipase-derived messengers in E-LTP are unknown at present. In addition, some disagreement exists in the literature concerning whether this mechanism is necessary for E-LTP (58). Thus, at present, this mechanism remains more in the category of interesting possibility versus established mechanism.

D. Section Summary: Mechanisms for Generating Persisting Signals in E-LTP

As was emphasized at the beginning of the chapter, the capacity to generate a persisting signal in response to a transient stimulus is the biochemical sine qua non of memory formation. In this section, we have seen several examples of these types of processes that have been proposed to be involved in the maintenance of early stages of LTP (see Table 2). These are the four best-characterized solutions to the problem of making a lasting signal in E-LTP, and these reactions serve as general prototypes for solutions to the problem of neuronal activity-dependent generation of molecular memory traces.

It is a useful exercise to perform a compare-and-contrast concerning these four documented mechanisms for molecular information storage (see Table 2). In the case of CaMKII, current models propose that Ca/CaM stimulation of the enzyme results in self-perpetuating inter-subunit autophosphorylation, which coupled with low phosphatase activity leads to a persisting level of active enzyme in the PSD. The read-out of this persisting signal potentially includes structural changes in

TABLE 2   Proposed Mechanisms for Generating Persisting Signals in E-LTP

Molecule	Mechanism	Role
CaMKII	Self-perpetuating autophosphorylation coupled with low phosphatase activity	Effector phosphorylation, Structural changes
Various PKCs	Direct, irreversible covalent modification by reactive oxygen species	Effector phosphorylation
PKC α/βII	Protected-site autophosphorylation resistant to phosphatase activity	Protection from down-regulation, Subcellular localization
PKMζ	De novo synthesis of a constitutively active kinase	Effector phosphorylation

the PSD and increased phosphorylation of target effectors. A second example is that various PKCs can undergo direct, irreversible covalent modification by reactive oxygen species. Oxidation of zinc finger domains in the enzyme leads essentially to irreversible activation of the enzyme, which is then free to phosphorylate target effectors. The third example may act in concert with this mechanism. Persistently activated PKC in cells is typically rapidly down-regulated as a homeostatic mechanism. However, PKC autophosphorylation leads to protection from down-regulation. When stimulated by calcium and DAG, PKC α/βII can undergo protected-site autophosphorylation at a site resistant to phosphatases, leading to a persisting signal that can help maintain the constitutively active kinase in the cell. Finally, in the case of PKMζ, de novo synthesis of a constitutively active kinase lacking the normal autoinhibitory domain leads to the presence of a persistently activated kinase in the cell. Overall, these are four unique and elegant biochemical solutions to the problem of making a lasting signal in response to a transient signal. In the next section, we will discuss the targets of these persisting signals that lead to enhanced synaptic transmission—the translation of the persisting signal into persisting effects at the synapse.

II. TARGETS OF THE PERSISTING SIGNALS

How is it that a persistently activated kinase or other persisting biochemical signal is converted to an enhancement of the coupling between two neurons at Schaffer-collateral synapses? This is the essential question concerning the mechanism of *expression* of E-LTP. Maintenance can be served by an autonomously active kinase, for example, but that persisting signal must be converted to some functional consequence at the synapse in order for synaptic potentiation to occur.

This is the issue we will focus on in this section. In considering the possible mechanisms for enhanced neuronal coupling, it is useful to think about the basics of synaptic transmission and postsynaptic responsiveness. There are three basic components of synaptic transmission—the release of neurotransmitter, the postsynaptic depolarization due to activation of ligand-gated ion channels, and the biophysical response of the postsynaptic membrane to that depolarization. Thus, potential sites for the expression of E-LTP include (1) the machinery of the presynaptic terminal involved in presynaptic calcium influx and the neurotransmitter release process, (2) the postsynaptic glutamate receptors plus their associated proteins, specifically receptors of the AMPA subtype involved in glutamatergic responses, and (3) the potassium and sodium channels that shape the postsynaptic response to glutamatergic receptor-mediated depolarization.

I will discuss each of these three categories of effectors separately as a means of organizing the following discussion, but it is important to remember that they do not operate in isolation nor are the mechanisms mutually exclusive. In fact, evidence exists that each of these three mechanisms participates in E-LTP expression, as we discussed in the chapters on LTP physiology. However, there is a much greater abundance and variety of information and results implicating glutamate receptor regulation in LTP, and much more is known about the mechanisms relevant to this category than the other two categories. Thus, we will direct more attention to this effector system than to the other two.

A. AMPA Receptors in E-LTP

The E-LTP-associated increase in synaptic strength, that is the increase in the EPSP, clearly results in part from increased levels of postsynaptic glutamate receptor activation (reviewed in reference 59). One set of mechanisms contributing to this phenomenon is fairly well understood—enhancement of AMPA receptor function. As both PKC and CaMKII are persistently activated in E-LTP and can affect AMPA receptor function as described below, a parsimonious explanation for the increased synaptic response postsynaptically in E-LTP is increased phosphorylation of AMPA receptors and their associated proteins by these kinases.

Three specific mechanisms for augmenting AMPA receptor function, mediated by CaMKII or PKC, have been implicated as playing a part in E-LTP (see Table 3). One mechanism is that the level of AMPA receptor phosphorylation is increased during E-LTP, phosphorylation at a site that can be phosphorylated by either CaMKII or PKC. Increased phosphorylation at this site results in increased receptor current

TABLE 3   Proposed Mechanisms for Augmenting AMPA Receptor Function in E-LTP

Mechanism	Likely Molecular Basis
Increased single-channel conductance	Direct phosphorylation of AMPA receptor alpha subunits by CaMKII or PKC
Increased steady-state levels of AMPAR	CaMKII (+ PKC?) phosphorylation of AMPA receptor-associated trafficking and scaffolding proteins
Insertion of AMPAR into silent synapses	CaMKII phosphorylation of GluR1-associated trafficking proteins

BOX 3

PI-3-KINASE AND E-LTP EXPRESSION

Sanna et al. recently reported that the activity of the PI-3-Kinase cascade is necessary for the expression of E-LTP in area CA1 (96). The essence of their findings is that PI-3-K and its target AKT are activated in E-LTP, and that PI-3-K inhibitors like LY294002 can block the expression of LTP (see Panel A). While the upstream regulators and downstream tarets of this cascade in E-LTP are mysterious at present, this finding represents an opportunity to introduce the basics of the PI-3-K cascade in the context of synaptic plasticity in area CA1.

PI-3-K is phosphatidylinositol-3-kinase, which synthesizes polyphosphoinositides (e.g., PIP3) in the plasma membrane. One of its principal targets is AKT (named for the transforming AKT8 retrovirus strain and also known as protein kinase B). By and large, this pathway has the attribute that it does not utilize readily diffusible second messengers, but rather relies on multiprotein signaling complexes and the translocation of activated proteins to various subcellular locales in order to achieve its effects. PI-3-K itself phosphorylates inositol-containing phospholipids, which subsequently activate AKT by binding to its pleckstrin homology (PH) domain (see Panel B).

To date, most work on PI-3-K/AKT in neurons has focused on its role as an

Continued

BOX 3—cont'd

PI-3-KINASE AND E-LTP EXPRESSION

anti-apoptotic signaling system that regulates neuronal cell death during development and promotes survival in adult neurons (97, 98). The study by Sanna et al. expands our appreciation of normal physiologic roles for the PI-3-K pathway in mediating synaptic plasticity in the adult CNS. Their work suggests that PI3K activity is one of the processes necessary for the ongoing expression of LTP

expressed physiologically. This appears to be one aspect of an emerging picture. For example, Kelly and Lynch (99) have found that long-term potentiation in the dentate gyrus involves PI-3-K as well. Importantly, these studies point out the continuing recognition of the wide diversity of signal transduction mechanisms necessary for complex neuronal information processing.

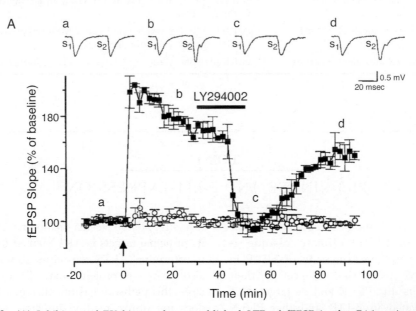

BOX 3 (A) Inhibitors of PI3-kinase abate established LTP of fEPSP in the CA1 region. Synaptic potentials were simultaneously monitored in two independent pathways [white circles, stimulus 1 (S1); black squares, stimulus 2 (S2)]. An inhibitor of PI3-kinase, LY294002 (100 μM), was applied 30 minutes after delivery of HFS to one of the two pathways (S2). Insets are representative traces of extracellular fEPSPs recorded at the times marked by lowercase letters. Each representative trace is an average of five responses. Graphs represent the mean-normalized fEPSP slopes plotted against time. Arrows indicate when tetanic stimulation to one pathway (black squares) was given at time 0. A transient 20-minute application of LY294002 30 minutes after LTP induction abated LTP in the potentiated pathway ($n = 7$) (*black squares*), but no change was seen in the untetanized pathway (white circles). Data reproduced from Sanna et al. (96).   *Continued*

BOX 3—cont'd

PI-3-KINASE AND E-LTP EXPRESSION

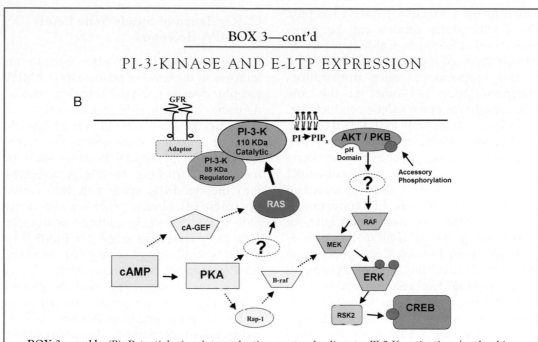

BOX 3, cont'd (B) Potential signal transduction routes leading to PI-3-K activation in the hippocampus Mechanisms coupling cAMP to PI-3-K are speculative but based on the available literature. Red circles represent the specific phosphorylation events that can be measured using available phospho-specific antibodies. Abbreviations: PI-3-K, phosphatidylinositol-3-kinase; PIPx, (poly) phosphorylated derivatives of phosphatidylinositol; pH domain, pleckstrin homology domain; RAS, the low-molecular weight G protein ras; GEF, guanine nucleotide exchange factor; PKA, cAMP-dependent protein kinase; GFR, growth factor receptor; RSK, ribosomal S6 kinase; CREB, cAMP response element binding protein; AKT/PKB, the kinase AKT, also known as protein kinase B; Rap-1, RAF, MEK, and ERK are all components of the extracellular signal-regulated kinase (ERK) cascade, a subfamily of the mitogen-activated protein kinases. Reproduced from Sweatt (97).

(60–62). A second proposed mechanism is that the steady-state level of membrane AMPA receptor protein is increased in a dynamic fashion by CaMKII through regulation of AMPA receptor trafficking and stabilization (9, 63). Finally, AMPA receptors can be inserted into previously "silent" synapses, increasing the strength of connections between two neurons in an essentially all-or-none fashion (reviewed in reference 64), and this mechanism has been proposed as contributing to E-LTP. In the next section, I will briefly review some of the mechanisms underlying these three processes, based on the current literature. The following discussion draws extensively from groundbreaking work in this area by the laboratories of Roberto Malinow, Rob Malenka, Tom Soderling, and Rick Huganir.

B. Direct Phosphorylation of the AMPA Receptor

AMPA receptors mediate the majority of fast synaptic transmission throughout the nervous system, including at Schaffer-collateral synapses in area CA1. Four homologous alpha subunits (GluR1–GluR4) combine in a mix-and-match fashion into a multiunit complex (likely tetrameric), which forms a functional AMPA receptor. The GluR1 alpha subunit can be phosphorylated at Ser831 by CaMKII or PKC in vitro, in cultured hippocampal neurons and in the hippocampal slice preparation. Phosphorylation of GluR1 at this site increases the receptor's ionic conductance, providing a direct route for CaMKII or PKC to enhance synaptic efficacy during LTP (65). In fact, in a key paper by Andres Barria and co-workers, phosphorylation of GluR1 at this site was shown to be increased in E-LTP (62). In addition, LTP induction is associated with increased conductance of AMPA receptors as well (61), which is consistent with increased phosphorylation at the Ser831 site. Thus, phosphorylation of GluR1 at Ser831 has been shown to occur in LTP, and this mechanism is sufficient to enhance synaptic transmission. Although most models for E-LTP posit the phosphorylation of Ser831 to be mediated by CaMKII, persistently active PKC could perform this role as well. An interesting variation on this idea is that CaMKII and PKC might be functionally redundant in E-LTP, each phosphorylating AMPA receptors and serving as a fail-safe mechanism for maintaining synaptic potentiation.

The AMPA receptor is also a substrate for PKA, and PKA phosphorylation likewise increases AMPA channel activity. In a fascinating series of studies by Hei-sung Lee in Rick Huganir's lab, regulation of AMPA receptors by PKA was found to predominantly be involved in de-depression of synaptic strength in area CA1 (66). These studies showed that potentiation and depotentiation revolved around the CaMKII/PKC phosphorylation site, while LTD and dedepression revolved around the PKA site. This important study thereby separated mechanisms for synaptic potentiation from mechanisms for synaptic depression by demonstrating that one process is not simply the reversal of the other. Similar recent work, using a different approach, from Dan Madison's lab has also supported this idea (67).

C. Regulation of Steady-State Levels of AMPA Receptors

Active CaMKII can also lead to an increase in the level of postsynaptic AMPA receptor density in hippocampal pyramidal neurons in culture. A wide variety of sophisticated studies by Robert Malinow's lab have shown that transfection of active CaMKII into pyramidal neurons leads to increased trafficking of AMPA receptors into the dendritic spine and into active synapses (64). Similar processes also occur with LTP induction in cultured neurons in vitro (68). Thus, one target for CaMKII in E-LTP is regulation of steady-state levels of AMPA receptors postsynaptically.

The mechanism for this increased trafficking and membrane insertion is under active investigation. It is known to be independent of Ser831 phosphorylation, clearly rendering this mechanism as distinct and separable from the mechanism described earlier for increasing current flow through the AMPA channel (68). Current models posit that one component of E-LTP is *activity-dependent* delivery of GluR1/2-containing AMPA receptors into the spine and postsynaptic density, a process distinct from a second constitutive pathway that delivers GluR2/3-containing receptors and maintains *baseline* synaptic transmission.

It is important to note that insertion of AMPA receptors into the postsynaptic membrane is not a mechanism for the *maintenance* of E-LTP. Postsynaptic membrane AMPA receptors turn over with a lifetime of about 15 minutes (69, 70). Thus, regulation of AMPA receptor insertion is an active process maintained by some other persisting signal. As mentioned previously, one relevant persisting signal is autophosphorylated, autonomously active CaMKII.

How is it that CaMKII increases steady-state levels of AMPA receptors? The mechanisms are currently under investigation and are complex. There also is not unanimity of opinion in this rapidly evolving area of research. What follows is a hybrid model drawn from the recent work on AMPA receptor trafficking referred to earlier, theoretical work by John Lisman and his colleagues, and findings from Michael Browning's laboratory. Although many investigators will likely disagree with some of the particulars, it will give a flavor of the current thinking about mechanisms for kinase regulation of AMPA receptor expression in E-LTP.

Figure 12 summarizes the model. Calcium influx through the NMDA receptor leads to activation of CaMKII and triggers membrane insertion of AMPA receptors. The calcium signal also causes CaMKII autophosphorylation, which as we discussed earlier leads to a self-perpetuating increase in autophosphorylated CaMKII. Autophosphorylated CaMKII binds with high affinity to the cytoplasmic domain of the NMDA receptor and to the actin-binding protein alpha-actinin. The actinin linkage couples the CaMKII/NMDA receptor complex to actin, and as we discussed in the last chapter actin filaments cross-link to AMPA receptors via a number of mechanism including by binding through the 4.1 protein and SAP97. Thus, by this mechanism, autophosphorylated CaMKII stabilizes AMPA receptors in the PSD by linking them to the more stable NMDA receptor complex.

An additional component of the model is that the calcium signal acting through persistently activated PKC and src leads to increased insertion of NMDA receptors in the postsynaptic membrane. This has been shown to occur with LTP-inducing stimulation by Grosshans, Clayton, Coultrap, and Browning (71). This second signal increases the number of NMDA receptor "anchors" in the PSD and, by this mechanism, contributes to elevating the steady-state level of AMPA receptors postsynaptically.

Notable components of the model distinguish it from Ser831 phosphorylation of AMPA receptors as a mechanism for increasing synaptic strength. First, it does not require CaMKII phosphorylation of AMPA receptors or indeed any other CaMKII substrate beside CaMKII itself—autophosphorylated CaMKII serves a structural not a catalytic role. Second, it involves a number of receptor-interacting proteins in the PSD that stabilize the presence of AMPA receptors. Third, it involves the cytoskeleton and thus could serve as a signaling system beyond simply regulating AMPA receptor function. Fourth, it involves

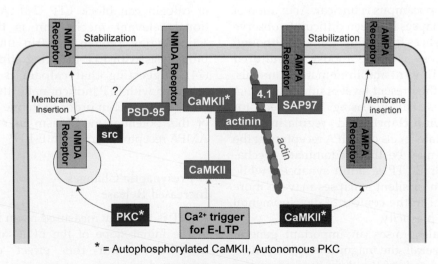

FIGURE 12   A model for glutamate receptor insertion and stabilization in E-LTP. See text for details. Adapted from Lisman and Zhabotinsky (9).

the NMDA receptor as well as the AMPA receptor, with the NMDA receptor serving as a PSD-organizing molecule. Finally, it involves parallel actions of PKC and CaMKII, as opposed to the two kinases converging on the same target phosphorylation site.

D. Silent Synapses

As we discussed in Chapter 4 on LTP physiology, de novo insertion of AMPA receptors is an additional potential mechanisms for enhanced synaptic strength in LTP. "Silent" synapses containing NMDA receptors but not functional AMPA receptors occur with reasonable frequency in prenatal and neonatal brain. NMDA receptor-dependent triggering of AMPA receptor insertion into silent synapses occurs in an activity-dependent fashion in neurons, likely by mechanisms quite similar to those described earlier for elevating AMPA receptor levels in the PSD. Thus, activation of silent synapses through AMPA receptor insertion is clearly a potential mechanism for E-LTP, and "AMPA-fication" of synapses occurs under a number of experimental conditions (reviewed in reference 64).

However, the quantitative contribution of silent synapse activation in LTP in the adult hippocampus is unclear. Activation of silent synapses has been difficult to observe in acute slices from adult animals, although the process is quite robust in cultured neurons in vitro and in immature animals. Thus, at the present level of understanding, it appears that increasing AMPA receptor ionic conductance and regulating the steady-state levels of AMPA receptors at the synapse may be the predominant mechanisms for E-LTP at adult synapses, while activation of silent synapses may be more important in the context of developmental synaptic plasticity.

This also raises an important general point. Overall, the magnitude of the contribution of each of the three mechanism for augmenting AMPA receptor function is

unclear as well. The extent of receptor insertion, stabilization, and phosphorylation are subject to many variables including the recent history of the synapse (see reference 67) and developmental age. Thus, there still is an open question concerning the precise mechanisms for enhancing AMPA receptor function, and different mechanisms may operate under a wide number of different experimental conditions and in different synaptic states in vivo.

E. Proteolysis

A final note is that proteolysis of cytoskeletal and AMPA receptor-associated proteins has also been proposed to play a role in the generation of enhanced synaptic strength. Michel Baudry and Gary Lynch have published a variety of evidence supporting their model that the calcium-activated protease calpain cleaves postsynaptic scaffolding and cytoskeletal proteins, and via this mechanism synaptic strength is enhanced. One specific mechanism that has been proposed is that the AMPA receptor interacting protein GRIP (72) is proteolyzed by calpain and that by this mechanism AMPA receptor function is enhanced. This idea is supported by the finding that inhibition of calpain can block LTP (73). An additional relevant mechanism is that the actin-binding protein spectrin undergoes proteolysis with LTP-inducing stimulation (74), suggesting that calpain is indeed activated with LTP induction. Further work will be required in order to define the role of this potential mechanism in elevating AMPA receptor function in E-LTP.

F. Presynaptic Changes— Increased Release

LTP is typically measured as an increase in the initial slope of the EPSP (or EPSP magnitude), and this effect can be subserved by an increase in postsynaptic receptor number or efficacy, as described previously, or by an increase in presynaptic neurotransmitter release, or both of these mechanisms together. The locus of LTP expression (pre- versus postsynaptic) has been widely debated and is a source of continuing controversy, as was described in Chapter 5. The evidence for postsynaptic changes in LTP seems quite convincing at this point, and not much argument about this aspect of LTP exists. The physiologic evidence for changes in neurotransmitter release is less convincing than that for changes in postsynaptic responsiveness in

my opinion, but many experts in this area disagree on the interpretation of the relevant data. However, there is much evidence indicative of a change in release presynaptically in E-LTP, and there is convincing biochemical evidence presynaptic changes do indeed occur in LTP. Thus, we will briefly discuss mechanism to account for lasting changes in the presynaptic compartment.

One of the most interesting and convincing physiologic studies on this topic was carried out by Dan Madison's laboratory (see Figure 13). Dan's lab has

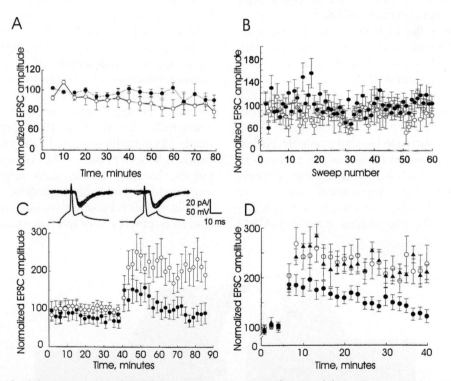

FIGURE 13   Selective reversal of E-LTP by a presynaptic protein kinase inhibitor. Presynaptic injection of the protein kinase inhibitor H-7 (100 μM) inhibits LTP but does not affect basal transmission. Controls, open circles; H-7, filled circles. (A) Monitoring basal transmission over a period of 80 minutes. Injection of H-7 into the presynaptic neuron did not suppress basal EPSC amplitudes compared with control ($n = 10$). (B) Responses to 1-Hz stimulation for 1 minute, such as those used to induced LTP, were unaffected by H-7 injection into the presynaptic cell. (C) Inhibitory effect of H-7 on LTP. The graph shows data from pairs in which the postsynaptic cell was obtained first with the amphotericin perforated patch technique, enabling basal transmission to be monitored for 40 minutes before pairing. After pairing there was some initial potentiation, but this decayed rapidly leaving no significant potentiation after 20 minutes. For H-7 experiments, $n = 7$; for control experiments $n = 17$. Inset, Sample sweeps from before and after pairing. (D) Summary of all H-7 experiments (both perforated patch and whole-cell mode) showing that LTP was reduced on average by H-7 (filled circles) when compared with controls (open circles and filled triangles). The baseline data in this panel have been truncated to the length of the experiments with the shortest baselines. Data and legend courtesy of Pavlidis, Montgomery, and Madison (75).

developed a very nice cell culture model system wherein they study LTP at synapses between CA3 pyramidal neurons in culture—synapses which appear to produce LTP quite similar to that at Schaffer-collateral synapses. The beauty of the system is that they can simultaneously have electrodes in both the presynaptic and postsynaptic neurons, giving unprecedented control over the presynaptic neuron, at least for mammalian CNS neurons. Using this preparation, Pavlides, Montgomery, and Madison (75) found that injection of the nonspecific protein kinase inhibitor H7 into the presynaptic neuron caused a selective reversal of E-LTP without perturbing baseline synaptic transmission.

What is the identity of this presynaptic kinase? Various evidence is consistent with the hypothesis that it is PKC. As described in the first section of this chapter, a variety of evidence indicates that persistently activated PKC is generated in LTP. More direct evidence that *presynaptic* PKC activity is increased is also available. As has been emphasized by one of the pioneers in this area, Aryeh Routtenberg, this is nicely illustrated by biochemical studies of LTP-associated increases in phosphorylation of the presynaptic protein GAP-43

(also known as B50, F1, and neuromodulin (76). There is very good biochemical evidence that PKC-mediated GAP-43 phosphorylation increases in LTP (32, 33, 77). GAP-43 is a calmodulin-binding protein similar to the protein neurogranin, which we discussed in the last chapter, and PKC phosphorylation of GAP-43 may increase presynaptic calmodulin levels and help facilitate neurotransmission by this mechanism (see Figure 14). In addition, a number of studies have shown that presynaptic PKC can increase neurotransmitter release by more direct effects on the release mechanism itself (37, 38, 78).

Taken together with data from Eric Klann's group showing persistent oxidative activation of PKC in E-LTP, these data allow a parsimonious model for retrograde signaling and facilitation of neurotransmitter release (see Figure 14). In this model, calcium-induced generation of reactive oxygen species postsynaptically allows retrograde signaling to PKC presynaptically. Persistently activated PKC presynaptically phosphorylates GAP-43 and other targets, leading to increased neurotransmitter release and synaptic potentiation.

This model is speculative, but the reader should not miss a very important point that

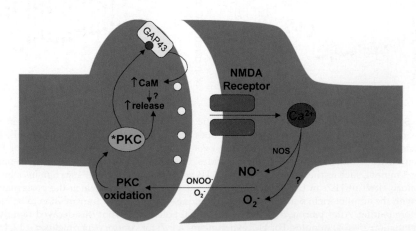

FIGURE 14 Retrograde signaling in E-LTP. Two potential presynaptic sites of PKC action are illustrated—direct effects on the release process and the calmodulin binding protein GAP43.

arises from the underlying data, which is independent of the particulars of the model. Consider the GAP-43 phosphorylation data together with other biochemical evidence from studies of other presynaptic proteins (79–83), plus the observations from Dan Madison's lab of presynaptic physiologic changes in their cultured neuron system. With these data in aggregate, a strong case can be made that NMDA receptor-dependent, postsynaptically induced *presynaptic* changes occur in LTP. The conclusion that can be drawn from these observations is profound; neurons in the CNS are capable of retrograde signaling. This conclusion stands independently of whether or not the particulars of the model are correct, or indeed independent of whether increased neurotransmitter release contributes to the expression of LTP. However it occurs and whatever its effects, retrograde signaling is an important component of the cell biological armamentarium available to the central neuron.

G. Postsynaptic Changes in Excitability?

As we have already discussed, LTP, as originally defined by Bliss and Lomo, is manifest as two physiologic components. The first component is an increase in synaptic strength, and the second component of LTP is referred to as EPSP-slope (E-S) potentiation. E-S potentiation is a general term used to refer to the postsynaptic cell having an increased probability of firing an action potential at a constant strength of synaptic input. E-S potentiation can be explained based on alterations in recurrent inhibitory connections in area CA1 (see Chapter 4). The other possibility is that E-S potentiation is a manifestation of increased excitability in the postsynaptic neuron, but the molecular mechanisms that could account for this aspect of LTP are completely mysterious at present. In an extension of the variety of mechanisms that we have been talking about in the context of AMPA receptor

regulation, one can hypothesize that persistently activated CaMKII or PKC could regulate potassium or sodium channels in order to increase excitability. Investigations to test whether such phenomena occur are currently under way, although these experiments are quite difficult due to the necessity of recording directly from CA1 pyramidal neuron dendrites after LTP induction. It also is important to remember that postsynaptic changes in voltage-dependent potassium and sodium channels might also alter the postsynaptic depolarization produced by AMPA receptor activation and by that mechanism contribute directly to EPSP potentiation as well as postsynaptic excitability.

III. DENDRITIC PROTEIN SYNTHESIS

In this final section we will begin to address issues related to the E-LTP to L-LTP transition. I include them in this chapter because they involve the generation of persisting signals, specifically the increased synthesis of proteins; thus, these mechanisms fit well within the general theme of this chapter. Also, there are data to suggest that regulation of protein synthesis may be a downstream target of some of the specific persisting signals involved in E-LTP, such as persistently activated PKC (see Figure 15), and these data fit in this chapter for that reason. However, these mechanisms also can be looked upon as part of the *induction process* for protein synthesis-dependent L-LTP, and thus serve as a transition to the next chapter where we talk about L-LTP as well. I also emphasize that these mechanisms are a gray area right now and are very much an area of ongoing discovery. Many aspects of the specific models and diagrams I will present in this section are speculative.

There was a resurgence of interest in this area when Kelsey Martin in Eric Kandel's laboratory published a seminal finding

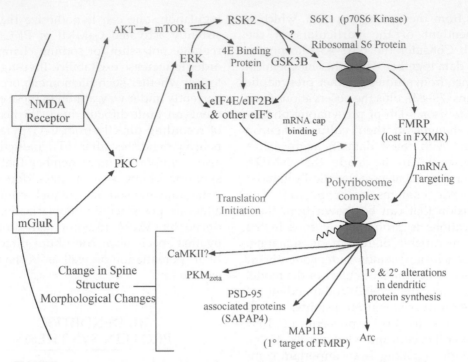

FIGURE 15 A model for activity-dependent regulation of local protein synthesis and spine morphological changes in LTP. See text for details and discussion.

demonstrating that localized dendritic protein synthesis is involved in synapse-specific potentiation of synaptic transmission in *Aplysia* sensory neurons (84). This discovery along with a variety of earlier findings led to the formulation of the model that local dendritic protein synthesis could provide a solution to the vexing problem of synapse-specificity for protein synthesis-dependent L-LTP. The conundrum was that L-LTP is dependent on protein synthesis, but dogma had it that protein synthesis happened exclusively in the rough ER in the *cell body*. The synapse specificity problem can be solved simply if there is activity-regulated protein synthesis limited to specific dendritic or synaptic regions. Formulation of the "local protein synthesis" model for L-LTP capitalized on earlier groundbreaking work from Ozzie Steward's group and Bill Greenough's group that indicated the existence of

dendritically localized protein synthesis machinery (polyribosomes).

Work from a wide variety of labs has supported the relevance of local protein synthesis to explaining synapse specificity of protein-synthesis-dependent LTP, and indeed to activity-dependent synaptic plasticity in the CNS in general. It is clear that there is activity-dependent regulation of protein synthesis for a variety of proteins, notably among them CaMKII (85), PKMζ (as described earlier), and Arc (see Box 1 in Chapter 3). It is also now quite clear that local, regulated protein synthesis occurs in dendrites (reviewed in references 86 and 87). Of course, the oft-replicated finding that protein synthesis inhibitors can block L-LTP is what precipitated the local protein synthesis model in the first place (1, 2).

How is local protein synthesis regulated in LTP? The mechanisms for regulating protein synthesis are themselves horrendously complicated, even without the added complexity of trying to understand how neuronal activity-dependent mechanisms might impinge upon them. Figure 15 and the following discussion summarizes a plethora of papers and reviews from the laboratories of Bill Greenough, Steve Warren, Erin Schuman, Ozzie Steward, Paul Worley, Cliff Abraham, and Eric Klann. It is a brief summary of some of the signal transduction mechanisms that are hypothesized to operate in the LTP-associated regulation of local protein synthesis in CA1 pyramidal neurons (86–88).

Protein synthesis must, of course, begin with the recognition of an mRNA by the ribosomal complex, which allows the intitiation of peptide chain elongation starting from the 5' end of the message. One mechanism for translational initiation involves the eukaryotic translation initiation factor 4e (eIF4e). Activated eIF4e associates with a number of co-activating proteins and this complex recruits the ribosome to the mRNA, which initiates the process of scanning for the AUG start codon. Activation of eIF4e is regulated by phosphorylation at one major site, Ser 209. The kinase likely to mediate this phosphorylation, at least based on the data available at present, is MNK1. MNK1 is mitogen-activated protein kinase-interacting-kinase 1 (MNK1). MNK1 is regulated by ERK MAPK, which as we have already discussed is involved in the induction of L-LTP.

Another target of ERK that may transduce a signal to the protein synthesis machinery is ribosomal S6 kinase 2 (RSK2). ERK directly phosphorylates and activates RSK2, which can then act upon the ribosome complex. While the role of RSK2 in regulating protein synthesis is not clear, both it and its target glycogen synthase kinase 3β (GSK3β) have been proposed to regulate protein synthesis through phosphorylation of ribosome-associated initiation factors (see Figure 15)—one specific candidate in this context is eIF2B (89). Thus, the ERK pathway has been proposed to regulate protein synthesis by a variety of mechanisms still being defined, but overall it is appealing to hypothesize a role for this cascade in regulating neuronal protein synthesis.

Another player implicated in regulating dendritic protein synthesis is PKC (90). Metabotropic glutamate receptors linked to PLC, of course, lead to PKC activation directly and ERK activation indirectly. Bill Greenough's group has found that metabotropic receptors via this pathway affect phosphorylation of ribosome-associated proteins (89). A parsimonious model integrating these findings is given in Figure 15, which shows one possible means of coupling glutamate receptors to protein synthesis in dendrites.

What are the messages regulated by this mechanism? One of the most interesting possibilities is FMRP. FMRP is the protein encoded by the fragile X mental retardation type 1 gene (91). FMRP is an mRNA binding protein that has both a nuclear localization signal and a nuclear export signal—it is hypothesized to be involved in trafficking of mRNAs. Moreover, FMRP colocalizes with polyribosomes in neuronal cell bodies and dendrites. FMRP knockout mice have altered dendritic spine morphology (in cortical neurons at least), which is consistent with a role for FMRP in regulating localized protein synthesis in dendrites. In addition, FMRP knockout animals exhibit alterations in mGluR-induced LTD at CA1 synapses (92). mGluR agonists also can regulate the synthesis of FMRP itself (90). Thus, one clear candidate as a target of local protein synthesis is FMRP, a protein involved in a human mental retardation syndrome. We will return to FMRP in Chapter 10 as well.

While FMRP is a *target* of the local synthesis machinery, as an mRNA binding protein localized to dendrites, it also likely contributes to *regulating* local protein synthesis as well. Two known targets of FMRP

BOX 4

SYNAPTIC TAGGING AND THE E-LTP/L-LTP TRANSITION

In 1997, Uwe Frey and Richard Morris published an interesting series of studies where they formulated the "synaptic tag" hypothesis of L-LTP induction (see reference 94 and figure). Without repeating the entirety of the details of their seminal paper and a variety of subsequent work in this area, the basic idea is as follows. L-LTP is dependent on protein synthesis and presumably on altered gene expression as well. How is it that one can have synapse specificity, which is known to occur with L-LTP, in the face of a certain central (nuclear) source of mRNA and potentially a central (rough ER) source of newly synthesized proteins? Frey and Morris proposed that local activity-regulated generation of persisting signals establishes a "synaptic tag" that marks synapses for potentiation when the synapse experiences an L-LTP-inducing stimulation.

The synaptic tag allows the capture of new gene products (mRNAs or proteins) sent out from the nucleus and cell body (also triggered by LTP-inducing stimulation), localizing these potentiating products at the appropriate synapses. Frey and Morris also showed in their original paper that the generation of the synaptic tag could be pharmacologically isolated from the more generalized induction of L-LTP. In other words, they could generate the tag in the absence of protein synthesis by giving E-LTP-inducing stimulation. Then, subsequent L-LTP-inducing stimulation at another set of synapses allowed the original group of synapses to capture the potentiating gene products. While the biochemical identity of the synaptic tag is unknown at present, any one of the variety of persisting post-translational modifications that we are discussing in this chapter are viable candidate mechanisms for contributing to the synaptic tag.

The synaptic tagging work of Frey and Morris also has another very important implication as a mechanism for generating long-lasting synaptic plasticity. Their findings imply that, after a cell has received an L-LTP-inducing strong stimulation, subsequent weaker stimuli can capture the L-LTP-inducing products at their synapses. Thus, a weaker stimulation, when following a strong stimulation, could produce L-LTP. This is a powerful mechanism for temporal integration of signals across time (95). Depending on the timing of the signals, at any particular time, a signal of a given strength may or may not trigger LTP depending on the prior recent "experience" of the cell.

I find this a fascinating finding, in part because this and similar mechanisms of temporal integration have the potential to explain one of the long-standing mysteries in learning and memory. As described in Chapter 2, a highly reproducible feature of learning across species and learning paradigms is the improved efficacy of "spaced" versus "massed" training. Ten training sessions separated by 15 minutes is much more effective in producing long-lasting and robust memory than ten training sessions back-to-back, for example. Synaptic tagging and other temporal integration mechanisms of this sort have the capacity to explain this phenomenon. Subsequent stimuli, when timed appropriately, can have stronger effects than they would otherwise. A weak signal, that normally might not cross the threshold for triggering change, can be converted to a long-lasting signal if it follows a previous training session. If the subsequent training

BOX 4—cont'd

SYNAPTIC TAGGING AND THE E-LTP/L-LTP TRANSITION

trials come too soon after the initial stimulus, the synaptic tag generated by the weak stimulus may have nothing to capture because the nuclear products have not diffused far enough to be captured. If the weak stimulus comes too late (i.e., the training is too spaced out), the genomic products will have been generated but not captured before they decayed. Thus, temporal integration mechanisms of this sort involving synaptic tagging and the generation of other persisting but transient signals allow for the cell to build an optimal time window for the efficacy of repeated stimuli.

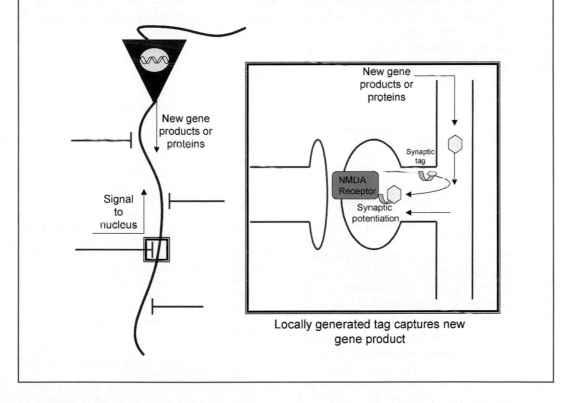

regulation are microtubule-associated protein 1B (MAP1B) and the PSD-95 associated protein SAPAP4. These cytoskeletal/scaffolding protein targets are a potential means by which FMRP might regulate spine structure.

Other well-known and extensively characterized products of local protein synthesis are CaMKII (85) and Arc (86).

While the synthesis of these proteins is probably not directly regulated by FMRP, they certainly may play an important role as targets of regulated protein synthesis in dendrites. As we have already discussed in various parts of this book, Arc mRNA and protein are selectively localized to active synapses, and Arc as a cytoskeleton-associated protein may serve a morphological/structural role. CaMKII, of course, is a dominant player in post-synaptic function and structure. Thus, while it is quite early to try to synthesize a complete model for the regulation and targets of local dendritic protein synthesis, it is not unreasonable to think that this process plays a key role in various processes including the regulation of spine structure, morphology, and PSD stabilization, as well as the regulation of signal transduction locally.

Finally, I should note that while for the present I am defining L-LTP as that phase of LTP dependent upon changes in both gene expression and protein synthesis, there are recent publications suggesting that there could be an intermediate phase of LTP dependent on altered protein synthesis but not altered gene expression (e.g., 93). This is certainly a reasonable idea, and, in the future, we may need to break down LTP into additional substages beyond E-LTP and L-LTP based on these criteria.

IV. CHAPTER SUMMARY

In this chapter, we explored several of the fundamentally important issues related to information storage in neurons. How is a persisting biochemical signal generated? How is that signal transmitted to an effector system to alter neuronal function? If there are multiple biochemical mechanisms for information storage, how might one mechanism transition into the next? In addressing these critical issues, a number of specific molecular mechanisms were proposed in the context of E-LTP at Schaffer-collateral synapses. Our models focused on persistent post-translational modifications as *maintenance* mechanisms, and on postsynaptic receptors as target *effectors* of these maintenance signals. Some of the models proposed may be wrong in their particulars, and likely some of the models are relevant to some types of LTP but not others. Future studies will refine and clarify these issues.

Nevertheless, the three decades-worth of studies on mechanisms of E-LTP stand as meaningful contributions to our understanding of the basics of molecular information storage in the nervous system. Much, much progress has been made in defining the basic biochemical mechanisms available to the neuron that allow it to generate a persisting signal and translate that signal into a persisting effect. This work also has begun to define the biochemical processes that can be used by *any* central synapse for augmenting the strength of its synaptic connections. Thus, investigations into the biochemistry of E-LTP have given us insights into the fundamental cell biology of the neuron.

References

1. Frey, U., Krug, M., Reymann, K. G., and Matthies, H. (1988). "Anisomycin, an inhibitor of protein synthesis, blocks late phases of LTP phenomena in the hippocampal CA1 region in vitro." *Brain Res.* 452:57–65.
2. Stanton, P. K., and Sarvey, J. M. (1984). "Blockade of long-term potentiation in rat hippocampal CA1 region by inhibitors of protein synthesis." *J. Neurosci.* 4:3080–3088.
3. Lu, K. P., Liou, Y. C., and Zhou, X. Z. (2002). "Pinning down proline-directed phosphorylation signaling." *Trends Cell Biol.* 12:164–172.
4. Duman, R. S., Terwilliger, R. Z., and Nestler, E. J. (1993). "Alterations in nitric oxide-stimulated endogenous ADP-ribosylation associated with long-term potentiation in rat hippocampus." *J. Neurochem.* 61:1542–1545.
5. Schuman, E. M., Meffert, M. K., Schulman, H., and Madison, D. V. (1994). "An ADP-ribosyltransferase as a potential target for nitric oxide action in hippocampal long-term potentiation." *Proc. Natl. Acad. Sci. USA* 91:11958–11962.
6. Lisman, J., Schulman, H., and Cline, H. (2002). "The molecular basis of CaMKII function in synaptic and behavioural memory." *Nat. Rev. Neurosci.* 3:175–190.
7. Strack, S., and Colbran, R. J. (1998). "Autophosphorylation-dependent targeting of calcium/calmodulin- dependent protein kinase II by the NR2B subunit of the *N*-methyl- D- aspartate receptor." *J. Biol. Chem.* 273:20689–20692.
8. Leonard, A. S., Lim, I. A., Hemsworth, D. E., Horne, M. C., and Hell, J. W. (1999). "Calcium/calmodulin-dependent protein kinase II is associated with the *N*-methyl-D-aspartate receptor." *Proc. Natl. Acad. Sci. USA* 96:3239–3244.

9. Lisman, J. E., and Zhabotinsky, A. M. (2001). "A model of synaptic memory: a CaMKII/PP1 switch that potentiates transmission by organizing an AMPA receptor anchoring assembly." *Neuron* 31:191–201.

10. Hvalby, O., Hemmings, H. C. Jr, Paulsen, O., Czernik, A. J., Nairn, A. C., Godfraind, J. M., Jensen, V., Raastad, M., Storm, J. F., Andersen, P., and Greengard, P. (1994). "Specificity of protein kinase inhibitor peptides and induction of long-term potentiation." *Proc. Natl. Acad. Sci. USA* 91:4761–4765.

11. Otmakhov, N., Griffith, L. C., and Lisman, J. E. (1997). "Postsynaptic inhibitors of calcium/calmodulin-dependent protein kinase type II block induction but not maintenance of pairing-induced long-term potentiation." *J. Neurosci.* 17:5357–5365.

12. Silva, A. J., Stevens, C. F., Tonegawa, S., and Wang, Y. (1992). "Deficient hippocampal long-term potentiation in alpha-calcium- calmodulin kinase II mutant mice." *Science* 257:201–206.

13. Hinds, H. L., Tonegawa, S., and Malinow, R. (1998). "CA1 long-term potentiation is diminished but present in hippocampal slices from alpha-CaMKII mutant mice." *Learn. Mem.* 5:344–354.

14. Mayford, M., Wang, J., Kandel, E. R., and O'Dell, T. J. (1995). "CaMKII regulates the frequency-response function of hippocampal synapses for the production of both LTD and LTP." *Cell* 81:891–904.

15. Chen, H. X., Otmakhov, N., Strack, S., Colbran, R. J., and Lisman, J. E. (2001). "Is persistent activity of calcium/calmodulin-dependent kinase required for the maintenance of LTP?" *J. Neurophysiol.* 85:1368–1376.

16. De Koninck, P., and Schulman, H. (1998). "Sensitivity of CaM kinase II to the frequency of Ca^{2+} oscillations." *Science* 279:227–230.

17. Poser, S., and Storm, D. R. (2001). "Role of Ca^{2+}-stimulated adenylyl cyclases in LTP and memory formation." *Int. J. Dev. Neurosci.* 19:387–394.

18. Roberson, E. D., and Sweatt, J. D. (1996). "Transient activation of cyclic AMP-dependent protein kinase during hippocampal long-term potentiation." *J. Biol. Chem.* 271:30436–30441.

19. Garthwaite, J., and Boulton, C. L. (1995). "Nitric oxide signaling in the central nervous system." *Annu. Rev. Physiol.* 57:683–706.

20. Kleppisch, T., Pfeifer, A., Klatt, P., Ruth, P., Montkowski, A., Fassler, R., and Hofmann, F. (1999). "Long-term potentiation in the hippocampal CA1 region of mice lacking cGMP-dependent kinases is normal and susceptible to inhibition of nitric oxide synthase." *J. Neurosci.* 19:48–55.

21. Bon, C. L., and Garthwaite, J. (2001). "Nitric oxide-induced potentiation of CA1 hippocampal synaptic transmission during baseline stimulation is strictly frequency-dependent." *Neuropharmacology* 40:501–507.

22. Selig, D. K., Segal, M. R., Liao, D., Malenka, R. C., Malinow, R., Nicoll, R. A., and Lisman, J. E. (1996). "Examination of the role of cGMP in long-term potentiation in the CA1 region of the hippocampus." *Learn. Mem.* 3:42–48.

23. Schuman, E. M., and Madison, D. V. (1991). "A requirement for the intercellular messenger nitric oxide in long-term potentiation." *Science* 254:1503–1506.

24. Arancio, O., Antonova, I., Gambaryan, S., Lohmann, S. M., Wood, J. S., Lawrence, D. S., and Hawkins, R. D. (2001). "Presynaptic role of cGMP-dependent protein kinase during long-lasting potentiation." *J. Neurosci.* 1:143–149.

25. Lovinger, D. M., Wong, K. L., Murakami, K., and Routtenberg, A. (1987). "Protein kinase C inhibitors eliminate hippocampal long-term potentiation." *Brain. Res.* 436:177–183.

26. Colley, P. A., Sheu, F. S., and Routtenberg, A. (1990). "Inhibition of protein kinase C blocks two components of LTP persistence, leaving initial potentiation intact." *J. Neurosci.* 10:3353–3360.

27. Malinow, R., Madison, D. V., and Tsien, R. W. (1988). "Persistent protein kinase activity underlying long-term potentiation." *Nature* 335:820–824.

28. Wang, J. H., and Feng, D. P. (1992). "Postsynaptic protein kinase C essential to induction and maintenance of long-term potentiation in the hippocampal CA1 region." *Proc. Natl. Acad. Sci. USA* 89:2576–2580.

29. Klann, E., Chen, S. J., and Sweatt, J. D. (1991). "Persistent protein kinase activation in the maintenance phase of long-term potentiation." *J. Biol. Chem.* 266:24253–24256.

30. Klann, E., Chen, S. J., and Sweatt, J. D. (1993). "Mechanism of protein kinase C activation during the induction and maintenance of long-term potentiation probed using a selective peptide substrate." *Proc. Natl. Acad. Sci. USA* 90:8337–8341.

31. Leahy, J. C., Luo, Y., Kent, C. S., Meiri, K. F., and Vallano, M. L. (1993). "Demonstration of presynaptic protein kinase C activation following long-term potentiation in rat hippocampal slices." *Neuroscience* 52:563–574.

32. Lovinger, D. M., Akers, R. F., Nelson, R. B., Barnes, C. A., McNaughton, B. L., and Routtenberg, A. (1985). "A selective increase in phosporylation of protein F1, a protein kinase C substrate, directly related to three day growth of long term synaptic enhancement." *Brain Res.* 343:137–143.

33. Gianotti, C., Nunzi, M. G., Gispen, W. H., and Corradetti, R. (1992). "Phosphorylation of the presynaptic protein B-50 (GAP-43) is increased during electrically induced long-term potentiation." *Neuron* 8:843–848.

34. Sacktor, T. C., Osten, P., Valsamis, H., Jiang, X., Naik, M. U., and Sublette, E. (1993). "Persistent activation of the zeta isoform of protein kinase C in the maintenance of long-term potentiation." *Proc. Natl. Acad. Sci. USA* 90:8342–8346.

35. Schwartz, J. H. (1993). "Cognitive kinases." *Proc. Natl. Acad. Sci. USA* 90:8310–8313.

36. Powell, C. M., Johnston, D., and Sweatt, J. D. (1994). "Autonomously active protein kinase C in the maintenance phase of N-methyl-D-aspartate receptor-independent long term potentiation." *J. Biol. Chem.* 269:27958–27963.

37. Malenka, R. C., Madison, D. V., and Nicoll, R. A. (1986). "Potentiation of synaptic transmission in the hippocampus by phorbol esters." *Nature* 321:175–177.

38. Malenka, R. C., Ayoub, G. S., and Nicoll, R. A. (1987). "Phorbol esters enhance transmitter release in rat hippocampal slices." *Brain Res.* 403:198–203.

39. Hvalby, O., Reymann, K., and Andersen, P. (1988). "Intracellular analysis of potentiation of CA1 hippocampal synaptic transmission by phorbol ester application." *Exp. Brain Res.* 71:588–596.

40. Hu, G. Y., Hvalby, O., Walaas, S. I., Albert, K. A., Skjeflo, P., Andersen, P., and Greengard, P. (1987). "Protein kinase C injection into hippocampal pyramidal cells elicits features of long term potentiation." *Nature* 328:426–429.

41. Abeliovich, A., Chen, C., Goda, Y., Silva, A. J., Stevens, C. F., and Tonegawa, S. (1993). "Modified hippocampal long-term potentiation in PKC gamma-mutant mice." *Cell* 75:1253–1262.

42. Weeber, E. J., Atkins, C. M., Selcher, J. C., Varga, A. W., Mirnikjoo, B., Paylor, R., Leitges, M., and Sweatt, J. D. (2000). "A role for the beta isoform of protein kinase C in fear conditioning." *J. Neurosci.* 20:5906–5914.

43. Goda, Y., Stevens, C. F., and Tonegawa, S. (1996). "Phorbol ester effects at hippocampal synapses act independently of the gamma isoform of PKC." *Learn. Mem.* 3:182–187.

44. Klann, E., and Thiels, E. (1999). "Modulation of protein kinases and protein phosphatases by reactive oxygen species: implications for hippocampal synaptic plasticity." *Prog. Neuropsychopharmacol. Biol. Psychiatry* 23:359–376.

45. Knapp, L. T., and Klann, E. (2002). "Potentiation of hippocampal synaptic transmission by superoxide requires the oxidative activation of protein kinase C." *J. Neurosci.* 22:674–683.

46. Sweatt, J. D., Atkins, C. M., Johnson, J., English, J. D., Roberson, E. D., Chen, S. J., Newton, A., and Klann, E. (1998). "Protected-site phosphorylation of protein kinase C in hippocampal long-term potentiation." *J. Neurochem.* 71:1075–1085.

47. Flint, A. J., Paladini, R. D., and Koshland, D. E. Jr. (1990). "Autophosphorylation of protein kinase C at three separated regions of its primary sequence." *Science* 249:408–411.

48. Orr, J. W., Keranen, L. M., and Newton, A. C. (1992). "Reversible exposure of the pseudosubstrate domain of protein kinase C by phosphatidylserine and diacylglycerol." *J. Biol. Chem.* 267:15263–15266.

49. Keranen, L. M., Dutil, E. M., and Newton, A. C. (1995). "Protein kinase C is regulated in vivo by three functionally distinct phosphorylations." *Curr. Biol.* 5:1394–1403.

50. Dutil, E. M., Keranen, L. M., DePaoli-Roach, A. A., and Newton, A. C. (1994). "In vivo regulation of protein kinase C by trans-phosphorylation followed by autophosphorylation." *J. Biol. Chem.* 269:29359–29362.

51. Zhang, J., Wang, L., Petrin, J., Bishop, W. R., and Bond, R. W. (1993). "Characterization of site-specific mutants altered at protein kinase C beta 1 isozyme autophosphorylation sites." *Proc. Natl. Acad. Sci. USA* 90:6130–6134.

52. Zhang, J., Wang, L., Schwartz, J., Bond, R. W., and Bishop, W. R. (1994). "Phosphorylation of Thr642 is an early event in the processing of newly synthesized protein kinase C beta 1 and is essential for its activation." *J. Biol. Chem.* 269:19578–19584.

53. Newton, A. C., and Koshland, D. E. Jr. (1987). "Protein kinase C autophosphorylates by an intrapeptide reaction." *J. Biol. Chem.* 262:10185–10188.

54. Osten, P., Valsamis, L., Harris, A., and Sacktor, T. C. (1996). "Protein synthesis-dependent formation of protein kinase Mzeta in long-term potentiation." *J. Neurosci.* 16:2444–2451.

55. Ling, D. S., Benardo, L. S., Serrano, P. A., Blace, N., Kelly, M. T., Crary, J. F., and Sacktor, T. C. (2002). "Protein kinase Mzeta is necessary and sufficient for LTP maintenance." *Nat. Neurosci.* 5:295–296.

56. Hrabetova, S., and Sacktor, T. C. (1996). "Bidirectional regulation of protein kinase M zeta in the maintenance of long-term potentiation and long-term depression." *J. Neurosci.* 16:5324–5333.

57. Williams, J. H., Errington, M. L., Lynch, M. A., and Bliss, T. V. (1989). "Arachidonic acid induces a long-term activity-dependent enhancement of synaptic transmission in the hippocampus." *Nature* 341:739–742.

58. O'Dell, T. J., Hawkins, R. D., Kandel, E. R., and Arancio, O. (1991). "Tests of the roles of two diffusible substances in long-term potentiation: evidence for nitric oxide as a possible early retrograde messenger." *Proc. Natl. Acad. Sci. USA* 88:11285–11289.

59. Scannevin, R. H., and Huganir, R. L. (2000). "Postsynaptic organization and regulation of excitatory synapses." *Nat. Rev. Neurosci.* 1:133–141.

60. Derkach, V., Barria, A., and Soderling, T. R. (1999). "Ca^{2+}/calmodulin-kinase II enhances channel conductance of alpha-amino-3-hydroxy-5-methyl-4-isoxazolepropionate type glutamate receptors." *Proc. Natl. Acad. Sci. USA* 96:3269–3274.

61. Benke ,T. A., Luthi, A., Isaac, J. T., and Collingridge, G. L. (1998). "Modulation of AMPA receptor unitary conductance by synaptic activity." *Nature* 393:793–797.

62. Barria, A., Muller, D., Derkach, V., Griffith, L. C., and Soderling, T. R. (1997). "Regulatory phosphorylation of AMPA-type glutamate receptors by CaM-KII during long-term potentiation." *Science* 276:2042–2045.

63. Shi, S. H. (2001). "Amersham Biosciences & Science Prize. AMPA receptor dynamics and synaptic plasticity." *Science* 294:1851–1852.

64. Malinow, R., and Malenka, R. C. (2002). "AMPA receptor trafficking and synaptic plasticity." *Annu. Rev. Neurosci.* 25:103–126.

65. Poncer, J. C., Esteban, J. A., and Malinow, R. (2002). "Multiple mechanisms for the potentiation of AMPA receptor-mediated transmission by alpha-Ca^{2+}/calmodulin-dependent protein kinase II." *J. Neurosci.* 22:4406–4411.

66. Lee, H. K., Barbarosie, M., Kameyama, K., Bear, M. F., and Huganir, R. L. (2000). "Regulation of distinct AMPA receptor phosphorylation sites during bidirectional synaptic plasticity." *Nature* 405:955–959.

67. Montgomery, J. M., and Madison, D. V. (2002). "State-dependent heterogeneity in synaptic depression between pyramidal cell pairs." *Neuron* 33:765–777.

68. Hayashi, Y., Shi, S. H., Esteban, J. A., Piccini, A., Poncer, J. C., and Malinow, R. (2000). "Driving AMPA receptors into synapses by LTP and CaMKII: requirement for GluR1 and PDZ domain interaction." *Science* 287:2262–2267.

69. Ehlers, M. D. (2000). "Reinsertion or degradation of AMPA receptors determined by activity-dependent endocytic sorting." *Neuron* 28:511–525.

70. Luscher, C., Xia, H., Beattie, E. C., Carroll, R. C., von Zastrow, M., Malenka, R. C., and Nicoll, R. A. (1999). "Role of AMPA receptor cycling in synaptic transmission and plasticity." *Neuron* 24:649–658.

71. Grosshans, D. R., Clayton, D. A., Coultrap, S. J., and Browning, M. D. (2002). "LTP leads to rapid surface expression of NMDA but not AMPA receptors in adult rat CA1." *Nat. Neurosci.* 5:27–33.

72. Lu, X., Wyszynski, M., Sheng, M., and Baudry, M. (2001). "Proteolysis of glutamate receptor-interacting protein by calpain in rat brain: implications for synaptic plasticity." *J. Neurochem.* 77:1553–1560.

73. Vanderklish, P., Bednarski, E., and Lynch, G. (1996). "Translational suppression of calpain blocks long-term potentiation." *Learn. Mem.* 3:209–217.

74. Vanderklish, P., Saido, T. C., Gall, C., Arai, A., and Lynch, G. (1995). "Proteolysis of spectrin by calpain accompanies theta-burst stimulation in cultured hippocampal slices." *Brain Res. Mol. Brain Res.* 32:25–35.

75. Pavlidis, P., Montgomery, J., and Madison, D. V. (2000). "Presynaptic protein kinase activity supports long-term potentiation at synapses between individual hippocampal neurons." *J. Neurosci.* 20:4497–4505.

76. Routtenberg, A. (1990). "Trans-synaptophobia." *Adv. Exp. Med. Biol.* 268:401–403.

77. Linden, D. J., Wong, K. L., Sheu, F. S., and Routtenberg, A. (1988). "NMDA receptor blockade prevents the increase in protein kinase C substrate (protein F1) phosphorylation produced by long-term potentiation." *Brain Res.* 458:142–146.

78. Parfitt, K. D., and Madison, D. V. (1993). "Phorbol esters enhance synaptic transmission by a presynaptic, calcium-dependent mechanism in rat hippocampus." *J. Physiol.* 471:245–268.

79. Ryan, T. A., Ziv, N. E., and Smith, S. J. (1996). "Potentiation of evoked vesicle turnover at individually resolved synaptic boutons." *Neuron* 17:125–134.

80. Malgaroli, A., Ting, A. E., Wendland, B., Bergamaschi, A., Villa, A., Tsien, R. W., and Scheller, R. H. (1995). "Presynaptic component of long-term potentiation visualized at individual hippocampal synapses." *Science* 268:1624–1628.

81. Zakharenko, S. S., Zablow, L., and Siegelbaum, S. A. (2001). "Visualization of changes in presynaptic function during long-term synaptic plasticity." *Nat. Neurosci.* 4:711–717.

82. Braun, J. E., and Madison, D. V. (2000). "A novel SNAP25-caveolin complex correlates with the onset of persistent synaptic potentiation." *J. Neurosci.* 20:5997–6006.

83. Antonova, I., Arancio, O., Trillat, A. C., Wang, H. G., Zablow, L., Udo, H., Kandel, E. R., and Hawkins, R. D. (2001). "Rapid increase in clusters of presynaptic proteins at onset of long-lasting potentiation." *Science* 294:1547–1550.

84. Martin, K. C., Casadio, A., Zhu, H., E. Y., Rose, J. C., Chen, M., Bailey, C. H., and Kandel, E. R. (1997). "Synapse-specific, long-term facilitation of aplysia sensory to motor synapses: a function for local protein synthesis in memory storage." *Cell* 91:927–938.

85. Ouyang, Y., Rosenstein, A., Kreiman, G., Schuman, E. M., and Kennedy, M. B. (1999). "Tetanic stimulation leads to increased accumulation of Ca(2+)/calmodulin-dependent protein kinase II via dendritic protein synthesis in hippocampal neurons." *J. Neurosci.* 19:7823–7833.

86. Steward, O., and Worley, P. F. (2001). "A cellular mechanism for targeting newly synthesized mRNAs to synaptic sites on dendrites." *Proc. Natl. Acad. Sci. USA* 98:7062–7068.

87. Steward, O., and Schuman, E. M. (2001). "Protein synthesis at synaptic sites on dendrites." *Annu. Rev. Neurosci.* 24:299–325.

88. Raught, B., Gingras, A. C., and Sonenberg, N. (2001). "The target of rapamycin (TOR) proteins." *Proc. Natl. Acad. Sci. USA* 98:7037–7044.

89. Angenstein, F., Greenough, W. T., and Weiler, I. J. (1998). "Metabotropic glutamate receptor-initiated translocation of protein kinase p90rsk to polyribosomes: a possible factor regulating synaptic protein synthesis." *Proc. Natl. Acad. Sci. USA* 95:15078–15083.

90. Greenough, W. T., Klintsova, A. Y., Irwin, S. A., Galvez, R., Bates, K. E., and Weiler, I. J. (2001). "Synaptic regulation of protein synthesis and the fragile X protein." *Proc. Natl. Acad. Sci. USA* 98:7101–7106.

91. Gao, F. B. (2002). "Understanding fragile X syndrome: insights from retarded flies." *Neuron* 34:859–862.

92. Huber, K. M., Gallagher, S. M., Warren, S. T., and Bear, M. F. (2002). "Altered synaptic plasticity in a mouse model of fragile X mental retardation." *Proc. Natl. Acad. Sci. USA* 99:7746–7750.

93. Raymond, C. R., Thompson, V. L., Tate, W. P., and Abraham, W. C. (2000). "Metabotropic glutamate receptors trigger homosynaptic protein synthesis to prolong long-term potentiation." *J. Neurosci.* 20:969–976.

94. Frey, U., and Morris, R. G. (1998). "Synaptic tagging: implications for late maintenance of hippocampal long-term potentiation." *Trends Neurosci.* 21:181–188.

95. Martin, S. J., Grimwood, P. D., and Morris, R. G. (2000). "Synaptic plasticity and memory: an evaluation of the hypothesis." *Annu. Rev.Neurosci.* 23:649–711.

96. Sanna, P. P., Cammalleri, M., Berton, F., Simpson, C., Lutjens, R., Bloom, F. E., and Francesconi, W. (2002). "Phosphatidylinositol 3-kinase is required for the expression but not for the induction or the maintenance of long-term potentiation in the hippocampal CA1 region." *J. Neurosci.* 22:3359–3365.

97. Sweatt, J. D. (2001). "Protooncogenes subserve memory formation in the adult CNS." *Neuron* 31:671–674.

98. Brunet, A., Datta, S. R., and Greenberg, M. E. (2001). "Transcription-dependent and -independent control of neuronal survival by the PI3K-Akt signaling pathway." *Curr. Opin. Neurobiol.* 11:297–305.

99. Kelly, A., and Lynch, M. A. (2000). "Long-term potentiation in dentate gyrus of the rat is inhibited by the phosphoinositide 3-kinase inhibitor, wortmannin." *Neuropharmacology* 39:643–651.

100. Silva, A. J., Stevens, C. F., Tonegawa, S., and Wang, Y. (1992). "Deficient hippocampal long-term potentiation in alpha-calcium-calmodulin kinase II mutant mice." *Science* 257:201–206.

101. Pettit, D. L., Perlman, S., and Malinow, R. (1994). "Potentiated transmission and prevention of further LTP by increased CaMKII activity in postsynaptic hippocampal slice neurons." *Science* 266:1881–1885.

102. Ouyang, Y., Kantor, D., Harris, K. M., Schuman, E. M., and Kennedy, M. B. (1997). "Visualization of the distribution of autophosphorylated calcium/calmodulin-dependent protein kinase II after tetanic stimulation in the CA1 area of the hippocampus." *J. Neurosci.* 17:5416–5427.

103. Malinow, R., Schulman, H., and Tsien, R. W. (1989). "Inhibition of postsynaptic PKC or CaMKII blocks induction but not expression of LTP." *Science* 245:862–866.

104. Wang, J. H., and Kelly, P. T. (1995). "Postsynaptic injection of CA^{2+}/CaM induces synaptic potentiation requiring CaMKII and PKC activity." *Neuron* 15:443–452.

105. Fukunaga, K., Stoppini, L., Miyamoto, E., and Muller, D. (1993). "Long-term potentiation is associated with an increased activity of Ca^{2+}/calmodulin-dependent protein kinase II." *J. Biol. Chem.* 268:7863–7867.

106. Matthies, H. Jr, Behnisch, T., Kase, H., Matthies, H., and Reymann, K. G. (1991). "Differential effects of protein kinase inhibitors on pre-established long-term potentiation in rat hippocampal neurons in vitro." *Neurosci. Lett.* 121:259–262.

107. Matthies, H., and Reymann, K. G. (1993). "Protein kinase A inhibitors prevent the maintenance of hippocampal long-term potentiation." *Neuroreport* 4:712–714.

108. Reymann, K. G., Brodemann, R., Kase, H., and Matthies, H. (1988). "Inhibitors of calmodulin and protein kinase C block different phases of hippocampal long-term potentiation." *Brain Res.* 461:388–392.

109. Reymann, K. G., Frey, U., Jork, R., and Matthies, H. (1988). "Polymyxin B, an inhibitor of protein kinase C, prevents the maintenance of synaptic long-term potentiation in hippocampal CA1 neurons." *Brain Res.* 440:305–314.

110. Blitzer, R. D., Wong, T., Nouranifar, R., Iyengar, R., and Landau, E. M. (1995). "Postsynaptic cAMP pathway gates early LTP in hippocampal CA1 region." *Neuron* 15:1403–1414.

111. Blitzer, R. D., Connor, J. H., Brown, G. P., Wong, T., Shenolikar, S., Iyengar, R., and Landau, E. M. (1998). "Gating of CaMKII by cAMP-regulated protein phosphatase activity during LTP." *Science* 280:1940–1942.

112. Winder, D. G., Mansuy, I. M., Osman, M., Moallem, T. M., and Kandel, E. R. (1998). "Genetic and pharmacological evidence for a novel, intermediate phase of long-term potentiation suppressed by calcineurin." *Cell* 92:25–37.

113. Frey, U., Huang, Y. Y., and Kandel, E. R. (1993). "Effects of cAMP simulate a late stage of LTP in hippocampal CA1 neurons." *Science* 260:1661–1664.

114. Chetkovich, D. M., and Sweatt, J. D. (1993). "NMDA receptor activation increases cyclic AMP in area CA1 of the hippocampus via calcium/calmodulin stimulation of adenylyl cyclase." *J. Neurochem.* 61:1933–1942.

115. Chetkovich, D. M., Gray, R., Johnston, D., and Sweatt, J. D. (1991). "N-methyl-D-aspartate receptor activation increases cAMP levels and voltage-gated Ca^{2+} channel activity in area CA1 of hippocampus." *Proc. Natl. Acad. Sci. USA* 88:6467–6471.

116. Chavez-Noriega, L. E., and Stevens, C. F. (1992). "Modulation of synaptic efficacy in field CA1 of the rat hippocampus by forskolin." *Brain Res.* 574:85–92.

117. Pockett, S., Slack, J. R., and Peacock, S. (1993). "Cyclic AMP and long-term potentiation in the CA1 region of rat hippocampus." *Neuroscience* 52:229–236.

118. Roberson, E. D. (1999). Roles for the cyclic AMP dependent protein kinase and superoxide in the induction of hippocampel long-term potentiation. *Eric Roberson, PhD Thesis.* Houston: Baylor College of Medicine.

119. English, J. D., and Sweatt, J. D. (1997). "A requirement for the mitogen-activated protein kinase Cascade in hippocampal long term potentiation." *J. Biol. Chem.* 272:19103–19106.

120. Atkins, C. M., Selcher, J. C., Petraitis, J. J., Trzaskos, J. M., and Sweatt, J. D. (1998). "The MAPK cascade is required for mammalian associative learning." *Nat. Neurosci.* 1:602–609.

121. Impey, S., Obrietan, K., Wong, S. T., Poser, S., Yano, S., Wayman, G., Deloulme, J. C., Chan, G., and Storm, D. R. (1998). "Cross talk between ERK and PKA is required for Ca^{2+} stimulation of CREB-dependent transcription and ERK nuclear translocation." *Neuron* 21:869–883.

122. English, J. D., and Sweatt, J. D. (1996). "Activation of p42 mitogen-activated protein kinase in hippocampal long term potentiation." *J. Biol. Chem.* 271:24329–24332.

123. Roberson, E. D., English, J. D., Adams, J. P., Selcher, J. C., Kondratick, C., and Sweatt, J. D. (1999). "The mitogen-activated protein kinase cascade couples PKA and PKC to cAMP response element binding protein phosphorylation in area CA1 of hippocampus." *J. Neurosci.* 19:4337–4348.

124. Verdaguer, N., Corbalan-Garcia, S., Ochoa, W. F., Fita, I., and Gomez-Fernandez, J. C. (1999). "Ca(2+) bridges the C2 membrane-binding domain of protein kinase Calpha directly to phosphatidylserine." *Embo. J.* 18:6329–6338.

125. Kolodziej, S. J., Hudmon, A., Waxham, M. N., and Stoops, J. K. (2000). "Three-dimensional reconstructions of calcium/calmodulin-dependent (CaM) kinase IIalpha and truncated CaM kinase IIalpha reveal a unique organization for its structural core and functional domains." *J. Biol. Chem.* 275:14354–14359.

126. Dineley, K. T., Weeber, E. J., Atkins, C., Adams, J. P., Anderson, A. E., and Sweatt, J. D. (2001). "Leitmotifs in the biochemistry of LTP induction: amplification, integration and coordination." *J. Neurochem.* 77:961–971.

127. Wong, S. T., Athos, J., Figueroa, X. A., Pineda, V. V., Schaefer, M. L., Chavkin, C. C., Muglia, L. J., and Storm, D. R. (1999). "Calcium-stimulated adenylyl cyclase activity is critical for hippocampus-dependent long-term memory and late phase LTP." *Neuron* 23:787–798.

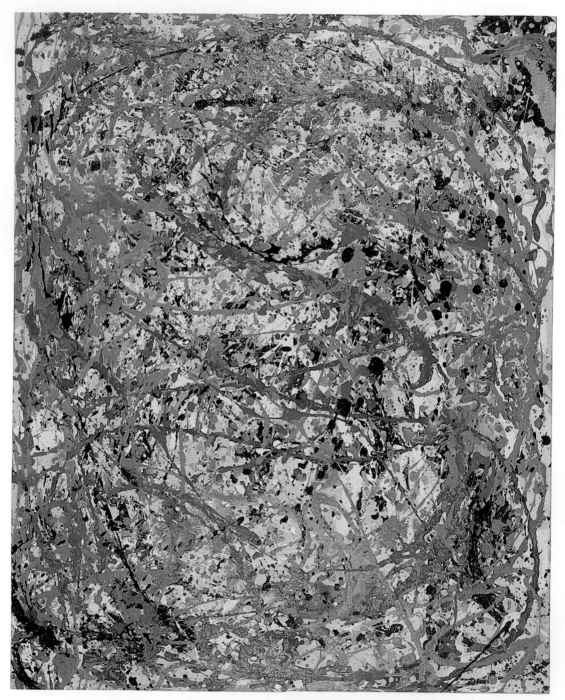

Genomic Regulation in Memory Formation
J. David Sweatt, Acrylic on canvas, 2002

8

Biochemical Mechanisms for Long-Term Information Storage at the Cellular Level

INTRODUCTION

In this chapter we will discuss the mechanisms unique to inducing and maintaining the long-lasting, late phase of LTP. This is an exciting, wide-open area of LTP research right now, one of those areas where it is clear that important work is underway but where the surface has just been scratched in terms of our understanding.

L-LTP is defined in terms of an enduring, protein synthesis-dependent form of synaptic potentiation in area CA1, as I will describe in more detail later. However, the phrase "L-LTP" is in some ways, and perhaps in its most meaningful way, an allegory of long-term memory in the behaving animal. The particular mechanisms that are being worked out to explain L-LTP

are likely to have impact far beyond understanding L-LTP at Schaffer/collateral and perforant-path synapses. This is one reason that this area of LTP research has a slightly different "feel" to it than the other areas we have been discussing (LTP physiology and E-LTP biochemistry, for example).

This area of LTP research is frequently discussed as an *analogue* of long-term memory as opposed to being limited to a description of a specific neuronal plasticity phenomenon. Many investigators study E-LTP in an effort to explain that specific phenomenon in physiologic and molecular terms, while frequently investigators studying L-LTP think of "L-LTP" as more of an umbrella term that encompasses gene regulation-dependent long-term plastic changes in the adult CNS. When I do an E-LTP experiment, I am doing an experiment to understand E-LTP. When I do an L-LTP experiment, I may be doing a more general experiment to understand the role of altered gene expression, protein synthesis, and structural changes in mediating long-term changes at synapses.

A couple of practical factors feed into this. One is that L-LTP experiments are hard to do. A hippocampal slice experiment to study L-LTP lasts about 7 hours, so you can do one experiment per slice rig per day, and as with any experiment that long there is the inevitably low yield. The alternative is to study L-LTP in vivo, which is of course also quite labor-intensive. Consequently, there have not been large numbers of L-LTP experiments published, and investigators in the area are more willing to mix results from various paradigms and preparations in order to gain insights into the phenomenon of interest. Thus, the unifying theme becomes the gene expression/protein synthesis aspect instead of the particulars of the experimental design itself. I will follow this philosophy in this chapter as well, and draw examples from outside the CA1 region of the hippocampus in several instances. In particular, many of the experiments I will draw from were performed using dentate gyrus.

A second practical consideration is that it seems obvious that understanding the regulation of gene expression in the adult CNS is going to be relevant to understanding long-term plasticity in some way, shape, or form. This gives workers in the area a little more license to investigate the regulation of gene expression per se, and to discuss it in the context of its likely relevance to L-LTP. This will, of course, change as we get a better definition of exactly which long-lasting synaptic phenomena are relevant in the behaving animal. But, for the present, we are in an early enough stage so that the fundamental synaptic processes that are subject to ongoing nucleus-dependent regulation are still being defined. We can often discuss them under the rubric L-LTP.

For the sake of balance, I should also point out that some investigators believe that all this discussion of gene expression is much ado about nothing, and that self-reinforcing protein-based mechanisms are sufficient to explain even life-long synaptic alterations. There is nothing wrong with this perspective from a theoretical standpoint. The question is whether or not evolution incorporated mechanisms of altered gene expression into the systems of long-lasting synaptic plasticity. This question is still under investigation. For this reason, I will start the chapter with a brief overview of the data indicating that altered gene expression is involved in triggering late stages of LTP.

The rest of the chapter will be divided into three additional sections. The first major section deals not only with NMDA receptor coupling to the genome but also with receptor-effector coupling mechanisms in the context of transcriptional regulation. We then will proceed in the second section to some identified gene targets in L-LTP and raise the issue of how the products of these genes get to the right synapses. Finally, I will speculate about likely read-outs of altered expression of these target genes— suggesting that these changes mediate structural and morphological changes in the neuron. The basic model for the third section is that altered expression of gene products gets translated into structural changes at the synaptic spine and altered connectivity of the neuron. Ultimately these changes are manifest as changes in the synaptic circuit in which the neuron resides.

In the context of our systematic nomenclature, in this chapter we will focus largely on the *induction* mechanisms of L-LTP, exploring how a triggering calcium signal gets converted into a genomic read-out. This is a fascinating area of current investigation and the area for which the most relevant data are available. The maintenance and expression mechanisms of L-LTP are still highly speculative at this point, and for this reason will be dealt with in less detail.

I. THE CASE FOR ALTERED GENE EXPRESSION IN L-LTP

In this section, I will make the case that there is a uniquely definable stage of LTP that we will call L-LTP. I will begin by describing three unique attributes of L-LTP that make it distinct from E-LTP. This will serve to define more precisely the form of synaptic plasticity that is under discussion. After that we can proceed to discuss L-LTP mechanisms per se.

First, L-LTP is defined as that phase of LTP that is dependent upon altered gene expression and protein synthesis for its *induction*. As we noted in the last chapter, "altered" is the key word here. In the limit, every cellular process depends upon ongoing gene expression and protein synthesis, if only to replenish mRNA and proteins as they turn over. What defines L-LTP is a requirement, for its induction, of *changes* in gene expression and protein synthesis, different from a pre-existing baseline.

The maintenance and expression mechanisms for L-LTP are still mysterious, and it is not clear if specifically altered gene expression is necessary for L-LTP *maintenance*. It is possible that the *ongoing* maintenance of altered levels of expression of specific genes is necessary for L-LTP maintenance, but this is not clear at this point. At a minimum, however, available data can be interpreted to indicate that alterations in gene and protein expression are necessary for the *induction* of L-LTP. Thus we will use this as the first and defining attribute of L-LTP for the purposes of the following discussion.

How then is L-LTP maintained? The working model of L-LTP maintenance that I will use posits a local, self-reinforcing alteration of protein synthesis and synaptic structure (broadly defined) as the

maintenance mechanism for L-LTP. I will speculate on some specific possibilities for molecular players in this scenario later in this chapter, and we will return to the issue in a more general sense in Chapter 12. The upshot of all this is that we will discuss hypothetical mechanisms involved in L-LTP maintenance that utilize persisting alterations in protein synthesis, but we will not discuss any scenario involving *persistent* changes in gene expression.

A second attribute of L-LTP is that it generally is induced, selectively, by multiple trains of tetanic stimuli or in some cases by more prolonged theta-type stimulation or stimulation paired with dopamine or other neuromodulators. The fact that L-LTP can be selectively induced with specific protocols suggests that unique molecular events are associated with its induction. Also, the unique L-LTP inducing stimuli serve a practical purpose in that one can design experiments to see what molecular events are uniquely associated with these stimuli.[1]

A third attribute of L-LTP is, of course, its "lateness." At the risk of sounding Clintonesque, it's hard to define exactly how late late is. Late LTP is generally held to be LTP beginning at about the 90-minutes post-tetanus time point. This is harder to nail down than you might think because there is not typically a precipitous drop-off of LTP at any specific time point even when L-LTP is blocked with protein synthesis inhibitors (see Figure 1). In addition, L-LTP is studied in a wide variety of preparations and at various temperatures, ranging from room temperature in in vitro slices to 37 degrees in intact animal in vivo recording. There's probably about a fivefold difference in the kinetics of most

---

[1] I need to note at this point that, regardless of the induction protocol used to generate the data we will be discussing in this chapter, all the data I will present concern NMDA receptor-dependent L-LTP. I will, however, intermingle data from Schaffer-collateral synapses with data from studies of the perforant path inputs to the dentate gyrus. I am taking this license in order to have an adequate body of literature to draw from.

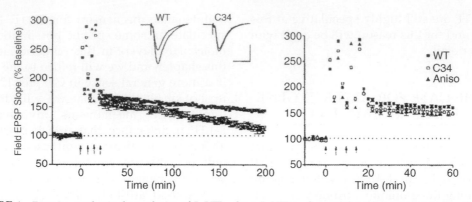

FIGURE 1 Protein synthesis dependence of L-LTP where L-LTP is disrupted in dominant negative CaMKIV transgenic mice. Late-phase LTP was induced by four trains of tetanic stimulation spaced by 5-minute intervals. The left panel illustrates the effects of application of the protein synthesis inhibitor anisomycin (filled triangles) and genetic suppression of CaMKIV (C34, open circles) on late-phase LTP. Note that later-developing stages of LTP are selectively lost. The right panel illustrates in greater detail the same data, focusing on the first 60 minutes of LTP. Filled triangles indicate L-LTP obtained with wild-type slices in the presence of anisomycin (Aniso). Superimposed representative EPSPs shown were recorded 5 minutes before and 3 hours after L-LTP induction. Calibration bars, 1 mV and 20 ms. As has been routinely observed, only modest effects of protein synthesis inhibitors are observed in E-LTP. Figure and legend adapted from Kang et al. (8).

biochemical reactions over that temperature range, so Late LTP may start at 3 hours at room temperature in vitro but at 36 minutes in an intact hippocampus in vivo. Of course, some in vivo experiments go for days to weeks as well, and what we monolithically call Late LTP is likely multiple processes. For these various reasons, I greatly prefer to define L-LTP mechanistically in terms of altered gene and protein expression, versus temporally in terms of any particular time point. Nevertheless, we are required to have in hand a reasonable functional definition of L-LTP for experimental purposes (how else to know if it is blocked?), and a working definition of L-LTP is synaptic potentiation in the 90-minutes to 4-hour time range.

With these attributes in mind, we can proceed to consider the case for altered gene expression in L-LTP. *Per usual*, we will consider this in the context of the block, measure, and mimic criteria (see Table 1). Thus, the hypothesis of a role for altered gene expression in L-LTP predicts that blocking changes in protein and RNA synthesis should block L-LTP induction,

that changes in gene and protein expression should occur with L-LTP-inducing stimulation, and that artificially increasing the synthesis of the appropriate genes should lead to an enhancement of synaptic transmission.[2]

Prediction One: blocking changes in protein and RNA synthesis should block L-LTP induction. In addition to the variety of experiments described in the last chapter demonstrating that protein synthesis inhibitors can block L-LTP (see Figure 1 for a recent example), it also is known that inhibition of RNA synthesis blocks L-LTP. Thus, actinomycin D application blocks

---

[2]An additional line of evidence discussed in the literature is based on deduction, and I will only mention it briefly here. L-LTP can last a *really* long time in vivo, and this implies altered gene expression at some level. This is because the lifetime of L-LTP *in vivo* encompasses many protein and mRNA half-lives, so the signals mediating that change surely at some level must impinge upon a genomic read-out. This is a compelling but not iron-clad argument because, as mentioned previously, the maintenance mechanism could be restricted to changes in protein synthesis, assuming an adequate baseline level of genomic read-out of the requisite mRNAs. We will return to this topic in the last chapter of the book.

TABLE 1   The Case for Gene Expression in L-LTP

Experiment Type	Finding	References
Block	Block of L-LTP with protein synthesis inhibitors	(76)
	Block of L-LTP with RNA synthesis inhibitors	(1, 2, 77)
	Loss of L-LTP with CREB knockouts	(3–5)
	Block of L-LTP with Arc antisense	(13)
	Loss of L-LTP with CaMKIV knockout	(7, 8, 78)
	Loss of L-LTP with zif268 knockout	(6)
Measure	Increased zif268/krox24 mRNA	(40)
	Increased krox20	(44)
	Increased expression of fos, jun IEG mRNAs	(40, 42, 43)
	Increased CREB phosphorylation	(24, 34, 35)
	Increased CRE read-out	(12, 79)
	Increased elk-1 phosphorylation	(35)
	Increased Arc/Arg3.1 mRNA expression	(13, 54, 59)
	Increased AMPA receptor protein	(51)
	Increased BDNF message	(46, 80)
	Increased tissue plasminogen activator message	(47)
	Increased C/EBP beta (in long-term memory)	(45)
	Increased HOMER	(11, 53, 72)
	Increased MAP kinase phosphatase-1	(35, 50)
	Increased SSAT message	(49)
	Increased MAP2 message	(81)
Mimic	Constitutively active CREB augments L-LTP induction	(14)

L-LTP induction (1, 2), although there are some differences in the particulars of the effect in the published reports.[3] Similarly, knocking out or inhibiting the transcription factor cAMP-Responsive Element Binding Protein (CREB) and homologous family members can block L-LTP induction, although again there is some disagreement in the reported effects (3–5). (Interpretation of the CREB knockout results is complicated because of compensatory mechanisms that occur with CREB knockouts, and

there is an apparent specificity of the effects on L-LTP that are dependent on the L-LTP induction paradigm used.) Finally, knocking out the transcriptional regulator zif268, whose message is increased with L-LTP-inducing stimulation, leads to a loss of L-LTP (6). Overall these results indicate that dynamic regulation of gene expression and RNA synthesis is necessary to elicit L-LTP.

There also are more inferential findings that are consistent with a necessity for transcriptional regulation for L-LTP induction. Knockout of CaMKIV, a calmodulin-dependent kinase that regulates the activity of the CREB/CREB Binding Protein complex, also leads to a loss of L-LTP (see references 7 and 8 and Figure 1). Given the prominent role of ERK in regulating gene

---

[3]Please keep in mind that although I am glibly stating that various processes are necessary for the induction of L-LTP, the same caveats that we discussed in Chapter 5 concerning designing experiments to distinguish between induction, maintenance, and expression of LTP also apply here. This is particularly relevant in the case of knockout mice and irreversible inhibitors like actinomycin D.

BOX 1

L-LTP DECAY IS AN ACTIVE PROCESS

If very long-lasting stages of L-LTP involve self reinforcing molecular mechanisms, then L-LTP should in theory be permanent. However, it is clear that L-LTP in vivo, although very long-lasting, does decay over time. How can one rationalize these two observations? One possibility is simply to say that even self-reinforcing mechanisms may not be flawless—any lack of fidelity in replicating the relevant molecules could lead to slow decay over time. This certainly is an important consideration that may apply to both LTP decay and behavioral forgetting. However, a novel and important recent finding from Desiree Villareal in Brian Derrick's lab suggests an alternate explanation. Desiree and Brian showed that NMDA receptor antagonists *block the decay* of L-LTP in the dentate gyrus in vivo (75; see figure). These findings indicate that the reversal of late stages of L-LTP is an active process, as might be expected if one had to break a self-perpetuating biochemical cycle. These investigators went on to show that the post-training NMDA receptor blockade also enhanced memory retention in an eight-arm radial maze spatial learning task—again, a finding consistent with the idea that synaptic plasticity is normally subserved by mechanisms with the capacity for self-perpetuation, that must be actively reversed for forgetting to occur.

How is the erasure of L-LTP achieved? The answer to this question is unknown, but the authors hypothesize that heterosynaptic

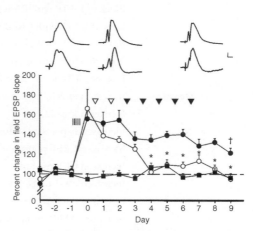

BOX 1 The NMDA receptor antagonist, CPP, blocks the decay of late-phase LTP. Effect of CPP or vehicle on LTP decay when administered 2 days after LTP induction (marked with IIIII). Water vehicle was administered to all animals 1 hour and 24 hours following LTP induction (white triangles). Forty-eight hours after LTP induction, CPP (black circles, $n = 4$) or the water vehicle (white circles, $n = 6$, pooled control data as in Figure 2) was administered daily for an additional 5 days (black triangles). Decay was observed in vehicle-treated animals as compared with the magnitude of LTP on day 2 (*$p < .05$). In CPP-treated animals, the magnitude of potentiated responses over the 3- to 7-day period of CPP administration did not differ significantly from the magnitude of LTP on day 2 (cross, $p < .05$). CPP was without effect on unpotentiated perforant path responses (black squares, $n = 3$). Insets show representative traces of perforant path–dentate baseline responses (left) and responses collected 1 hour (middle) and 7 days (right) following LTP induction for vehicle and CPP-treated animals. Scale bar, 5 ms, 0.5 mV. Reproduced from Villarreal et al. (75).

expression, it is intriguing that ERK activation is necessary for L-LTP (9–12). However, these data are suggestive but not direct evidence for a necessity for changes in gene expression in L-LTP.

A final piece of more direct "block" evidence comes from investigating expression of the immediate early gene (IEG) Arc. Arc mRNA is normally present at low levels, and is up-regulated by L-LTP-inducing

---

BOX 1—cont'd

L-LTP DECAY IS AN ACTIVE PROCESS

LTD underlies the phenomenon (75). The idea is that when neighboring synapses undergo LTP, other inactive synapses in the same neuron are simultaneously depressed. This has been directly demonstrated to occur experimentally and to be NMDA receptor-dependent. The general idea is that ongoing formation of new memories triggers a cellular trade-off, causing the erasure of previously stored information. The evolutionary advantage to this might be that it prevents the driving of synapses to cell-wide

saturation, exhausting the capacity of the system for ongoing change. This, of course, would lead to an overall degradation of memory capacity over time.

Regardless, these fascinating observations demonstrate a fact that is counter-intuitive for most of us. Memories seem frustratingly fragile and fleeting based on our personal experience. However, it appears that our brain actively works to make them that way, directly participating in their ongoing erasure.

---

stimulation. Inhibition of Arc message with antisense to that message leads to an attenuation of L-LTP (13). This finding suggests a necessity for Arc up-regulation in L-LTP. Because Arc is one of the genes known to be up-regulated with L-LTP-inducing stimulation, this is additional evidence for a requirement for altered gene expression in the induction of L-LTP.

Overall while the data from the block approach are not airtight, published results are consistent with a necessity for altered regulation of gene expression in L-LTP induction. Again, as mentioned in the last chapter, a variety of published results have shown that protein synthesis inhibitors block L-LTP induction, which is also supportive of the hypothesis.

Prediction two: Changes in gene and protein expression should occur with L-LTP-inducing stimulation. A wide range of published experiments demonstrate that alterations in gene expression occur with L-LTP-inducing stimulation. The following mRNAs have been documented to increase after L-LTP-inducing stimulation: zif268/krox24, krox20, Arc, fos and related proteins, BDNF, C/EBP, MAP2, HOMER,

and GluR1 AMPA receptor (see Table 1 for references, with apologies for any I might have missed). In addition, phosphorylation of the transcription factors CREB and elk-1 are known to increase with L-LTP, again indicative of an acute activation of transcriptional regulation. In an elegant series of studies, Soren Impey in Dan Storm's lab demonstrated increased read-out of CREB-regulated genes with L-LTP. Soren engineered a CRE-driven beta-galactosidase-expressing transgenic mouse that allows monitoring of CREB-mediated gene expression. Use of this mouse allowed a direct demonstration of a CRE-mediated increase in gene expression with LTP-inducing stimulation. Thus, overall the data supporting the measure approach are quite solid and indicative of a role for altered gene expression in L-LTP.

Prediction three: Artificially increasing the synthesis of the appropriate genes should lead to an enhancement of synaptic transmission. This is, of course, a virtually impossible prediction to test given our present state of understanding. Appropriately designing the experiments would mean that one would have the capacity to regulate the precise L-LTP-associated genes and have them be appropriately targeted, which is, of course, considerably beyond the present level of technology and knowledge. However, in a rough approximation, Kandel's group has engineered a mouse that inducibly expresses a constutively active version of the CREB transcription factor in the dorsal hippocampus (14). Hippocampal slices from these mice exhibit a decreased threshold for L-LTP induction. This observation is in agreement with the idea that altered CREB-mediated gene expression is involved in L-LTP induction.

II. SIGNALING MECHANISMS

We now turn our attention to discussing the mechanisms by which L-LTP-associated changes in gene expression are achieved. How does the L-LTP-triggering calcium elevation at the synaptic spine get a signal to the nucleus? In the following section, I will summarize a variety of studies investigating this question. Leading groups in this area are the laboratories of Dan Storm, Dick Tsien, Eric Kandel, Susumu Tonegawa, Alcino Silva, Tim Bliss, and Jocelyn Caboche—the following summary draws extensively from the findings, thoughts, and models from these various groups as well as work from my own lab.

By way of introduction let me point out that what we are talking about for the remainder of this chapter is a complex multistage process. Of course, the core signal transduction component is calcium activation of kinase cascades that phosphorylate transcription factors and thereby regulate gene expression. However, many other signals get integrated into this basic process. There are pathways controlling nuclear translocation of transcription factors and kinases. "Transcription factors" should really be thought of as multiprotein complexes that integrate a variety of signals in order to compute whether gene expression should be altered. A single gene can integrate the output of multiple transcriptional regulatory elements. After the gene is transcribed, mRNA processing and trafficking mechanisms are subject to additional layers of regulation. Translation of the mRNA into protein is subject to regulation as we discussed in the last chapter. In L-LTP, there are likely multiple waves of altered gene expression, in part because one category of regulated genes codes for transcription factors, which when expressed can lead to secondary alterations in gene expression. There are mysterious but clearly extant mechanisms for temporal and spatial integration of signals in the nucleus. There are mechanisms for controlling gene expression that involve relief of inhibitory constraints, such as histone acetylation. Transcriptional repressors also impinge upon mechanisms for expression of target genes, and these are themselves subject to regulation.

Clearly a detailed description of all these processes is beyond the scope of a single book chapter. What I will do here is distill the essential processes into a working model of how gene expression is regulated in L-LTP, limiting myself to those processes where there are direct experimental data linking them to activity-dependent synaptic plasticity in area CA1 and the dentate gyrus.

It may be helpful to break down L-LTP-related mechanisms for regulating gene expression into the following basic components of L-LTP to help organize your thinking:

1. A core signal transduction cascade linking calcium to the transcription factor CREB
2. Modulatory influences that impinge upon this cascade
3. Additional transcription factors besides CREB that may be involved
4. Genes targeted in L-LTP
5. mRNA targeting and transport

Of course, the altered mRNA expression must be converted into a physiologic read-out by some mechanism, giving us a more hypothetical sixth category:

6. Effects of the gene products on synaptic structure

I will organize the remainder of the chapter around these six topics.

A. A Core Signal Transduction Cascade Linking Calcium to the Transcription Factor CREB

Introduction to Gene Transcription

Genes are stretches of DNA that have the capacity to code for a functional protein. Transcription of the DNA into a protein-encoding mRNA begins with a transcriptional promoter complex binding to a TATA sequence (TATA box) in the DNA sequence, which promotes association of the RNA polymerase II complex with the DNA and transcription at the transcription start site (see references 15 and 16 and Figure 2). This transcription machinery is regulated by transcription factors that bind to upstream *regulatory elements* (REs), that is, DNA sequences that the transcription factors specifically recognize. The transcription factors and their associated co-activators bind to their REs and enable gene transcription of the downstream target gene. Transcription factor activity is regulated by a variety of post-translational processes including phosphorylation, redox state, ubiquitination, and degradation of associated inhibitory proteins. *Co-activators* whose activity is typically necessary for the transcription factor per se to be active usually bind to the promoter complex and/or acetylate histones locally to free up DNA for transcription.

A diagram of the basic structure of the CREB transcriptional complex is given in Figure 2 for reference purposes. A more realistic picture of CREB bound to the DNA double helix is given in Figure 3. The CRE (5'-TGACGTCA-3') is the DNA sequence identified by CREB. The activity of CREB is regulated by phosphorylation at Ser 133, which can be phosphorylated by PKA, CaMKII and CaMKIV, and RSK2 (among many others). This phosphorylation event,

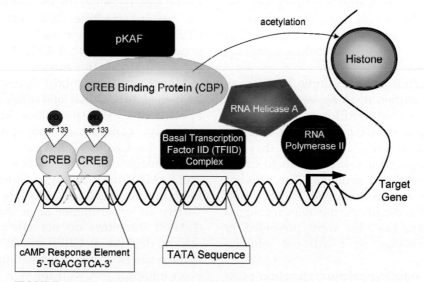

FIGURE 2 The CREB/CRE gene regulation system. Phosphorylated CREB recruits a supramolecular complex to the CyclicAMP response element in DNA, triggering increased expression of downstream target genes. CBP, an accessory to CREB, facilitates gene expression by modulation of RNA polymerase activity and histone acetylation. Adapted from Shaywitz and Greenberg, (16).

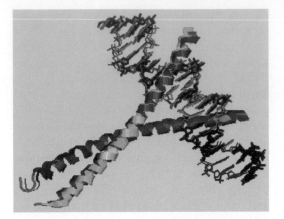

FIGURE 3   Crystal structure of CREB bound to the CRE. Data obtained from the Brookhaven National Protein Structure Data Bank and rendered with Rasmol. Figure courtesy of Jennifer Gatchel.

however, is not sufficient for transcriptional activation; binding of *CREB Binding Protein* (CBP) is also necessary. CBP binding and activation is itself regulated by phosphorylation; in particular, phosphorylation and activation by CaMKIV is relevant in the present context. CBP does a number of things—it binds to phosphorylated CREB, it helps bridge CREB to the promoter complex structurally, and it is a *Histone Acetyl Transferase* (HAT) enzyme that acetylates histone lysine residues to free up bound DNA.

I use CREB as an example because, as described earlier, it, along with the *Serum Response Element* (SRE)-recognizing transcription factor *elk-1*, has been directly implicated in L-LTP. How is it that the calcium trigger for L-LTP signals to CREB and its associated proteins? The relevant pathways are summarized in Figure 4. Most of the details of the relevant signal transduction cascades were presented in the last chapter, so I will not reiterate them here.

L-LTP-inducing calcium elevation postsynaptically activates Adenlyl Cyclase I/ VIII and via B-raf activates MEK (reviewed in reference 17). In addition, as described in the last chapter, ras-coupled receptors and

PKC-coupled receptors also can feed into this pathway. The product of MEK activation, dually phosphorylated ERK (ppERK) is then translocated into the nucleus. This nuclear translocation of ppERK is a regulated process—both BDNF and PKA can control this translocation by mechanisms that are still being investigated. Active ERK in the nucleus is most likely coupled to CREB phosphorylation via activation of a member of the pp90rsk family of S6 kinases, RSK2. Ser133 of CREB is not a substrate for ERK; ERK's effect is indirect through activating RSK2. Phosphorylation of Ser133 by RSK2 recruits the CREB binding protein, CBP, to the initiator complex and thereby promotes transcription. CBP activation is itself regulated by CaMKIV phosphorylation, and most likely both CBP activation by CaMKIV and ERK regulation of RSK2/CREB are necessary events for L-LTP induction (see 7, 18).

This model is consistent with a wide variety of evidence demonstrating that AC knockouts, inhibition of PKA and ERK, and loss of CaMKIV function all lead to loss of L-LTP (see reference 19 and Table 1). Also, the various positive data demonstrating CREB phosphorylation and CRE-mediated gene expression with L-LTP, described in Table 1, motivate this model.

However, one might wonder what happened to CaMKII and PKA phosphorylation of CREB, since these kinases are perfectly capable of phosphorylating Ser133 in CREB. The short answer is that available data do not indicate that PKA and CaMKII have access to CREB, at least in rat hippocampus and dentate gyrus. A variety of experiments have shown that CaMKII inhibitors do not affect synaptic activity-dependent CREB phosphorylation in these systems. In fact, if anything CaMKII is an inhibitor of CREB through phosphorylation at a site other than Ser133.

Also, Eric Roberson and others in my lab showed that PKA cannot cause elevated CREB phosphorylation without going

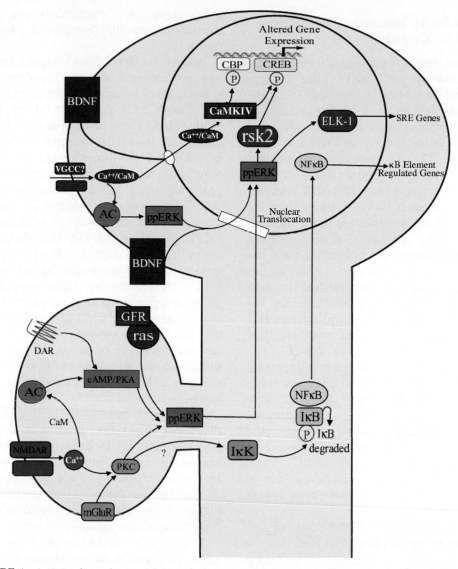

FIGURE 4   Activity-dependent regulation of gene expression in neurons. See text for details and discussion.

through the ERK cascade (20). Activation of PKA by application of forskolin to hippocampal slices results in ERK activation in area CA1, and this manipulation also elicits increased CREB phosphorylation. Eric and his colleagues determined the effects of MEK inhibition on forskolin stimulation of CREB phosphorylation in area CA1, and, surprisingly, the MEK inhibitor U0126 completely blocked CREB phosphorylation in response to forskolin application. While this was unexpected, this effect has been confirmed by Lu, Kandel, and Hawkins (21) and the data are consistent with additional work by Impey et al. (12). Thus, these data demonstrate that activation of MAPK results in increased CREB phosphorylation in area CA1; interestingly, these data also indicate that the cAMP pathway utilizes the MAPK cascade as an obligatory intermediate in regulating CREB phosphorylation in area CA1.

B. Modulatory Influences That Impinge Upon This Cascade

One of the most important co-regulators of this cascade is CaMKIV. Mice (or hippocampal slices) deficient in CaMKIV signaling have deficits in L-LTP, hippocampal CREB phosphorylation, and CREB-mediated gene expression (see Figure 1 and references 7, 8, and 22). As mentioned previously, CaMKIV acts by phosphorylating Ser301 in CBP, co-regulating the CREB/CBP complex (7). Regulation of CaMKIV likely depends on calmodulin translocation to the nucleus, an interesting attribute that may confer a capacity for temporal integration onto the nuclear read-out of cellular calcium signals (23). The pathways for nuclear calcium signaling are still being worked out, but they may be initiated by local calcium flux at the cell body coupled with ancillary signals from the synapse (24–26). The bottom line of all this is that it is important to remember that increased CREB phosphorylation at Ser133 is not sufficient to give altered gene expression—an additional CaMKIV-mediated signal through the CREB co-activator CBP is necessary for altered gene expression as well (7). Thus, the ERK and CaMKIV pathways act in concert to trigger L-LTP-associated altered gene expression.

The growth factor BDNF also triggers modulatory mechanisms that feed into the CREB regulation cascade. BDNF is released with L-LTP inducing stimulation (27, 28) and likely contributes to L-LTP induction by two means (see Figure 4). First, it may act via ras to help to activate the MEK/ERK pathway directly, a mechanism for augmenting ERK-dependent gene expression (29). In addition, BDNF by mechanisms still being worked out controls ERK translocation into the nucleus, providing a gate-keeping role for triggering L-LTP (30). This BDNF-dependent regulation of ppERK translocation to the nucleus is necessary for L-LTP to be induced, conferring an additional signal integration mechanism onto the system. This mechanism also likely contributes to BDNF-induced plasticity per se (31).

Additional modulatory signal integration mechanisms also can operate at the *synaptic* level by augmenting activation of the ERK/CREB pathway. Many possibilities along these lines have already been discussed in earlier chapters when we talked about the numerous complexities of regulating the level of calcium achieved postsynaptically with LTP-inducing stimulation. One specific example that has received attention experimentally is regulation of L-LTP induction by DA (32). Dopamine coapplication during theta-frequency synaptic activity augments the induction of L-LTP. In the mouse hippocampus this pathway appears to be particularly important for generating CREB-dependent L-LTP (5). DA may augment NMDA receptor activation by way of the cAMP gate as we discussed in the last chapter, or may enhance ERK activation by elevating cAMP levels, or both.

In addition, nitric oxide acting through the cGMP-dependent protein kinase may also modulate L-LTP induction by impinging upon CREB phosphorylation (21). However, this pathway appears to operate in parallel to the pathway outlined in Figure 4, as opposed to influencing it directly or indirectly.

Finally, it is important to note that a static diagram such as Figure 4 cannot adequately convey some of the kinetic complexities that are known to exist in this system. Work from Gang-yi Wu, Karl Dieisseroth, and others in Dick Tsien's lab has shown that there are important temporal integration mechanisms that play a role in activity-dependent nuclear signaling in hippocampal neurons (23; reviewed along with other interesting aspects of this system in references 25 and 33). Specifically, repeated stimuli lead to a prolonged activation of the ERK/CREB pathway, a mechanism that is likely relevant in the system computing whether to trigger altered gene expression and L-LTP. There also exists in pyramidal neurons a "fast" CaMKIV-dependent signaling mechanism direct to CREB, which depends on activation of L-Type calcium channels (24). The role of this mechanism in L-LTP induction is still under investigation. It is possible that these two pathways act sequentially to give the biphasic CREB phosphorylation that has been observed with L-LTP-inducing stimulation (34). Regardless, it is clear that a number of temporal factors impinge upon the CREB transcriptional regulation pathway with L-LTP-inducing stimulation; these factors likely are controlled by distinct activity-dependent signaling mechanism such as L-channel activation and NMDA receptor-dependent events (26).

C. Additional Transcription Factors Besides CREB That May Be Involved in L-LTP Induction

The activation and nuclear translocation of ERK can lead to the activation of several transcription factors besides CREB, such as Elk-1 and c-Myc. Historically prominent among the transcription factors regulated by ERK is Elk-1, which when phosphorylated at multiple sites by ERK cooperates with serum response factor (SRF) to drive transcription of serum response element (SRE)-controlled genes. Elk-1 phosphorylation increases with L-LTP-inducing stimulation, a mechanism that likely triggers SRE-mediated changes in gene expression (35). One specific candidate target for this pathway is the transcription factor zif268, whose expression is mediated by Elk-1/SRE-dependent processes. In addition, the target gene Arc/Arg3.1 may also be regulated by this pathway independently of CREB (36).

A final pathway potentially contributing to L-LTP induction is the NFkB pathway (15, 37; see Figure 4). Nuclear Factor kappa B (NFkB) is a transcription factor that normally resides in the cytoplasm, bound to an inhibitory partner IkB (Inhibitor of kappa B). NFkB is activated when the kinase IkB Kinase (IKK) phosphorylates IkB, which leads to loss of IkB by ubiquitin-mediated proteolysis. The free, active NFkB can then translocate to the nucleus and effect transcription of its target genes. Inhibition of NFkB activity leads to a reduction of L-LTP (38), and Ari Routtenberg's group has demonstrated NFkB activation with LTP–inducing stimulation (39). The mechanism of NFkB activation in LTP is unclear at this time, however interesting possible mechanisms include activation by reactive oxygen species like superoxide, direct phosphorylation of IkB by PKC, or indirect activation of IKK by PKC.

D. Gene Targets in L-LTP

This is one of the most fascinating aspects of L-LTP investigation, and an area where we have just started to scratch the surface in uncovering the relevant players. Identifying the gene targets of activity-dependent transcriptional regulation in L-LTP specifically, and in long-term memory generally, will be a watershed event in our understanding the molecular basis of memory. Clearly, identifying the genes whose expression changes with LTP (and learning) will give us needed clues concerning how very long-lasting changes in synaptic function are achieved in the CNS.

I already have listed the known gene targets in L-LTP as part of the measure-related experiments supporting a role for altered gene expression in L-LTP (see Table 1). In this section, I will reorganize the list along some functional lines. The take-home message from this section is threefold. First, we clearly are at an early stage with these studies because not many candidates have been identified. Second, where target genes have been identified the functions of their gene products suggest that there are many complex post-gene-read-out layers of signal transduction involved in L-LTP. Third, even with the paucity of targets that

BOX 2

NEUROGENESIS IN THE ADULT CNS

As if the processes for establishing and maintaining long-term memory weren't already complicated enough, recent findings indicate that hitherto unanticipated mechanisms also may play a role. Specifically, neurogenesis has entered the picture. When I was a young scientific sprout, the dogma was that there is no new generation of neurons in the adult CNS. However, fascinating recent results have shown that neurogenesis does indeed continue into the adult, particularly in the dentate gyrus. One key publication by Fred Gage and his colloborators showed specifically that new neurons are generated in the adult *human* brain (73). How might one be able to ascertain this fact? Cancer patients sometimes receive treatment with the drug Bromo-deoxy Uridine (BrdU). It selectively affects dividing cells by being incorporated into their DNA upon de novo DNA synthesis. Therefore, an ancillary aspect of this is that BrdU selectively labels freshly divided cells. Post-mortem analysis of the brains of cancer patients that had received BrdU as a chemotherapeutic treatment revealed that indeed new dentate granule cells are produced in an ongoing fashion in the adult human brain.

Are these newly generated cells important for memory? Recent work by Tracy Shors, Elizabeth Gould, and their collaborators has indicated that these new cells are necessary for memory formation, in rodents at a minimum. They have shown that both Morris water maze training and trace eye-blink conditioning lead to enhanced neurogenesis in rats (see reference 74 and figure). Moreover, inhibiting neurogenesis attenuates memory formation in these same paradigms. This fascinating paradigm shift, while at an early stage, promises to change fundamentally the types of options we need to consider when formulating models for long-term memory.

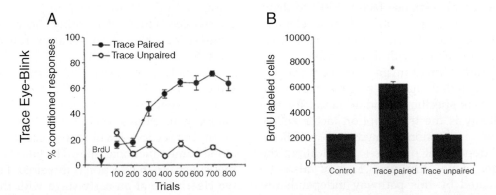

BOX 2   Learning that requires the hippocampus, but not other types of learning or a similar experience in the absence of overt learning, increases the numbers of adult-generated hippocampal granule neurons in the dentate gyrus. (A) Acquisition of the trace eye-blink conditioned response (trace paired) and the unpaired condition (trace unpaired). (B) Total numbers of BrdU-labeled cells in the dentate gyrus of these animals following trace conditioning (trace paired). These animals received BrdU injections 1 week before training and were perfused 24 hours after the last day of training. Bars represent mean ± standard error ($n = 6$). *significant difference ($p < .01$) from other groups.   *Continued*

BOX 2—cont'd

NEUROGENESIS IN THE ADULT CNS

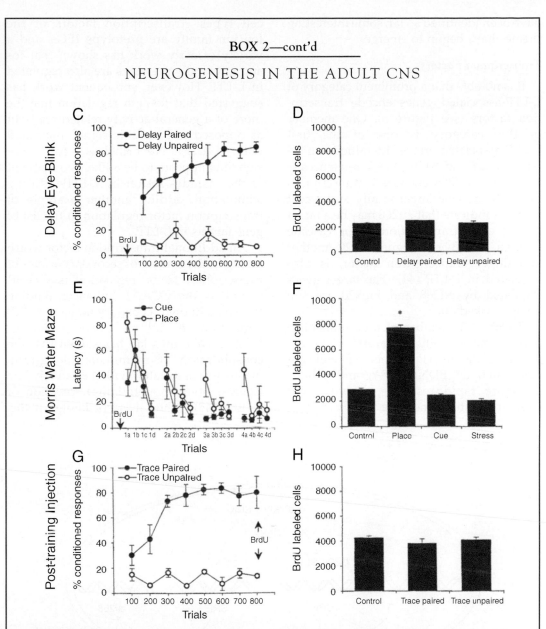

BOX 2, cont'd   (C) Acquisition of the delay eye-blink conditioned response (delay paired) and the unpaired condition (delay unpaired). (D) Total numbers of BrdU-labeled cells in the dentate gyrus of these animals following delay conditioning. These animals received BrdU injections 1 week before training and were perfused 24 hours after the last day of training. (n = 5–6). (E) Acquisition of place and cue learning in the Morris water maze. (F) Total numbers of BrdU-labeled cells in the dentate gyrus of these animals following spatial (place) or cue (cue) training. These animals received BrdU injections 1 week before training and were perfused 24 hours after the last day of training (n = 6). (G) Acquisition of the trace eye-blink conditioned response (trace paired) and the unpaired condition (trace unpaired) from animals injected with BrdU on the last day of training after all animals had reached learning criterion. These animals were perfused 24 hours after the BrdU injection. (H) Total numbers of BrdU-labeled cells in the dentate gyrus of these animals following trace conditioning (trace paired) (n = 5–6). Reproduced from Gould, Beylin, Tanapat, Reeves, and Shors (74).

have been identified so far, some interesting themes have begun to emerge.

Transcription Factors

It is notable that a prominent category of L-LTP-associated genes encode transcription factors (see Figure 5). One member of this category is one of the first L-LTP-associated genes identified: zif268 (aka krox24 and NGFI-A; see references 6, 11, 40–43). Zif268 encodes a transcription factor of the zinc finger family, and recent findings indicate that zif268 may be a target of the elk-1 transcription factor cascade (35). The zif268 homologue krox20, another zinc-finger transcription factor, is also regulated in L-LTP (44). The target genes regulated by zif268 and krox20 are still being worked out.

Zif268 is a member of the "immediate early gene" family of proteins, as are many of the L-LTP targets we will discuss such as BDNF, t-PA, and others. IEGs are rapid response, activity- and signal-regulated genes in a wide variety of cell types. Transcription factors of the fos/jun family are prototype IEGs, and a variety of early work has shown that fos and jun family members are also regulated in L-LTP. However, subsequent work has suggested that fos/jun regulation may be more of a general activity-related read-out as opposed to a specific signal associated with L-LTP. Nevertheless, fos/ jun signaling appears to be a likely component of the cascades set off by L-LTP-inducing stimulation, adding another example of transcription factor regulation to the list of gene targets in L-LTP.

An additional transcription factor worth noting in the context of secondary waves of transcription factor regulation is C/EBP. C/EBP is the CCAAT Enhancer Binding Protein, a known secondary target of CREB regulation in *Aplysia* sensory neurons. Cristina Alberini's lab has shown that the consolidation of mammalian long-term memory is associated with a relatively late (several hours post-training) elevation of C/EBP (45). While it is not known if this

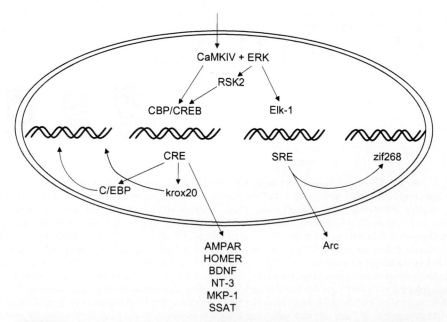

FIGURE 5   Transcriptional regulation pathways controlling the expression of synaptic plasticity-associated genes. See text for discussion.

occurs with L-LTP, these interesting findings support the idea that late waves of altered gene expression contribute to memory consolidation involving hippocampal neurons.

Thus, we see that at least two (zif268 and krox 20) and probably several more transcription factor-encoding genes are up-regulated in L-LTP. Overall, these findings that transcription factors are targets of the gene expression system of L-LTP and long-term memory suggest that plasticity-associated gene regulation will be quite complex. The findings indicate the likelihood that the initial triggering of altered gene expression with L-LTP-inducing stimulation sets off secondary waves of altered gene expression. The potential for exponential expansion of altered gene expression in L-LTP, along with combinatorics for secondary signals impinging on these mechanisms, appears somewhat daunting. However, parsing out these complex pathways will be necessary to answer a fundamental question in biology—how neuronal cell surface activity impinges upon the genome.

Signaling Molecules

A second category of L-LTP-associated genes encode signaling molecules. As with the transcription factors regulated in L-LTP, increased production of signaling molecules and regulators of signal transduction cascades suggest the triggering of a variety of post-genome secondary effects by L-LTP-inducing stimulation.

One of the most interesting molecules in this category is BDNF, which we have already discussed several times. BDNF gene expression increases with L-LTP-inducing stimulation, along with that of a related growth factor, Neurotrophin-3 (46). This likely occurs via CRE-regulated expression as the BDNF gene has the necessary sequence in its upstream region. BDNF is particularly intriguing because, as we have already discussed, it is a modulator of LTP induction and is furthermore capable of triggering lasting increases in synaptic strength in its own right. Thus increased BDNF expression could play a role in modulating subsequent plasticity in a temporal integration fashion, or itself trigger lasting plastic change. In the limit, BDNF, which couples to the ERK/CREB cascade, could trigger a self-perpetuating feedback mechanism for maintaining increased synaptic strength perpetually. Even though this idea is quite speculative, it provides an appealing example of a potential self-reinforcing mechanism that could survive protein turnover and last the lifetime of the animal.

Another signaling molecule gene regulated by L-LTP-inducing stimulation codes for tissue Plasminogen Activator (t-PA). t-PA is a secreted protease that has the capacity to modulate the extracellular matrix structure. t-PA knockout mice have defects in L-LTP (47). t-PA could potentially serve in a long-term regulatory role through increasing active products in the extracellular space via its known role of converting pro-hormones into hormones. Another molecule that has been proposed to play a similar role is Matrix Metalloprotease-9 (MMP-9), whose gene is regulated in an activity-dependent fashion and which cleaves extracellular matrix molecules (48). Both t-PA and MMP-9 might also play a role in regulating the structure of the synaptic region as well.

In the last chapter, we discussed the fact that polyamines like spermine and spermidine can directly modulate NMDA receptor function. In this context, it is interesting to note that a synthetic enzyme that is involved in their production, SSAT (spermidine/spermine N1-acetyltransferase), is also up-regulated in L-LTP (49). This potentially provides yet another positive feedback signal that might be used by the neuron for long-term temporal integration. However, lest we get too carried away with the positive feedback loop concept, I note that not all gene targets in L-LTP will promote subsequent activity-dependent plasticity.

The MAP Kinase Phosphatase MKP-2 also is up-regulated in L-LTP. This dual-specificity phosphatase dephosphorylates phospho-ERK, providing a potential negative feedback mechanism limiting activation of the ERK/CREB pathway (35, 50).

Thus, no clear model for the role of L-LTP-associated genes affecting signal transduction emerges at this time. However, some interesting possibilities exist, and, as I mentioned earlier, the available data are consistent with diverse secondary effects downstream of altered gene regulation. As with the transcription factor category of targets, the regulation of signaling molecules with L-LTP similarly suggests that complicated cascades of biochemical sequelae will be triggered by L-LTP-inducing stimulation.

Structural Proteins

In contrast to the signaling molecules described earlier, the few structural proteins that have been identified as targets in L-LTP bring us refreshingly back around to tried-and-true functional players in synaptic transmission. Most straightforward in this context is the AMPA receptor itself (51). Mike Browning's group has shown that L-LTP is associated with increased AMPA receptor synthesis at the protein level (although the genetic basis for this has not been worked out). This translates in a conceptually straightforward way into a mechanism for increasing synaptic strength.

The metabotropic receptor scaffolding protein HOMER has also been identified as a gene regulated in L-LTP (11, 52, 53). This is interesting because this protein is a part of the synaptic spine structural complex interacting with metabotropic glutamate receptors, as we discussed in Chapter 6. In addition, mGluRs have been implicated as controlling dendritic spine protein synthesis as we discussed in the last chapter, and increased HOMER expression might play a role in facilitating or regulating local protein synthesis as one component of a mechanism for maintaining increased synaptic strength.

This last idea is not as far-fetched as it might sound considering that another target of L-LTP-associated gene expression is involved in the same types of processes— Arc. We have already discussed Arc in the context of local dendritic protein synthesis (see Chapter 7 and reference 54 for a review). Arc mRNA is rapidly induced by LTP-inducing stimulation. Moreover, as we will discuss in the next section, this mRNA is selectively localized to recently active synaptic regions and is subject to selective expression by local protein synthesis mechanisms. Arc is a cytoskeleton-associated protein that may be involved in stabilizing structural changes at potentiated synapses, as inhibition of Arc synthesis disrupts maintenance of LTP (13).

Thus, it is palatable to think that increased expression of AMPA receptors, HOMER, and Arc might contribute to a stable increase in synaptic strength as a mechanism for L-LTP expression. As more pieces of the puzzle become available, the applicability of this model will become clear.

While we are at a very early stage with these types of studies, some tantalizing themes have begun to emerge from the identified gene targets in L-LTP. First, transcription factors are up-regulated, suggesting that secondary waves of gene expression will be involved in L-LTP induction and maintenance. Second, structural proteins at the synapse appear to be targets that are up-regulated, suggesting that the hypothesis that altered gene expression is a component of triggering and maintaining long-term structural changes at the synapse in L-LTP (55, 56). We will return to this idea in more general terms in the last section of the chapter. Finally, signaling molecules and modulators of plasticity-related signal transduction mechanisms are targets of altered gene expression in L-LTP. Specifically, both positive and negative feedback mechanisms are triggered with L-LTP-inducing stimulation.

Particularly intriguing molecules in this context are molecules like BDNF, which themselves are capable of triggering long-term change and promoting activity-dependent long-term change. This suggests the interesting idea that positive feedback mechanisms that provide a self-reinforcing component necessary for maintaining synaptic potentiation perpetually might be triggered. We will return to this idea in a theoretical context in the last chapter of the book.

E. mRNA Targeting and Transport

L-LTP, a protein-synthesis-dependent phenomenon, can be selectively induced at particular synapses, or at least particular dendritic regions (see Box 4 in the last chapter, for example). Considering these data leads us to the hypothetical necessity for localization of newly synthesized mRNAs (or proteins) at recently activated synapses, so that the altered mRNA expression necessary for L-LTP be manifest appropriately at these potentiated synapses. This brings us to the final question that we will think about in the context of the cell biology of L-LTP. How is it that the new gene products get expressed at the right place among the multitude of synapses in a pyramidal neuron dendritic tree? It is known that L-LTP is synapse-specific—how is it that the gene products get targeted to the right synapses in order to increase synaptic strength appropriately?

This process is still mysterious but is actively under investigation. However, several useful insights are already available, in large part from studies of regulation of induction and expression of the mRNA for Arc/Arg3.1. The research groups of Deitmar Kuhl, Paul Worley, and Ozzie Steward have pioneered this area of investigation, and the following discussion derives largely from their work.

It is useful to think of the Arc messenger RNA as a prototype for studying the regulation of the distribution of new gene products in the neuron (reviewed in references 57 and 58). As we have already discussed, Arc/Arg3.1 was discovered as a gene product induced by activity in general and LTP in particular (13, 54, 59). Arc, like many of the other L-LTP-associated gene products we have been discussing, is an immediate early gene. Like the other IEGs, its increased expression is transient, which facilitates experimental study because there is a low pre-stimulus level of its mRNA. Finally and most importantly, once Arc mRNA is expressed, the mRNA is selectively localized to active synapses, or synapses that have been potentiated (see Figure 6). Thus, Arc regulation likely represents a microcosm of activity-dependent, selectively targeted gene products in the neuron.

Returning to our original question, how is it that mRNAs end up at the right synapses? Two broad possibilities present themselves. One possibility is that mRNAs leave the nucleus with "addresses" that send them to the right spot. The second possibility is that mRNAs are sent throughout the neuron and are selectively captured at the appropriate synapses. Studies of Arc indicate that the second scenario is the correct one. Newly synthesized Arc mRNA is distributed throughout the dendrites, presumably by diffusion but also potentially by mRNA carrier proteins associated with the cytoskeleton. The Arc mRNA is then "captured," or concentrated, at active synapses.

Thus, the targeting process appears to be not just locally initiated and controlled, but also dependent upon biochemical processes restricted to a particular synaptic region. The mRNA is not targeted specifically to a predefined dendritic region as it leaves the nucleus. There is no address on the mRNA when it leaves the nucleus—the mRNA is sent out globally and sequestered locally. If this is the general mechanism for neuronal mRNA targeting (and there is no reason to think it isn't), this type of mechanism eliminates an enormously complex trafficking problem. mRNAs do not have to

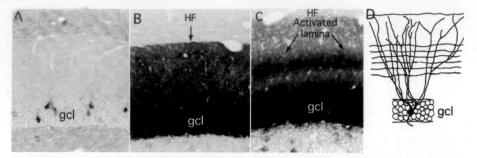

FIGURE 6   Activity-dependent Arc expression and dendritic localization. Newly synthesized Arc mRNA is selectively targeted to dendritic domains that have been synaptically activated. The photomicrographs illustrate the distribution of Arc mRNA as revealed by in situ hybridization in (A) nonactivated dentate gyrus; (B), 2 hours after a single electroconvulsive seizure and (C), and after delivering high-frequency trains to the medial perforant path over a 2-hour period. Note the uniform distribution of Arc mRNA across the dendritic laminae after an ECS and the prominent band of labeling in the middle molecular layer after high-frequency stimulation of the perforant path. (D) Schematic illustration of the dendrites of a typical dentate granule cell and the pattern of termination of medial perforant path projections. HF, hippocampal fissure; gcl, granule cell layer. Figure from Steward and Worley, (57).

have to be pre-addressed—local demands can dictate their disposition.

An additional implication of this finding is that induction signals from the dendrites to the nucleus, such as those processes we discussed in Section II.A, can be "unaddressed" as well. The synapse-to-nucleus signal does not have to have a return address on it, a signal arriving at the genome can originate from any synapse or dendritic region and its point of origin is immaterial. The genome simply has to respond appropriately to the signal with an increased readout, and local activity-dependent mechanisms in the dendrites will assure that the right synapses capture the product.

The mechanism for the appropriate capture of mRNAs at potentiated synapses is unknown, but the basic phenomenon is, of course, highly reminiscent of the synaptic tagging observation described in the last chapter (Box 4). As we discussed earlier, a parsimonious model for synaptic capture is to simply invoke persisting signals already localized at potentiated synapses, such as autonomously active CaMKII or PKC, as the root of the capture signal. A similar

mechanism has already been proposed to operate in site-specific facilitation of *Aplysia* sensory neuron synapses by Wayne Sossin and his colleagues (60). This idea is speculative but is appealing because it allows for a straightforward transition of E-LTP into L-LTP at predefined synapses.

One aspect of the targeting and capture mechanism that seems clear is that an mRNA binding protein of some sort must be involved. After all, a priori it is clear that an mRNA must bind to something in order to have its diffusion restricted to a particular domain. Several interesting candidate molecules are known mRNA binding proteins and thus might participate in mRNA capture at dendrites (reviewed in references 58 and 61). One appealing possibility is the fragile X mRNA binding protein (FMRP) that we discussed in the last chapter. Activity-dependent synthesis of FMRP might provide a mechanism for mRNA capture. Another candidate that at a minimum is involved in dendritic mRNA trafficking (if not synapse-specific localization) is the staufen protein (62). Staufen is an mRNA binding protein localized to dendrites that is involved in mRNA targeting in a variety of systems. A final possibility is the cytoplasmic polyadenylation element binding proteins (CPEB, *not* to be confused with the transcription factor C/EBP; see (33). The CPEBs are mRNA binding proteins that also regulate translation of mRNAs. Again, I emphasize that the mechanisms for targeting are unknown and that these are just possibilities that have been identified as potential players.

Though the mechanisms are unknown, it is clear that the specifically localized Arc mRNA is converted into a localized increase in Arc protein. There is no need to invoke a specific mechanism for this—it can simply be accomplished by local protein synthesis as we discussed at the end of the last chapter in the context of dendritic protein expression. Arc might be handled by the same mechanisms that are used for the synthesis of proteins from mRNAs that are expressed constitutively such as CaMKII and MAP2.

What is it that the Arc protein does once it is made at the right synapses? Although the function of Arc is unknown, there are tantalizing clues. It is known from various studies that Arc is part of the NMDAR supramolecular complex that we discussed in Chapter 5. Also, Arc is known to be a cytoskeleton-associated protein, which is part of how it got its name (*Activity-regulated cytoskeleton-associated protein*). Thus, Arc may be part of a local receptor-complex stabilizing structure, or even a component of the specific NMDAR/AMPAR stabilizing mechanism that was described in the last chapter in Figure 12. This is, of course, speculative, but it at least allows the possibility of directly translating an increase in Arc protein into an increase in synaptic strength. Many additional components of the synapse are almost certainly involved as well. Specifically relevant in this context is the observation from Michael Browning's group of increased synthesis of AMPA receptor protein in L-LTP (51).

However, in summary, Arc is an interesting proof-of-principle molecule.

Studies of Arc have demonstrated that activity-dependent mechanisms of mRNA localization exist in neurons. They have given important initial insights into some of the strategies the neuron uses to solve the problem of targeting altered gene products to the right synapses, and highlight an important role for localized protein synthesis at activated synapses. What remains is to figure out the detailed biochemical mechanisms for these processes and to increase our understanding of how local protein synthesis gets converted into potentiated synaptic transmission locally. Also, it is clear that identifying the molecular identity of the "synaptic tag" is a high priority, in order to understand the bridging mechanisms for the E-LTP to L-LTP transition.

F. Effects of the Gene Products on Synaptic Structure

Consideration of Arc as a molecule contributing to L-LTP also introduces a number of very important considerations about constraints on maintenance mechanisms for very long-lasting L-LTP. The half-life of the Arc protein is a few hours—think about the implications of this fact. The Arc message increases transiently (about $1/2$ hour) and returns to a low basal level. The mRNA is concentrated at the right synapses and translated into protein, which is broken down with a half-life of a few hours. In the absence of Arc mRNA, which has already decayed to basal levels, this protein cannot be replenished. Thus, if Arc (or any other protein with similar regulation and kinetics) participates in synaptic potentiation, this mechanism can only allow potentiation to be maintained for less than a day. Induction of Arc or any similar protein is clearly not a maintenance mechanism for very long-lasting events.

This type of thought experiment is prima facie evidence that there are multiple phases of L-LTP, because LTP is clearly able to be maintained for many days in vivo.

Any Arc-dependent process will have decayed within about 5 protein half-lives, or something on the order of 24 hours at most. Some other molecular process must maintain later stages of L-LTP in vivo.

Even though we have discussed this concept specifically in the context of Arc because it is well-studied and known to be necessary for L-LTP (13), the generalization applies to any protein involved in very long-lasting effects in neurons. This consideration highlights the fact that triggering altered gene expression and protein synthesis is likely an *induction* mechanism for long-lasting changes, but not necessarily a *maintenance* mechanism. All proteins have a finite half-life, thus maintaining long-lasting change requires an ongoing process. As we will discuss in the last chapter of the book, in biochemical systems the route for achieving persisting effects in the face of breakdown and resynthesis of the component molecules involved is via a self-reinforcing chemical reaction. This is a controlled positive feed-back loop wherein the activated molecule promotes its own resynthesis.

Given the constraint of protein turnover, how is it that you get really long-lasting changes in synaptic strength in L-LTP? I will speculate wildly here about how this might happen, looking to the studies of L-LTP that we have been discussing for clues. The model I will present has two components: a change in synaptic structure that results from altered expression of structural proteins and a positive feedback mechanism to maintain these changes in the face of protein turnover.

The Structural Change

I am going to leave the structural change ill-defined. It could be an increased number of AMPA receptors at a pre-existing spine, with its multitudinous receptor binding partners and cytoskeletal/PSD associations. It could be a new spine that splits off by spine fission, as has been proposed by a number of investigators (reviewed in 56). It

could be the growth of entirely new spines from the dendritic shaft (55, 56, 63–65). These are variations on the same issue from a biochemical perspective—doubling the surface area of a spine is basically placing the same demand on the protein synthetic machinery as splitting off a second spine or growing a new spine from the dendrite. It's not that the question of which of these actually happens is uninteresting, or that they are even functionally identical, it's just that for the purposes of the present discussion they are equivalent in their impact. However, for ease of presenting the model, I will just take the case of increasing the postsynaptic size (equivalent to an increased number of receptors) in a pre-existing spine.

The mechanisms we talked about in Sections II.C and II.E have gotten us to the point of having a spine with increased AMPA receptor protein, hypothetically through Arc-dependent signaling mechanisms. What happens when the Arc signal decays and all of the newly synthesized AMPA receptors and the like are undergoing continual breakdown and resynthesis? The new, larger PSD complex must have some way to perpetuate itself in its new, larger, state. This requires some ongoing feedback signal that says "stay big." This could happen by any of a number of specific mechanisms, but this basic point is the important concept for this section of the chapter. *Maintaining an increased synaptic connection over many protein half-lives, in the face of complete breakdown and resynthesis of all the protein components that make up that synapse, requires a self-reinforcing maintenance signal.*

The specific mechanisms for this self-perpetuating signal are completely unknown at this point. The possibilities fall into two broad categories. One possibility is that there is an ongoing activity integration mechanism that keeps the size of the synapse scaled to its pre-existing level. Variations of this idea are such things as a mechanism integrating the average spine

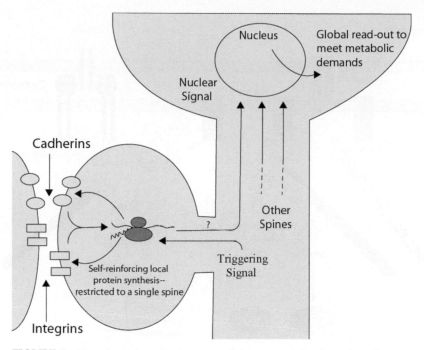

FIGURE 7 Hypothetical mechanisms contributing to activity-dependent changes in synaptic structure. Both local effects and nuclear signaling are likely involved in triggering and maintaining very long-term structural changes in synaptic spines. See text for additional discussion.

calcium level (which would vary depending on the net synaptic activity; it would be larger in a potentiated synapse) or a mechanism reading out the amount of receptor amino termini present and maintaining it at a constant level. These are just specific examples for illustrative purposes, there are, of course, many other possibilities.[4]

The second general possibility is that a unique molecule is introduced into a potentiated synapse that makes a unique signal that is self-perpetuating. This

molecule must, of course, have the capacity to in parallel increase synaptic size through impinging on protein synthesis, the receptor insertion machinery, and the like.

I have a modest preference for this second model because there are some appealing specific candidate molecules that can perform this function, that have been implicated experimentally as playing a role in L-LTP. These are the cell adhesion molecules, specifically the integrins and cadherins (see Figures 7 and 8). While I will not belabor the case for these molecules because my entire model for long-lasting LTP is so speculative, there are a number of appealing findings in this context. First, blocking the function of either cadherins or integrins blocks L-LTP (67–71). Second, this category of molecules functions in transducing signals from one cell directly to another, allowing for direct presynaptic-to-postsynaptic communication. Third,

---

[4]One of the advantages of the spine fission/new spine models is that the necessity for this type of scaling mechanism is obviated. A synapse, once formed, must simply keep making itself unless it gets a new signal to go away. However, I don't prefer this idea at present because it requires that a doubling of synaptic strength involves a doubling of the number of synaptic spines. Quantitatively large morphological changes such as this have not generally been observed to date, although there are clearly examples of increased synaptic contacts with L-LTP inducing stimulation (reviewed in reference 66).

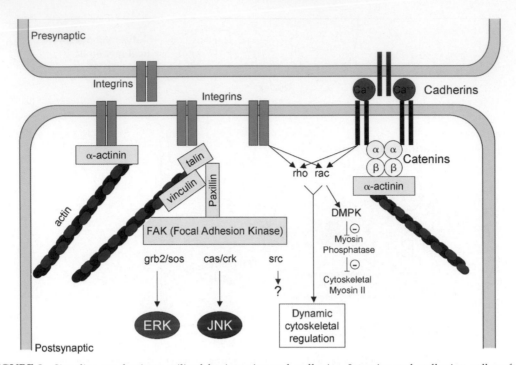

FIGURE 8 Signaling mechanisms utilized by integrins and cadherins. Integrins and cadherins, cell surface adhesions molecules, are prominent regulators of the cytoskeleton. Both families of molecules serve as cytoskeletal anchors and also regulate various signal transduction mechanisms. One role of activating these signal transduction processes is dynamically to regulate cytoskeletal structure and function. Via other pathways such as ERK, they might regulate local protein synthesis.

integrins couple to MAPK cascades in many cells to trigger local changes at the submembranous compartment, similar to what would be required for allowing them to communicate locally with the protein synthesis machinery at synapses. This local control of protein synthesis could allow for both pleiotropic effects on synaptic function and for self-reinforcing stimulation of their own synthesis. ERK coupling could be also used to communicate with the genome if that were necessary, for example for allowing the nucleus to integrate total metabolic needs for ongoing gene expression across a large number of synapses. Fourth, these molecules classically function in regulating cell morphology by controlling the cytoskeleton (reviewed in reference 72; see Figure 8); in fact, in most cells, the molecules are involved in maintaining long-lasting morphological differentiation.

Thus, while the case for integrins and cadherins in maintaining long-lasting synaptic change is somewhat circumstantial at this point, these molecules appear to have all the attributes necessary to serve as self-perpetuating signals at dendritic spines.

Thus, the basic model for maintaining perpetual synaptic strengthening is as follows. Specific integrin and cadherin molecules have their mRNA expression increased and targeted to the right synapse à la Arc. The synthesis and insertion of these molecules into a synapse (where they did not previously exist) leads to the following consequences: morphological changes and increased contact with the presynaptic terminal; enhanced ongoing AMPA receptor insertion; and localized self-stimulation of their ongoing synthesis and membrane insertion via stimulation of

ERK or other signal transduction pathways. This last point fulfils the requirement for generating a self-perpetuating signal that can outlast the triggering events and maintain the potentiated state indefinitely.

While I have presented this brief model using specific molecules as examples, please keep in mind that the model is more in the vein of a thought experiment than a specific hypothesis. It serves to illustrate some of the important functions that must be subserved in maintaining a life-long change in synaptic strength, especially the necessity of a self-perpetuating signal that can impinge upon synaptic transmission. I happen to think that the specific candidate molecules I outlined are appealing possibilities, but they are after all just candidates.

III. SUMMARY

In this chapter, we talked about those molecular mechanisms that are uniquely involved in triggering long-lasting and very long-lasting changes in synaptic transmission in the hippocampus. We focused most of our attention on how a signal gets from the synapse to the genome, highlighting the PKA/ERK/RSK/CREB pathway as a principal player in L-LTP. We also touched upon the intriguing problem of how altered gene expression becomes manifest at just the appropriate synapse, looking at Arc mRNA as a prototype molecule.

One of the important ideas that emerged from this chapter was that we need to keep in mind that the available data support the model that altered gene expression is an *induction* mechanism for L-LTP. The question of whether altered gene expression contributes to the maintenance of L-LTP is still, by and large, an open one at present.

We also talked about how changes in gene expression get manifest as changes at the synapse. We in actuality developed two different models for how this happens. The first was based on increased AMPA

receptors and associated proteins at the synapse, dependent upon a triggering event such as Arc arrival at the synapse. These changes then manifested themselves as an increased synaptic strength. This proposed mechanism is a fairly straightforward read-out of increased production of synaptic components with Arc-like molecules serving as a nucleating event.

However, considering the limitations of proteins like Arc with a half-life of a few hours led us to conclude that later stages of "L-LTP" must involve additional processes. In response to this consideration, we formulated a speculative model for how self-perpetuating changes in local protein synthesis might underlie weeks-long or life-long synaptic changes.

This final section of the chapter brought us back to the issue raised at the very beginning of the chapter, that is, considering "L-LTP" as an analogue of forms of long-term memory that depend on changes in gene expression for their induction. It is very important to remember that the types of synaptic changes we have discussed in this chapter are functionally manifest as an alteration in the properties of a neuronal *circuit* in the CNS. Clearly, self-perpetuating molecular changes are necessary for very long-lasting effects, but the lasting effects are not the entirety of the memory. The maintenance of the synaptic change *in the context of the circuit* is what constitutes the memory. The self-perpetuating synaptic change is the mechanism for the maintenance of the memory.

Thus, we see an interesting parallel between L-LTP and long-term memory. Throughout the last three chapters we have made the important molecular distinction between mechanisms for the induction, maintenance, and expression of LTP. We need to make an equally important distinction between the mechanisms for the induction, maintenance, and expression of memory. The induction of memory is learning. The maintenance of long-term memory is self-perpetuating synaptic change in the context of a specific circuit. The expression of memory is the recall of the memory by sending activity through the circuit. Just as it is important to keep in mind the molecular distinctions between the induction, maintenance, and expression of LTP, it is important to keep in mind the molecular distinctions between the induction, maintenance, and expression of long-term memory.

This was an essential point that was made in Chapter 1, where a comparison was made between current learning and memory theory and the changes that need to be made in light of a better understanding of the molecular processes involved in synaptic plasticity. If you have made it this far in the book you have made it through about 75,000 words concerning the gory details of LTP physiology, biochemistry, and molecular biology. You might find it interesting to go back and reread Chapter 1 in light of all the new information you have under your belt.

This analogy between L-LTP and long-term memory is important and valid independently of whether the particular molecular mechanisms for L-LTP that we have been talking about are actually used in the behaving animal for memory itself. That does not mean that this is an uninteresting question, however! In the next chapter we will talk about the evidence for and against a role for LTP specifically in hippocampus-dependent memory formation. We also will discuss the corollary question of whether LTP has accurately modeled memory, that is, are the molecular processes involved in LTP the molecular processes involved in memory?

References

1. Nguyen, P. V., Abel, T., and Kandel, E. R. (1994). "Requirement of a critical period of transcription for induction of a late phase of LTP." *Science* 265:1104–1107.
2. Frey, U., Frey, S., Schollmeier, F., and Krug, M. (1996). "Influence of actinomycin D, a RNA synthesis inhibitor, on long-term potentiation in rat hippocampal neurons in vivo and in vitro." *J. Physiol.* 490 (3):703–711.
3. Bourtchuladze, R., Frenguelli, B., Blendy, J., Cioffi, D., Schutz, G., and Silva, A. J. (1994). "Deficient long-term memory in mice with a targeted mutation of the cAMP-responsive element-binding protein." *Cell* 79:59–68.
4. Gass, P., Wolfer, D. P., Balschun, D., Rudolph, D., Frey, U., Lipp, H. P., and Schutz, G. (1998). "Deficits in memory tasks of mice with CREB mutations depend on gene dosage." *Learn. Mem.* 5:274–288.
5. Pittenger, C., Huang, Y. Y., Paletzki, R. F., Bourtchouladze, R., Scanlin, H., Vronskaya, S., and Kandel, E. R. (2002). "Reversible inhibition of CREB/ATF transcription factors in region CA1 of the dorsal hippocampus disrupts hippocampus-dependent spatial memory." *Neuron* 34:447–462.
6. Jones, M. W., Errington, M. L., French, P. J., Fine, A., Bliss, T. V., Garel, S., Charnay, P., Bozon, B., Laroche, S., and Davis, S. (2001). "A requirement for the immediate early gene Zif268 in the expression of late LTP and long-term memories." *Nat. Neurosci.* 4:289–296.
7. Impey, S., Fong, A. L., Wang, Y., Cardinaux, J. R., Fass, D. M., Obrietan, K., Wayman, G. A., Storm, D. R., Soderling, T. R., and Goodman, R. H. (2002). "Phosphorylation of CBP mediates transcriptional activation by neural activity and CaM kinase IV." *Neuron* 34:235–244.
8. Kang, H., Sun, L. D., Atkins, C. M., Soderling, T. R., Wilson, M. A., and Tonegawa, S. (2001). "An important role of neural activity-dependent CaMKIV signaling in the consolidation of long-term memory." *Cell* 106:771–783.
9. English, J. D., and Sweatt, J. D. (1996). "Activation of p42 mitogen-activated protein kinase in hippocampal long term potentiation." *J. Biol. Chem.* 271:24329–24332.
10. English, J. D., and Sweatt, J. D. (1997). "A requirement for the mitogen-activated protein kinase cascade in hippocampal long term potentiation." *J. Biol. Chem.* 272:19103–19106.
11. Rosenblum, K., Futter, M., Voss, K., Erent, M., Skehel, P. A., French, P., Obosi, L., Jones, M. W., and Bliss, T. V. (2002). "The role of extracellular regulated kinases I/II in late-phase long-term potentiation." *J. Neurosci.* 22:5432–5441.
12. Impey, S., Obrietan, K., Wong, S. T., Poser, S., Yano, S., Wayman, G., Deloulme, J. C., Chan, G., and Storm, D. R. (1998). "Cross talk between ERK and PKA is required for Ca²⁺ stimulation of CREB-dependent transcription and ERK nuclear translocation." *Neuron* 21:869–883.
13. Guzowski, J. F., Lyford, G. L., Stevenson, G. D., Houston, F. P., McGaugh, J. L., Worley, P. F., and Barnes, C. A. (2000). "Inhibition of activity-dependent arc protein expression in the rat

hippocampus impairs the maintenance of long-term potentiation and the consolidation of long-term memory." *J. Neurosci.* 20:3993–4001.

14. Barco, A., Alarcon, J. M., and Kandel, E. R. (2002). "Expression of constitutively active CREB protein facilitates the late phase of long-term potentiation by enhancing synaptic capture." *Cell* 108:689–703.

15. Brivanlou, A. H., and Darnell, J. E. Jr. (2002). "Signal transduction and the control of gene expression." *Science* 295:813–818.

16. Shaywitz, A. J., and Greenberg, M. E. (1999). "CREB: a stimulus-induced transcription factor activated by a diverse array of extracellular signals." *Annu. Rev. Biochem.* 68:821–861.

17. Poser, S., and Storm, D. R. (2001). "Role of Ca^{2+}-stimulated adenylyl cyclases in LTP and memory formation." *Int. J. Dev. Neurosci.* 19:387–394.

18. Kornhauser, J. M., Cowan, C. W., Shaywitz, A. J., Dolmetsch, R. E., Griffith, E. C., Hu, L. S., Haddad, C., Xia, Z., and Greenberg, M. E. (2002). "CREB transcriptional activity in neurons is regulated by multiple, calcium-specific phosphorylation events." *Neuron* 34:221–233.

19. Ohno, M., Frankland, P. W., Chen, A. P., Costa, R. M., and Silva, A. J. (2001). "Inducible, pharmacogenetic approaches to the study of learning and memory." *Nat. Neurosci.* 4:1238–1243.

20. Roberson, E. D., English, J. D., Adams, J. P., Selcher, J. C., Kondratick, C., and Sweatt, J. D. (1999). "The mitogen-activated protein kinase cascade couples PKA and PKC to cAMP response element binding protein phosphorylation in area CA1 of hippocampus." *J. Neurosci.* 19:4337–4348.

21. Lu, Y. F., Kandel, E. R., and Hawkins, R. D. (1999). "Nitric oxide signaling contributes to late-phase LTP and CREB phosphorylation in the hippocampus." *J. Neurosci.* 19:10250–10261.

22. Ho, N., Liauw, J. A., Blaeser, F., Wei, F., Hanissian, S., Muglia, L. M., Wozniak, D. F., Nardi, A., Arvin, K. L., Holtzman, D. M., Linden, D. J., Zhuo, M., Muglia, L. J., and Chatila, T. A. (2000). "Impaired synaptic plasticity and cAMP response element-binding protein activation in Ca^{2+}/calmodulin-dependent protein kinase type IV/Gr-deficient mice." *J. Neurosci.* 20:6459–6472.

23. Mermelstein, P. G., Deisseroth, K., Dasgupta, N., Isaksen, A. L., and Tsien R. W. (2001). "Calmodulin priming: nuclear translocation of a calmodulin complex and the memory of prior neuronal activity." *Proc. Natl. Acad. Sci. USA* 98:15342–15347.

24. Deisseroth, K., Bito, H., and Tsien, R. W. (1996). "Signaling from synapse to nucleus: postsynaptic CREB phosphorylation during multiple forms of hippocampal synaptic plasticity." *Neuron* 16:89–101.

25. Deisseroth, K., and Tsien, R. W. (2002). "Dynamic multiphosphorylation passwords for activity-dependent gene expression." *Neuron* 34:179–182.

26. Dudek, S. M., and Fields, R. D. (2002). "Somatic action potentials are sufficient for late-phase LTP-related cell signaling." *Proc. Natl. Acad. Sci. USA* 99:3962–3967.

27. Gooney, M., and Lynch, M. A. (2001). "Long-term potentiation in the dentate gyrus of the rat hippocampus is accompanied by brain-derived neurotrophic factor-induced activation of TrkB." *J. Neurochem.* 7:1198–1207.

28. Hall, J., Thomas, K. L., and Everitt, B. J. (2000). "Rapid and selective induction of BDNF expression in the hippocampus during contextual learning." *Nat. Neurosci.* 3:533–535.

29. Yin, Y., Edelman, G. M., and Vanderklish, P. W. (2002). "The brain-derived neurotrophic factor enhances synthesis of Arc in synaptoneurosomes." *Proc. Natl. Acad. Sci. USA* 99:2368–2373.

30. Patterson, S. L., Pittenger, C., Morozov, A., Martin, K. C., Scanlin, H., Drake, C., and Kandel, E. R. (2001). "Some forms of cAMP-mediated long-lasting potentiation are associated with release of BDNF and nuclear translocation of phospho-MAP kinase." *Neuron* 32:123–140.

31. Ying, S. W., Futter, M., Rosenblum, K., Webber, M. J., Hunt, S. P., Bliss, T. V., and Bramham, C. R. (2002). "Brain-derived neurotrophic factor induces long-term potentiation in intact adult hippocampus: requirement for ERK activation coupled to CREB and upregulation of Arc synthesis." *J. Neurosci.* 22:1532–1540.

32. Matthies, H., Becker, A., Schroeder, H., Kraus, J., Hollt, V., and Krug, M. (1997). "Dopamine D1-deficient mutant mice do not express the late phase of hippocampal long-term potentiation." *Neuroreport* 8:3533–3535.

33. Wu, L., Wells, D., Tay, J., Mendis, D., Abbott, M. A., Barnitt, A., Quinlan, E., Heynen, A., Fallon, J. R., and Richter, J. D. (1998). "CPEB-mediated cytoplasmic polyadenylation and the regulation of experience-dependent translation of alpha-CaMKII mRNA at synapses." *Neuron* 21:1129–1139.

34. Schulz, S., Siemer, H., Krug, M., and Hollt, V. (1999). "Direct evidence for biphasic cAMP responsive element-binding protein phosphorylation during long-term potentiation in the rat dentate gyrus in vivo." *J. Neurosci.* 19:5683–5692.

35. Davis, S., Vanhoutte, P., Pages, C., Caboche, J., and Laroche, S. (2000). "The MAPK/ERK cascade targets both Elk-1 and cAMP response element-binding protein to control long-term potentiation-dependent gene expression in the dentate gyrus in vivo." *J. Neurosci.* 20:4563–4572.

36. Waltereit, R., Dammermann, B., Wulff, P., Scafidi, J., Staubli, U., Kauselmann, G., Bundman, M., and Kuhl, D. (2001). "Arg3.1/Arc mRNA induction by Ca^{2+} and cAMP requires protein kinase A and mitogen-activated protein kinase/extracellular regulated kinase activation." *J. Neurosci.* 21:5484–5493.

37. Mattson, M. P., Culmsee, C., Yu, Z., and Camandola, S. (2000). "Roles of nuclear factor kappaB in neuronal survival and plasticity." *J. Neurochem.* 74:443–456.

38. Albensi, B. C., and Mattson, M. P. (2000). "Evidence for the involvement of TNF and NF-kappaB in hippocampal synaptic plasticity." *Synapse* 35:151–159.

39. Meberg, P. J., Kinney, W. R., Valcourt, E. G., and Routtenberg, A. (1996). "Gene expression of the transcription factor NF-kappa B in hippocampus: regulation by synaptic activity." *Brain Res. Mol. Brain Res.* 38:179–190.

40. Cole, A. J., Saffen, D. W., Baraban, J. M., and Worley, P. F. (1989). "Rapid increase of an immediate early gene messenger RNA in hippocampal neurons by synaptic NMDA receptor activation." *Nature* 340:474–476.

41. Wisden, W., Errington, M. L., Williams, S., Dunnett, S. B., Waters, C., Hitchcock, D., Evan, G., Bliss, T. V., and Hunt, S. P. (1990). "Differential expression of immediate early genes in the hippocampus and spinal cord." *Neuron* 4:603–614.

42. Abraham, W. C., Dragunow, M., and Tate, W. P. (1991). "The role of immediate early genes in the stabilization of long-term potentiation." *Mol. Neurobiol.* 5:297–314.

43. Abraham, W. C., Mason, S. E., Demmer, J., Williams, J. M., Richardson, C. L., Tate, W. P., Lawlor, P. A., and Dragunow, M. (1993). "Correlations between immediate early gene induction and the persistence of long-term potentiation." *Neuroscience* 56:717–727.

44. Williams, J., Dragunow, M., Lawlor, P., Mason, S., Abraham, W. C., Leah, J., Bravo, R., Demmer, J., and Tate, W. (1995). "Krox20 may play a key role in the stabilization of long-term potentiation." *Brain Res. Mol. Brain Res.* 28:87–93.

45. Taubenfeld, S. M., Wiig, K. A., Monti, B., Dolan, B., Pollonini, G., and Alberini, C. M. (2001). "Fornix-dependent induction of hippocampal CCAAT enhancer-binding protein [beta] and [delta] Co-localizes with phosphorylated cAMP response element-binding protein and accompanies long-term memory consolidation." *J. Neurosci.* 21:84–91.

46. Patterson, S. L., Grover, L. M., Schwartzkroin, P. A., and Bothwell, M. (1992). "Neurotrophin expression in rat hippocampal slices: a stimulus paradigm inducing LTP in CA1 evokes increases in BDNF and NT-3 mRNAs." *Neuron* 9:1081–1088.

47. Huang, Y. Y., Bach, M. E., Lipp, H. P., Zhuo, M., Wolfer, D. P., Hawkins, R. D., Schoonjans, L., Kandel, E. R., Godfraind, J. M., Mulligan, R., Collen, D., and Carmeliet, P. (1996). "Mice lacking the gene encoding tissue-type plasminogen activator show a selective interference with late-phase long-term potentiation in both Schaffer collateral and mossy fiber pathways." *Proc. Natl. Acad. Sci. USA* 93:8699–8704.

48. Szklarczyk, A., Lapinska, J., Rylski, M., McKay, R. D., and Kaczmarek, L. (2002). "Matrix metalloproteinase-9 undergoes expression and activation during dendritic remodeling in adult hippocampus." *J. Neurosci.* 22:920–930.

49. Ingi, T., Worley, P. F., and Lanahan, A. A. (2001). "Regulation of SSAT expression by synaptic activity." *Eur. J. Neurosci.* 13:1459–1463.

50. Qian, Z., Gilbert, M., and Kandel, E. R. (1994). "Temporal and spatial regulation of the expression of BAD2, a MAP kinase phosphatase, during seizure, kindling, and long-term potentiation." *Learn. Mem.* 1:180–188.

51. Nayak, A., Zastrow, D. J., Lickteig, R., Zahniser, N. R., and Browning, M. D. (1998). "Maintenance of late-phase LTP is accompanied by PKA-dependent increase in AMPA receptor synthesis." *Nature* 394:680–683.

52. Kato, A., Ozawa, F., Saitoh, Y., Hirai, K., and Inokuchi, K. (1997). "vesl, a gene encoding VASP/Ena family related protein, is upregulated during seizure, long-term potentiation and synaptogenesis." *FEBS Lett.* 412:183–189.

53. Matsuo, R., Murayama, A., Saitoh, Y., Sakaki, Y., and Inokuchi, K. (2000). "Identification and cataloging of genes induced by long-lasting long-term potentiation in awake rats." *J. Neurochem.* 74:2239–2249.

54. Steward, O., and Worley, P. F. (2001). "Selective targeting of newly synthesized Arc mRNA to active synapses requires NMDA receptor activation." *Neuron* 30:227–240.

55. Bolshakov, V. Y., Golan, H., Kandel, E. R., and Siegelbaum, S. A. (1997). "Recruitment of new sites of synaptic transmission during the cAMP-dependent late phase of LTP at CA3-CA1 synapses in the hippocampus." *Neuron* 19:635–651.

56. Luscher, C., Nicoll, R. A., Malenka, R. C., and Muller, D. (2000). "Synaptic plasticity and dynamic modulation of the postsynaptic membrane." *Nat. Neurosci.* 3:545–550.

57. Steward, O., and Worley, P. F. (2001). "A cellular mechanism for targeting newly synthesized mRNAs to synaptic sites on dendrites." *Proc. Natl. Acad. Sci. USA* 98:7062–7068.

58. Steward, O., and Schuman, E. M. (2001). "Protein synthesis at synaptic sites on dendrites." *Annu. Rev. Neurosci.* 4:299–325.

59. Link, W., Konietzko, U., Kauselmann, G., Krug, M., Schwanke, B., Frey, U., and Kuhl, D. (1995). "Somatodendritic expression of an immediate early gene is regulated by synaptic activity." *Proc. Natl. Acad. Sci. USA* 92:5734–5738.

60. Khan, A., Pepio, A. M., and Sossin, W. S. (2001). "Serotonin activates S6 kinase in a rapamycin-sensitive manner in Aplysia synaptosomes." *J. Neurosci.* 21:382–391.

61. Raught, B., Gingras, A. C., and Sonenberg, N. (2001). "The target of rapamycin (TOR) proteins." *Proc. Natl. Acad. Sci. USA* 98:7037–7044.

62. Tang, S. J., Meulemans, D., Vazquez, L., Colaco, N., and Schuman, E. (2001). "A role for a rat homolog of staufen in the transport of RNA to neuronal dendrites." *Neuron* 32:463–475.

63. Engert, F., and Bonhoeffer, T. (1999). "Dendritic spine changes associated with hippocampal long-term synaptic plasticity." *Nature* 399:66–70.

64. Maletic-Savatic, M., Malinow, R., and Svoboda, K. (1999). "Rapid dendritic morphogenesis in CA1 hippocampal dendrites induced by synaptic activity." *Science* 283:1923–1927.

65. Toni, N., Buchs, P. A., Nikonenko, I., Bron, C. R., and Muller, D. (1999). "LTP promotes formation of multiple spine synapses between a single axon terminal and a dendrite." *Nature* 402:421–425.

66. Yuste, R., and Bonhoeffer, T. (2001). "Morphological changes in dendritic spines associated with long-term synaptic plasticity." *Annu. Rev. Neurosci.* 24:1071–1089.

67. Bozdagi, O., Shan, W., Tanaka, H., Benson, D. L., and Huntley, G. W. (2000). "Increasing numbers of synaptic puncta during late-phase LTP: N-cadherin is synthesized, recruited to synaptic sites, and required for potentiation." *Neuron* 28:245–259.

68. Tang, L., Hung, C. P., and Schuman, E. M. (1998). "A role for the cadherin family of cell adhesion molecules in hippocampal long-term potentiation." *Neuron* 20:1165–1175.

69. Chun, D., Gall, C. M., Bi, X., and Lynch, G. (2001). "Evidence that integrins contribute to multiple stages in the consolidation of long term potentiation in rat hippocampus." *Neuroscience* 105:815–829.

70. Kramar, E. A., Bernard, J. A., Gall, C. M., and Lynch, G. (2002). "Alpha3 integrin receptors contribute to the consolidation of long-term potentiation." *Neuroscience* 110:29–39.

71. Bliss, T., Errington, M., Fransen, E., Godfraind, J. M., Kauer, J. A., Kooy, R. F., Maness, P. F., and Furley, A. J. (2000). "Long-term potentiation in mice lacking the neural cell adhesion molecule L1." *Curr. Biol.* 10:1607–1610.

72. Juliano, R. L. (2002). "Signal transduction by cell adhesion receptors and the cytoskeleton: functions of integrins, cadherins, selectins, and immunoglobulin-superfamily members." *Annu. Rev. Pharmacol. Toxicol.* 42:283–323.

73. Eriksson, P. S., Perfilieva, E., Bjork-Eriksson, T., Alborn, A. M., Nordborg, C., Peterson, D. A., and Gage, F. H. (1998). "Neurogenesis in the adult human hippocampus." *Nat. Med.* 4:1313–1317.

74. Gould, E., Beylin, A., Tanapat, P., Reeves, A., and Shors, T. J. (1999). "Learning enhances adult neurogenesis in the hippocampal formation." *Nat. Neurosci.* 2:260–265.

75. Villarreal, D. M., Do, V., Haddad, E., and Derrick, B. E. (2002). "NMDA receptor antagonists sustain LTP and spatial memory: active processes mediate LTP decay." *Nat. Neurosci.* 5:48–52.

76. Frey, U., Krug, M., Reymann, K. G., and Matthies, H. (1988). "Anisomycin, an inhibitor of protein synthesis, blocks late phases of LTP phenomena in the hippocampal CA1 region in vitro." *Brain Res.* 452:57–65.

77. Nguyen, P. V., and Kandel, E. R. (1997). "Brief theta-burst stimulation induces a transcription-dependent late phase of LTP requiring cAMP in area CA1 of the mouse hippocampus." *Learn. Mem.* 4:230–243.

78. Wei, F., Qiu, C. S., Liauw, J., Robinson, D. A., Ho, N., Chatila, T., and Zhuo, M. (2002). "Calcium calmodulin-dependent protein kinase IV is required for fear memory." *Nat. Neurosci.* 5:573–579.

79. Impey, S., Mark, M., Villacres, E. C., Poser, S., Chavkin, C., and Storm, D. R. (1996). "Induction of CRE-mediated gene expression by stimuli that generate long-lasting LTP in area CA1 of the hippocampus." *Neuron* 16:973–982.

80. Gartner, A., and Staiger, V. (2002). "Neurotrophin secretion from hippocampal neurons evoked by long-term-potentiation-inducing electrical stimulation patterns." *Proc. Natl. Acad. Sci. USA* 99:6386–6391.

81. Roberts, L. A., Large, C. H., Higgins, M. J., Stone, T. W., O'Shaughnessy, C. T., and Morris B. J. (1998). "Increased expression of dendritic mRNA following the induction of long-term potentiation." *Brain Res. Mol. Brain Res.* 56:38–44.

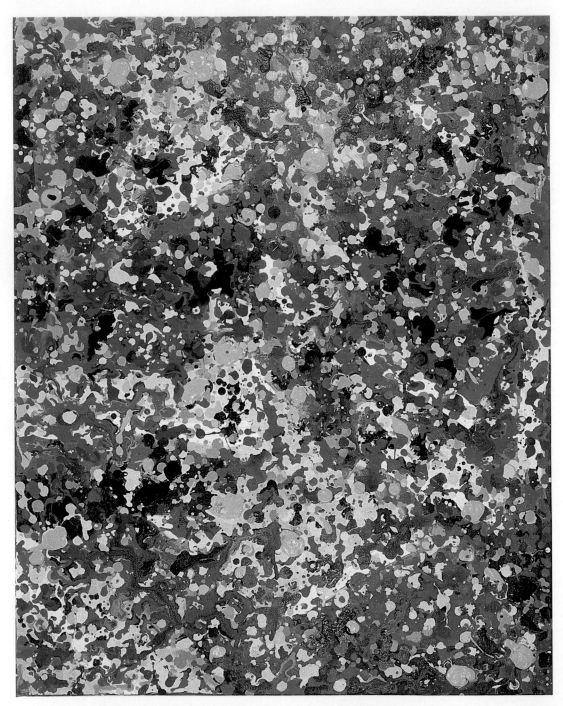

Transgenic Approaches to Understanding Memory
J. David Sweatt, Acrylic on canvas, 2002

LTP Does Not Equal Memory

In 1998 Chuck Stevens wrote a review that asked the question, "Does LTP = Memory?" Neither Chuck nor most investigators in the field considered that a *literal* yes might be the answer to this question, but it nicely captured one of the central issues in current research in learning and memory, that is, what is the role of LTP in the behaving animal (1).

I like Chuck's rhetorical construct so much that I am going to use it as the organizing framework for this chapter. Thus, we will ask the question: does LTP = memory? The answer to this question clearly is no, as I mentioned above, because it is an extremely stringent statement. It only takes one example of inequivalency to falsify the statement. Are we then just treating the question as a straw-man construct, easily knocked down?

No, because exploring the reasons *why* the answer is no is a useful way to review the literature concerning the role for hippocampal LTP specifically as a mechanism contributing to memory. In this way, we can discuss a number of issues concerning whether LTP is one of those processes that the brain actually uses as a mechanism subserving memory formation. For example, in several cases there has been a clear dissociation of hippocampal LTP from memory of specific sorts, and considering these examples is instructive. However, there also are many cases where LTP has been directly implicated as playing a role in hippocampus-dependent memory formation, and we will discuss these as well.

In this chapter we also will specifically formulate the idea that hippocampal LTP is not a mechanism for memory per se, but rather a mechanism serving as a hippocampal information buffer, contributing to memory consolidation in the cortex. We also will tie LTP in with multimodal information processing by the hippocampus and discuss the idea of LTP serving as a short-term information storage mechanism locally within the hippocampus.

In some brain areas for some specific forms of learning, LTP may actually equal memory, and we will touch on this idea as well. What I mean by LTP equaling memory in this case is that, in some forms of learning, LTP specifically may be the mechanism that serves to store a change in a behaviorally relevant circuit, and potentiation of that circuit then manifests itself as a behavioral memory. The specific example I am referring to is amygdalar LTP and cued fear conditioning. We will briefly review the considerable and impressive data extant linking LTP with cued fear conditioning as an example of a situation where LTP may "equal" memory.

Another way to disprove the equivalency of memory and LTP is to find an example of something else that equals memory, but that does not equal LTP. Thus, for example, you can make the case that LTP does not equal memory because LTD equals memory. We will draw an example of this sort by looking at eye-blink conditioning and cerebellar LTD, where there is very nice evidence that LTD contributes to a behavioral read-out of memory. We also will use this system as a good excuse to review quickly a little of the biochemistry of LTD in Purkinje cells. It makes a nice compare-and contrast at the biochemical level with hippocampal LTP.

A final theme of this chapter is that the analogy between L-LTP and long-term memory is important and valid independent of whether LTP itself is used in the behaving animal for memory storage per se. Intrinsic to many of the issues we will discuss in this chapter is the question of whether LTP has accurately modeled memory, that is, has investigating the

molecular processes involved in LTP given us insights into the molecular processes involved in memory in the behaving animal? In my opinion, the answer to this question is a resounding yes—perhaps the most important outcome of three decades of investigations into the molecular basis of LTP. This is an important overarching theme to keep in mind as we review throughout the chapter many experimental approaches that address the relationship of LTP to memory formation.

I. LTP DOES NOT EQUAL MEMORY

The "strong" hypothesis that LTP *equals* memory makes a number of predictions. We can frame these in the general form that we have been using throughout the book—block, mimic, and measure. Thus,

The block experiment—agents that block LTP should block memory formation. A corollary of this is that agents that enhance LTP should enhance memory.

The mimic experiment—inducing LTP in the right place in the brain should cause a behavioral change indistinguishable from learned behavior. A variation of this idea is that saturating LTP at the right synapses should interfere with memory formation utilizing those synapses—a behavioral variation of an "occlusion" experiment.

Finally, the measure experiment—when an animal learns, LTP should be observable in its CNS. A variation of this prediction is that molecular events associated with LTP induction should be observable in the animal's CNS in association with memory formation.

In this chapter I will provide a brief overview of the available data testing whether LTP = Memory, using these categories of experiments as the organizing basis for the chapter.

I should note before I begin that the discussion will not be exhaustive because this topic has received considerable attention already in the literature. Obviously, this has been one of the hottest topics around since the first report of LTP by Bliss and Lomo. I have listed several reviews evaluating the role of LTP in memory formation in the references (2–5). In particular, I point you to the recent review from Richard Morris's group as an additional reading (2)—it is executed with the typical depth and clarity that Richard brings to his varied efforts.[1]

A. The Block Experiment

Many, many experiments that touch on the issue of whether experimental manipulations that block LTP also block learning and memory have been published. For our purposes here, I am going to focus on experiments using genetic manipulation of mice because this type of experimental approach has several appealing aspects. For one thing, this is a fairly absolute manipulation—either the gene is there or it isn't. Dosages and efficacy are not nearly as much a concern with knockout and transgenic animals, versus drug studies, although, of course, cellular compensation and compensatory changes in homologous gene expression levels are a caveat to the approach (see Box 1). Another reason I like genetic manipulation experiments for our purposes is that, in almost every case, the LTP experiments and the behavior experiments were done side by side in the same lab group and using the same animals. Even in those cases where background strain effects or molecular compensation are factors, molecularly identical or even individually identical animals were used for both the LTP and the behavior studies in essentially every case. The LTP and behavior studies are then as directly comparable as can be achieved as a practical matter.

In our thought experiment, we are going to posit that hippocampal LTP *equals* hippocampus-dependent memory. If LTP gets better, memory should get better. If

---

[1] I wrote this chapter in July 2002. When I started to write this chapter, I accumulated all the relevant references I could find, and one in particular stuck out —the review by Martin, Grimwood, and Morris "Synaptic Plasticity and Memory: An Evaluation of the Hypothesis" (2). I had never read it (sorry Richard), and I set it aside. It was clear from reading the abstract that it dealt with many of the same issues that I was going to be dealing with in this chapter, and I wanted to conduct an exercise using it. I wrote this chapter without referring to the Martin et al. review, and after writing the chapter I went back and read Martin et al. as a compare-and-contrast exercise to see how my thinking compared to theirs. Part of my rationale was that it has been my experience that two people assessing the same question independently tend to come up with a broader range of ideas than if one leads and the other follows. Thus, I didn't want to deny myself the opportunity of potentially coming up with different ideas than Richard and his colleagues.

After drafting the chapter and going back to read their review my response was twofold. First, I was astonished at the degree of similarity in how they had organized their thinking and writing about the topic, relative to my own writing in this chapter. I took this as a good sign. Second, I was relieved that my thinking on the general role of LTP in memory was in line with theirs. It's nice to have your thoughts match up with one of the leading scholars and thinkers in the field, in this case Richard Morris. The congruence is perhaps not surprising because, of course, I have read most of Richard's primary publications in the area, and his work has always greatly influenced me.

I promised myself that I would not go back and substantially change the chapter after reading Martin et al., and I was able to adhere to that. Nevertheless, after reading their review I added a couple of mutants to Table 1 that I had missed and modified the section on the "mimic" experiment based on the historical clarification available in Martin et al. Also, I went back to Chapter 7 and added some discussion to the synaptic tagging Box because reading Martin et al. highlighted in my mind the potential role of synaptic tagging in temporal integration.

I relate this anecdote for three reasons. First, one of the responsibilities of a scholarly writer is to acknowledge priority in publication, which is certainly applicable here. The second purpose is to acknowledge the profound influence that Richard has had on my thinking and everyone else's in the field. He has been and continues to be a pioneering experimentalist and thinker on the issue of the role of synaptic plasticity in memory formation. Finally, I relate the story because I think that this sort of exercise is a very interesting and edifying experience, and that students should attempt it routinely. Pick a review by one of the leaders in your field and "blindly" outline how you would write a review on the same topic. Go back and compare your outline with their review. What holes did you have in your outline? Are your ideas on the important topics and future directions similar to theirs? Did you think of anything that they didn't?

One day, when you're an old guy like me, you can enjoy the luxurious fun of having your exercises published in a book, such as happened in this case.

LTP gets worse, memory should get worse. To test these predictions, I surveyed the available literature and found those publications where both LTP and spatial memory had been assessed in a knockout or transgenic animal. Generally speaking, the LTP studied is NMDA receptor-dependent (with one exception), in Area CA1 mostly (but also dentate gyrus in some cases), and induced with 100-Hz stimulation or theta-frequency stimulation. The memory paradigms are almost all either Morris water maze or contextual fear conditioning. I tried, to the best of my ability, to eliminate strains where pronounced structural deficits or neurodegenerative

processes occurred—this eliminated a number of disease models, for example.

About 50 different molecules were knocked out, genetically inhibited, or aberrantly expressed in the studies I surveyed.[2] I have arranged the results of the survey

---

[2]This is about 0.1–0.2 % of the genome, amazingly enough. Moreover, as a practical matter, it is difficult to find publications for animals that had no phenotype in either LTP or memory, so many of these that exist would have been missed. In addition, embryonic lethality or mutations that cause gross pathological changes are eliminated from consideration. Thus, Table 1 may in fact represent a reasonably broad sampling of the genome, at least for those genes that are experimentally tractable using these approaches.

BOX 1

MOUSE TRAPS—CAVEATS TO THE USE OF KNOCKOUT ANIMALS

Sometime in 1995, Joey English discovered that ERK MAP kinases are activated with LTP-inducing stimulation. Because no inhibitor of ERK activation that would allow testing the necessity of the phenomenon for LTP induction was available at that time, I broached the issue with Joey of generating ERK knockout mice. I'll never forget Joey's response: "Those animals will never make it past the eight-cell stage." Here it is eight years later, and still no ERK2 knockout animal is available, so Joey may well have been correct. His point was that some signal transduction processes are so fundamentally important for general cellular regulation that you will never be able to obtain a knockout mouse missing those components.

This is just one example of a number of caveats to using the knockout/transgenic mouse approaches in neurobiology. In fact, the overall complexity of the CNS and the

functions it serves make this the worst-case scenario for the application of genetic engineering technology. Of course, it's also the most interesting, important, and powerful application of the technology! Given this Catch-22, it is widely recognized these days that in most cases we must simply bite the bullet and go ahead and use genetically modified animals wherever possible, keeping in mind the important caveats that go along with the approach. In the table I've listed some of the documented pitfalls to the approach. Please note that the table is not comprehensive, simply illustrative.

I've also added a brief section on some established ways around known traps. These include some of the emerging technologies that allow inducible genetic deletions and/or brain-subregion specific manipulations, in order to get around some of the problems listed in the first part of the table.

BOX 1—cont'd

MOUSE TRAPS—CAVEATS TO THE USE
OF KNOCKOUT ANIMALS

TABLE Box 1

Caveat	Example Molecule	Example Effect	LTP/Memory Present?
Nonspecific effects	ERK2	ES cell lethal?	No
	NMDAR1	Dead	No
	Fyn	Deformed hippocampus	No
	CaMKII	Epileptic	No
Compensatory effects	PKC-gamma	Rescue of LTP depending on stimulation protocol	No/yes
	CREB	Compensatory up-regulation of homologous proteins	Yes
Redundancy	nNOS/eNOS/both	No single-knockout affect	Yes/yes/no
	AC1/AC8/both	No single-knockout affect	Yes/yes/no
Variability	mGluR1	Variable results between groups	Yes and no
	rasGRF	Variable results between groups	No
Lack of effect	PKA RII-beta	Disappointing lack of	Yes
	Synapsin	Disappointing lack of	Yes
Background strain effects	CREB, others (see Table 1)	Influence of mouse strain (129, C57, etc) on phenotype	
Successful alternate strategies	CaMKII inducible kinase	Overexpressing the molecule instead of knocking it out	
	NMDAR1 regional KO	Subregion-specific knockout to avoid embryonic lethality	
	Inducible CREB dominant negative	Allows development in the presence of a needed molecule	
	BDNF, fyn rescue	In vitro application of a missing molecule to rescue its function	
	thr286 CaMKII mutant	Point mutant transgenic for increased molecular selectivity	
	MEK partial dominant negative	Partial suppression of a critical gene	
	Floxed gene plus inducible regional CRE recombinase expression	Theoretically allows the inducible regional knockout of any gene	
	Back-crossing 6–10 generations	Places the knockout in a more consistent background strain	

in Table 1. Any experimental outcome could include enhanced, unchanged, or diminished LTP, and enhanced, unchanged or diminished memory, giving us a nine-compartment matrix. A quick glance at Table 1 reveals that of the nine possible combinations, eight are represented in the literature.[3] What this means is that LTP and memory have been dissociated from each other in almost every conceivable fashion. LTP can be decreased and memory enhanced. Hippocampus-dependent memory deficits can occur with no discernable effect on LTP.

Does this mean that LTP is not involved in hippocampus-dependent memory formation? Certainly not. There are ways to rationalize each of the outcomes and maintain the hypothesis that LTP is involved in memory, as I will discuss later. Most of the explanations are variations of either (1) compensation by multiple, redundant memory systems or (2) measurement of the wrong type of LTP. However, what Table 1 does make clear, and the first point of the exercise, is that hippocampal LTP does not *equal* hippocampal memory. There is no one-to-one correspondence between LTP and memory.

One must bring to bear subtlety of thinking when considering the role of LTP in memory. There will be no direct quantitative or even qualitative relationship between LTP measured experimentally and memory measured experimentally—that is already abundantly clear from the available literature. This probably seems like a statement of the obvious to anyone who is an active researcher in the area. However,

I am constantly amazed at the extent to which the general scientific audience is surprised when results from an LTP experiment do not "match up" with results from a behavior experiment. I think that those of us who work on LTP and behavior perhaps have not done a very good job of conveying this point in our publications.

In terms of testing the hypothesis of a *role* for LTP in memory (versus an equivalency), the most damning observations probably are those examples where LTP is completely lost and there is no effect on hippocampus-dependent memory formation. A specific example of this finding is the GluRA knockout mouse (see reference 7 and Figure 1), but there are several other similar observations in the literature. If LTP is lost and there is no effect on memory, that seems like a pretty hard spot to wiggle out of. Nevertheless, there are important caveats to interpreting these observations. For example, overtraining the animals could lead to memory formation by an alternate route that is not normally utilized. Or perhaps the particular learning paradigm is not measuring the relevant type of memory. (This is likely the case in the GluRA knockout animal; see reference 8.) Conversely, perhaps the physiology paradigm is not measuring the relevant form of LTP, or LTP in the relevant brain region. These are all issues that must be taken into consideration when interpreting these results.

The point here is not to flip-flop around like a politician and evade the question but rather to make two points. First, the discussion illustrates several specific issues that must be considered when interpreting experimental results comparing LTP with behavior, such as the multitude of experimental variables for both LTP and behavior. The second point is that, as I mentioned at the outset of the section, we have to bring some subtlety of thinking to bear on the question of the role of LTP in memory. The available data already make it clear that there will be no one-to-one correspondence of LTP to memory. We must begin to

---

[3]The ninth position, LTP unchanged and memory enhanced, can also be filled in by stepping slightly outside the bounds of the table. There are examples in the literature of two mouse strains that have equivalent LTP in vitro but that differ in their spatial learning capacity. As this is not a genetic manipulation in the same sense as a knockout or transgenic mouse line, I did not include this example in the chart. If anyone knows of other interesting mouse lines that dissociate LTP and memory, please let me know.

TABLE 1 LTP and Memory in Genetic Mouse Models

LTP

		Increased	No Change	Decreased
Memory	Increased	Nociception receptor (66) Ryanodine receptor-3 (67, 68) Telencephalin (69) S100 B (70) NR2B Transgenic (71, 72) Calcineurin (inhibited) (73)		Heparin-binding growth-associated molecule (transgenic) (74)
	No Change	Mas protooncogene (75) IP$_3$Kinase (76)	PKCγ (mild effects reported) (77, 78) ERK1 (6, 79) ApoE (80) Dystrophin (81)	Kv1.4 (82) NO synthase (83, 84) GluRA (7) t-PA (85) Trk B receptor +/− (86) CaMKIV/Gr (87) Phosphatase Inhibitor 1 (88) Thy-1 (89, 90)
	Decreased	Heparin-binding growth-associated molecule (knockout) (74) LIM Kinase (Williams syndrome) (91) Fragile X2 protein (92) PSD-95 (93)	5HT1A receptor (94) Cav2.3 channel (95) PKCβ (9) Ataxin-1 (96) L1 adhesion molecule (97) Truncated TrkB receptors (98) Kv1.1 (99)	CaMKII (100–102) CREB (104, 105) BDNF (106–109) mGluR1 (111) NMDAR (32, 112) NMDAR tail mutants (32, 112) AC1/8 double knockout (115) TrkB receptor −/− (86) Integrin-associated protein (118) t-PA (119) NT-4 (121) PACAP receptor 1(mossy fiber LTP) (125) Acid-sensing ion channel (126) Mitochondrial VDAC (128) Ras GRF (130) Neurofibromatosis Type 1 (103) Angelman syndrome gene (ubiquitin ligase) (110) Extracellular superoxide dismutase (transgenic) (113) SOD1 (transgenic) (116) Zif268 (114) Constitutively active CaMKII (29, 117) CREB/ATF family transcription factors (120) CaMKIV (122) PKA (123, 124) Inbred mouse lines—CBA and DBA (127) Calbindin/ D28 (129)

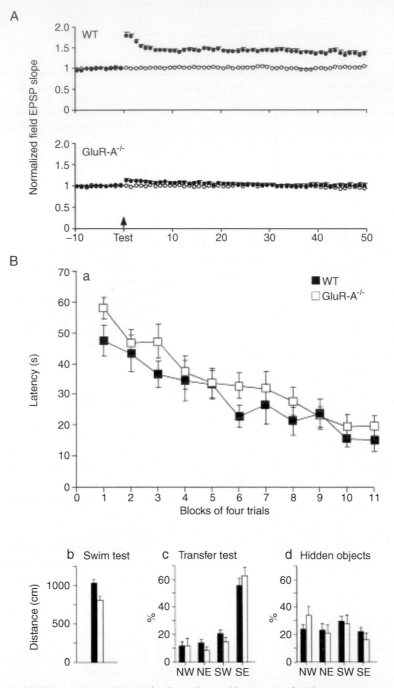

FIGURE 1 Loss of LTP does not correlate with a loss of spatial learning in the Morris water maze. (A) Summary graphs of extracellular fEPSP slopes evoked in the tetanized (filled circles) and untetanized (open circles) pathways from slices of wild-type (WT; $n = 5$–17; five mice) and GluR-A deficient mice ($n = 20$; six mice). Data were obtained in bicuculline methochloride (10 mM) and 4 mM Ca^{2+} and Mg^{2+}. Arrow, time of tetanic stimulation. (B) Spatial learning. (a) In a Morris water maze the mean latency ($\pm$ SEM) to escape from the pool to the submerged platform (eight trials per day in blocks of four) is presented as a function of trial block for male wild-type ($n = 19$) (filled squares) and GluR-A$-/-$ ($n = 21$) (open squares) mice. (b) Swim test gives the mean distance covered by the two genotypes in 50 s in the pool without a platform before training. (c) In a transfer test after trial block 10, the platform was removed and wild-type and GluR-A$-/-$ mice were allowed to search for 60 seconds. Both groups searched selectively in the target quadrant (SE). Ordinate, percent time spent in each quadrant. (d) Quadrant preference was not observed when distal visual cues were invisible in the transfer test. Figure and Legend reproduced from Zamanillo et al. (7).

entertain alternative ways of thinking about how LTP fits into the larger issue of how memory happens.

Some of the other dissociations of LTP and memory that are illustrated in Table 1 are fairly easily explained. No change in LTP with an attendant memory deficit can be explained simply by the presence of a deficit in another relevant brain region. A likely example of this is the PKC beta knockout mouse characterized by Ed Weeber in my lab (9). These animals have a pronounced contextual fear-conditioning deficit but no hippocampal LTP deficit. However, PKC beta is prominently expressed in the basolateral nucleus of the amygdala, and the knockout animals have a deficit in cued fear conditioning. Thus, their deficit in the hippocampus-dependent memory paradigm is easily explained as being the result of a defect in amygdalar plasticity. A similar rationale can be applied to other findings where memory is affected without an attendant change in hippocampal LTP.

Similarly, one can explain animals that exhibit an enhancement of LTP with an attendant memory deficit in a fairly straight-forward fashion. Any manipulation that perturbs LTP may disrupt the plastic capacity of the entire hippocampal system. An aberrantly high net baseline synaptic transmission caused by a lifelong over-expression of LTP may be functionally equivalent to a hippocampal lesion. In a more specific scenario, if hippocampal synapses are driven to saturation as a result of excessively robust LTP capacity, this may occlude the plasticity necessary for memory formation. We will return shortly to this as a specific type of experimental manipulation. The observation that saturating LTP artificially causes memory deficits is, in fact, interpreted as being consistent with a role for LTP in memory formation.

Thus, we have seen from our analysis of Table 1 that LTP clearly does not equal memory. One should not be surprised when experimental analysis reveals that hippocampal LTP and hippocampus-dependent memory are not co-varying. Nevertheless, further consideration of the experimental observations reveals that the data can be interpreted in ways that are consistent with a *role* for LTP in memory formation of various sorts. LTP does not equal memory, but it is still quite the viable candidate as a mechanism contributing to memory. Moreover, while hypothesis testing is not a democratic process, it is somewhat reassuring that in the vast majority of the cases so far there has been good agreement between effects of genetic manipulation on hippocampal LTP and their attendant effects on hippocampus-dependent memory.

Finally, I should note that we have so far dealt with only one specific variation of the block experiment, wherein genetic engineering is used as the experimental tool. The armamentarium is not limited to this single bullet—many drug infusion studies have addressed the question of whether blocking LTP blocks memory formation as well. Many of these have been reviewed in the excellent paper by Martin et al. (2), and in general the findings are quite supportive of a role for LTP in hippocampus-dependent memory. Later in the chapter, I will return to a couple of specific, and seminal, findings from Richard Morris's lab using this approach.

B. The Mimic Experiment

The mimic experiment is a fascinating thought experiment. In one specific variation, we would take an animal, place electrodes in its hippocampus, and use defined LTP-inducing stimulation patterns to place a memory in its CNS for the location of a food reward. Placing the stimulated but otherwise naïve animal into a maze with a hidden food pellet would reveal that the animal could proceed directly to the reward – this despite never having received any direct experience concerning the location of the reward. A positive outcome in an experiment of this sort would be strongly supportive of the hypothesis of a role for LTP in memory formation.

The principal thing that we can say about the mimic experiment is that we are nowhere near being able to execute it at our present level of understanding and technology, at least for behaviors relevant to the hippocampus. Consider for a moment what the proper design and implementation of the experiment would entail. First, we would have to know the precise neuronal circuit underlying the behavior and how those circuits tied into the hippocampus. The details of the circuit would have to be known down to the level of the specific synapses involved in the hippocampus, if such is the case (perhaps the hippocampus never specifies synapses on a predetermined basis but rather allocates synaptic resources for computation on the fly). We would have to know that potentiating those synapses would translate into the formation of the relevant behavioral pattern—that is, that synaptic potentiation there would translate into the appropriate change in neuronal circuit properties somewhere down the line (it seems unlikely that the hippocampus is directly "in-line" as part of a circuit *directly* mediating a behavior). We would have to be able to induce LTP selectively at the relevant synapses with pinpoint accuracy. Overall, this is an experiment unlikely to be achievable anytime soon and perhaps never depending on how exactly the hippocampus operates.

Nevertheless, spending some time considering the mimic experiment is quite useful in my opinion for several reasons. It helps define what it is that we don't understand about the hippocampus—highlighting important areas of future pursuit. It also emphasizes the importance of being able to do this type of experiment in those memory paradigms where it is beginning to be practicable, such as in amygdala- and cerebellum-dependent memory paradigms (see references 10 and 11).

The mimic experiment also has import beyond the memory field, testing an important prediction of the general model driving all contemporary neuroscience. I am referring to the general theory that changes in the CNS *mediate* behavioral change, a point for which there substantial correlative evidence but scant direct evidence. Considering the mimic experiment also impinges upon the critical issues of the neural basis of consciousness—after all, the animal presumably is unable to distinguish real experience from artificially implanted experience. Thus, considering the mimic experiment brings us face to face with some of the key issues confronting modern neurobiology and philosophy. All in all, it is an obdurate topic of great significance.

Given the technical incapacity to execute the mimic experiment, what approaches of this sort are we left with? A very important variation of this idea that has been previously attempted by several pioneering labs and executed lately with great sophistication is the "occlusion" variant. The rationale here is that if we can go in and saturate LTP in the hippocampus, further naturally occurring LTP is not possible; thus, learning deficits should arise because of the lost capacity of the hippocampus to trigger its necessary synaptic plasticity.

Pioneering studies using this approach were executed by Bruce McNaughton and Carol Barnes's groups, which indicated that saturating hippocampal LTP produced learning deficits (12, 13). A more recent collaborative study by the Moser/Morris consortium has confirmed and solidified the original conclusions (14). The studies from both groups used a similar rationale and approach, although there were appreciable and significant differences in the technical execution of the studies and the types of data analysis brought to bear. Regardless, the overall conclusions were the same—saturating LTP at the perforant path inputs to the dentate gyrus leads to a loss of the capacity for hippocampus-dependent memory formation (Figure 2). These data strongly support the hypothesis that synaptic changes of a sort similar or identical to LTP are necessary for memory formation in vivo.

What distinguishes this experiment from the block experiment? At one level, they use the same approach, certainly. However, the appeal of the occlusion variation is that all changes are brought about by synaptic activity occurring endogenously. The only molecules brought into play are those normally and already in existence in the animal. The blocking manipulation utilizes the animal's own axons, neurotransmitters, and synapses. Overall the experiment has a much more physiologic "feel" to it.

Thus, while the mimic experiment is not now and may never be practical for hippocampus-dependent memory formation, its cousin the occlusion experiment has provided some satisfaction. The findings also are complementary to and consistent with the variety of inhibitor and gene-engineering experiments that we have already discussed. The conclusion from these disparate studies is that LTP or a very similar phenomenon is necessary for hippocampus-dependent memory formation. In the next section, we turn our attention to the issue of whether LTP or something similar in fact happens when the animal learns.

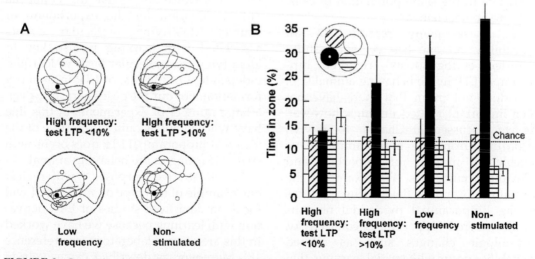

FIGURE 2   Saturating hippocampal LTP occludes Morris water maze learning. Four groups of animals were tested. Two groups were controls that received no LTP-inducing stimulation (nonstimulated and low frequency). Another group received LTP-inducing stimulation, but that did not saturate LTP (high-frequency test LTP > 10%). The final group, which exhibited saturated LTP (test LTP < 10%) had learning deficits. (A) Records of the search pattern of a representative animal from each group during the final spatial probe test (60 seconds). (B) Time spent inside a circle (radius of 35 cm) around the platform position (black bar) and in corresponding, equally large zones in the three other pool quadrants (diagonally striped, horizontally striped, and white bars) during the final spatial probe test (60 seconds). The dotted line indicates the chance level. Error bars indicate SEM. Reproduced from Moser et al. (14).

C. The Measure Experiment

While not as prohibitively difficult as the mimic experiment, the measure experiment is nevertheless a tough nut to crack. In the ideal experiment, we would be able to put stimulating and recording electrodes into the hippocampus, have the animal learn, and then directly measure an increased strength of synaptic connections in situ attendant with the memory formation. This would demonstrate that indeed LTP is occurring with memory formation in the behaving animal.

However, the practical constraints on executing this experiment are legion. What behavioral paradigm do you use? At what time point during learning do you expect LTP to happen? What hippocampal subregion do you record from? Are a significant fraction of the synapses in that region potentiated with a single learning experience? Might LTP formation be counterbalanced by simultaneous LTD elsewhere in the same population of cells, yielding no net change?

For these many reasons, in all probability, no one has yet successfully recorded endogenously triggered hippocampal LTP in the behaving animal (15). This does not mean that there have not been important related findings, however. As we discussed in Chapter 3, in vivo recordings from the hippocampus have revealed a number of important and relevant occurrences. For example, the formation of place field firing patterns among hippocampal pyramidal neurons implies altered hippocampal connectivity. Physiologic changes such as altered excitability occur with spatial learning, that are consistent with the induction and maintenance of LTP-like phenomena. Endogenous learning-related firing patterns are consistent with the occurrence of LTP-triggering high-frequency synaptic activity. Moser et al. also have directly observed synaptic potentiation in the dentate gyrus with learning (16, 17); however, the observable potentiation is fairly short-lived. Thus, the lack of capacity to observe LTP in the hippocampus with spatial learning has not been demonstrated directly, but a circumstantial case can be made that it happens. To the chagrin of us hippocampal types, the occurrence of LTP in amygdala-dependent learning has been nailed down (see Box 2).

If we cannot observe LTP directly using physiologic approaches, are there alternate ways to get at the "measure" question? A similar, molecular approach has been utilized in a variety of instances. The general rationale for these studies is that if one can identify specific molecular events associated with LTP induction and show that those same events occur in the behaving animal with hippocampus-dependent learning, then the inference can be made that LTP has indeed happened in vivo. It is worth noting that this is not the only motivation for the experiment, of course. Identifying molecular events associated with learning is also key to identifying the molecular basis of learning independent of the role of LTP in memory formation. For our purposes here, however, a large number of experiments in this line have worked out as quite supportive of the idea that hippocampal LTP does occur with spatial learning in the behaving animal.

For illustrative purposes I will review one example of this type of approach. I will focus on data from studies of ERK activation with learning because we have worked in this area in my laboratory (see reference 18). Moreover, as described extensively in prior chapters, a number of studies have shown that ERK is necessary for LTP induction. It also is clearly activated with LTP-inducing stimuli, allowing one to treat it as a biochemical marker of LTP induction.

Text continued on pg. 279

BOX 2

LTP MAY EQUAL MEMORY IN THE AMYGDALA

In 1997, two groups broke through a long-standing barrier by directly demonstrating the occurrence of LTP in association with behavioral training in animals (55, 56). Thus, the amygdala became the envy of hippocampologists everywhere. These studies were particularly compelling because in this system there is appreciable understanding of the structure of the relevant circuits and how they map onto the behavior (see Panel A).

The behavioral system under study by both groups was cued fear conditioning, which we discussed as a popular rodent learning paradigm in Chapter 2. In this paradigm, the animal learns to associate an auditory cue (the CS) with an aversive foot shock (the US). The US normally elicits a spectrum of defensive, fear-associated behaviors such as immobile posture (freezing), tachycardia, and increased respiration—these are the unconditioned response (UR). As with all associative learning, after CS-US pairing the CS becomes enabled to elicit the UR, and after fear-conditioning training, the auditory cue elicits the same spectrum of defensive and physiologic responses as the foot shock did previously.

The relevant pathways involve the amygdala. The tone CS is transduced to the lateral nucleus of the amygdala via both thalamic and cortical relays (see Panel A). The shock pathway also triggers activity in the lateral nucleus via a strong input, the pathway that mediates triggering the reflex defensive behaviors. Pairing of the cue with the US somehow allows the CS to co-opt the reflex pathway and trigger the defensive responses on its own.

How does this happen? Pat Shinnick-Gallagher's group and Joe LeDoux's group have both performed experiments indicating that pairing of the strong US signal with the weaker CS input to the lateral nucleus of the amygdala leads to LTP of the CS input (55–57). This LTP results in the augmentation or unmasking of a latent circuit—the CS is now able to trigger the entire spectrum of defensive behaviors because the CS input is now sufficiently strong (Panel A, right half). This strong CS input is able to activate the lateral nucleus cells and trigger the conditioned response.

The key findings by both groups involved directly measuring LTP production in the amygdala in response to behavioral training. The two groups took distinct and complementary approaches to looking for LTP in response to fear conditioning training. McKernan and Shinnick-Gallagher used an ex vivo approach (55). These investigators trained animals and assessed the presence of LTP in amygdala slices prepared acutely, using electrical stimulation of synaptic inputs to the lateral nucleus from the medial geniculate nucleus (see Panel B). LeDoux's colleagues used in vivo recording techniques with implanted electrodes (see Panel C and reference 56). They monitored field responses from the amygdala in response to presentation of the tone cue—directly monitoring population neuronal responses to an environmental signal. Both approaches yielded the same conclusion—synaptic potentiation of CS inputs into the amygdala is occurring with fear-conditioning training.

Continued

BOX 2—cont'd

LTP MAY EQUAL MEMORY
IN THE AMYGDALA

Subsequent work by several groups has indicated that the relevant LTP is probably of a mixed etiology. It appears that both NMDA receptor-dependent and independent LTP is involved. Moreover, a number of sophisticated molecular studies are underway probing the biochemical basis of LTP in the amygdala. Thus far, the forms of LTP involved appear to be indistinguishable from those types we have been discussing in the context of hippocampal synaptic plasticity.

Overall, this work suggests that LTP at the CS-lateral nucleus synapses is sufficient to mediate the alteration in behavior. The papers are landmark publications in the history of the learning and memory field— the first demonstrations of LTP triggered in vivo by environmental signals. It thus is clear that LTP can happen in vivo, with endogenously occurring, natural patterns of neuronal firing, triggered by salient environmental signals.

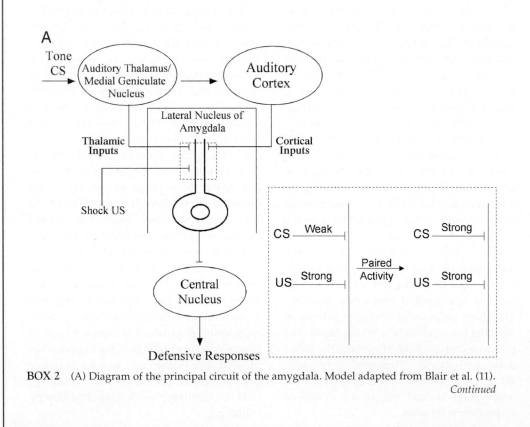

BOX 2   (A) Diagram of the principal circuit of the amygdala. Model adapted from Blair et al. (11).

Continued

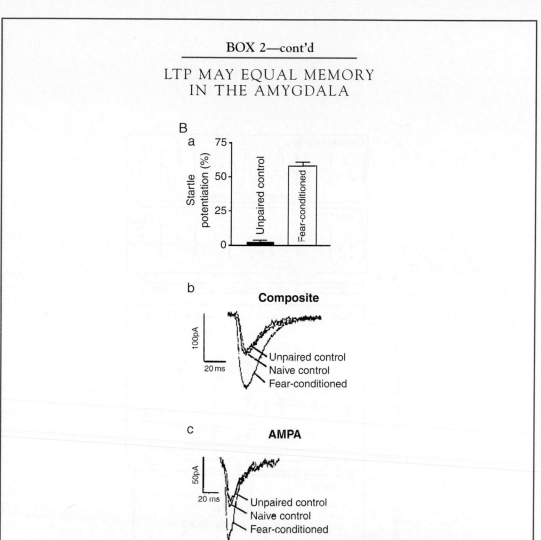

BOX 2—cont'd

LTP MAY EQUAL MEMORY
IN THE AMYGDALA

BOX 2, cont'd   (B) Fear-conditioning results in potentiation of evoked EPSCs in the amygdala. (a) Plot of percent startle potentiation in fear-conditioned and unpaired control animals. (b) Composite EPSCs in amygdala neurons in trained and untrained animals, evoked with constant input stimulations of 9V. (c) AMPA receptor-mediated EPSCs evoked with input stimulations of 9 V. Reproduced from McKernan and Shinnick-Gallagher (55). (C) The effect of paired and unpaired training on CS-evoked field potentials and behavior. Sessions are numbered 1–7; one session occurred per day, except that sessions 3 and 4 occurred on the same day. (a) CS-evoked field potentials from a conditioned rat (top) and a control rat (bottom), covering the full time course of the experiment. Quantitative analysis was performed on the first negative (downward)-going deflection (dot). Previous studies of these waveforms have concentrated on this feature because it has the shortest latency, is reliably present, coincides with local evoked unit activity, shows experience-dependent plasticity, and reflects transmission from the auditory thalamus to the amygdala. The other components of the waveform visible in these examples are not reliably present across trials and subjects, and little is known about their origin and mechanisms.

Continued

Continued

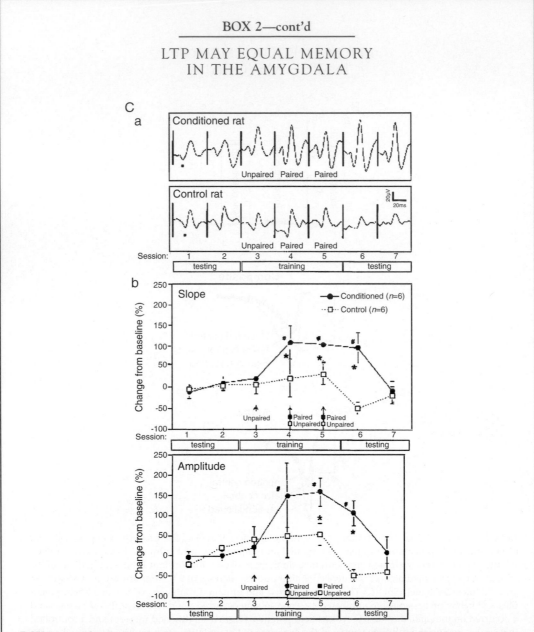

BOX 2—cont'd

LTP MAY EQUAL MEMORY IN THE AMYGDALA

BOX 2, cont'd (b) Fear-conditioning increases the slope and amplitude of CS-EPs, but unpaired training does not. Slope and amplitude of the negative-going potential are normalized as a percentage of the mean values before training (sessions 1 and 2). The normalized slope and amplitude of the evoked potentials were evaluated statistically with two-factor ANOVAs with group (conditioned, control) as the between-subjects factor and experimental session as within subject factor. A significant group–session interaction was observed for both measures ($p < .05$). Significant differences of post hoc analyses are indicated ($p < .05$). Error bars, = s.e.m. Reproduced from Rogan, Staubli and LeDoux (56).

Thus, this led us to ask the question: does ERK activation occur in the hippocampus with hippocampus-dependent learning? If so, it is evidence that LTP has occurred in the hippocampus in association with memory formation. Coleen Atkins addressed this issue in an impressive series of studies that were part of her Ph.D. thesis project in my laboratory. Coleen, working with Joel Selcher, found that contextual fear conditioning results in the activation of ERK in the hippocampus (19). Coleen and Joel trained animals with a contextual fear-conditioning protocol, pairing five foot shocks with a novel context, and then assayed the hippocampus for changes in ERK phosphorylation 1 hour post-training. They observed a significant increase in hippocampal ERK2 activation in trained animals 1 hour after contextual fear conditioning, as measured using a phospho-site-specific antibody (see Figure 3).

Identical sham-training of the animals (by placing them in the fear-conditioning apparatus in the same manner as the trained animals, but without being shocked), resulted in no change in ERK2 activation. To control for potential changes in ERK2 activation due to the shock itself, animals were placed in the fear-conditioning box and immediately shocked. This protocol elicits no learning in response to the context, nor did it result in increased ERK activation. These control experiments indicate that the increase in ERK activation during training is not a nonspecific response to the context, handling, or foot shock alone.

To test whether another associative conditioning paradigm also led to ERK activation, Coleen and Joel paired a tone and shock three times in the unique context and then assayed for hippocampal ERK activation. This protocol resulted in robust associative conditioning to both the cue and context as well as a significant increase in ERK activation at 1 hour post-training, indicating that the ERK MAPK cascade is activated during cued-plus-contextual fear conditioning. Delivery of the tone alone in

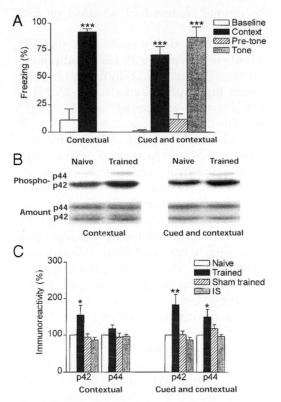

FIGURE 3 Fear-conditioning results in associative learning and ERK MAPK activation. (A) Animals were trained using a contextual fear conditioning protocol, and pre-training baseline freezing behavior (baseline) was compared to freezing when the animals were placed in the context on testing day (context, $n = 6$, $p < .001$, Student's t-test). For the cue and contextual protocol, baseline freezing behavior (baseline; pre-tone) was compared to freezing behavior when placed in the context on testing day (context, $n = 5$, $p < .001$, ANOVA) or when placed in a novel context with tone presentation (tone, $n = 5$, $p < .001$, ANOVA). (B) Representative western blots of MAPK phosphorylation levels and amounts from naïve and trained animals. This phospho-site-specific MAPK antibody detects the covalent modifications (phospho-Thr202 and Tyr204) that cause activation of MAPK. (C) Densitometric analysis for MAPK activation 1 hour after training (contextual, $n = 10$ for p42, $n = 11$ for p44; cued and contextual, $n = 14$ for p42, $n = 13$ for p44), sham training (contextual, $n = 6$ for p42, $n = 5$ for p44; cued and contextual, $n = 9$ for both) and immediate shocking (IS, $n = 8$ for both). Phospho-p44 MAPK levels in trained animals were markedly lower relative to phospho-p42 MAPK levels, indicating a fairly selective activation of p42 MAPK (p42 MAPK = ERK2, p44 MAPK = ERK1. No changes in total MAPK amounts were observed 1 hour after training. $*p < .05$; $**p < .01$; $***p < .001$. Data reproduced from Atkins et al. (19).

the unique context had no effect on ERK activation.

These data demonstrate that the ERK cascade is activated with fear conditioning, just as it is with LTP-inducing stimulation in hippocampal area CA1 (20, 21). Is this learning-associated effect NMDA receptor-dependent as it is in LTP? Administration of the NMDA receptor antagonist MK801 to animals prior to training resulted in an attenuation of learning with both protocols, and also attenuated ERK activation when the hippocampi were assayed 1 hour after training with the contextual fear conditioning protocol or the cued and contextual fear conditioning protocol (19). These data indicate a necessity for NMDA receptor activation for the learning-associated ERK activation and are consistent with the hypothesis that LTP or a similar phenomenon is causing the stimulation of hippocampal ERK.

Having observed activation of ERK in response to behavioral associative conditioning using the fear-conditioning paradigm, it was of interest to determining if a blockade of ERK activation could cause a blockade of learning in this situation. Again, this would be reminiscent of the necessity of ERK activation for LTP to be triggered (21). Fortunately, the MEK inhibitor SL327 can be administered intraperitoneally and will achieve effective concentrations in the CNS. Administration of SL327 either before or immediately after behavioral training led to a blockade of learning, (i.e., the animals exhibited essentially no contextual or cued fear conditioning) (19). These data strongly support the hypothesis that ERK activation is a necessary component of the biochemical cascades utilized to establish behavioral plasticity and are consistent with the general hypothesis that LTP is involved in contextual memory formation.

One limitation to the experiments described above using SL327 is that the drug is administered intraperitoneally and thus inhibits MEK throughout the animal. In a significant refinement, Schafe et al. (22)

and Ohno et al. (23) provided additional strong evidence that MEK activation is required for contextual fear conditioning. These investigators infused MEK inhibitors into the CNS and observed selective blockade of long-term but not short-term fear conditioning. Also, Walz et al. (24, 25), using a similar approach of cortical and limbic infusion of PD98059, observed significant effects of MEK inhibition on step-down inhibitory avoidance, a learning paradigm with similarities to associative fear conditioning. Overall these studies, combined with those by Atkins et al, (19), provide convincing evidence of a necessity for ERK activation in mammalian contextual learning.

Learning in the Morris water maze is also associated with hippocampal ERK activation. In pioneering studies, Pramod Dash's laboratory (26) nicely demonstrated ERK activation in the hippocampus when animals underwent Morris maze training, directly demonstrating that ERK activation occurs in the hippocampus during spatial learning (Figure 4). These same investigators used MEK inhibitor infusion into the hippocampus to demonstrate a necessity for hippocampal ERK activation for spatial memory formation. This necessity for ERK activation later was confirmed by Selcher et al. (27) using SL327 in mice (see Figure 5). The effects of MEK inhibition were selective for the hidden platform test, while no effect was seen in the visible platform; these data indicate that the MEK inhibition did not nonspecifically interfere with the animal's physical ability to execute the task. Thus, similar to fear conditioning, spatial learning in rodents involves ERK activation in the CNS, an effect that is necessary for the formation of lasting memories.

These data directly investigating ERK activation with spatial learning are a specific example of a variation on the "measure" experiment. ERK activation is triggered with LTP in an NMDA receptor-dependent fashion, and the same molecular event occurs with spatial learning in the animal. These observations are consistent with the

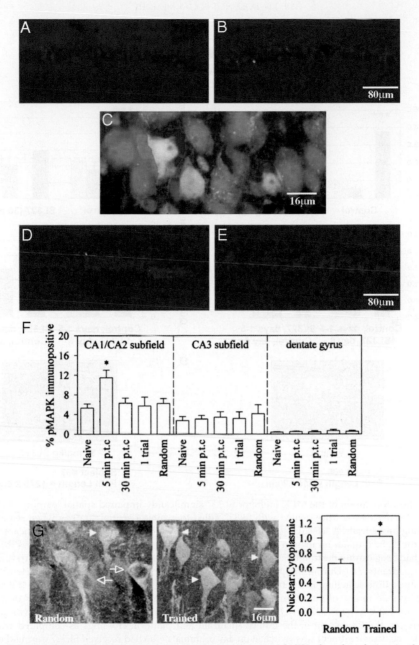

FIGURE 4 Behavioral training in the Morris water maze increases MAPK phosphorylation in the CA1/CA2 subfields of the dorsal hippocampus. Representative photomicrographs for phospho-MAPK immunoreactivity in the CA1/CA2 subfields of dorsal hippocampi (1.0 mm from the dorsal tip) from (A) naïve and (B) 5-minutes post-training animals. Training to criterion increases the number of immunopositive cells for phospho-MAPK as compared with naive controls. (C) Laser confocal image, indicating that the phospho-MAPK-positive cells (red) are also immunoreactive for a neuron-specific nuclear antigen (green). Areas with overlapping immunofluorescences appear yellow. Representative photomicrographs for MAPK immunoreactivity from (D) a naïve and (E) a 5-minutes post-training animal. (F) Summary showing percentage of neurons staining positive for phosphorylated MAPK in the dorsal hippocampus from the control and experimental groups. The data are represented as the mean ± SEM (n = 5 for each group). (G) Representative laser confocal images from a randomized platform and an animal trained to criterion and killed 5 minutes later, showing increased numbers of CA1/CA2 pyramidal neurons with nuclear staining for phospho-MAPK as a result of training. The open and closed arrows indicate neurons with weak or strong phospho-MAPK nuclear immunoreactivity, respectively. The bar graph shows the nuclear to cytoplasmic ratio for phospho-MAPK immunofluoroscence. *$p < .05$; p.t.c., posttraining to criterion. Data and figure reproduced from Blum, Moore, Adams, and Dash (26).

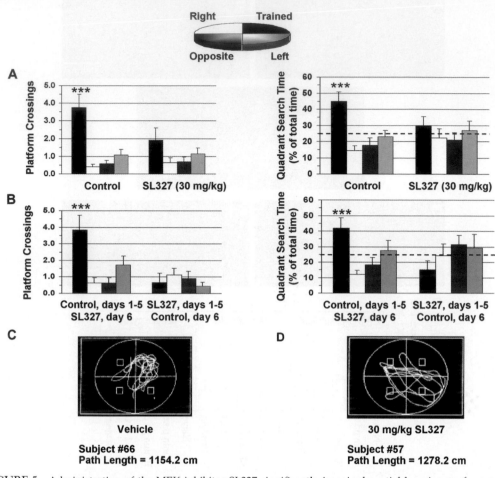

FIGURE 5 Administration of the MEK inhibitor SL327 significantly impaired spatial learning performance in the Morris water maze task. Mice treated with SL327 failed to exhibit a spatial strategy when searching for the platform during probe trials. A selective search strategy is one in which the subjects spend significantly more time searching in the trained quadrant than in the other three quadrants. The subjects must also cross the area where the platform had been during the training sessions significantly more often than they cross the corresponding areas in the other quadrants. (A) During the probe trials on days 4 and 5, mice treated with vehicle ($n = 13$) spent significantly more time searching in the trained quadrant and crossed the platform area in the trained quadrant more frequently than in any of the alternate quadrants. However, mice injected with an inhibitor of ERK MAP kinase activation (30 mg/kg SL327, $n = 11$) did not exhibit a selective search strategy. There was no significant difference between the time spent in the trained quadrant and platform crossings as compared with the other quadrants. (B) The drug treatment was switched on day 6; animals who had received SL327 during the first 5 days now received vehicle and vice versa. The vehicle-trained mice ($n = 11$) still exhibited a selective search strategy after injection with SL327 on day 6. SL327-trained mice ($n = 9$) who were administered vehicle on day 6, did not display a selective search strategy. (***) Significantly larger ($p < .01$) than all three of the other quadrants. Panels C and D. (C) Representative probe trial of a vehicle-treated mouse. The swim path trace shown here provides an excellent example of a selective search. This particular subject was trained with the platform located in the northeast quadrant. During the probe trial, this mouse spent 56% of the time in the correct quadrant and crossed the exact area where the platform had been nine times. (D) Representative probe trial of an SL327-treated mouse. This trace does not represent a selective search. This mouse was trained with the platform in the northwest quadrant, but during the probe trial, the subject crossed this platform area only once and spent 32% of the time in this quadrant (vs. 34% in the opposite quadrant). Adapted from Selcher et al. (27).

TABLE 2   Molecular Markers for LTP

Biochemical Marker	Occurs With What Type of LTP	Occurs With What Type of Behavior	Necessary for LTP?	Necessary for Behavior?
ERK activation	multiple	Contextual conditioning (131)	Yes	Yes
		Water maze		Yes
CaMKII autophosphorylation	SC/CA1	Contextual conditioning (131)	Yes	Yes
PKC activation	multiple	Contextual conditioning (131)	Yes	Yes
CRE activation	multiple	Contextual conditioning (132)	Yes	Yes
		Passive avoidance		?
Arc expression	multiple	Water maze (133–135)	Yes	Yes
		Novel environment learning		?
BDNF expression	Multiple	Contextual conditioning (136)	Yes	?
Increased glu release	PP/dentate	Operant conditioning (137–139)	?	?
Increased glu uptake	SC/CA1	Contextual conditioning (140)	?	?

hypothesis that LTP occurs in vivo with memory formation. There also have been quite a number of other experiments of exactly the same sort, demonstrating that LTP-associated molecular events occur in the hippocampus and other parts of the CNS with learning (see Table 2). I focused on ERK activation as a specific example of this general category of experiment because it is the system with which I am most familiar.

Thus, while it has not been possible so far to directly demonstrate LTP physiologically in association with spatial learning, biochemical "markers" for LTP induction such as ERK activation, CaMKII activation, PKC activation, glutamate release, and altered gene expression (see Table 2) *have* been demonstrated to occur with spatial learning. That such a broad spectrum of molecular changes occurs with both LTP in vitro and spatial learning in vivo strongly suggests that LTP is indeed occurring in the hippocampus with hippocampus-dependent memory formation.

Molecular Events in LTP Versus Memory Formation—Some Dissociation in Time Courses

One additional comment is worth making in the context of biochemical markers for LTP. The data are consistent with the hypothesis that LTP is occurring in vivo, as various investigations have found that biochemical mechanisms occurring in LTP are valid predictors of biochemical changes associated with and necessary for associative learning. In a number of studies, however, different time courses for LTP-associated molecular changes versus learning-associated changes have been observed. For example, in our studies of protein kinase activation with LTP and contextual fear conditioning, we found different time courses for MAPK, PKC, and α-CaMKII activation during LTP versus fear conditioning (Figure 6). MAPK is activated within 2 minutes of LTP induction and returns to baseline levels of activation within 1 hour. PKC undergoes a similar time course of activation as α-CaMKII, both

Kinase	Contextual Conditioning			Cue and Contextual Conditioning		
	1 min	1 h	2 h	1 min	1 h	2 h
p42 MAPK	-9 ± 12 (8)	54 ± 27 (10)	-3 ± 9 (7)	-16 ± 5 (7)	83 ± 28 (14)	19 ± 8 (10)
p44 MAPK	-3 ± 5 (8)	18 ± 10 (11)	-5 ± 5 (8)	-3 ± 6 (7)	50 ± 21 (13)	13 ± 11 (10)
PKC	-7 ± 5 (8)	*25 ± 15 (11)	-5 ± 11 (7)	11 ± 23 (7)	25 ± 11 (12)	10 ± 11 (10)
α-CaMKII	-2 ± 7 (8)	7 ± 11 (11)	8 ± 10 (7)	-3 ± 16 (7)	13 ± 23 (14)	47 ± 20 (10)

FIGURE 6   Percent change in phosphorylation from control for each protein kinase. Number of animals used are in parentheses. All protein phosphorylation measurements were normalized to corresponding protein kinase amounts. Shaded boxes are statistically significant. The asterisk (*) denotes a nonsignificant ($p = .1$) increase in autophosphorylated PKC 1 hour after contextual conditioning. Table reproduced from Atkins et al. (19).

becoming activated 2–5 minutes after LTP is induced and lasting for at least 1 hour. In our behavior studies, we observed that MAPK, PKC, and α-CaMKII are activated in the hippocampus at later time points than what has been observed during hippocampal LTP. Specifically, all three kinases were activated in vivo at a time point about 1 hour later than would have been expected if LTP had occurred immediately upon training. Similar differences in the time course of activation of protein kinases in the amygdala with cued fear conditioning have also been observed (28).

This raises the interesting possibility that LTP in vivo in the relevant brain areas is happening after training but after some period of time delay. This raises three issues. One, it implies that some memory trace must be present that holds the relevant information in the CNS before it triggers LTP in the hippocampus. Second, it suggests that LTP might be involved in memory consolidation versus learning per se, an idea that we will return to in the next section. Regardless, it raises the third issue of when it is that LTP actually happens in vivo after a learning event—maybe it's later than most people think.

The important caveat to this is that at present we do not know how a 100-Hz, 1-second tetanic stimulation of hippocampal slices relates to an associative pairing of

stimuli in a behaving animal. Thus, the temporal sequence of the biochemical events underlying learning and LTP may be the same, yet shifted to alternative kinetics during associative learning. The final alternative is that the protein kinase activation that occurs with associative training may be a result of mechanisms distinct from those recruited in LTP.

Regardless, the most parsimonious interpretation of these data with ERK, CaMKII, CREB, and the like is that they support the hypothesis that LTP is actually occurring in the CNS. In addition, they raise the important point that LTP accurately *models* memory. Studies of LTP led to the identification of CaMKII, CREB, ERK, and a vast array of other molecules as potential players in mammalian learning and memory. LTP-derived insights led to the formulation of the hypotheses that these molecules might be involved in memory in the behaving animal. I am confident that there will be many more examples of this truism as time progresses. The fact that LTP does not equal memory does not diminish the importance of studying LTP to help us understand memory. The fact that LTP is likely directly involved in memory formation is very important. But regardless, LTP retains its utility as a tool to gain molecular insights into the likely processes involved in memory formation as well.

A Role for LTP in Hippocampal Information
Processing, Short-Term Information Storage
in the Hippocampus, and Consolidation
of Long-Term Memory

If LTP does not equal memory, then what does it equal? We will address this question next. In brief, current thinking among workers in the area is that LTP is obligatorily involved in hippocampus-dependent memory formation, of course. However, LTP does not *equate* to memory, but it is one of those processes *contributing* in an essential way to memory formation. It is a component mechanism utilized by the hippocampus to allow it to perform its multitudinous functions. It is a physiologic and molecular tool that allows the hippocampus to do what it needs to do. Specifically, recent work on this issue suggests a role for LTP or related processes in several of the important roles of the hippocampus that we have already discussed: in information processing, as a temporary memory store, and in long-term memory consolidation. Laboratories that have contributed monumentally to formulating current thinking in this area include those of Tim Bliss, Richard Morris, Eric Kandel, and Susumu Tonegawa.

In the next section, I will review several key studies that support a role for LTP in these three hippocampus-dependent processes. Please note this important caveat: I am going to treat hippocampal NMDA receptor-dependence as being equivalent to hippocampal LTP-dependence for illustrative purposes. This is a bit of a stretch, but not too much of one in my opinion. For example, despite decades of investigation, no one has observed that NMDA receptors function in baseline synaptic transmission in the hippocampus. The only known physiologic role of the NMDA receptor in the hippocampus is triggering LTP. Thus, manipulations that selectively block the NMDA receptor appear to be selective for blocking LTP induction but not background neuronal activity in the hippocampus (but see also reference 2). Loss of NMDA

receptor function by various manipulations in general does not appear to cause derangement of overall activity in the hippocampal circuit, but rather it causes a selective loss of the capacity to trigger changes in synaptic strength.

An additional consideration is that equating NMDA receptor function with the triggering of synaptic change is about as close as we can get right now in terms of practicable experiments. Equating NMDA receptor activation with LTP or similar phenomena is not flawless by any means, but it is a tool that we have at our disposal that allows testing of specific predictions of a role for LTP in memory formation and information processing in the hippocampus. Loss of NMDA receptor function may cause additional effects besides loss of LTP. Loss of LTD and derangement of the postsynaptic molecular infrastructure are two prominent exceptions to keep in mind. However, loss of a particular hippocampal function upon loss of NMDA receptor function is at least consistent with the hypothesis of a role for NMDA receptor-dependent LTP in that phenomenon.

The other thing to keep in mind is that while I will focus on NMDA receptor-related studies, these are by no means are the only relevant data. Many other manipulations that block LTP also affect memory formation, consolidation, and hippocampal information processing (see reference 29 for example). The NMDA receptor manipulation is simply the one I will use for our present purposes to give an example of the types of experiments that have formed current thinking in this area.

II. ROLES FOR LTP

A. Hippocampal Information Processing

This specific role harkens back to the extensive discussion we had in Chapters 4–6 concerning the capacity of LTP to serve as a memory trace that is triggered when certain associative events have occurred. For example, we talked about how back-propagating action potentials coupled with neuromodulatory neurotransmitter receptor activation plus synaptic glutamate could give three-way coincidence detection.

This type of molecular information processing, resulting in a persisting change (LTP) can function to allow temporary storage of information integrated from a wide variety of sensory inputs. A principal example of this may be in learning complex visuo-spatial tasks such as the Morris water maze. These types of mechanisms can also allow the monitoring of the emotional valence of an experience, or assessment of the attentive state of the animal. In broad terms, these mechanisms likely contribute to the role of the hippocampus in making multimodal associations and storing these associations for some period of time.

For illustrative purposes I'll describe a few experiments supporting this idea of a role for NMDA receptor-dependent LTP in these types of information processing.

One relevant paradigm is the formation of pyramidal neuron place fields. It is clear that LTP is not necessary for hippocampal place field formation (30–33). However, molecular disruptions that block LTP formation do have consistent effects on place fields. Specifically, loss of LTP is associated with a decreased stability of place fields (33). There also are effects on the spatial specificity of place fields and the coordinated firing of pyramidal neurons that have the same place fields (30). Overall, these data provide one explanation for the loss of hippocampus-dependent spatial learning in animals deficient in LTP. The effects on place fields specifically are consistent with the idea that NMDA receptor-dependent LTP is necessary in forming an accurate and lasting representation of complex visuo-spatial environments.

NMDA receptor-dependent LTP in area CA1 of the hippocampus also appears to be necessary for multimodal associative learning (34). Mice can learn to form complex associations among three different odor cues in order to make predictions about food rewards. In one type of task, mice must learn that odor A + B is different from odor B + C is different from odor C + A. Mice deficient in NMDA receptor-dependent LTP in area CA1 are deficient in making the types of complex multiple associations necessary to efficiently execute this task (34). Thus, LTP appears to be necessary for the formation of relational memories involving complex associative information processing.

A final and fascinating recent example illustrates that NMDAR-dependent processes are necessary for reconstituting spatial locations using partial visual cues (35). In these experiments, NMDA receptors were selectively eliminated in hippocampal area CA3 using genetic engineering approaches. Mice deficient in NMDA receptor-dependent LTP in area CA3 can learn the Morris water maze normally but exhibit a deficiency in being able to recall the hidden platform location when they are primed for recollection using a partial set of visual cues. In other words, animals are selectively deficient in recalling a spatial location when some of the training-associated visual stimuli are removed. These deficits are associated with a similar derangement of place cell activity in a partial-cue environment. These findings indicate that hippocampal LTP is involved in the animal forming a complete and unified representation of a complex set of visual stimuli.

Two important experiments using infusion of the NMDA receptor antagonist APV into the CNS also bear directly on this idea—in fact, these two papers from Richard Morris's lab are seminal findings that both shaped our general thinking in the area and served as a foundation for much of the later work in this area. In a pioneering study, Richard and his colleagues found that intraventricular infusions of APV, at concentrations that block LTP induction, block spatial learning

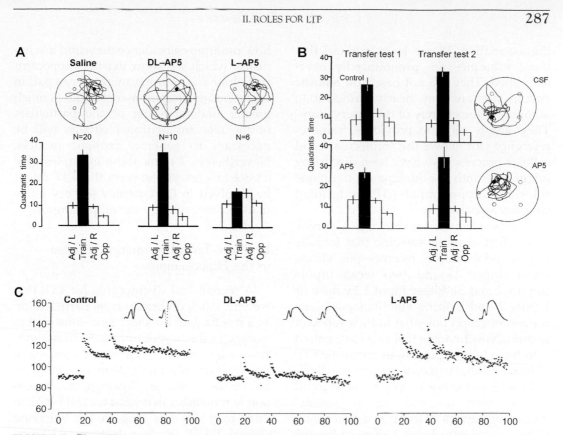

FIGURE 7 The NMDA receptor antagonist D AP5 (i.e., APV) blocks learning in the Morris water maze. These data are from the landmark paper by Richard Morris and his colleagues (111), demonstrating that infusion into the CNS of DL-AP5 (an active mixture) but not the control, inactive enantiomer L-AP5 blocks learning in the water maze task. (A) This panel illustrates that pre-training infusion of DL-AP5 blocks learning of a spatially selective search strategy for locating the hidden platform. (B) This panel illustrates that post-training blockade of NMDA receptors does not affect memory recall. (C) This panel illustrates that the same infusion protocol leads to effective blockade of NMDA receptor-dependent LTP in the dentate gyrus. See text for additional discussion.

in the water maze (see reference 36 and Figure 7). A few years later Richard shocked us by revealing that this effect was not the result of a loss of the capacity of the animal to learn the spatial relationship of the hidden platform to the visual cues (37). Rather, NMDA receptor blockade appears to block the capacity of the animal to learn the task, that is to learn that there is a consistent relationship between the spatial cues and the hidden platform, and that they can use spatial cues to predict where the platform will be located. The NMDA receptor (and by inference LTP) is not necessary for spatial learning per se—it is necessary for learning more complex relationships

about spatial information. These pioneering data are in nice agreement with the more recent work indicating that NMDA receptor-dependent processes are necessary for an animal to reconstitute a special representation from partial visual stimuli (35).

How might NMDA receptor-dependent LTP contribute to multimodal information processing in the hippocampus? This is certainly not clear at present. However, one can imagine a couple of ways in which the cellular and molecular properties of LTP induction might contribute to the processing of complex associations and the establishment of a lasting representation of the association. Please keep in mind that these examples are pronouncedly over-simplified. They are not based on realistic circuits nor are they nearly sufficient to account for the entirety of the observations. They simply serve to provide a frame of reference for how the molecular and cellular processes we have been discussing might enter into our thinking about unique roles for hippocampal LTP in forming complex associations.

Two possibilities are shown in Figure 8. In the first example imagine that initially a pyramidal neuron receives one strong input (Input 1) and two weak inputs (Inputs 2 and 3). Either Input 1 by itself or Inputs 2 and 3 firing simultaneously can trigger an action potential in their follower neuron. Now imagine that you have paired activity in Input 1 plus Input 2, causing LTP at Input 2. Similarly, you get paired activity of Input 1 and Input 3 and get LTP at Input 3. Now Inputs 1, 2, and 3 are all "strong" inputs and capable of firing an action potential. Consequently, Input 2 alone or Input 3 alone can reconstitute the response that previously required both Inputs 2 and 3.

A second example is conceptually similar. Imagine that a pyramidal neuron receives a strong input (Input 1), a modulatory input such as ACh (Input 2) and a weak input (Input 3). Input 1 triggers a back-propagating action potential, which ACh modulation of dendritic K channels allows to propagate into the distal dendrites. This back-propagating action potential is paired with Input 3, causing LTP at this site. Input 3 is now sufficient to cause an action potential on its own and give a readout equivalent to Input 1. Thus, Input 3, by virtue of its association with a salience signal (ACh in this example), is now uniquely able to trigger the same response as Input 1.

As I emphasized earlier, these examples are not realistic models to try to account for the complex behavioral changes described in the earlier parts of this section. They are merely simple examples to give an idea of how multiple coincidence detection mechanisms, which we know exist in hippocampal pyramidal neurons, might play a part in representing complex associations. A much greater understanding of the particulars of the relevant neuronal circuits will be necessary to generate realistic models. Nevertheless, I think these examples give a taste of a few of the ways that LTP might be involved in the complex sensory information processing by the hippocampus.

B. Short-Term Information Storage in the Hippocampus

A second and distinct role for LTP that we will touch on briefly is its participation as a mechanism for short-term information storage in the hippocampus. At first blush, this may seem oxymoronic—*long-term* potentiation as a mechanism for *short-term* information storage. However, it's important to remember that what we call E-LTP in vitro may not last long in the behaving animal. E-LTP or other decremental forms of LTP may only last 15 minutes in vivo owing to the increased rates of reaction of the underlying biochemistry at 37°C. Moreover, there is no reason to think that LTP might not be established and then specifically erased after its role was finished. These two considerations bring to mind the findings by Moser et al. (16, 17), where they observed learning-associated synaptic potentiation in vivo that lasted for about 15 minutes or so.

One experimental observation that specifically prompts our concluding that LTP is involved in short-term information storage in the hippocampus is the finding that NMDA receptor activation is necessary for trace fear conditioning. Huerta et al. (38) used their sophisticated engineered mouse lacking NMDA receptors in area CA1 in order to probe the role of the hippocampus and NMDA receptor-dependent processes in time-dependent learning. The specific paradigm that they used was trace fear conditioning. They found that the

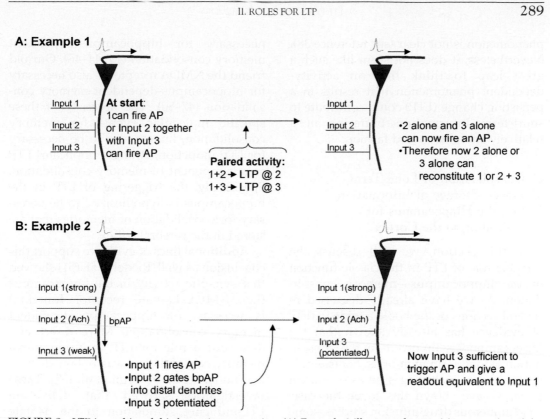

A: Example 1

Input 1
Input 2
Input 3

At start:
1can fire AP
or Input 2 together
with Input 3
can fire AP

Paired activity:
1+2 → LTP @ 2
1+3 → LTP @ 3

Input 1
Input 2
Input 3

•2 alone and 3 alone
can now fire an AP.
•Therefore now 2 alone or
3 alone can
reconstitute 1 or 2 + 3

B: Example 2

Input 1(strong)
Input 2 (Ach)   bpAP
Input 3 (weak)

•Input 1 fires AP
•Input 2 gates bpAP
into distal dendrites
•Input 3 potentiated

Input 1(strong)
Input 2 (Ach)
Input 3
(potentiated)

Now Input 3 sufficient to
trigger AP and give a
readout equivalent to Input 1

FIGURE 8 LTP in multimodal information processing. (A) Example 1 illustrates how pairing synaptic activity of strong plus weak activity can allow a single input to achieve the same effect that formerly required its activity plus another input. Associative activity allows a single input to represent subsequently either an entirely different input from its original meaning or a partial re-presentation of an original stimulus to reconstitute the entire original effect. (B) Example 2 illustrates how an excitatory input (Input 1) coupled with a modulatory input (ACh in this example) allows a different input (Input 3) to trigger a new response. The new response to Input 3 is now functionally equivalent to the original response to Input 1. See text for additional discussion.

introduction of even a brief 30-second delay between CS and US presentation rendered the learning dependent upon hippocampal NMDA receptors. These data strongly suggest that one role for LTP in area CA1 is the temporary storage of information so that events can be associated over time.

In an earlier work, Richard Morris made a conceptually similar observation indicating a role for NMDA receptor-dependent processes in short-term information storage. Richard trained animals in delayed match-to-place task and found that the extent of NMDA receptor dependency varied based on the length of the delay period between stimulus and match (37).

Again, these data indicate a role for LTP or similar processes in temporary information storage.

The general idea coming out of studies of this sort is that LTP or a similar process in the hippocampus is involved in the storage of *episodes* of experience for brief periods of time (see references 38–41). This allows that the episode can be processed into the appropriate temporal context (i.e., what came before, what came after) so that associations can be made between one event or sequence of events and another. As with the other roles for LTP that we have been discussing, the precise function that LTP might play in contributing to this phenomenon is not clear (see reference 38). Nevertheless, it does not seem like such a great leap to think that an activity-dependent phenomenon that results in a persisting change (LTP) could contribute to short-term information buffering in a relatively straightforward fashion.

C. Consolidation of Long-Term Memory—Storage of Information Within the Hippocampus for Downloading to the Cortex

In this section, we will discuss the possible role of LTP in the classic function of the hippocampus—memory consolidation. As we have already discussed in several sections of the book, a wide variety of evidence has already shown that the hippocampus is involved in the consolidation of long-term memories. For example lesion studies including studies of human patients have shown this to be the case. Also numerous drug infusion studies, some of which will be described later, have shown a role for the hippocampus in memory consolidation. A key point with the drug infusion studies is that drugs can be infused into the hippocampus *post-training* and interfere with long-term memory formation. Appreciation of the significance of this was what led to the distinction of hippocampal memory consolidation as a distinct process from the initial events triggering memory formation.

A number of different experiments have shown that hippocampal protein synthesis and mRNA synthesis is necessary for the consolidation of long-term memories (42, 43). In fact, these same studies make it clear that multiple stages of protein-synthesis-dependent cellular processes are required for memory consolidation, as injection of protein synthesis inhibitors at different time points after training can lead to disruption of memory consolidation.

Moreover, specific molecular processes such as ERK activation, CREB activation, Arc induction, and C/EBP induction are

necessary for hippocampus-dependent memory consolidation (19, 44–46). Our old friend the NMDA receptor is also necessary for hippocampus-dependent memory consolidation (47–50). The necessity of these specific molecular events for memory consolidation, known also to be necessary for LTP induction, strongly implicates LTP as a component of memory consolidation. Specifically, the triggering of LTP in the hippocampus is hypothesized to be necessary for consolidation of memories that are stored in the cerebral cortex.

Additional lines of evidence support this conclusion as well. Riedel et al. (51) showed that synaptic activity in the hippocampus (i.e., AMPA/kainate receptor function) is necessary for hippocampus-dependent memory consolidation. More direct evidence for a role for LTP in hippocampal memory consolidation was obtained in an additional study by Brun et al. (52). These investigators showed that delivering LTP-inducing stimulation to the dentate gyrus, *after* training, led to disruption of memory consolidation. This effect was blocked by NMDA receptor blockade, demonstrating that the triggering of LTP or a related phenomenon, as opposed to network firing, is what is disrupting the consolidation.

Thus, taken together there is a substantial body of direct and indirect findings that indicate that LTP is participating in the consolidation of hippocampus-dependent memory formation. The relevant LTP is occurring in the hippocampus, and it is triggering changes downstream in cortical targets of the hippocampus that store the memory. We will return to a broad-brush-stroke model of how this might happen a little later.

It is important to note that the relevant LTP is probably not triggered immediately, and may even be triggered multiple times as part of the consolidation of a single memory. NMDA receptor antagonist studies make it clear that an NMDA receptor–independent mechanisms exists

BOX 3

CEREBELLAR LONG-TERM DEPRESSION

Workers in the cerebellum might state that LTP does not equal memory because LTD equals memory. Specifically, LTD of synaptic connections in the cerebellar cortex has been demonstrated to play a role in two important forms of learned behavior: adaptation of the vestibulo-ocular reflex (VOR) and eye-blink conditioning (reviewed in references 10 and 58).

As we discussed in Chapter 2, classical conditioning of the eye-blink response in rabbits uses delivery of a neutral stimulus such as a tone paired with a mild aversive stimulus such as an airpuff delivered to the surface of the eye (Panel A). With repeated

pairings, animals learn that the tone predicts the air-puff, and they will learn to "blink" when the tone is delivered by itself; a learned protective response involving co-opting a reflex pathway. Eye-blink conditioning sounds simple but is actually fairly complex. For example, the "blink" is really more than a blink; it is an elaborate programmed motor response involving a number of muscle groups that cause eyeball retraction and closure of the eyelid. The animals also can learn precisely the temporal relationship between tone and air-puff. They automatically adjust their "blink" to slightly precede when the air-puff would be

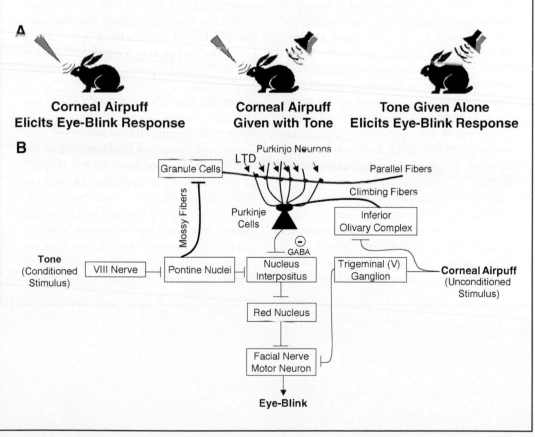

A

Corneal Airpuff Elicits Eye-Blink Response

Corneal Airpuff Given with Tone

Tone Given Alone Elicits Eye-Blink Response

B

Continued

BOX 3—cont'd

CEREBELLAR LONG-TERM DEPRESSION

delivered. Trace eye-blink conditioning (CS followed by an intervening time delay) is hippocampus-dependent, while delay conditioning (no intervening time delay) is hippocampus-independent, so additional circuits outside the cerebellum clearly can come into play.

Adaptation of the VOR is even more complicated (59). Shake your head back and forth while you are looking at this *word*. You are amazingly good at keeping your eyes pointed at exactly the right spot as your head goes back and forth. This seems simple, but remember that you are precisely moving both your left and right eyes to exactly counterbalance your head movements. (To get a feel for what it would be like to live without a VOR, hold your finger out at arm's length and stare at your fingertip. Now rotate your entire upper body back and forth—(there is quite a difference!). The VOR detects signals from your vestibular system semicircular canals (that read-out head movement) and allows triggering of the appropriate eye muscle contractions to hold the eye position constant in space. To complicate matters further, this reflex is of necessity subject to adaptation. If your eye movements are not holding the visual field constant for some reason (e.g., damage to your oculomotor system or to the eye muscles themselves, or even a new pair of eyeglasses that change your focal point), the system adapts to the change and modifies the VOR to appropriate for your new state. This depends on complicated signals from the visual cortex that provide information concerning constancy of the visual percept—obviously not a trivial matter.

Clearly synaptic plasticity at a single type of synapse cannot account for all of the elaborate behavioral changes underlying eye-blink conditioning and adaptation of the VOR. However, a wide variety of evidence from pharmacologic, genetic, lesioning, and physiologic recording studies has indicated an important role in these processes for LTD at parallel fiber-to-Purkinje cell synapses in the cerebellar cortex. This LTD in the cerebellar cortex has been extensively studied, and shortly I will highlight a few of its properties and present a simplified version of how it might participate in eye-blink conditioning.

Parallel fiber LTD in the cerebellum is a persistent, input-specific decrease in the efficacy of synaptic transmission between the parallel fibers and Purkinje cells in the cerebellar cortex (see Panel B). It is induced by low-frequency co-activation of climbing fibers and parallel fiber inputs to Purkinje neurons. *Climbing fibers* are highly potent inputs onto Purkinje neurons—a single climbing fiber matches to only one Purkinje neuron, and its activation is sufficient to trigger an action potential in its specific

BOX 3—cont'd

CEREBELLAR LONG-TERM DEPRESSION

follower Purkinje neuron. Climbing fibers originate in brain stem nuclei and are involved in processing sensory signals, such as sending a signal to the cerebellar cortex that an eye-blink has been triggered by a puff of air on the cornea. *Parallel fibers* originate from cerebellar granule cells, which are a major cell type in the cerebellum. Parallel fibers carry information such as auditory signals—(e.g., information that an auditory cue has been received). Thus, via this part of the circuit a coincidence of auditory cue (parallel fibers) and air-puff (climbing fibers) can lead to a depression of parallel fiber inputs onto the Purkinje neurons. This is activity-dependent synaptic plasticity, manifest as a synaptic weakening.

How does this synaptic depression translate into a behavioral change? The Purkinje neurons are the only output neurons from the cerebellar cortex—they provide the net output of the cerebellum and are involved in modulating a wide variety of motor movements including those involved in eye movement and the eye blink. Purkinje neurons use GABA as their neurotransmitter; thus, they are inhibitory. LTD at their parallel fiber inputs leads to a net loss of inhibitory output onto motor pattern generators downstream. In the case of eye-blink conditioning, this loss of inhibition causes a net enhancement of a pre-existing connection between tone-activated neurons and follower neurons

that when unmasked can trigger an eye-blink (see VIIIth nerve inputs in Panel B). This connection is normally inhibited in a feed-forward fashion by the Purkinje cell output from the cerebellar cortex and, thus, is inactive. Loss of the Purkinje cell inhibitory input allows unmasking of the connection between the tone-activated cells and the blink pattern generator cells. Thus, the tone is then able to trigger the eye-blink response on its own. The conditioned stimulus (tone) now triggers the conditioned response (eye-blink), in classical conditioning parlance.

It is important to keep in mind that this is a great oversimplification of the cellular basis of eye-blink conditioning. Nevertheless, it allows us to make several important points. First, this is a specific example of the generalization that associative learning involves the unmasking of latent circuits, ones already in existence in the CNS but that become effective in triggering behavior as a result of the plasticity of their synaptic inputs (see Box 2 and Figure 8 as well). Second, it illustrates that learning does not have to be dependent upon strengthening synapses—depressing synapses is an equally effective mechanism for memory formation. A positive or negative behavioral change can be mediated by either a positive or negative change in synaptic strength, it all simply depends on the circuit in which the neuron is imbedded.

for storing information for a few minutes to an hour or so post-training (33, 47, 48). Short-term contextual fear conditioning for example, is intact in the face of NMDA receptor blockade. Some memory trace that is *not* NMDA receptor-dependent LTP is keeping it there. So information is being stored somehow, and it is perfectly reasonable to hypothesize that this information is converted to an LTP trace after some period(s) of delay. This specific idea would be consistent with the delayed manifestation of molecular markers for LTP induction, such as ERK activation, that we discussed previously.

To reiterate, many studies make it clear that all relevant LTP-like phenomena are not immediately triggered by environmental stimulation during the learning phase. Many post-training infusion experiments demonstrate that signal transduction mechanisms, such as ERK activation and NMDA receptor activation, necessary for LTP induction, can be unperturbed at the time of training but still be necessary for long-term memory formation. Thus, there is some delay before the LTP-associated events are necessary for memory formation. These events are not triggered immediately by the environmental stimuli— post-training infusion effects make it clear that the environmental signals set up a memory trace that subsequently triggers LTP or a similar phenomenon.

On the other hand, this does not mean that the acute signals do not trigger LTP as well. The short-term storage/information processing mechanism that we described in Sections II.A and II.B are hypothesized to utilize E-LTP as we discussed. It's just important to keep in mind the distinction that LTP may be contributing to one type of process during learning or at early stages while it contributes to memory consolidation at later stages. Post-training inhibitor effects simply mean that another round of plasticity similar or identical to LTP must also be triggered for long-term memory to be formed.

A Model for LTP in Consolidation of Long-Term Memory

The upshot of the hypothesized role of LTP in memory consolidation is that *hippocampal* LTP is not a long-term memory storage mechanism—it is a memory buffer. The long-term storage of hippocampus-dependent memories occurs downsteam of the hippocampus in various regions of the cortex. In these final few paragraphs, I will present a thumbnail sketch of how LTP might participate in cortical memory consolidation. Once again, I emphasize that this is not a sophisticated or realistic model—it is an illustrative example of how LTP in the hippocampus could lead to long-term changes downstream in the cortex.

The basics of the model are based on what we have seen thus far: that LTP serves to maintain information in the hippocampus, represented as a pattern of synaptic weights, during the process of memory consolidation. The output of the potentiated circuit, manifest as a result of these altered synaptic strengths, triggers long-lasting changes in the cortex and the formation of long-term memory. The "model" will simply be an elaboration of this basic idea, but with a few more specifics added.[4]

---

[4]The model draws inspiration from a recent lively series of exchanges between Joe Tsien and Richard Morris. Joe Tsien has promulgated the idea of ongoing synaptic reinforcement in the hippocampus, LTP-dependent, as a contributing factor for memory consolidation (50). His idea is that ongoing NMDA receptor-dependent synaptic plasticity, over a fairly long period of time (days to weeks), is necessary for long-term memory consolidation. However, this hypothesis has met with some skepticism and rebuttal (49). As such, it remains for now in the "interesting but controversial" category. Nevertheless, synaptic activity in the hippocampus clearly is necessary for memory consolidation, based on the finding that AMPA/kainite receptor blockers infused into the hippocampus can block memory consolidation. This is consistent with the idea that activity through the altered synaptic weights (resulting from LTP) is necessary for memory consolidation at downstream target sites (51, 52). My model is more in line with the Richard Morris model than the Joe Tsien model because it does not involve any ongoing production of LTP in the hippocampus as part of the memory consolidation process.

BOX 4

THE MOLECULES OF LTD

Recent studies have given a number of important insights into the molecular mechanisms underlying cerebellar LTD. Cerebellar LTD induction requires mGluR and AMPAR activation, and postsynaptic Ca^{2+} influx through voltage-gated Ca^{2+} channels (reviewed in reference 10). The mGluR activation produces DAG, which subsequently along with calcium activates PKC. This PKC activation is necessary for the induction of cerebellar LTD (60), as has been shown in a variety of inhibitor studies, and PKC activators mimic LTD (i.e., they cause synaptic depression).

In an interesting mirror image of hippocampal LTP, AMPAR *internalization* appears to underly cerebellar LTD. Interference with clathrin endocytosis blocks the induction of cerebellar LTD, and induction of AMPAR internalization produces an LTD that occludes stimulus-induced LTD (61, 62). PKC phosphorylates the GluR2/3 AMPA receptor at serine 880 (serine 885 in GluR3), and this phosphorylation decreases the binding of the GluR to glutamate receptor-interacting protein/AMPAR binding protein (GRIP/ABP) (63). As we have already discussed, GRIP is a PDZ domain containing protein, which serves as an adaptor to cross-link AMPAR to other neuronal proteins including cytoskeletal elements. Thus, LTD requires PKC phosphorylation of the GluR2/3 receptors, which regulates intereactions with several PDZ domain-containing proteins and apparently controls their rate of internalization.

Although the mechanisms are unclear at this point, there also are different molecular stages of cerebellar LTD. Later stages of LTD are blocked by protein synthesis inhibitors, just like hippocampal LTP. Also, late LTD is dependent upon CREB activation, a process that is dependent on CaMKIV activation (64, 65).

Again, these molecular studies allow us to make generalizations about the molecular basis of learning and memory. The same signal transduction processes (PKC in this case) can lead to either synaptic strengthening or weakening depending on the cellular context in which that process is imbedded. Signal transduction mechanisms are used for information processing at synapses, detecting cell surface signals and translating them into the appropriate change in cellular properties. Finally, that multiple molecular mechanisms trigger biochemical processes of differing durations is the rule rather than the exception.

In Figure 9 is a simplified diagram of the hippocampus—only area CA1 is specified to any extent. The hippocampus receives "sensory input" and neuromodulatory "arousal/attention/emotion" signals. These are simply a lumping together of the various inputs to the hippocampus and area CA1 that we have discussed extensively in previous chapters. The "consolidation signal" designates activity that is triggered externally or internally as part of the consolidation process—it basically represents the AMPA/kaninate receptor-dependent activity that is known to be necessary for memory consolidation. The consolidation signal could also involve several neuromodulatory systems, as Jim McGaugh's work has highlighted.

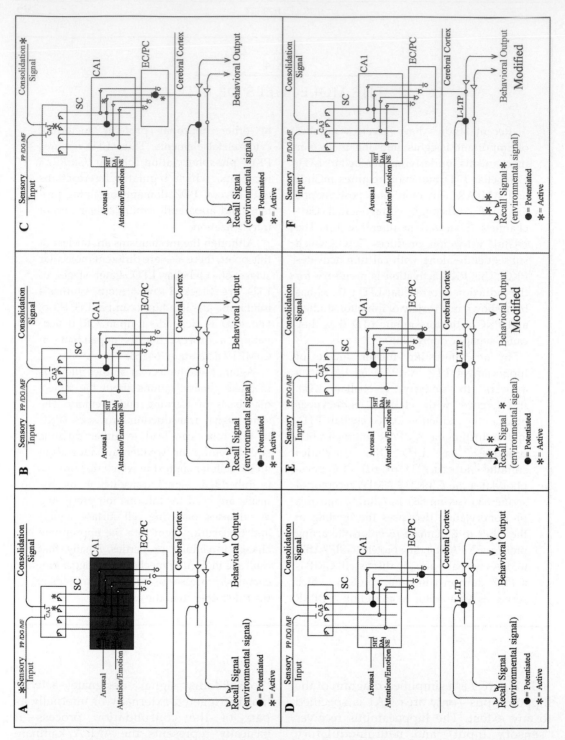

FIGURE 9 A simple model for how LTP might participate in memory consolidation. See text for discussion. (A) Activity in a sensory input plus activation of an ACh input into area CA1 (142). PP/DG/MF = inputs via the perforant path, dentate gyrase, and mossy fiber Pathway. EC/PC = entorhinal cortex / perirhinal cortex. Note also that a recall signal routed through the cerebral cortex elicits a given pre-training behavioral output. (B) LTP at a set of synapses in area CA1. (C) A consolidation signal played through the potentiated pathway results in synaptic potentiation in downstream synapses, including in the cerebral cortex. (D) L-LTP is now established at specific synapses in the cortex. (E) Sending a recall signal through the modified cortical synapses elicits a modified behavioral output. (F) Even when synaptic potentiation is lost in the hippocampus and its immediate targets, the modified behavior persists.

The output from area CA1 goes to the entorhinal cortex and perirhinal cortex and these are treated in block fashion as a way-station to the cerebral cortex. The entirety of the cerebral cortex is reduced to two neurons in the model, which is about how many functioning cortical neurons I have left after a long day of writing.

When memory is to be assessed, the cortex receives a "recall signal"—you might imagine this as an environmental signal such as being asked the question, "What is the capital of Alabama?" Before training, your "behavioral output" is the answer "Birmingham." After training and the ministrations of your hippocampus, your behavioral output is altered, and your answer becomes "Montgomery."

How might the hippocampus bring about this change, capitalizing (so to speak) on its capacity for LTP? You receive sensory input in the form of new information, such as the preceding sentence, manifest as the firing of hippocampal neurons. The importance of the information is clear, so your hippocampal synapses receive a blast of neuromodulatory neurotransmitter (i.e., your professor just told you that the question will be on the exam). The simultaneous activity of neuronal projections into area CA1 and the neuromodulatory signal leads to the formation of LTP at one (for our purposes) of your Schaffer/collateral synapses. These events are diagrammed in Figure 9A, B.

If you are going to store this new information long enough to make it to the test next week, your hippocampus has to receive the "consolidation signal" (Figure 9C). This relays neuronal activity through the hippocampus, including your newly potentiated CA1 synapse. This heightened firing of one of your CA1 pyramidal neurons is manifest as a potentiation of synapses downstream in the entorhinal cortex/perirhinal cortex, and ultimately potentiation of a synapse downstream of there in one of your two functioning cortical neurons (Figure 9D).

The potentiated synapse in your cerebral cortex is the result of a very long-lasting variety of LTP.[5] The potentiated cortical synapse participates in a network of neurons storing information. Its potentiated state leads to an altered behavioral output when its circuit receives a recall signal (Figure 9E). Your cortical circuit stays altered long past the duration of the potentiation in the hippocampus (Figure 9F). Hippocampal synapses are free to relax back to their original state—the hippocampus after all is not storing the memory long-term, just participating in consolidating the memory in the cortex. Thus, your hippocampal synapses return to an unpotentiated state, but their potentiation was an absolute requirement for storing the memory in the cortex.

Now exam day arrives, and your behavior has been modified appropriately as a result of sensory input—in this case the correct information concerning the capital of Alabama. You receive the recall signal— "What is the capital of Alabama?" Your two functioning cortical neurons fire and give the modified behavioral output— "Montgomery." You make a 100 on the test and go on to get your Ph.D. in Neuroscience—all because of a little hippocampal LTP.

Please keep in mind that the model is deliberately oversimplified. I made it up using the absolute minimum number of components that I could, simply to illustrate the basic idea of a role for the hippocampus in cortical memory consolidation. Nevertheless, it is an interesting exercise to expand upon the model yourself. What happens if you potentiate two synapses in the hippocampus? What

---

[5]This aspect of the model is probably accurate. Long-lasting memory storage in the cortex may well involve LTP or LTP-like processes as well (53, 54). Ultra-long-term LTP of the sort we discussed at the end of the last chapter may be the mechanism for cortical information storage, triggered by the potentiated outputs of the hippocampus and entorhinal cortex.

constraints do you place on the model if you only allow yourself to use homosynaptic LTP? How can you increase the complexity of the information processing capacity if you add more details to the dentate gyrus/CA3 region? Exploring these various options, while still keeping the model quite simple, is an edifying exercise in the power of synaptic plasticity in information processing.

III. SUMMARY

LTP does not equal memory. Rather, it is a critical *component* of the complicated process of memory formation. It seems to me now that I have written this chapter that the case for LTP or a similar phenomenon in memory formation is surprisingly strong! A very broad range of studies supports the hypothesis that hippocampal LTP is involved in triggering consolidation of memories in the cortex. It's important to keep in mind the subtleties of the hippocampal/cortical memory system. In addition, a second take-home message of this chapter is that hippocampal LTP need not be constrained to contributing to this single process. A powerful mechanism of activity-dependent synaptic plasticity such as LTP, particularly one that has the capacity for detecting three- or four-way coincidence events, has likely been adapted to multiple roles in the hippocampus and elsewhere in the brain. Specifically, we have discussed the likelihood that hippocampal LTP contributes to the formation of complicated associations and abstract spatial constructs, and that LTP may serve as part of a short-term memory buffer for trace associative conditioning.

In the next two chapters, we will discuss how these processes may be going awry in human learning and memory disorders, specifically human mental retardation syndromes and Alzheimer's disease.

Recent work in these areas has made clear the importance of understanding the molecular basis of LTP and memory formation in the biomedical realm. Far from being esoteric investigations into the minutia of synaptic plasticity, studies of LTP and the molecular basis of memory are giving important insights of great relevance to the human condition.

References

1. Stevens, C. F. (1998). "A million dollar question: does LTP = memory?" *Neuron* 20:1–2.
2. Martin, S. J., Grimwood, P. D., and Morris, R. G. (2000). "Synaptic plasticity and memory: an evaluation of the hypothesis." *Annu. Rev. Neurosci.* 3:649–711.
3. Izquierdo, I., and Medina, J. H. (1997). "Memory formation: the sequence of biochemical events in the hippocampus and its connection to activity in other brain structures." *Neurobiol. Learn. Mem.* 68:285–316.
4. Roman, F. S., Truchet, B., Marchetti, E., Chaillan, F. A., and Soumireu-Mourat, B. (1999). "Correlations between electrophysiological observations of synaptic plasticity modifications and behavioral performance in mammals." *Prog. Neurobiol.* 58:61–87.
5. Maren, S. (1999). "Long-term potentiation in the amygdala: a mechanism for emotional learning and memory." *Trends Neurosci.* 22:561–567.
6. Mazzucchelli, C, Vantaggiato, C, Ciamei, A, Fasano, S, Pakhotin, P, Krezel, W, Welzl, H., Wolfer, D. P., Pages, G., Valverde, O., Marowsky, A., Porrazzo, A., Orban, P. C., Maldonado, R., Ehrengruber, M. U., Cestari, V., Lipp, H. P., Chapman, P. F., Pouyssegur, J., and Brambilla, R. (2002). "Knockout of ERK1 MAP kinase enhances synaptic plasticity in the striatum and facilitates striatal-mediated learning and memory." *Neuron* 34:807–820.
7. Zamanillo, D., Sprengel, R., Hvalby, O., Jensen, V., Burnashev, N., Rozov, A., Kaiser, K. M., Koster, H. J., Borchardt, T., Worley, P., Lubke, J., Frotscher, M., Kelly, P. H., Sommer, B., Andersen, P., Seeburg, P. H., and Sakmann, B. (1999). "Importance of AMPA receptors for hippocampal synaptic plasticity but not for spatial learning." *Science* 284:1805–1811.
8. Reisel, D., Bannerman, D. M., Schmitt, W. B., Deacon, R. M., Flint, J., Borchardt, T., Seeburg, P. H., and Rawlins, J. N. (2002). "Spatial memory dissociations in mice lacking GluR1." *Nat. Neurosci.* 5:868–873.

9. Weeber, E. J., Atkins, C. M., Selcher, J. C., Varga, A. W., Mirnikjoo, B., Paylor, R., Leitges, M., and Sweatt, J. D. (2000). "A role for the beta isoform of protein kinase C in fear conditioning." *J. Neurosci.* 20:5906–5914.

10. Ito, M. (2001). "Cerebellar long-term depression: characterization, signal transduction, and functional roles." *Physiol. Rev.* 81:1143–1195.

11. Blair, H. T., Schafe, G. E., Bauer, E. P., Rodrigues, S. M., and LeDoux, J. E. (2001). "Synaptic plasticity in the lateral amygdala: a cellular hypothesis of fear conditioning." *Learn. Mem.* 8:229–242.

12. Castro, C. A., Silbert, L. H., McNaughton, B. L., and Barnes, C. A. (1989) "Recovery of spatial learning deficits after decay of electrically induced synaptic enhancement in the hippocampus." *Nature* 342:545–548.

13. McNaughton, B. L., Barnes, C. A., Rao, G., Baldwin, J., and Rasmussen, M. (1986). "Long-term enhancement of hippocampal synaptic transmission and the acquisition of spatial information." *J. Neurosci.* 6:563–571.

14. Moser, E. I., Krobert, K. A., Moser, M. B., and Morris, R. G. (1998). "Impaired spatial learning after saturation of long-term potentiation." *Science* 281:2038–2042.

15. Moser, E., Mathiesen, I., and Andersen, P. (1993). "Association between brain temperature and dentate field potentials in exploring and swimming rats." *Science* 259:1324–1326.

16. Moser, E., Moser, M. B., and Andersen, P. (1993). "Synaptic potentiation in the rat dentate gyrus during exploratory learning." *Neuroreport* 5:317–320.

17. Andersen, P., Moser, E., Moser, M. B., and Trommald, M. (1996). "Cellular correlates to spatial learning in the rat hippocampus." *J. Physiol. Paris* 90:349.

18. Adams, J. P., and Sweatt, J. D. (2002). "Molecular psychology: roles for the ERK MAP kinase cascade in memory." *Annu. Rev. Pharmacol. Toxicol.* 42:135–163.

19. Atkins, C. M., Selcher, J. C., Petraitis, J. J., Trzaskos, J. M., and Sweatt, J. D. (1998). "The MAPK cascade is required for mammalian associative learning." *Nat. Neurosci.* 1:602–609.

20. English, J. D., and Sweatt, J. D. (1996). "Activation of p42 mitogen-activated protein kinase in hippocampal long term potentiation." *J. Biol. Chem.* 271:24329–24332.

21. English, J. D., and Sweatt, J. D. (1997)."A requirement for the mitogen-activated protein kinase cascade in hippocampal long term potentiation." *J. Biol. Chem.* 272:19103–19106.

22. Schafe, G. E., Nadel, N. V., Sullivan, G. M., Harris, A., and LeDoux, J. E. (1999). "Memory consolidation for contextual and auditory fear conditioning is dependent on protein synthesis, PKA, and MAP kinase." *Learn. Mem.* 6:97–110.

23. Ohno, M., Frankland, P. W., Chen, A. P., Costa, R. M., and Silva, A. J. (2001). "Inducible, pharmacogenetic approaches to the study of learning and memory." *Nat. Neurosci.* 4:1238–1243.

24. Walz, R., Roesler, R., Barros, D. M., de Souza, M. M., Rodrigues, C., Sant'Anna, M. K., Quevedo, J., Choi, H. K., Neto, W. P., DeDavid e Silva, T. L., Medina, J. H., and Izquierdo, I. (1999). "Effects of post-training infusions of a mitogen-activated protein kinase kinase inhibitor into the hippocampus or entorhinal cortex on short- and long-term retention of inhibitory avoidance." *Behav. Pharmacol.* 10:723–730.

25. Walz, R., Roesler, R., Quevedo, J., Sant'Anna, M. K., Madruga, M., Rodrigues, C., Gottfried, C., Medina, J. H., and Izquierdo, I. (2000). "Time-dependent impairment of inhibitory avoidance retention in rats by posttraining infusion of a mitogen-activated protein kinase kinase inhibitor into cortical and limbic structures." *Neurobiol. Learn. Mem.* 73:11–20.

26. Blum, S., Moore, A. N., Adams, F., and Dash, P. K. (1999). "A mitogen-activated protein kinase cascade in the CA1/CA2 subfield of the dorsal hippocampus is essential for long-term spatial memory." *J. Neurosci.* 19:3535–3544.

27. Selcher, J. C., Atkins, C. M., Trzaskos, J. M., Paylor, R., and Sweatt, J. D. (1999). "A necessity for MAP kinase activation in mammalian spatial learning." *Learn. Mem.* 6:478–490.

28. Schafe, G. E., Atkins, C. M., Swank, M. W., Bauer, E. P., Sweatt, J. D., and LeDoux, J. E. (2000). "Activation of ERK/MAP kinase in the amygdala is required for memory consolidation of pavlovian fear conditioning." *J. Neurosci.* 20:8177–8187.

29. Rotenberg, A., Mayford, M., Hawkins, R. D., Kandel, E. R., and Muller, R.U. (1996). "Mice expressing activated CaMKII lack low frequency LTP and do not form stable place cells in the CA1 region of the hippocampus." *Cell* 87:1351–1361.

30. McHugh, T. J., Blum, K. I., Tsien, J. Z., Tonegawa, S., and Wilson, M. A. (1996). "Impaired hippocampal representation of space in CA1-specific NMDAR1 knockout mice." *Cell* 87:1339–1349.

31. Tsien, J. Z., Chen, D. F., Gerber, D., Tom, C., Mercer, E. H., Anderson, D. J., Mayford, M., Kandel, E. R., and Tonegawa, S. (1996). "Subregion- and cell type-restricted gene knockout in mouse brain." *Cell* 87:1317–1326.

32. Tsien, J. Z., Huerta, P. T., and Tonegawa, S. (1996). "The essential role of hippocampal CA1 NMDA receptor-dependent synaptic plasticity in spatial memory." *Cell* 87:1327–1338.

33. Kentros, C., Hargreaves, E., Hawkins, R. D., Kandel, E. R., Shapiro, M., and Muller, R. V. (1998). "Abolition of long-term stability of new hippocampal place cell maps by NMDA receptor blockade." *Science* 280:2121–2126.

34. Rondi-Reig, L., Libbey, M., Eichenbaum, H., and Tonegawa, S. (2001). "CA1-specific *N*-methyl-D-aspartate receptor knockout mice are deficient in solving a nonspatial transverse patterning task." *Proc. Natl. Acad. Sci. USA* 98:3543–3548.

35. Nakazawa, K., Quirk, M. C., Chitwood, R. A., Watanabe, M., Yeckel, M. F., Sun, L. D., Kato, A., Carr, C. A., Johnston, D., Wilson, M. A., and Tonegawa, S. (2002). "Requirement for hippocampal CA3 NMDA receptors in associative memory recall." *Science* 297:211–218.

36. Davis, S., Butcher, S. P., and Morris, R. G. (1992). "The NMDA receptor antagonist D-2-amino-5-phosphonopentanoate (D-AP5) impairs spatial learning and LTP in vivo at intracerebral concentrations comparable to those that block LTP in vitro." *J. Neurosci.* 12:21–34.

37. Bannerman, D. M., Good, M. A., Butcher, S. P., Ramsay, M., and Morris, R. G. (1995). "Distinct components of spatial learning revealed by prior training and NMDA receptor blockade." *Nature* 378:182–186.

38. Huerta, P. T., Sun, L. D., Wilson, M. A., and Tonegawa, S. (2000). "Formation of temporal memory requires NMDA receptors within CA1 pyramidal neurons." *Neuron* 25:473–480.

39. Morris, R. G. (1996). "Further studies of the role of hippocampal synaptic plasticity in spatial learning: is hippocampal LTP a mechanism for automatically recording attended experience?" *J. Physiol. Paris* 90:333–334.

40. Morris, R. G., and Frey, U. (1997). "Hippocampal synaptic plasticity: role in spatial learning or the automatic recording of attended experience?" *Philos. Trans. R. Soc. Lond. B. Biol. Sci.* 352:1489–1503.

41. Shapiro, M. L., and Eichenbaum, H. (1999). "Hippocampus as a memory map: synaptic plasticity and memory encoding by hippocampal neurons." *Hippocampus* 9:365–384.

42. Igaz, L. M., Vianna, M. R., Medina, J. H., and Izquierdo, I. (2002). "Two time periods of hippocampal mRNA synthesis are required for memory consolidation of fear-motivated learning." *J. Neurosci.* 22:6781–6789.

43. Grecksch, G., and Matthies, H. (1980). "Two sensitive periods for the amnesic effect of anisomycin." *Pharmacol. Biochem. Behav.* 12:663–665.

44. Guzowski, J. F., Lyford, G. L., Stevenson, G. D., Houston, F. P., McGaugh, J. L., Worley, P. F., and Barnes, C. A. (2000). "Inhibition of activity-dependent arc protein expression in the rat hippocampus impairs the maintenance of long-term potentiation and the consolidation of long-term memory." *J. Neurosci.* 20:3993–4001.

45. Guzowski, J. F., and McGaugh, J. L. (1997). "Antisense oligodeoxynucleotide-mediated disruption of hippocampal cAMP response element binding protein levels impairs consolidation of memory for water maze training." *Proc. Natl. Acad. Sci. USA* 94:2693–2698.

46. Taubenfeld, S. M., Milekic, M. H., Monti, B., and Alberini, C. M. (2001). "The consolidation of new but not reactivated memory requires hippocampal C/EBPbeta." *Nat. Neurosci.* 4:813–818.

47. Kim, J. J., Fanselow, M. S., DeCola, J. P., and Landeira-Fernandez, J. (1992). "Selective impairment of long-term but not short-term conditional fear by the *N*-methyl-D-aspartate antagonist APV." *Behav. Neurosci.* 106:591–596.

48. Steele, R. J., and Morris, R. G. (1999). "Delay-dependent impairment of a matching-to-place task with chronic and intrahippocampal infusion of the NMDA-antagonist D-AP5." *Hippocampus* 9:118–136.

49. Day, M., and Morris, R. G. (2001). "Memory consolidation and NMDA receptors: discrepancy between genetic and pharmacological approaches." *Science* 293:755.

50. Shimizu, E., Tang, Y. P., Rampon, C., and Tsien, J. Z. (2000). "NMDA receptor-dependent synaptic reinforcement as a crucial process for memory consolidation." *Science* 290:1170–1174.

51. Riedel, G., Micheau, J., Lam, A. G., Roloff, E., Martin, S. J., Bridge, H., Hoz, L., Poeschel, B., McCulloch, J., and Morris, R. G. (1999). "Reversible neural inactivation reveals hippocampal participation in several memory processes." *Nat. Neurosci.* 2:898–905.

52. Brun, V. H., Ytterbo, K., Morris, R. G., Moser, M. B., and Moser, E. I. (2001). "Retrograde amnesia for spatial memory induced by NMDA receptor-mediated long-term potentiation." *J. Neurosci.* 21:356–362.

53. Rioult-Pedotti, M. S., Friedman, D., and Donoghue, J. P. (2000). "Learning-induced LTP in neocortex." *Science* 290:533–536.

54. Rioult-Pedotti, M. S., Friedman, D., Hess, G., and Donoghue, J. P. (1998). "Strengthening of horizontal cortical connections following skill learning." *Nat. Neurosci.* 1:230–234.

55. McKernan, M. G., and Shinnick-Gallagher, P. (1997). "Fear conditioning induces a lasting potentiation of synaptic currents in vitro." *Nature* 390:607–611.

56. Rogan, M. T., Staubli, U. V., and LeDoux, J. E. (1997). "Fear conditioning induces associative long-term potentiation in the amygdala." *Nature* 390:604–607.

57. Rogan, M. T., and LeDoux, J. E. (1995). "LTP is accompanied by commensurate enhancement of auditory-evoked responses in a fear conditioning circuit." *Neuron* 15:127–136.

58. Carey, M., and Lisberger, S. (2002). "Embarrassed, but not depressed: eye opening lessons for cerebellar learning." *Neuron* 35:223–226.

59. Sparks, D. Personal Communication.

60. De Zeeuw, C. I., Hansel, C., Bian, F., Koekkoek, S. K., van Alphen, A. M., Linden, D. J., and Oberdick, J. (1998). "Expression of a protein kinase C inhibitor in Purkinje cells blocks cerebellar LTD and adaptation of the vestibulo-ocular reflex." *Neuron* 20:495–508.

61. Man, H. Y., Lin, J. W., Ju, W. H., Ahmadian, G., Liu, L., Becker, L. E., Sheng, M., and Wang, Y. T. (2000). "Regulation of AMPA receptor-mediated synaptic transmission by clathrin-dependent receptor internalization." *Neuron* 25:649–662.

62. Wang, Y. T., and Linden, D. J. (2000). "Expression of cerebellar long-term depression requires postsynaptic clathrin-mediated endocytosis." *Neuron* 25:635–647.

63. Xia, J., Chung, H. J., Wihler, C., Huganir, R. L., and Linden, D. J. (2000). "Cerebellar long-term depression requires PKC-regulated interactions between GluR2/3 and PDZ domain-containing proteins." *Neuron* 28:499–510.

64. Ahn, S., Ginty, D. D., and Linden, D. J. (1999). "A late phase of cerebellar long-term depression requires activation of CaMKIV and CREB." *Neuron* 23:559–568.

65. Linden, D. J. (1996). "A protein synthesis-dependent late phase of cerebellar long-term depression." *Neuron* 17:483–490.

66. Manabe, T., Noda, Y., Mamiya, T., Katagiri, H., Houtani, T., Nishi, M., Noda, T., Takahashi, T., Sugimoto, T., Nabeshima, T., and Takeshima, H. (1998). "Facilitation of long-term potentiation and memory in mice lacking nociceptin receptors." *Nature* 394:577–581.

67. Balschun, D., Wolfer, D. P., Bertocchini, F., Barone, V., Conti, A., Zuschratter, W., Missiaen, L., Lipp, H. P., Frey, J. U., and Sorrentino, V. (1999). "Deletion of the ryanodine receptor type 3 (RyR3) impairs forms of synaptic plasticity and spatial learning." *Embo. J.* 18:5264–5273.

68. Futatsugi, A., Kato, K., Ogura, H., Li, S. T., Nagata, E., Kuwajima, G., Tanaka, K., Itohara, S., and Mikoshiba, K. (1999). "Facilitation of NMDAR-independent LTP and spatial learning in mutant mice lacking ryanodine receptor type 3." *Neuron* 24:701–713.

69. Nakamura, K., Manabe, T., Watanabe, M., Mamiya, T., Ichikawa, R., Kiyama, Y., Sanbo, M., Yagi, T., Inoue, Y., Nabeshima, T., Mori, H., and Mishina, M. (2001). "Enhancement of hippocampal LTP, reference memory and sensorimotor gating in mutant mice lacking a telencephalon-specific cell adhesion molecule." *Eur. J. Neurosci.* 13:179–189.

70. Nishiyama, H., Knopfel, T., Endo, S., and Itohara, S. (2002). "Glial protein S100B modulates long-term neuronal synaptic plasticity." *Proc. Natl. Acad. Sci. USA* 99:4037–4042.

71. Tang, Y. P., Shimizu, E., Dube, G. R., Rampon, C., Kerchner, G. A., Zhuo, M., Liu, G., and Tsien, J. Z. (1999). "Genetic enhancement of learning and memory in mice." *Nature* 401:63–69.

72. Tang, Y. P., Wang, H., Feng, R., Kyin, M., and Tsien, J. Z. (2001). "Differential effects of enrichment on learning and memory function in NR2B transgenic mice." *Neuropharmacology* 41:779–790.

73. Malleret, G., Haditsch, U., Genoux, D., Jones, M. W., Bliss, T. V., Vanhoose, A. M., Weitlauf, C., Kandel, E. R., Winder, D. G., and Mansuy, I. M. (2001). "Inducible and reversible enhancement of learning, memory, and long-term potentiation by genetic inhibition of calcineurin." *Cell* 104:675–686.

74. Pavlov, I., Voikar, V., Kaksonen, M., Lauri, S. E., Hienola, A., Taira, T., and Rauvala, H. (2002). "Role of Heparin-Binding Growth-Associated Molecule (HB-GAM) in Hippocampal LTP and Spatial Learning Revealed by Studies on Overexpressing and Knockout Mice." *Mol. Cell. Neurosci.* 20:330–342.

75. Walther, T., Balschun, D., Voigt, J. P., Fink, H., Zuschratter, W., Birchmeier, C., Ganten, D., and Bader, M. (1998). "Sustained long term potentiation and anxiety in mice lacking the Mas protooncogene." *J. Biol. Chem.* 273:11867–11873.

76. Jun, K., Choi, G., Yang, S. G., Choi, K. Y., Kim, H., Chan, G. C., Storm, D. R., Albert, C., Mayr, G. W., Lee, C. J., and Shin, H. S. (1998). "Enhanced hippocampal CA1 LTP but normal spatial learning in inositol 1,4,5-trisphosphate 3-kinase(A)-deficient mice." *Learn. Mem.* 5:317–330.

77. Abeliovich, A., Paylor, R., Chen, C., Kim, J. J., Wehner, J. M., and Tonegawa, S. (1993). "PKC gamma mutant mice exhibit mild deficits in spatial and contextual learning." *Cell* 75:1263–1271.

78. Abeliovich, A., Chen, C., Goda, Y., Silva, A. J., Stevens, C. F., and Tonegawa, S. (1993). "Modified hippocampal long-term potentiation in PKC gamma-mutant mice." *Cell* 75:1253–1262.

79. Selcher, J. C., Nekrasova, T., Paylor, R., Landreth, G. E., and Sweatt, J. D. (2001). "Mice lacking the ERK1 isoform of MAP kinase are unimpaired in emotional learning." *Learn. Mem.* 8:11–19.

80. Anderson, R., Barnes, J. C., Bliss, T. V., Cain, D. P., Cambon, K., Davies, H. A., Errington, M. L., Fellows, L. A., Gray, R. A., Hoh, T., Stewart, M., Large, C. H., and Higgins, G. A. (1998). "Behavioural, physiological and morphological analysis of a line of apolipoprotein E knockout mouse." *Neuroscience* 85:93–110.

81. Sesay, A. K., Errington, M. L., Levita, L., and Bliss, T. V. (1996). "Spatial learning and hippocampal long-term potentiation are not impaired in mdx mice." *Neurosci. Lett.* 211:207–210.

82. Meiri, N., Sun, M. K., Segal, Z., and Alkon, D. L. (1998). "Memory and long-term potentiation (LTP) dissociated: normal spatial memory despite CA1 LTP elimination with Kv1.4 antisense." *Proc. Natl. Acad. Sci. USA* 95:15037–15042.

83. Bannerman, D. M., Chapman, P. F., Kelly, P. A., Butcher, S. P., and Morris, R. G. (1994). "Inhibition of nitric oxide synthase does not impair spatial learning." *J. Neurosci.* 14:7404–7414.

84. Son, H., Hawkins, R. D., Martin, K., Kiebler, M., Huang, P. L., Fishman, M. C., and Kandel, E. R. (1996). "Long-term potentiation is reduced in mice that are doubly mutant in endothelial and neuronal nitric oxide synthase." *Cell* 87:1015–1023.

85. Huang, Y. Y., Bach, M. E., Lipp, H. P., Zhuo, M., Wolfer, D. P., Hawkins, R. D., Schoonjans, L., Kandel, E. R., Godfraind, J. M., Mulligan, R., Collen, D., and Carmeliet, P. (1996). "Mice lacking the gene encoding tissue-type plasminogen activator show a selective interference with late-phase long-term potentiation in both Schaffer collateral and mossy fiber pathways." *Proc. Natl. Acad. Sci. USA* 93:8699–8704.

86. Minichiello, L., Korte, M., Wolfer, D., Kuhn, R., Unsicker, K., Cestari, V., Rossi-Arnaud, C., Lipp, H. P., Bonhoeffer, T., and Klein, R. (1999). "Essential role for TrkB receptors in hippocampus-mediated learning." *Neuron* 24:401–414.

87. Ho, N., Liauw, J. A., Blaeser, F., Wei, F., Hanissian, S., Muglia, L. M., Wozniak, D. F., Nardi, A., Arvin, K. L., Holtzman, D. M., Linden, D. J., Zhuo, M., Muglia, L. J., and Chatila, T. A. (2000). "Impaired synaptic plasticity and cAMP response element-binding protein activation in Ca^{2+}/calmodulin-dependent protein kinase type IV/Gr-deficient mice." *J. Neurosci.* 20:6459–6472.

88. Allen, P. B., Hvalby, O., Jensen, V., Errington, M. L., Ramsay, M., Chaudhry, F. A., Bliss, T. V., Storm-Mathisen, J., Morris, R. G., Andersen, P., and Greengard, P. (2000). "Protein phosphatase-1 regulation in the induction of long-term potentiation: heterogeneous molecular mechanisms." *J. Neurosci.* 20:3537–3543.

89. Errington, M. L., Bliss, T. V., Morris, R. J., Laroche, S., and Davis, S. (1997). "Long-term potentiation in awake mutant mice." *Nature* 387:666–667.

90. Nosten-Bertrand, M., Errington, M. L., Murphy, K.P., Tokugawa, Y., Barboni, E., Kozlova, E., Michalovich, D., Morris, R. G., Silver, J., Stewart, C. L., Bliss, T. V., and Morris, R. J. (1996). "Normal spatial learning despite regional inhibition of LTP in mice lacking Thy-1." *Nature* 379:826–829.

91. Meng, Y., Zhang, Y., Tregoubov, V., Janus, C., Cruz, L., Jackson, M., Lu, W. Y., MacDonald, J. F., Wang, J. Y., Falls, D. L., and Jia, Z. (2002). "Abnormal spine morphology and enhanced LTP in LIMK-1 knockout mice." *Neuron* 35:121–133.

92. Gu, Y., McIlwain, K. L., Weeber, E. J., Yamagata, T., Xu, B., Antalffy, B. A., Reyes, C., Yuva-Paylor, L., Armstrong, D., Zoghbi, H., Sweatt, J. D., Paylor, R., and Nelson, D. L. (2002). "Impaired conditioned fear and enhanced long-term potentiation in Fmr2 knock-out mice." *J. Neurosci.* 22:2753–2763.

93. Migaud, M., Charlesworth, P., Dempster, M., Webster, L. C., Watabe, A. M., Makhinson, M., He, Y., Ramsay, M. F., Morris, R. G., Morrison, J. H., O'Dell, T. J., and Grant, S. G. (1998). "Enhanced long-term potentiation and impaired learning in mice with mutant postsynaptic density-95 protein." *Nature* 396:433–439.

94. Sarnyai, Z., Sibille, E. L., Pavlides, C., Fenster, R. J., McEwen, B. S., and Toth, M. (2000). "Impaired hippocampal-dependent learning and functional abnormalities in the hippocampus in mice lacking serotonin(1A) receptors." *Proc. Natl. Acad. Sci. USA* 97:14731–14736.

95. Kubota, M., Murakoshi, T., Saegusa, H., Kazuno, A., Zong, S., Hu, Q., Noda, T., and Tanabe, T. (2001). "Intact LTP and fear memory but impaired spatial memory in mice lacking Ca(v)2.3 (alpha(IE)) channel." *Biochem. Biophys. Res. Commun.* 282:242–248.

96. Matilla, A, Roberson, E. D., Banfi, S., Morales, J., Armstrong, D. L., Burright, E. N., Orr, H. T., Sweatt, J. D., Zoghbi, H. Y., and Matzuk, M. M. (1998). "Mice lacking ataxin-1 display learning deficits and decreased hippocampal paired-pulse facilitation." *J. Neurosci.* 18:5508–5516.

97. Bliss, T., Errington, M., Fransen, E., Godfraind, J. M., Kauer, J. A., Kooy, R. F., Maness, P. F., and

Furley, A. J. (2000). "Long-term potentiation in mice lacking the neural cell adhesion molecule L1." *Curr. Biol.* 10:1607–1610.

98. Saarelainen, T., Pussinen, R., Koponen, E., Alhonen, L., Wong, G., Sirvio, J., and Castren, E. (2000). "Transgenic mice overexpressing truncated trkB neurotrophin receptors in neurons have impaired long-term spatial memory but normal hippocampal LTP." *Synapse* 38:102–104.

99. Meiri, N., Ghelardini, C., Tesco, G., Galeotti, N., Dahl, D., Tomsic, D., Cavallaro, S., Quattrone, A., Capaccioli, S., Bartolini, A., and Alkon, D. L. (1997). "Reversible antisense inhibition of Shaker-like Kv1.1 potassium channel expression impairs associative memory in mouse and rat." *Proc. Natl. Acad. Sci. USA* 94:4430–4434.

100. Silva, A. J., Stevens, C. F., Tonegawa, S., and Wang, Y. (1992). "Deficient hippocampal long-term potentiation in alpha-calcium-calmodulin kinase II mutant mice." *Science* 257:201–206.

101. Silva, A. J., Paylor, R., Wehner, J. M., and Tonegawa, S. (1992). "Impaired spatial learning in alpha-calcium-calmodulin kinase II mutant mice." *Science* 257:206–211.

102. Hinds, H. L., Tonegawa, S., and Malinow, R. (1998). "CA1 long-term potentiation is diminished but present in hippocampal slices from alpha-CaMKII mutant mice." *Learn. Mem.* 5:344–354.

103. Costa, R. M., Federov, N. B., Kogan, J. H., Murphy, G. G., Stern, J., Ohno, M., Kucherlapati, R., Jacks, T., and Silva, A. J. (2002). "Mechanism for the learning deficits in a mouse model of neurofibromatosis type 1." *Nature* 415:526–530.

104. Bourtchuladze, R., Frenguelli, B., Blendy, J., Cioffi, D., Schutz, G., and Silva, A. J. (1994). "Deficient long-term memory in mice with a targeted mutation of the cAMP-responsive element-binding protein." *Cell* 79:59–68.

105. Gass, P., Wolfer, D. P., Balschun, D., Rudolph, D., Frey, U., Lipp, H. P., and Schutz, G. (1998). "Deficits in memory tasks of mice with CREB mutations depend on gene dosage." *Learn. Mem.* 5:274–288.

106. Korte, M., Carroll, P., Wolf, E., Brem, G., Thoenen, H., and Bonhoeffer, T. (1995). "Hippocampal long-term potentiation is impaired in mice lacking brain-derived neurotrophic factor." *Proc. Natl. Acad. Sci. USA* 92:8856–8860.

107. Patterson, S. L., Abel, T., Deuel, T. A., Martin, K. C., Rose, J. C., and Kandel, E. R. (1996). "Recombinant BDNF rescues deficits in basal synaptic transmission and hippocampal LTP in BDNF knockout mice." *Neuron* 16:1137–1145.

108. Linnarsson, S., Bjorklund, A., and Ernfors, P. (1997). "Learning deficit in BDNF mutant mice." *Eur. J. Neurosci.* 9:2581–2587.

109. Montkowski, A., and Holsboer, F. (1997). "Intact spatial learning and memory in transgenic mice with reduced BDNF." *Neuroreport* 8:779–782.

110. Jiang, Y. H., Armstrong, D., Albrecht, U., Atkins, C. M., Noebels, J. L., Eichele, G., Sweatt, J. D., and Beaudet, A. L. (1998). "Mutation of the Angelman ubiquitin ligase in mice causes increased cytoplasmic p53 and deficits of contextual learning and long-term potentiation." *Neuron* 21:799–811.

111. Aiba, A., Chen, C., Herrup, K., Rosenmund, C., Stevens, C. F., and Tonegawa, S. (1994). "Reduced hippocampal long-term potentiation and context-specific deficit in associative learning in mGluR1 mutant mice." *Cell* 79:365–375.

112. Sprengel, R., Suchanek, B., Amico, C., Brusa, R., Burnashev, N., Rozov, A., Hvalby, O., Jensen, V., Paulsen, O., Andersen, P., Kim, J.J., Thompson, R.F., Sun, W., Webster, L. C., Grant, S. G., Eilers, J., Konnerth, A., Li, J., McNamara, J. O., and Seeburg, P. H. (1998). "Importance of the intracellular domain of NR2 subunits for NMDA receptor function in vivo." *Cell* 92:279–289.

113. Thiels, E., Urban, N. N., Gonzalez-Burgos, G. R., Kanterewicz, B. I., Barrionuevo, G., Chu, C. T., Oury, T. D., and Klann, E. (2000). "Impairment of long-term potentiation and associative memory in mice that overexpress extracellular superoxide dismutase." *J. Neurosci.* 20:7631–7639.

114. Jones, M. W., Errington, M. L., French, P. J., Fine, A., Bliss, T. V., Garel, S., Charnay, P., Bozon, B., Laroche, S., and Davis, S. (2001). "A requirement for the immediate early gene Zif268 in the expression of late LTP and long-term memories." *Nat. Neurosci.* 4:289–296.

115. Wong, S. T., Athos, J., Figueroa, X. A., Pineda, V. V., Schaefer, M. L., Chavkin, C. C., Muglia, L. J., and Storm, D. R. (1999). "Calcium-stimulated adenylyl cyclase activity is critical for hippocampus-dependent long-term memory and late phase LTP." *Neuron* 23:787–798.

116. Gahtan, E., Auerbach, J. M., Groner, Y., and Segal, M. (1998). "Reversible impairment of long-term potentiation in transgenic Cu/Zn-SOD mice." *Eur. J. Neurosci.* 10:538–544.

117. Bejar, R, Yasuda, R, Krugers, H, Hood, K, and Mayford, M. (2002). "Transgenic calmodulin-dependent protein kinase II activation: dose-dependent effects on synaptic plasticity, learning, and memory." *J. Neurosci.* 22:5719–5726.

118. Chang, H. P., Lindberg, F. P., Wang, H. L., Huang, A. M., and Lee, E. H. (1999). "Impaired memory retention and decreased long-term potentiation in integrin-associated protein-deficient mice." *Learn. Mem.* 6:448–457.

119. Calabresi, P., Napolitano, M., Centonze, D., Marfia, G. A., Gubellini, P., Teule, M. A., Berretta, N., Bernardi, G., Frati, L., Tolu, M., and Gulino, A. (2000). "Tissue plasminogen activator controls multiple forms of synaptic plasticity and memory." *Eur. J. Neurosci.* 12:1002–1012.

120. Pittenger, C., Huang, Y. Y., Paletzki, R. F., Bourtchouladze, R., Scanlin, H., Vronskaya, S., and Kandel, E. R. (2002). "Reversible inhibition of CREB/ATF transcription factors in region CA1 of the dorsal hippocampus disrupts hippocampus-dependent spatial memory." *Neuron* 34:447–462.

121. Xie, C. W., Sayah, D., Chen, Q. S., Wei, W. Z., Smith, D., and Liu, X. (2000). "Deficient long-term memory and long-lasting long-term potentiation in mice with a targeted deletion of neurotrophin-4 gene." *Proc. Natl. Acad. Sci. USA* 97:8116–8121.

122. Kang, H., Sun, L. D., Atkins, C. M., Soderling, T. R., Wilson, M. A., and Tonegawa, S. (2001). "An important role of neural activity-dependent CaMKIV signaling in the consolidation of long-term memory." *Cell* 106:771–783.

123. Abel, T., Nguyen, P. V., Barad, M., Deuel, T. A., Kandel, E. R., and Bourtchouladze, R. (1997). "Genetic demonstration of a role for PKA in the late phase of LTP and in hippocampus-based long-term memory." *Cell* 88:615–626.

124. Rotenberg, A., Abel, T., Hawkins, R. D., Kandel, E. R., and Muller, R. U. (2000). "Parallel instabilities of long-term potentiation, place cells, and learning caused by decreased protein kinase A activity." *J. Neurosci.* 20:8096–8102.

125. Otto, C., Kovalchuk, Y., Wolfer, D. P., Gass, P., Martin, M., Zuschratter, W., Grone, H. J., Kellendonk, C., Tronche, F., Maldonado, R., Lipp, H. P., Konnerth, A., and Schutz, G. (2001). "Impairment of mossy fiber long-term potentiation and associative learning in pituitary adenylate cyclase activating polypeptide type I receptor-deficient mice." *J. Neurosci.* 21:5520–5527.

126. Wemmie, J. A., Chen, J., Askwith, C. C., Hruska-Hageman, A. M., Price, M. P., Nolan, B. C., Yoder, P. G., Lamani, E., Hoshi, T., Freeman, J. H. Jr, and Welsh, M. J. (2002). "The acid-activated ion channel ASIC contributes to synaptic plasticity, learning, and memory." *Neuron* 34:463–477.

127. Nguyen, P. V., Abel, T., Kandel, E. R., and Bourtchouladze, R. (2000). "Strain-dependent differences in LTP and hippocampus-dependent memory in inbred mice." *Learn. Mem.* 7:170–179.

128. Weeber, E. J., Levy, M., Sampson, M. J., Anflous, K., Armstrong, D. L., Brown, S. E., Sweatt, J. D., and Craigen, W. J. (2002). "The role of mitochondrial porins and the permeability transition pore in learning and synaptic plasticity." *J. Biol. Chem.* 277:18891–18897.

129. Molinari, S., Battini, R., Ferrari, S., Pozzi, L., Killcross, A. S., Robbins, T. W., Jouvenceau, A., Billard, J. M., Dutar, P., Lamour, Y., Baker, W. A., Cox, H., and Emson, P. C. (1996). "Deficits in memory and hippocampal long-term potentiation in mice with reduced calbindin D28K expression." *Proc. Natl. Acad. Sci. USA* 93:8028–8033.

130. Brambilla, R., Gnesutta, N., Minichiello, L., White, G., Roylance, A. J., Herron, C. E., Ramsey, M., Wolfer, D. P., Cestari, V., Rossi-Arnaud, C., Grant, S. G., Chapman, P. F., Lipp, H. P., Sturani, E., and Klein, R. (1997). "A role for the Ras signalling pathway in synaptic transmission and long-term memory." *Nature* 390:281–286.

131. Bach, M. E., Hawkins, R. D., Osman, M., Kandel, E. R., and Mayford, M. (1995). "Impairment of spatial but not contextual memory in CaMKII mutant mice with a selective loss of hippocampal LTP in the range of the theta frequency." *Cell* 81:905–915.

132. Impey, S., Smith, D. M., Obrietan, K., Donahue, R., Wade, C., and Storm, D. R. (1998). "Stimulation of cAMP response element (CRE)-mediated transcription during contextual learning." *Nat. Neurosci.* 1:595–601.

133. Richter-Levin, G., Thomas, K. L., Hunt, S. P., and Bliss, T. V. (1998). "Dissociation between genes activated in long-term potentiation and in spatial learning in the rat." *Neurosci. Lett.* 251:41–44.

134. Guzowski, J. F., McNaughton, B. L., Barnes, C. A., and Worley, P. F. (1999). "Environment-specific expression of the immediate-early gene Arc in hippocampal neuronal ensembles." *Nat. Neurosci.* 2:1120–1124.

135. Guzowski, J. F., Setlow, B., Wagner, E. K., and McGaugh, J. L. (2001). "Experience-dependent gene expression in the rat hippocampus after spatial learning: a comparison of the immediate-early genes Arc, c-fos, and zif268." *J. Neurosci.* 21:5089–5098.

136. Hall, J., Thomas, K. L., and Everitt, B. J. (2000). "Rapid and selective induction of BDNF

expression in the hippocampus during contextual learning." *Nat. Neurosci.* 3:533–535.

137. Laroche, S., Errington, M. L., Lynch, M. A., and Bliss, T. V. (1987). "Increase in [3H]glutamate release from slices of dentate gyrus and hippocampus following classical conditioning in the rat." *Behav. Brain Res.* 25:23–29.

138. Richter-Levin, G., Canevari, L., and Bliss, T. V. (1995). "Long-term potentiation and glutamate release in the dentate gyrus: links to spatial learning." *Behav. Brain Res.* 66:37–40.

139. Richter-Levin, G., Canevari, L., and Bliss, T. V. (1998). "Spatial training and high-frequency stimulation engage a common pathway to enhance glutamate release in the hippocampus." *Learn. Mem.* 4:445–450.

140. Levenson, J., Weeber, E., Selcher, J. C., Kategaya, L. S., Sweatt, J. D., and Eskin, A. (2002). "Long-term potentiation and contextual fear conditioning increase neuronal glutamate uptake." *Nat. Neurosci.* 5:155–161.

141. Morris, R. G. (1989). "Synaptic plasticity and learning: selective impairment of learning rats and blockade of long-term potentiation in vivo by the *N*-methyl-D-aspartate receptor antagonist AP5." *J. Neurosci.* 9:3040–3057.

142. Cobb, S. R., Bulters, D. O., Suchak, S., Riedel, G., Morris, R. G., and Davies, C. H. (1999). "Activation of nicotinic acetylcholine receptors patterns network activity in the rodent hippocampus." *J. Physiol.* 518 (Pt 1):131–140.

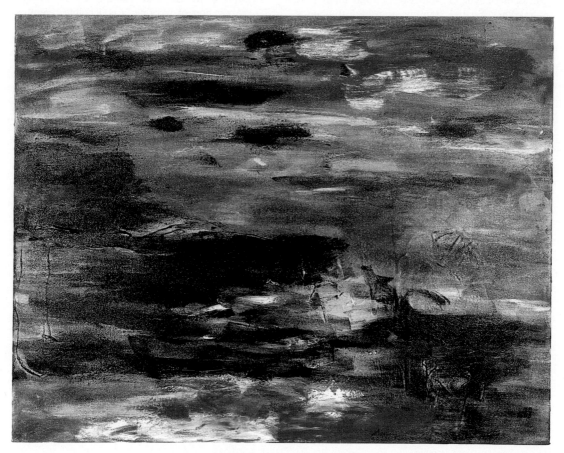

Mental Retardation Syndromes
J. David Sweatt, Acrylic on canvas, 2002

10

Inherited Disorders of Human Memory

Mental Retardation Syndromes

As we discussed in the first chapter, our great capacity for learning and remembering plays an enormous role in forming our human potential. Moreover, our personal experiences, where we have learned and remembered specific items and events, define us as individuals. These truths are nowhere more evident than when we consider individuals with pronounced learning and memory deficits, present from birth. In this chapter, we consider human mental retardation syndromes and their underlying molecular basis. In some intellectually satisfying instances, we will actually be able to tie mechanisms for these disorders back into fundamental mechanisms for synaptic plasticity and learning that we have already discussed.[1]

There is another point that is important to make in the context of this chapter. Of all the various areas of cognitive neurobiology, the field of learning and memory has advanced the farthest into studies at the molecular level, based on a reductionist approach of using model systems simpler than the human. But how can one bridge the enormous distance from specific molecules to *human* cognition? Over the past few years, a number of groups, including research teams at Baylor College of Medicine, UCLA, Johns Hopkins University, and the University of Illinois to name a few specific examples, have undertaken to bridge this gap by studying naturally occurring human mental retardation syndromes. The philosophy of the approach is to use identified human genetic mutations that result in mental retardation and learning disorders as an entrée to beginning to understand the molecular basis of human

---

[1]Parts of this chapter are adapted from Weeber and Sweatt (1).

cognition. As a practical matter, this translates into taking an identified human gene linked to a mental retardation syndrome and making knockout and transgenic mouse models. These models are then used to generate insights into the underlying molecular and cellular basis for the defect. The rationale is that this gives one insights into the analogous "knockout humans" and hence gives insights into the molecular neurobiology of human cognitive processing. Some specific examples of mental retardation syndromes where this approach has been applied are given in Table 1.

Even though this approach is at a very early stage, it is interesting that different studies of this sort have already begun to converge on two common signal transduction cascades as being involved in human learning and memory: the ras/ERK cascade and its associated upstream regulators and downstream targets (see Figure 1) and the CaMKII system. In the first section of this chapter, I will describe exciting recent findings implicating dysfunction of the ras/ERK cascade in human mental retardation syndromes. I should emphasize that several of the ideas I will present in this section, where I present potential mechanistic links between various different human mental retardation syndromes, are at best educated guesses. However, I simply cannot resist beginning to synthesize a unified picture of critical molecular events in human learning. This extends perfectly the sorts of studies we have been discussing where learning was studied in rodent models.

In the second section of this chapter, I will discuss recent findings from my lab and Alcino Silva's lab implicating CaMKII in a form of human mental retardation. In the final section, I will discuss fragile X retardation syndromes, and we will see yet another instance of the basic studies of synaptic plasticity running head-on into studies of a human learning disorder. In this last section I will highlight work from Bill Greenough's lab, among others' that has begun to tie mechanisms of local

dendritic protein synthesis in with molecular mechanisms of fragile X mental retardation type 1.

Before getting down to the serious business of this chapter, I want to relate a personal anecdote that illustrates the funny way that things sometime evolve in science. Alcino Silva and I are of the same scientific generation and, as such, have been competitors in a certain sense—we both set out as naïve, optimistic young scientists to "solve memory," of course ideally before anyone else did. While I'm oversimplifying, Alcino basically staked his claim with CaMKII and I grabbed MAP kinases, each of us working on basic mechanisms of synaptic plasticity and memory that were described earlier in this book. Essentially as side projects, Alcino started working on neurofibromatosis mental retardation and my lab started working on Angelman Mental Retardation Syndrome (AS). In the first section of this chapter, I will describe work from Alcino's lab, highlighting the likely importance of MAP kinase in human memory, based on his studies of Neurofibromatosis. In the second section I am going to describe studies from my lab suggesting the importance of CaMKII in human memory, based on our studies of the Angelman Syndrome. In my mind, these are very satisfying examples of how following the clues that Nature gives us will always lead us to common ground.

I. NEUROFIBROMATOSIS, COFFIN-LOWRY SYNDROME, AND THE RAS/ERK CASCADE

Neurofibromatosis is an autosomal-dominant disease that exhibits a variety of clinical features, principally neurofibromas, or benign tumors of neural origin. Other characteristics can include skin discoloration (café au lait spots) and skeletal malformation. The gene that causes neurofibromatosis when mutated in humans is the neurofibromatosis type 1 oncogene, NF1. NF1 is distinct from the gene coding for a

TABLE 1   Mouse Models of Human Mental Retardation Syndromes

Human Mental Retardation Syndromes	Gene Product	Potential Targets	Mouse Model		References
			Learning Defects?	LTP Change?	
Neurofibromatosis	Neurofibromin 1 (NF1)	ras/ ERK, adenylyl cyclase, cytoskeleton	+	+	Costa et al. (4, 39) Tong et al. (9)
Coffin-Lowry Syndrome	Ribosomal S6 kinase2 (rsk2)	CREB, ribosomal S6 protein	+	?	Dufresne et al. (12); Harum et al. (13)
Angelman Syndrome	Ubiquitin ligase (E6AP)	p53 tumor suppressor protein, others?	+	+	Jiang et al. (40)
Fragile X mental retardation 1	FMR1 protein (RNA binding proteins)	Protein synthesis machinery, mRNA targeting, spine structure	+ (strain dependent)	?	Bardoni et al. (17)
Fragile X mental retardation 2	FMR2 protein (putative transcription factor)	Unknown— gene expression	+	+	Gu et al. (41)
Rett Syndrome	Methyl-CpG binding protein 2 (MeCP$_2$)	Transcriptional repressors— regulation of unknown genes	?	?	Shahbazian et al. (23)
Myotonic dystrophy	Dystrophin protein kinase (DMPK)	Na$^+$ channels, Tau many others	?	?	Mistry et al. (42)
Down Syndrome (Trisomy 21)	DS critical locus	Multiple genes including DYRK1A and SOD	+	+	Siarey et al. (36)
	DYRK1A (minibrain kinase homolog)	Unknown	+	?	Altafaj et al. (35)
	Superoxide dismutase (SOD)	Superoxide dependent processes—redox regulation of PKC, ras, transcription factors	+	+	Gahtan et al. (43)
Williams Syndrome	WS critical locus: LIMK-1 Elastin Syntaxin 1A FKBP6 EIFH4	Cytoskeleton, extracellular matrix, spine morphology	+	+	Morris and Mervis (44)

second type of neurofibroma-related gene, NF2, which causes a different type of neurofibromatosis.

Heterozygous NF1 mutations result in human mental retardation in about 50% of cases. The heterogeneity of mutations in the NF1 gene is likely to contribute to its lack of complete penetrance for various phenotypes including the mental retardation phenotype. Thus, while *neurofibromatosis* was initially identified and named for the neurofibroma tumor phenotype, the genetic mutation also causes *mental retardation* in humans (2, 3).

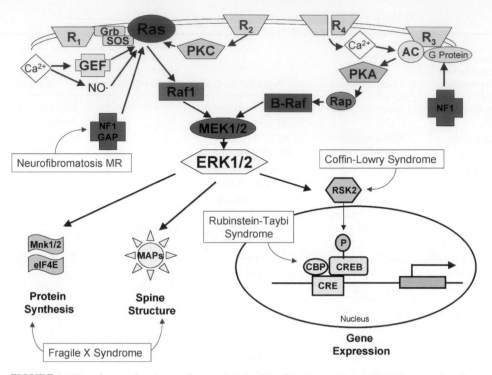

FIGURE 1   Signal transduction pathways involved in learning and memory. See text for discussion and additional definitions. R1 = growth factor receptor tyrosine kinases; R2 = phospholipase C coupled receptors; R3 = adenylyl cyclase coupled receptors; R4= ligand-gated calcium channels. MAPs = Microtubulin associated proteins. CBP = CREB binding protein. CRE = cAMP response element. Figure reproduced from Weeber and Sweatt (1).

The product of the NF1 gene is neuro-fibromin, a multidomain molecule that has the capacity to regulate several intracellular processes, including the ERK MAP kinase cascade, adenylyl cyclase, and cytoskeletal assembly. In vivo human neurofibromin is expressed as the product of four different mRNA splice variants, and the type I and type II variants are abundantly expressed in the brain. Alternative splicing of exon 23a in the gene results in the type I and type II variants; type II neurofibromin includes the 23a exon product while type I does not. In a sophisticated study using knockout mouse technology, Alcino Silva and his colleagues based at UCLA identified the 23a exon product as being critical for learning (4). Mice lacking the 23a product exhibited learning problems but no apparent developmental abnormalities nor

tumor predisposition, thus implicating the 23a-encoded protein domain as being involved in learning. The 23a-encoded domain of neurofibromin type I protein contributes to regulating the GAP (GTPase activating protein) domain of NF1, a domain that regulates interaction with the NF1 target ras (5, 6). As was described in Chapter 4, ras is a low-molecular-weight G protein coupled to downstream activation of the ERK cascade (see Figures 1 and 2).

In considering that the learning-associated exon of NF1 controlled its GAP activity, Alcino and his group proposed that loss of NF1 regulation of ras, specifically hyper-activation of ras, caused the learning disorder phenotype in Nf1 exon 23a−/− animals. However, because of the complexities of NF1 protein function, and indeed even the complexities of how the 23a exon

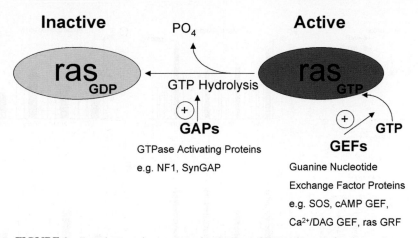

FIGURE 2   Regulation of ras activity by GAPs and GEFs. See text for discussions. Figure reproduced from Weeber and Sweatt (1). Adapted from Sweatt (45).

product might itself regulate GAP activity in NF1, the conclusion was inferential. Thus, it was necessary to come up with an independent line of evidence that the NF-1 mutation-associated learning deficits were indeed due to mis-regulation of ras. In impressive follow-up studies published in *Nature*, Rui Costa in Alcino's lab directly tested their hypothesis that ras hyper-activation caused learning deficiencies in NF1-deficient animals. In this series of studies, they used the classical genetic approach of diminishing ras function through heterozygous ras gene deletion, as well as using a pharmacologic inhibitor of ras activity in vivo to probe for interactions of the NF1 gene product with the ras pathway (7, 39).

The mouse model that they used was an NF1 knockout mouse with a heterozygous deficiency. Costa et al. assessed learning using the Morris water maze paradigm, which as we have already discussed, measures hippocampus-dependent spatial learning. They observed that heterozygous NF1-deficient animals exhibited deficits in the Morris maze task, as assessed using a probe trial and by quantitating quad-rant search time. Thus, as expected, heterozygous NF1-deficient mice mimicked aspects of the human learning defects associated with NF1 deficiency. Prior studies by another group (8) had shown directly that loss of NF1 led to aberrant activation of the ras/ERK cascade, specifically that NF1 heterozygous deficiency animals exhibited increased ras/ERK activity in non-neuronal cells. This observation directly suggested that alterations is ras activity occurred in these mice and, thus, could be causative of the learning phenotype, as Costa et al. had hypothesized based on their earlier studies with exon 23a-deficient mice.

To test this idea Costa et al. crossed NF1 heterozygous knockout animals with animals deficient in ras, reasoning appro-priately that if hyperactive ras caused the NF1+/− learning phenotype, then geneti-cally diminishing ras activity should rescue the animals to normal learning behavior. Costa et al. identified both N-ras and K-ras heterozygous deficiencies as rescuing the learning defect in NF1+/− mice (see Figure 3). These data strongly implicate ras, specifically N-ras and K-ras, as down-stream effectors of NF1 in vivo. Moreover, these findings implicate hyperactivation of this pathway as the cause of learning deficiencies in NF1-deficient mammals, including, of course, the human.

In all studies using animal models constitutively deficient in a gene product, it

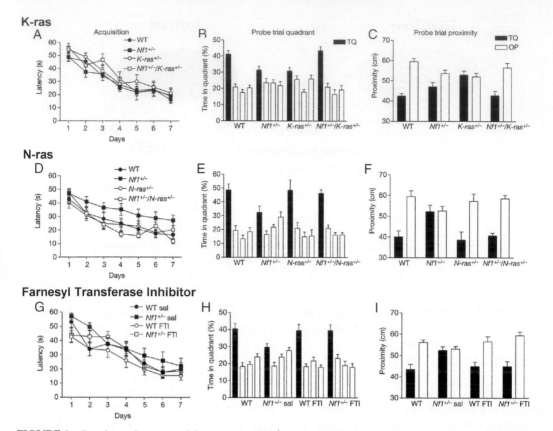

FIGURE 3 Ras-dependent spatial learning in Nf1$^{+/-}$ animals. These data illustrate that learning deficits of Nf1$^{+/-}$ mice are ras-dependent. Results shown are from the hidden version of the water maze for the Nf1$^{+/-}$/K-ras$^{+/-}$ population, $n = 11$ (wild type (WT), $n = 24$; Nf1$^{+/-}$, $n = 15$; K-ras$^{+/-}$, $n = 15$). (A) Latency to get to the platform over days. (B) Percent time spent in each quadrant during a probe trial. (C) Average proximity to the exact position where the platform was during training, compared with proximity to the opposite position in the pool. Panels D–F illustrate acquisition, percent time in quadrant, and proximity data for the Nf1$^{+/-}$/N-ras$^{+/-}$ population (WT, $n = 10$; Nf1$^{+/-}$, $n = 10$; N-ras$^{+/-}$, $n = 7$; Nf1$^{+/-}$/N-ras$^{+/-}$, $n = 9$). Panels G–I illustrate data obtained with acute pharmacologic inhibition of ras by use of a farnesyl transferase inhibitor (FTI). Acquisition, percent time in quadrant, and proximity data for the different genotypes and treatments during the FTI rescue experiment (WT + $_{FTI}$, $n = 19$; WT$_{saline}$, $n = 18$; Nf1$^{+/-}$$_{FTI}$, $n = 18$; Nf1$^{+/-}$$_{saline}$, $n = 18$). Quadrants are training quadrant (TQ), adjacent right, adjacent left and opposite quadrant (OP). Figure reproduced from Costa et al. (39).

is important to distinguish between the acute, ongoing need for the activity of the gene product versus a developmental necessity for the same protein. Alcino and his collaborators addressed this issue by acutely administering a farnesyl transferase inhibitor (which inhibits ras activity by disrupting its membrane association) and demonstrating that transient inhibition of ras in adult animals rescued the learning phenotype in NF1 heterozygous animals. Of course, farnesyl transferases act on other proteins besides ras, so a caveat to this experiment is the possibility of the inhibitor affecting other targets besides ras. However, their interpretation of a need for acute ras-dependent processes for adult learning and memory is also consistent with the wide variety of additional evidence we have already discussed implicating the ras/ERK cascade in learning.

Costa et al. next used their NF1+/− animal models to assess hippocampal long-term potentiation, using theta-burst

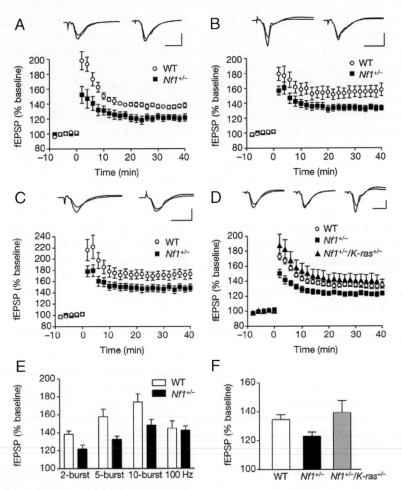

FIGURE 4   Ras-dependent LTP deficits in Nf1+/− animals. In panels A through D, neurofibromin 1 heterozygous deficiency animals exhibit LTP deficits for a variety of LTP induction protocols. Panel d illustrates that K-ras heterozygous deficiency rescues the Nf1-associated LTP deficit, indicating that it results from an overactivation of ras. For each panel, percentage of baseline field EPSP is plotted over time. (A) Two-burst induction protocol (wild-type (WT), $n = 5$; Nf1+/−, $n = 8$). (B) Five-burst induction protocol (WT, $n = 7$; Nf1+/−, $n = 8$). (C) Ten-burst induction protocol (WT, $n = 7$; Nf1+/−, $n = 11$). (D) Two-burst induction protocol ras rescue experiment, where heterozygous deficiency of K-ras rescues the LTP in Nf1-deficient animals. Thus, LTP deficits in Nf1+/− mice are ras-dependent (WT, $n = 13$; Nf1+/−, $n = 13$; Nf1+/−/K-ras+/−, $n = 8$). Representative traces are shown from left to right for WT, Nf1+/−, and Nf1+/−/K-ras+/−. Horizontal bar, 10 ms; vertical bar, 1 mV. (E) Summary of the amount of LTP measured 40 minutes after induction under the different stimulation protocols. (F) LTP measured 40 minutes after induction in the Nf1+/−/K-ras+/− rescue experiment is comparable to wild-type. Data, figure, and legend reproduced from Costa et al. (39).

stimulation. They found deficits in theta-burst LTP in NF1-deficient animals which, like the learning defects, were rescued by heterozygous deletion of ras (see Figure 4). One twist to the story is that Costa et al. found that alterations in GABAergic function are likely involved in the LTP phenotype, specifically GABAergic feed-forward inhibitory neurons in area CA1 that regulate cellular excitability and the likelihood of LTP induction under some conditions such as theta-burst stimulation. They observed that blocking this system rescued the effects of NF1 deficiency on

LTP, suggesting that NF-1 functioned to control this GABAergic system and, through this mechanism control the likelihood of LTP induction. They also directly observed enhanced GABAergic function in the NF1+/− animals in whole-cell recording of GABA inputs onto CA1 pyramidal neurons. Thus, the critical locus of NF1 function may be GABAergic interneurons. However, in additional, more recent studies, Alcino's group has also observed derangement of LTP in the pyramidal neurons of area CA1, using other types of LTP induction protocols that don't involve GABAergic interneurons. Thus, there is also an effect of NF1/ras in pyramidal neuron dendrites.

Having found that diminishing ras function led to a rescue of the phenotype, we are compelled to ask: what is the target of ras that leads to these derangements? As described in Chapter 4, ras regulates the MEK/ERK MAPK cascade in hippocampal neurons, and Ingram et al. (8) had previously reported elevated ERK activity in NF1-deficient animals. Thus, the most likely target is the raf/MEK/ERK signal transduction cascade. Moreover, other work by Alcino's research team has also nicely demonstrated an interaction of ras with the ERK cascade, using an approach they termed pharmacogenetics. They found that mice heterozygous for a null mutation of the K-ras gene (K-ras$^{+/-}$) showed normal hippocampal ERK activation, LTP, and contextual conditioning in a conditioned place preference task. However, treatment with a low dose of MEK inhibitor, ineffective in wild-type controls, blocked MAPK activation, LTP, and contextual learning in K-ras$^{+/-}$ mutants. These data strongly indicated that K-Ras is upstream of MEK/ERK signaling in hippocampus, and that acute activation of this pathway is involved in synaptic plasticity and memory.

Aside from direct ras/ERK cascade regulation another potential function of NF1 is regulating adenylyl cyclase; Tong et al. demonstrated that NF1 also regulates adenylyl cyclase in mammalian neurons (see reference 9 and Figure 1). They showed that neuropeptide and G-protein-stimulated adenylyl cyclase activity were reduced in mice completely deficient in NF1 activity. Even though the effects on adenylyl cyclase seen by Tong et al. were selective for animals with homozygous deletions of NF1, it is certainly worthwhile to consider that attenuation of subtle forms of regulation of adenylyl cyclase might play a role in learning deficits in heterozygous NF1-deficient animals as well. Of course, adenylyl cyclase also is upstream of the ERK MAP kinase cascade in hippocampal neurons (see Figure 1). Thus, NF1 may couple to erk via two pathways in the hippocampus, and both these effects may contribute to dysregulation of ERK in NF1-deficient mice and humans.

One of the targets of ERK in the hippocampus is CREB, and, as we have discussed, this molecule has been widely implicated in learning and memory in many species. ERK couples to CREB through the intervening kinase ribosomal S6 kinase (RSK2), which phosphorylates CREB at ser133 just like PKA. As I described in Chapter 7, in the mammalian hippocampus, it has been found that PKA cannot elicit CREB phosphorylation without going through ERK, thus ERK/RSK2 is an obligatory step in PKA regulation of CREB-mediated gene expression in mammalian hippocampal neurons (10, 11). The important implication of this in the present context is that rsk2 is the gene disrupted in human Coffin-Lowry Mental Retardation Syndrome (12, 13). Thus, the same pathway implicated in studies of Neurofibromatosis Mental Retardation, ERK/RSK2/CREB, has also been implicated as being involved in human learning and memory in an independent line of studies (see also Box 1).

Overall, while our current thinking is likely oversimplified, it is interesting that two different human mental retardation syndromes impinge upon the same signal transduction cascade, the ras/ERK/CREB cascade, which is coupled to regulation of gene expression in neurons. As we discussed earlier, it is noteworthy that this

---

BOX 1

RUBINSTEIN-TAYBI SYNDROME

Another mental retardation syndrome associated with the PKA/ERK/CREB pathway is Rubinstein-Taybi Syndrome (RTS). RTS patients have some facial abnormalities, broad big toes and thumbs, and mental retardation. The RTS gene has been mapped to chromosome 16 and identified as CREB Binding Protein (CBP). As described earlier, CBP is a transcriptional co-activator with CREB that obligatorily participates with phospho-CREB to regulate gene expression downstream of the CRE (20). CBP is a Histone Acetyl Transferase (HAT), and one mechanism through which CBP promotes gene expression is histone acetylation, which promotes exposure of DNA for transcription. CBP's loss of this HAT function likely is one important contributing factor in RTS, through derangements of the normal mechanisms controlling CREB-mediated gene expression. A partial knockout mouse model in which CBP activity is lost also exhibits learning deficiencies (20), which is similar to several other mental retardation syndromes that are highlighted in this chapter (see Table 1).

---

same cascade has been implicated in learning and memory in a wide variety of different species—it is now safe in my opinion to add the human to the list.

It also is interesting to speculate about another potential downstream target of the ERK cascade, the protein synthesis machinery (see Figure 1). This target is appealing given the widespread documentation that we have discussed concerning a role for protein synthesis in learning. As was described in Chapter 7, ERK is known to regulate protein synthesis by regulating the activity of eIF4E via the intervening kinase mnk. Also, a known role for RSK2, the Coffin-Lowry Syndrome gene product, is regulation of protein synthesis. It is intriguing to consider protein synthesis as a potential target downstream of the gene products for Neurofibromatosis and Coffin-Lowry Syndrome because the Fragile X Mental Retardation type 1 (FMR1) gene product (FMRP) likely contributes to regulating protein synthesis as well (14); we will discuss this in Section III. This potentially would tie yet a third human mental retardation gene product, the Fragile X Protein, into a common signaling/regulatory cascade.

It is notable that no mutation in any of the core signaling components of the ras/ERK cascade (ras, raf, mek, and ERK) has been identified as linked to human learning disorders to date. I think that it is unlikely that this will ever be the case because, as we have already discussed, the role of these enzymes is in no way limited to learning and memory—this pathway was discovered as one of the core signaling components controlling cell division. Loss of the core signal transduction cascade quite likely could result in cellular lethality. Mutations in modulators of the ras/ERK cascade such as NF1, of course, can lead to viable animals. In the specific case of the neurofibromatosis gene, the gene was initially discovered as an oncogene, which when mutated leads to uncontrolled cell division in specific cells. Subsequent work led to the discovery of its role in regulating ras-dependent processes, which is, of course, consistent with the fundamental role of the ras/ERK cascade in regulating cell division.

In thinking about these disparate roles of the ras/ERK cascade in both learning and cell division, it is interesting to consider that in the early 1970s President Nixon declared a "war on cancer", which in part led to increased cancer funding and great progress in understanding the regulation of mammalian cell division. Also, a great number of oncogenes were discovered in this era, which were named for the cancers with which they are associated. If Nixon had instead declared a "war on mental retardation," I find it interesting to think that cancer biologists might now be scratching their heads, wondering what all these learning-related genes were doing regulating cell division.

II. ANGELMAN SYNDROME

The use of traditional (i.e., non-inducible) knockout mouse models to try to study the signal transduction events involved in synaptic plasticity and memory has been widely and legitimately criticized because of the great confound of secondary effects of loss of the gene. In particular, developmental derangements can contribute to any observed phenotype, and there is a real concern that the effect of loss of the gene product is not an indication of the protein having any necessary role in an acute, learning-related signal transduction event. Need for caution in interpreting these types of experiments is highlighted by the numerous demonstrations that these types of developmental and secondary effects do occur in knockout animals.

However, this weakness in the context of one type of experiment is a strength of knockout models in another context. In making a model of a human inherited (i.e., genetic) disorder such as a mental retardation syndrome, one wishes to have the defect present from the point of conception, as is typically the case for the analogous human. The generation of secondary molecular and developmental effects is desirable in that they model the same secondary effects that are likely to occur in the human. Thus, a strength of the

knockout approach in mouse models of human mental retardation is that, by characterizing the knockout mice, one can gain insights into the entire range of molecular and anatomical effects that contribute to the human learning disorder.

In this section, we will be discussing a mouse model for human Angelman Mental Retardation Syndrome. Current thinking in the area is that the Angelman gene product is not itself directly involved in signaling events necessary for learning and memory (although it is too early to really rule this out!), but that secondary changes in targets of the gene product lead to disruption of signaling events necessary for memory. Tracking down these secondary changes has been an interesting "detective story" that Ed Weeber in my laboratory has been pursuing in collaboration with Yong-hui Jiang and Art Beaudet in the Genetics Department here at Baylor College of Medicine. While we are only part of the way there, our recent results suggest that one culprit in Angelman Syndrome is dysregulation of CaMKII.

Angelman Syndrome is a fairly rare (~1/15,000) but severe human learning and behavioral disorder characterized by four principal features: (1) developmental delay and pronounced mental retardation: (2) near or total absence of the capacity for language and speech; (3) motor dysfunction; (4) an abnormally cheerful disposition, propensity for laughter, and cheerful affect. In addition, a history of seizures often presents. The principal features of Angelman Syndrome led to the unfortunate use of the description "Happy Puppet Syndrome" for these patients at one point in time.

As with most mental retardation syndromes the underlying genetic etiology is mixed, in large part due to heterogeneity of deletion mutations that can lead to the disorder. Despite this complexity, recent efforts have identified the gene for Angelman Syndrome as UBE3A, which codes for the E6-AP ubiquitin ligase. E6-AP is an E3 ubiquitin ligase, which covalently attaches

BOX 2

DOWN'S SYNDROME

Mental retardation can arise not only from loss or derangement of the function of a gene product but also from aberrant over-production of a gene product. One example of mental retardation in this category is Down's Syndrome. Down's Syndrome results not from a genetic mutation but from aber-rant chromosome duplication, specifically duplication of one copy of chromosome 21. For this reason, Down's Syndrome is also referred to as Trisomy 21. Because of this unique mechanism, Down's Syndrome is not a heritable disorder in the usual sense—it arises as an epigenetic phenomenon as part of the initial stages of chromosome replication during oocyte generation or oocyte fertilization.

Thus, Down's Syndrome arises as a result of the overproduction of proteins encoded by the genes on chromosome 21. Obviously the molecular basis of the syndrome is quite complex because of the plethora of gene products potentially involved. However, portions of chromosome 21 (region q22.2 specifically) that are critical for the development of Down's Syndrome have been identified. This region is referred to as the Down's Syndrome "critical locus" or "critical region." In part, this region was identified by characterizing Down's Syndrome patients who had not undergone complete duplication of chromosome 21. It is not clear at present precisely which genes in the critical region (or combination of genes) results in Down's Syndrome, and this is an area of active research at present.

Two genes on chromosome 21 are receiving particular attention at this point, because they are interesting in the context of known signal transduction mechanisms that we have been discussing as related to learning and memory. These are DYRK1 and superoxide dismutase (SOD, see refer-ences 35–37). DYRK1 is the human homo-logue to *Drosophila* minibrain kinase, which was identified in that species as a nervous system development-related gene. DYRK1 is homologous to members of the MAP kinase superfamily. The targets and mecha-nisms for regulation of DYRK1/minibrain kinase are unclear at present but are under active investigation. SOD is another inter-esting candidate. As we discussed in Chapters 6 and 7, superoxide has been implicated as a signaling molecule in hippocampal LTP, which is hypothesized to act through its capability to lead to autonomous PKC activation. Thus the interesting model arises that part of the defects in Down's Syndrome are due to overexpression of SOD and attenuation of superoxide signaling in the nervous system. In fact, transgenic animal models have indicated that this is a viable hypothesis, as SOD-overproducing mice have deficits in LTP and hippocampus-dependent memory formation.

A final chromosome 21 gene worth noting is the gene for amyloid precursor protein (APP). As we will discuss in more detail in Chapter 11, overproduction of the APP-derived product amyloid beta peptide likely leads to Alzheimer's Disease. Gene duplication of the APP gene in Down's Syndrome patients leads to overproduction of amyloid beta peptide, and unfortunately almost all Down's Syndrome patients who live past the age of 35 develop Alzheimer's Disease-like pathology as well.

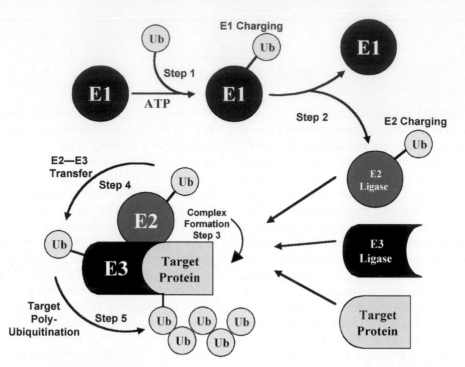

FIGURE 5   The ubiquitination pathway. Covalent association of an E1 subunit with a single ubiquitin (Ub) molecule results in the ATP-dependent activation of Ub (Step 1). Ub is then transferred to an E2 subunit (Step 2). Association of the E2 and/or E3 plus the target protein results in the formation of a complex (Step 3). Complex formation results in the transfer of Ub by E2 either directly to the target protein or through the transfer of the Ub to an E3 (Step 4). E3 transfers successive UB molecules to the target protein forming poly-UB chains (Step 5). Reproduced from Weeber and Sweatt (46).

the low-molecular-weight protein ubiquitin to substrate proteins (see Figure 5), a complex process involving other proteins that serve as intermediates and modulators of the final ubiquitination step. Ubiquitination, of course, by and large serves to control trafficking of proteins to the proteasome for degradation. However it is important to keep in mind that new functions for ubiquitination are being discovered. These new features play a signal transduction role conceptually similar to other post-translational processes like phosphorylation.

The Angelman Syndrome E6-AP E3 ligase is one member of a large family of around 60 different E3 ligases, each of which has different substrate selectivities. The E6-AP protein has a very restricted substrate specificity—known substrates include the p53 tumor suppressor protein,

E6-AP itself, and one additional protein of unknown function.

Expression of the UBE3A gene, in both human and mouse, exhibits a phenomenon called *imprinting*. Imprinting is a general term to describe epigenetic phenomena that can result in silencing the expression of a particular gene. In the case of the UBE3A gene, imprinting, through complex mechanisms that are not entirely clear at this point, results in selective silencing of the paternal copy of the gene in the hippocampus and cerebellum. The upshot of this is that the maternal copy of the gene is selectively expressed in these brain subregions. Thus, offspring who inherit a defective copy of UBE3A from their mother have a selective loss of the E6-AP ubiquitin ligase in their hippocampus and cerebellum. Put in genetics jargon, maternal deficiency (m–/p+) results in a subregion specific

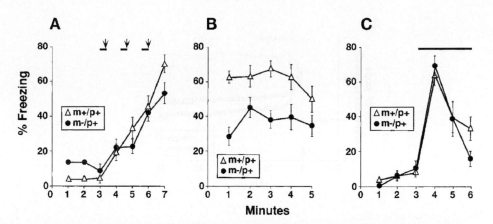

FIGURE 6 Selective deficit in context-dependent fear conditioning in ubiquitin ligase maternal deficiency mice. The E6AP ubiquitin ligase gene (the Angelman Syndrome gene) exhibits imprinting such that the maternal copy of the gene is selectively expressed in the hippocampus. Offspring of a female mouse deficient in the E6AP ubiquitin ligase thus have a selective hippocampal loss of the E6AP subtype of E3 ubiquitin ligase. In these experiments, wild-type mice or maternal deficiency mice were assessed for both contextual (Panel B) or cued (Panel C) fear conditioning 24 hours after training (Panel A). The same group of maternal deficiency mice (n = 12) and wild-type mice (n = 12) were assessed for both context- and tone-dependent freezing. (A) Wild-type and maternal deficiency mice showed comparable freezing during and after the tone and foot shock were administered. (B) Context dependent fear conditioning: Maternal deficiency mice displayed significantly less freezing than wild-type when returned to the test chamber 24 hours later. Significant p values (< .001 were seen at each sampling period and for the total data by X^2 test. (C) Tone-dependent fear conditioning: Maternal deficiency mice and wild-type mice showed comparable freezing when presented with the tone in a novel context immediately after context-dependent testing. Tone is shown by horizontal bar and shock is indicated by arrows. Data and figures reproduced from Jiang et al. (40). Copyright Cell Press.

knockout of E6AP in both the mouse and human. Angelman Syndrome patients have a rare defect—a brain subregion-selective loss of a specific protein. This imprinting pattern and subregion-selective defect is, of course, consistent with the deficits observed in these patients, which selectively involve learning and motor control. It seems clear on its face that understanding the underlying pathology of Angelman Syndrome patients will give insights into the effects of hippocampal lesions in the human, much like studies of other patients such as H. M. have done. In the case of Angelman Syndrome patients, however, the lesion is genetic and not anatomical—in fact, there appear to be no discernable anatomical malformations in the CNS of AS patients. In Angelman Syndrome patients, the defect is, of course, also present from birth, in contrast to lesions such as those experienced by H. M.

After Kishino et al. discovered that the UBE3A gene was the Angelman Syndrome gene, Yong-hui Jiang in Art Beaudet's lab at Baylor College of Medicine developed ube3a knockout mice in order to generate a murine model for Angelman Syndrome. Yong-hui, who was a graduate student at the time, came down the hall to my lab to undertake a behavioral and electrophysiologic characterization of his interesting mice. He studied the maternal deficiency mice, as opposed to other types of heterozygous or homozygous knockout animals, in order to model the human syndrome most accurately. Yong-hui discovered that mice with a maternal deficiency in ube3a ubiquitin ligase exhibited a selective deficit in contextual fear conditioning, consistent with the selective loss of *hippocampal* ubiquitin ligase due to the maternal imprinting (see reference 15 and Figure 6). The same mice did not exhibit any deficit in

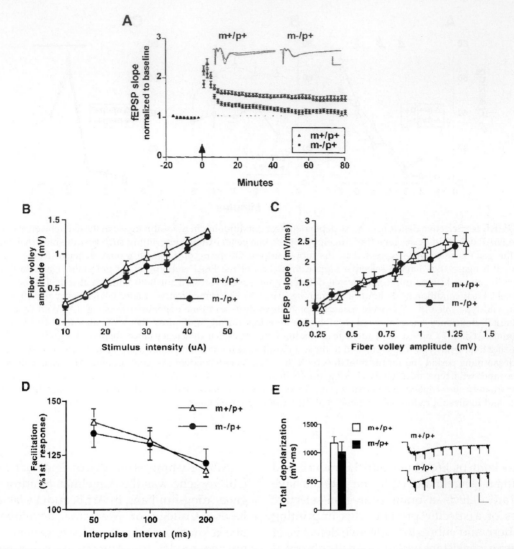

FIGURE 7   Impairment of hippocampal LTP in ubiquitin ligase maternal deficiency mice. (A) Summary of field potential recordings from the CA1 region (mean ± SEM) from wild-type (n = 17 slices, 11 animals) and E6AP maternal deficiency mice (14 slices, 6 animals). Baseline measurements were taken for at least 20 minutes to confirm stability. Stimulation intensity was adjusted for responses that were ~50% of the maximal fEPSP. Two 100-Hz, 1-second stimuli were given at time 0. Each point is a 2-minute average of six individual fEPSP measurements. The inset presents extracellular field recordings from a representative experiment during a basline interval and 60 minutes after induction of LTP for a wild-type (m+/p+) and a maternal deficiency (m−/p+) slice. Scale bars for inset, 2 mV and 4 ms. (B & C) Baseline synaptic responses were similar for maternal deficiency and wild-type mice. Plots of fiber volley amplitude versus stimulus strength and fEPSP slope versus fiber volley amplitude revealed no difference between wild-type and maternal deficiency mice. Results shown are from nine slices for wild-type and eight slices for maternal deficiency mice. (D) Paired-pulse facilitation is not impaired in maternal deficiency mice. The magnitude of the second response is presented as a percentage of the first response. Results shown are from five slices for wild-type and seven slices for maternal deficiency animals. (E) Responses to tetanic stimulation are not different between maternal deficiency and wild-type mice. Total depolarization (the integral of the tetanic depolarization response) is presented for wild-type (n = 6, upper trace) and maternal deficiency (n = 6, lower trace) animals. Scale bars for inset, 2 mV and 90 ms. Reproduced from Jiang et al. (40).

cued conditioning. This serves as a nice positive control for the animals having normal capacity in the amygdala-dependent, hippocampus-independent component of the task.

In addition, hippocampal slices prepared from maternal deficiency mice exhibited a loss of long-term potentiation of Schaffer/collateral inputs in area CA1, but normal stimulus-response relationships and paired-pulse facilitation (see Figure 7). Thus, the hippocampus-dependent learning deficit apparently can be accounted for by a selective loss of LTP in the hippocampus — a striking finding considering that hippocampal baseline synaptic transmission, short-term plasticity, and hippocampal anatomy all appear normal in these mice.

In a broad sense these findings implicate the ubiquitin/proteosome pathway in mammalian associative learning and hippocampal long-term potentiation. This represents an interesting parallel to a variety of evidence demonstrating a role for the ubiquitin pathway in long-term facilitation and long-term memory in *Aplysia*. In this system, long-term behavioral sensitization is in part subserved by ubiquitin-mediated proteolysis of PKA regulatory subunits, which elicits long-term increases in PKA activity and long-term facilitation of neurotransmitter release (see Box 3). In the future, it will be interesting to determine to what extent the roles of the ubiquitin system in mammals parallels those in *Aplysia*.

BOX 3

THE UBIQUITIN SYSTEM PLAYS A ROLE IN SYNAPTIC PLASTICITY AND MEMORY IN *APLYSIA*

Eric Kandel and his colleagues—Jimmy Schwartz, Vince Castellucci, Jack Byrne, and Bob Hawkins, along with many others— have used the simple marine mollusk *Aplysia californica* to great effect to study the behavioral attributes and cellular and molecular mechanisms of learning and memory. Much (but by no means all) of the work in *Aplysia* has been geared toward understanding the basis of sensitization in this animal. *Aplysia* has on its dorsum a respiratory gill and siphon complex, which is normally extended when the animal is in the resting state. If the gill or siphon is lightly touched (or experimentally, squirted with a Water-Pic), a defensive withdrawal reflex is elicited in order to protect the gill from potential damage. This defensive withdrawal reflex can undergo both habituation

(by repeated light stimuli) and sensitization. Sensitization occurs when the animal receives an aversive stimulus, for example a modest tail-shock experimentally. After sensitizing stimulation, the animal exhibits a more robust, longer-lasting gill withdrawal in response to the identical light touch or water squirt.

Initial progress in this system came by way of beginning to understand the neuronal circuitry underlying the defensive withdrawal reflex and the associated modulatory inputs from the tail. One appeal of the *Aplysia* experimental system was the relatively simple nervous system in the animal, allowing the tracing of significant parts of the circuitry underlying the behavior using electrophysiology techniques. This circuit tracing was greatly facilitated

Continued

BOX 3—cont'd

THE UBIQUITIN SYSTEM PLAYS
A ROLE IN SYNAPTIC PLASTICITY
AND MEMORY IN *APLYSIA*

by the enormous (relatively speaking) size of the neurons in *Aplysia*, allowing for easy microelectrode recording from specific, identified neurons in the animal's CNS.

A greatly simplified description of the circuitry underlying sensitization of the gill- and siphon-withdrawal reflex in *Aplysia* is as follows (we will cover this in more detail in Chapter 12). The touch to the gill and siphon complex stimulates siphon sensory neurons, which make direct and indirect connections (via interneurons) to gill motor neurons. The gill motor neurons stimulate muscles in the gill and siphon complex that mediate the defensive withdrawal reflex. The tail shock impinges upon this circuit by way of tail sensory neurons, which make direct contacts (and indirect contacts by way of interneurons) with the presynaptic terminals of the siphon sensory neurons.

It was soon realized that plasticity at the siphon sensory neuron/gill motor neuron synapse is one critical locus contributing to sensitization in the animal—one of the first demonstrations of the importance of synaptic plasticity in learning and memory. A predominant component of plasticity at this synapse is increased neurotransmitter release from the siphon sensory neurons. Thus, tail shock and the attendant activity in tail sensory neurons and associated interneurons leads to release of modulatory neurotransmitters onto the siphon sensory neuron presynaptic terminal, increasing the release of neurotransmitter from these cells and augmenting the defensive withdrawal reflex. These observations highlighted the role of *presynaptic facilitation* of neurotransmitter release as a mechanism for memory in this system.

Although all of the modulatory neurotransmitters involved in presynaptic facilitation in *Aplysia* sensory neurons are not yet identified, one important player is 5-Hydroxytryptamine (5HT, serotonin). Serotonin is released onto a subset of the siphon sensory neurons by a serotonergic tail sensory neuron stimulated by tail shock. In fact, serotonin application to siphon sensory neurons elicits the vast majority of the physiologic responses contributing to presynaptic facilitation of neurotransmitter release and sensitization in the animal.

As mentioned previously, sensitization in *Aplysia* exhibits both short-term and long-term forms. Similarly, in sensory neurons, serotonin application can lead to either short-term or long-term facilitation of neurotransmitter release. Single (5-minute) applications of serotonin give facilitation that lasts only a few minutes; repeated (5 × 5 minutes over the course of an hour) applications give facilitation lasting at least 24 hours.

What happens when the sensory neuron sees repeated applications of serotonin, which elicit long-lasting synaptic facilitation? Although many mechanistic details have not yet been worked out, several key steps resulting from 5HT application have been identified. The long-lasting elevation of cAMP leads to PKA activation and subsequent phosphorylation of CREB, and one of the genes whose activity CREB regulates controls an important pathway for the ubiquitination of specific proteins. The ubiquitin pathway is recruited to cause proteolytic degradation of one subunit of PKA, the PKA regulatory subunit (21, 22). Loss of regulatory subunits results in a

---

BOX 3—cont'd

THE UBIQUITIN SYSTEM PLAYS A ROLE IN SYNAPTIC PLASTICITY AND MEMORY IN *APLYSIA*

decrease in the overall ratio of regulatory to catalytic subunits, promoting an excess of free, active catalytic subunits and a persistent increase in PKA activity. By this clever mechanism, a chain of events is set in motion whereby a biochemical effect is established in the cell that outlasts the initial, triggering elevation of the second messenger cAMP. The PKA will remain activated until compensatory resynthesis of new regulatory subunit occurs, or until the catalytic subunit is degraded. Interestingly, although the mechanism has not yet been worked out, recent evidence indicates that the DAG-responsive effector PKC also is persistently activated after serotonin stimulation of sensory neurons. Available evidence indicates that the persistent activation of PKA underlies an intermediate stage of facilitation, lasting on the order of many hours after the triggering applications of serotonin are finished. Interestingly, pioneering work on this mechanism was performed using sensitization training in animals, emphasizing the strong likelihood of this mechanism contributing to the underlying cellular basis for the change in the animal's behavior. We will return to the *Aplysia* system in greater detail in Chapter 12. For the present, it represents an interesting example of regulation of synaptic plasticity by the ubiquitin system, and thus an interesting parallel to the identification of a role for ubiquitination in memory based on studies of Angelman Syndrome.

To the extent that deficiencies in the mouse model for Angelman Syndrome reflect those in human Angelman Syndrome patients, Yong-hui's data suggest that defects in hippocampal long-term potentiation may underlie the learning defects exhibited in Angelman Syndrome. Angelman mice have normal synaptic transmission, short-term plasticity, and hippocampal morphology. Anatomical studies of humans indicate that their hippocampal morphology is similarly normal. Thus, Angelman Syndrome humans appear to have a selective deficit in synaptic plasticity with normal baseline function based on their anatomical characterization and extrapolating from the mouse model findings. Because the UBE3A gene is imprinted, AS patients likely have this loss of synaptic plasticity restricted to their hippocampus (and cerebellum). Thus, these patients appear to have a very precise and selective lesion, in contrast to patients such as H. M. where there is extensive and imprecise anatomical derangement and, of course, loss of anatomical connections to and from the hippocampus. To the best of our ability to determine what is happening in the human based on studies of the mouse model, selective deficits in hippocampal long-term synaptic plasticity are what lead to the profound learning and memory deficits of Angelman Syndrome. In my mind, this is one of the most important findings to come out of this work.

What are the targets of the E6-AP ubiquitin ligase pathway that lead to this striking memory dysfunction? One possibility, as mentioned previously, is that this E3 ligase is serving as a signal transduction pathway that modulates downstream targets acutely. Although this is a possibility, there is no direct evidence to suggest this at present, and a much more parsimonious hypothesis is that the E6-AP is playing the more traditional role of controlling the level of target proteins by sending them to the proteasome. In this scenario, loss of E6-AP will secondarily lead to elevations in the levels of downstream targets resulting from loss of this mechanism for their degradation. At present, we prefer this hypothesis of secondary effects to increase the levels of downstream targets, although it is certainly always necessary to keep an open mind.

In considering this hypothesis, I note that it does not immediately lead to a lot of specific possibilities. The E6AP E3 ligase apparently has a very restricted set of substrates, as mentioned earlier, so not many candidates come to mind as downstream targets. One known substrate is the p53 tumor suppressor. In fact, maternal deficiency mice exhibit altered levels of p53 in hippocampal pyramidal neurons, so this is one potential mechanism. Disappointingly, however, p53 function is difficult to tie in to synaptic plasticity based on our present state of knowledge. In short, nothing specific about the function of p53 suggests how it could lead to a derangement of LTP and memory.

To try to address the problem in a different way, Ed Weeber in my lab decided to test for derangements in the signal transduction mechanisms that we already knew were involved in normal memory formation. In collaboration with Yong-hui and Art Beaudet, Ed set about using hippocampal tissue from the Angelman mouse model in Western blotting screens, to see if any candidate molecules know to function in LTP could be identified. To make a long story very short, after looking at a wide variety of specific proteins and protein kinases, we found an alteration in hippocampal CaMKII.

The alteration was in Thr286 autophosphorylation, not total protein level, which was quite surprising to us because we had expected the loss of proteolysis of a target protein to lead to an increase in the level of that protein. Nevertheless, Ed observed that hippocampal extracts from Angelman mice exhibited a selective increase in Thr286 autophosphorylation with no change in total protein.

Based on the known property of Thr286 autophosphorylation to render the kinase autonomously active, we next tested these hippocampal extracts for increases in CaMKII activity. In fact, to our further surprise in these studies, we found that Angelman mice had *decreased* CaMKII activity. Further studies in collaboration with Ype Elgersma and Alcino Silva indicated the answer to this mystery. These studies showed that there was aberrant hyperphosphorylation of CaMKII at the inhibitory site, thr305/306. This increased inhibitory autophosphorylation is the likely mechanism through which there is a diminution of CaMKII activity in Angelman hippocampus.

Is this single molecular change, increased autophosphorylation at thr305, sufficient to cause Angelman Syndrome? In a complementary series of studies, Alcino's lab converged on this same hypothesis using a transgenic point mutant animal that mimicked hyperphosphorylation at the 305 site, a transgenic animal expressing a thr-to-asp CaMKII point mutant. Their motivation for generating this animal arose from their years of work investigating the details of CaMKII function and phosphorylation in synaptic plasticity and memory. Strikingly, the data from Alcino's lab indicated that the 305 hyperphosphorylation is indeed sufficient to give an LTP and learning phenotype reminiscent of Angelman syndrome. Thus, approaching a problem from two very different viewpoints, my lab and Alcino's once again converged on a common answer.

We do not know the basis of the hyperphosphorylation. Our current working hypothesis, which is very speculative, is that E6AP regulates the level of some protein(s) that controls phosphatase activity, perhaps a phosphatase inhibitor. This would link up proteolysis, which presumably controls the steady-state level of some protein in the cell, with the phosphorylation increase that we have observed. As mentioned earlier, we certainly at this point cannot rule out the involvement of a more acute, signal—transduction type process wherein ubiquitination acutely controls a target's catalytic activity.

Overall these data strongly indicate that the normal function of the CaMKII cascade is necessary for human synaptic plasticity and memory. Specifically, these findings implicate the subtle derangement of regulatory mechanisms for CaMKII in the pronounced memory dysfunction of Angelman Syndrome. As was the case with studies of neurofibromatosis and the ras/ERK cascade, once again decades of study of the basic signal transduction mechanisms for synaptic plasticity and memory converged with studies of human mental retardation.

III. FRAGILE X SYNDROMES

A. Fragile X Mental Retardation Syndrome Type 1

In the late 1980s, an interesting new mechanism for gene disruption was discovered as an outgrowth of studies investigating the genetic basis of human degenerative CNS disorders—the *triplet repeat* mechanism. The essential discovery was that in humans there are repetitive DNA sequences, specifically CGG or similar trinucleotide sequences, that can expand in length (i.e., number of CGG repeats) from generation to generation. In general, once a triplet repeat sequence in or around a gene reaches a critical length, normal expression of the gene product is disrupted. Thus, from one generation to the next a family can go from normal

expression of a gene product to loss of that same gene due to triplet repeat expansion.

In another variation of triplet repeat-based disorders, the loss of gene function is not precipitous. For example, in a number of neurodegenerative disorders, the family exhibits *anticipation*, which refers to a progressive decrease in age-of-onset for the disorder from generation to generation. The decrease in age-of-onset is highly correlated with the length of the triplet repeat expansion.

The exact mechanisms by which triplet repeats disrupt gene expression and gene product function are complex and subject to vigorous investigation at present. If the CGG triplet repeat lies within a coding region of a gene, it can result in the expression of a protein product containing polyglutamine. The presence of the polyglutamine stretch can, of course, disrupt the normal function of the protein in which it resides. Alternatively, the expression in cell of polyglutamine itself can be toxic, essentially (or theoretically even directly) resulting in a toxic "gain of function" gene product. Again, the exact mechanisms by which cellular expression of polyglutamine-containing proteins in neurons leads to neurodegeneration is unclear at present and represents an active area of investigation.

There also are a number of ways the presence of triplet repeats has been found to affect gene expression. In myotonic dystrophy, the disorder in which triplet repeats were first identified, the mechanism appears to be due to disruption of the function of upstream regulatory DNA sequences that control expression of a protein kinase referred to as dystrophin protein kinase (a.k.a. DMPK, see Figure 8 of chapter 8), although other genes may also be affected.

For other triplet repeat-based disorders the mechanism is also caused by the loss of gene/protein expression, but through more complex mechanisms (see Box 4). One example in this category is fragile X mental retardation type 1 (14, 16, 17). Fragile X

BOX 4
_____

RETT SYNDROME

Rett Syndrome is an unusual disorder in girls that manifests itself as an age-dependent progressive decline in cognitive function starting after the first year of life. Among its attributes are diminished brain size, mental retardation, the development of stereotyped hand-wringing movements, and ultimately autism-like features. The gene for Rett Syndrome is on the X chromosome, and embryonic lethality in males (which, of course, have only one copy of the X chromosome) likely leads to the syndrome being selectively observed in girls. However, recent findings of Rett gene mutations in boys may lead to identification of a new homologous syndrome in males.

The Rett gene encodes methyl-CpG binding protein 2 (MECP2, see reference 23). As discussed in the main text, DNA methylation plays a role in transcriptional silencing of genes, and MECP is a protein that binds to methylated DNA sequencing and contributes to suppressing the expression of genes in the vicinity. Thus, loss of MECP2 leads to aberrant expression of genes that are normally silent. There is, of course, the potential that a large number of genes are affected secondarily to loss of MECP2, and experiments are underway to determine target genes of this pathway. Studies in this area are also giving important new insights into the mechanisms involved in DNA methylation-associated transcriptional silencing.

---

mental retardation syndrome, often abbreviated FRAXA, is one of the most common and debilitating forms of human mental retardation, with a frequency of occurrence in the 1/2,000 range. The FMR1 gene promoter region in normal humans has 5–50 CGG repeats, which do not adversely affect gene expression. Expansion of the repeats into the 200-repeat range leads to loss of gene expression, and the mechanism for this gene loss is complex (see Figure 8). With expanded repeat number, the FMR1 gene promoter region undergoes DNA methylation at C residues of CpG dinucleotides, resulting in gene silencing. Of course, loss of gene transcription leads to loss of mRNA and protein synthesis. Again, the means by which DNA methylation leads to transcriptional repression is an active and important area of research (see Box 4). Current models highlight the importance of methyl-CpG binding proteins and

their recruitment of histone deacetylation mechanisms as a component of the gene silencing process.

The product of the FMR1 gene is referred to as FMRP, the fragile X mental retardation protein. Although the function of this protein is still being investigated, several studies have indicated that FMRP is an RNA binding protein. As we have already discussed, a current model proposes that FMRP regulates protein synthesis by binding a variety of mRNA species (see Chapters 7 and 8). Moreover, Bill Greenough's group at the University of Illinois has found that FMRP function is necessary for metabotropic glutamate receptor regulation of protein synthesis in synaptoneurosomes, or pinched-off dendritic/presynaptic processes (14). Other studies have also indicated derangements of dendritic spine numbers and morphology in Fragile X tissue samples and in a fragile X mouse

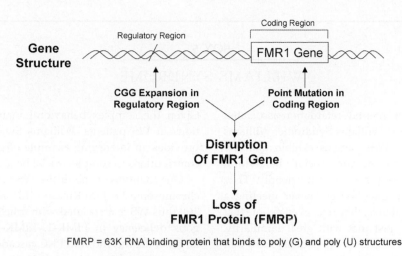

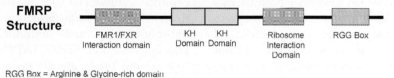

FIGURE 8   A model for Fragile X Mental Retardation Syndrome. Triplet repeats in the regulatory region, or mutations in the coding region, of the FMR1 gene lead to (among other things) a loss of the FMR1 gene product, FMRP. FMRP is an RNA binding protein proposed to be involved in dendritic mRNA localization and local protein synthesis (see text for additional discussion).

model (see also Box 5 and reference 18). Thus, while studies in this area are still at a relatively early stage, the intriguing hypothesis is emerging that FMRP plays a key role in local protein synthesis in dendrites, and, by disrupting this process, leads to the learning derangements of fragile X. As the potential role of FMRP in dendritic protein synthesis was discussed in detail in Chapter 7, I won't reiterate the particulars here. Suffice it to say that once again we see an example of how detailed studies of the molecular mechanisms of synaptic plasticity have converged with studies of a human learning disorder.

B. Fragile X Mental Retardation Type 2

Fragile X mental retardation type 2 (FMR2), similar to the case with FMR1, results from expansion and methylation of a CCG trinucleotide repeat located in exon 1 of the X-linked FMR2 gene, which results in transcriptional silencing. While the FMR1 syndrome and FMR2 mental retardation share a similar name and mechanism of mutation, FMR2 (a.k.a. FRAXE) is "nonsyndromic" (see Box 6). Also, in contrast to the profound mental retardation of FMR1, loss of the FMR2 gene product is associated with a milder mental impairment. Among those with the FMR2 phenotype, delays in language development are particularly prominent, and some FMR2 patients also have behavioral deficits, such as attention deficit, hyperactivity, and autistic-like behavior. Also in contrast to Fragile X type 1, which is likely the most common form of mental retardation, expansion of the FMR2-associated CCG repeat is quite rare, with an incidence estimated at less than 1:50,000.

Expansion and methylation of a CCG repeat in the 5' untranslated region (UTR)

BOX 5

WILLIAMS SYNDROME

Another mental retardation-associated syndrome is Williams Syndrome. Williams Syndrome (WS) patients exhibit an interesting idiosyncratic social behavioral syndrome—they are overly friendly. They have been described as "never meeting a stranger", that is, they treat even people that they have just met with great familiarity. Behavioral studies of WS patients show that they manifest an abnormal positive bias toward unknown individuals (24). They also exhibit spatio-visual processing deficits and mild to severe mental retardation. Williams Syndrome arises from deletions in chromosome 7 that typically include multiple genes.

Given the complex behavioral manifestations in WS patients, Williams Syndrome provides an interesting example of genetic contributions to complex social behaviors.

One identified gene in the WS locus on chromosome 7 is LIM Kinase 1 (LIMK-1; 25, 26), thus WS is associated with a heterozygous deficiency in LIMK-1. LIMK-1 is a target of the rac, rho, and PKC cascades that controls cytoskeletal organization (see figure). LIMK-1 exerts its effects through phosphorylating and inhibiting Actin Depolymerization Factor (ADF)/cofilin. ADF/cofilin binds directly to actin and promotes actin depolymerization. Thus,

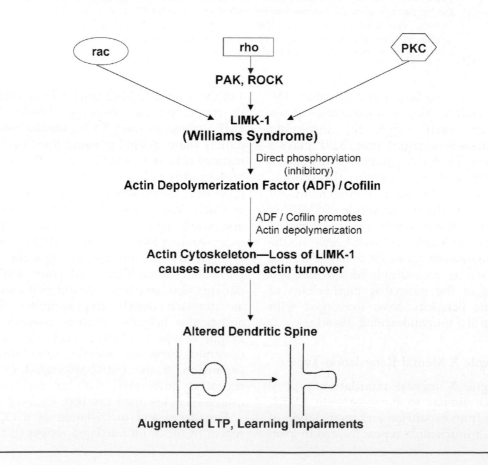

BOX 5—cont'd

WILLIAMS SYNDROME

the LIMK-1 pathway is one of the specific mechanisms whereby the rho system regulates cytoskeletal structure.

LIMK-1 homozygous knockout mice, as might be expected, have alterations in actin microfilaments owing to derangements of actin turnover (27). They also manifest altered dendritic spine morphology at Schaffer-collateral synapses in the hippocampus. Specifically, they have fewer actin microfilaments than the normally actin-dense spines, and the dendritic spines in LIMK-1 knockout mice lack the normal bulbous ending that dendritic spines exhibit. There are no apparent alterations in synaptic number or baseline synaptic function, however. Like FMR2 knockout mice, LIMK-1 knockouts exhibit LTP that saturates at a higher level than controls—a higher maximal level of potentiation is achieved with repetitive LTP-inducing stimulation.

This alteration in synaptic plasticity is associated with impaired learning as well. Specifically, LIMK-1 knockouts show a decrease in their capacity to "unlearn" the location of a hidden platform in a Morris water maze task after they have learned that a platform is associated with a particular location. This is assessed using a platform reversal variation of the water maze, where the hidden platform is moved to a new location after the animal has been repeatedly trained with the platform in one place. The effects on LTP and dendritic spine morphology in the LIMK-1 knockout mouse suggest a possible basis for the cognitive effects in Williams Syndrome. They also point to the growing understanding of the importance of morphological regulation in learning and synaptic plasticity, including apparently those processes occurring in the human CNS.

of exon 1 of FMR2 is the most common lesion and results in the reduction of FMR2 gene expression. The product of FMR2 is a novel member of a family of proteins, and the gene encodes a 1311 amino acid protein with a predicted molecular mass of 141 kDa. As described in the next paragraph, the current hypothesis for the function of the FMR2 protein is that the protein functions as a transcription factor or transcriptional regulator. Adult brain expression studies using Northern blots in mice show high expression of fmr2 (the mouse homologue) in hippocampus and amygdala.

As already mentioned, even though the function of FMR2 has yet to be directly determined, FMR2 is hypothesized to be transcriptional activator. It shares significant homology (20–35% amino acid identity) with three autosomal genes: AF4,

LAF4, and AF5Q31. All four proteins of the FMR2 family share several highly similar regions that are homologous to functional motifs involved in transcriptional regulation. The proteins also exhibit features of proteins involved in transcriptional regulation, such as being rich in serine and proline. In fact, FMR2 protein family members AF4 and LAF4 have been shown experimentally to have a capacity for transcriptional transactivation, but this has not yet been tested directly for FMR2 itself.

David Nelson's laboratory at Baylor College of Medicine developed a murine Fmr2 gene knockout model for FRAXE (19). Mice lacking Fmr2 showed impairment of both contextual and cued fear conditioning, suggesting a similarity of learning deficiencies in the mouse and human. The contextual fear impairment was found to be

BOX 6

NONSYNDROMIC X-LINKED MENTAL RETARDATION

There are a variety of different forms of mental retardation that are not "syndromic," or linked to a specific and consistent spectrum of clinical features other than cognitive impairment, and there have been a number of different genes identified as contributing to these nonsyndromic forms of mental retardation. Some of the interesting genes on the X chromosome that have been associated with mental retardation include the L1 neural cell adhesion molecule and three different genes involved in the rho signal transduction cascade (28–31). Rho stands for ras homologue, which like ras is a low-molecular-weight G protein linked to a variety of downstream targets (see figure and reference 32). While the details of the molecular components of this cascade in neurons are still being worked out, three different members of this general cascade have been identified as loci for mental retardation. These include the rho target PAK3 (p21-activated kinase; 31, 33) and the rho guanine nucleotide exchange factors ARHGEF6 (30) and oligophrenin 1 (OPHN1, 34). In general, the

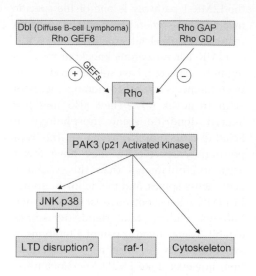

rho cascades control cytoskeleton arrangement, cell migration, and gene expression. Current working models for the rho cascade-associated mental retardation, as well as the retardation associated with L1 protein deficiency, hypothesize the involvement of derangements of cell migration and neuronal process extension.

time-dependent. Fmr2 knockout mice displayed significantly less conditioned fear in the 24-hour delay context test; however, levels of contextual fear conditioning were similar between Fmr2-deficient and wild-type control mice when the test occurred 30 minutes after training. These findings indicate that the Fmr2-deficient mice learn to associate the shock with the training context and can remember the context over a short delay interval, but that these same mice have impaired conditioned fear that is delay-dependent. Overall, these

data indicate that the FMR2 protein may play a role in the memory consolidation process for contextual memory.

Ironically, long-term potentiation in area CA1 was found to be *enhanced* in hippocampal slices of Fmr2 knockout compared to their wild-type littermates (see Figure 9). Thus, this knockout is an example of an animal model of human mental retardation with impaired learning and memory performance and *increased* LTP, as we discussed in Chapter 9. These findings highlight the importance of keeping

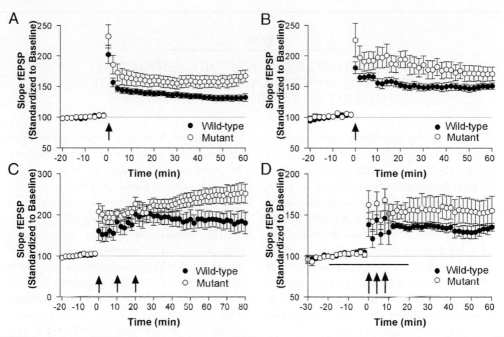

FIGURE 9   Enhanced LTP in Fmr2 knockout mice. (A) Fmr2 knockout hippocampal slices showed enhanced LTP compared with wild-types after a modest LTP-inducing protocol consisting of a single set of tetani while maintaining slices at 25°C [60 minutes after tetanus: n (KO, male) = 9, 167 ± 9%; n (WT, male) = 14, 132 ± 6%; p = .003]. (B) Enhanced LTP in Fmr2 knockout hippocampal slices is present after a single set of tetanic stimulation while maintaining slices at 32°C [60 minutes after tetanus: n (KO, male) = 6, 170 ± 11%; n (WT, male) = 6, 150 ± 5%; p = .14]. (C) Fmr2 knockout mice maintain the enhanced LTP after three sets of HFS at 32°C [60 minutes after tetanus: n (KO, male) = 7, 244 ± 18%; n (WT, male) = 5, 189 ± 20%; p = .020]. (D) In the presence of the NMDA receptor antagonist AP-5 (50 μM), Fmr2 knockout mice showed NMDA-independent LTP compared with wild types after three trains of 200-Hz stimulation for 1 second separated by 4 minutes at 32°C [60 minutes after tetanus: n (KO, male) = 6, 155 ± 8%; n (WT, male) = 6, 135 ± 4%; p = .038]. Reproduced from Gu et al. (41).

in mind that increases in LTP may be a fundamental mechanism that leads to impaired cognitive processing, just like loss of LTP.

It is interesting to speculate and consider what the role of the FMR2 protein, a presumed transcriptional regulator, may be doing in LTP and memory. As shown in Figure 9, FMR2 appears to somehow control a "ceiling" for the maximum amount of LTP that can be induced—loss of FMR2 leads to an increased maximum potentiation. It is intriguing to consider that transcriptional regulation by FMR2 might somehow be involved in limiting the overall amount of potentiation that can be achieved, although this idea is, of course, highly speculative.

Regardless, the mechanism of enhanced LTP in Fmr2 knockout mice is not clear at this moment. The studies of Wu et al. indicate that the enhancement of LTP in Fmr2 knockout mice is not entirely dependent on NMDA receptor-dependent processes, as NMDA receptor-independent LTP was also augmented (see Figure 9). Most mice with abnormal LTP have been created by knockout of postsynaptic receptors, scaffolding proteins, or protein kinases, while FMR2 is a nuclear protein, a member of a new family of putative transcription factors. It will be interesting in the future to begin to parse out more directly the role of the FMR2 protein in controlling synaptic plasticity.

BOX 7

NURTURE VERSUS NATURE: ENRICHED ENVIRONMENTS CAN HELP OVERCOME INHERITED LEARNING DISORDERS

Coffin-Lowry Syndrome, neurofibromatosis mental retardation, and fragile X syndrome—these devastating forms of mental retardation arise from defects in genes whose normal functioning is critical for learning and memory. From the moment of conception, children with these disorders face an uphill battle to overcome their inherited disadvantage. Can their environment help compensate for their being short-changed by Nature? Studies by Joe Tsien and his colleagues at Princeton University suggest that there is indeed cause for hope.

Tsien and colleagues capitalized on genetic engineering to construct a general mouse model for inherited learning defects—they created a mouse strain missing the NMDA receptor. In an additional refinement, Tsien and colleagues engineered their mouse so that the NMDA receptor was selectively lost in the hippocampus. As expected, in behavioral tests, these mice demonstrated a decrease in learning capacity in several tasks linked to hippocampal function, such as identifying new foodstuffs appropriately, recognizing objects, and recognizing their environment (38).

The investigators then set out to determine if enriching the animals' environment could help compensate for their inborn loss of learning capacity. In their studies, they made the important discovery that raising these animals in an environment rich in sensory stimuli, toys, and opportunities for exploration resulted in a significant improvement in their learning capacity. These results are one of the most convincing demonstrations to date that an enriched environment can help overcome learning deficiencies, even those deficiencies arising from defects in the genetic hard-wiring of an individual.

IV. SUMMARY

In this chapter, we have covered a topic of pronounced importance—disorders of human cognition, specifically related to memory formation. We saw three examples of convergence of basic memory research with clinical investigation, highlighting neurofibromatosis mental retardation, Angelman Syndrome, and Fragile X mental retardation. It is quite striking how the detailed analysis of the basic signal transduction mechanisms underlying rodent learning and memory have converged upon many of the same molecular systems recently identified using human genetic characterization approaches in the study of mental retardation syndromes. I am cautiously optimistic that this convergence will ultimately lead to an improvement of the human condition, by identifying new therapeutic approaches to treating mental retardation.

On the abstract, intellectual side, the findings we have covered in this chapter also have interesting cognitive neurobiological implications. It appears that the last decades of parsing the esoteric details of synaptic plasticity and rodent memory mechanisms may well have lived up to its promise. In my opinion, it is not too early to begin to think of the types of mechanisms we have been covering in this book in the context of giving insights into human cognitive processing as well. The convergence of human and basic studies onto the same molecular cascades suggests that, indeed, we may be in the process of generating insights into the molecular basis of human cognition.

This line of thinking raises an interesting issue as well: the distinction between a developmental necessity for the gene products versus an acute, ongoing necessity as part of the signal transduction mechanisms subserving cognition. Many of the mutations we have discussed do not lead to gross morphological changes in the human CNS. Moreover, mouse studies, where available, indicate that baseline synaptic transmission is normal after loss of these gene products. These observations are consistent with a necessity for an *ongoing* need for the gene products in human learning and memory. In addition, in the case of both the ERK/CREB/CBP system and the CaMKII system, there is direct evidence from animal studies that acute inhibition of these systems in adults is *sufficient* to cause learning deficiencies. These types of considerations suggest a rethinking of our outlook on human learning disorders, changing from the traditional view of them as purely developmental problems to a new view of them as cognitive deficiencies. This sea-change in outlook may be one of the most important outcomes of new and ongoing discoveries concerning the basic signal transduction processes subserving learning and memory.

References

1. Weeber, E. J., and Sweatt, J. D. (2002). "Molecular neurobiology of human cognition." *Neuron* 33:845–848.
2. Ozonoff, S. (1999). "Cognitive impairment in neurofibromatosis type 1." *Am. J. Med. Genet.* 89:45–52.
3. Silva, A. J., Frankland, P. W., Marowitz, Z., Friedman, E., Lazlo, G., Cioffi, D., Jacks, T., and Bourtchuladze, R. (1997). "A mouse model for the learning and memory deficits associated with neurofibromatosis type I." *Nat. Genet.* 15:281–284.
4. Costa, R. M., Yang, T., Huynh, D. P., Pulst, S. M., Viskochil, D. H., Silva, A. J., and Brannan, C. I. (2001). "Learning deficits, but normal development and tumor predisposition, in mice lacking exon 23a of Nf1." *Nat. Genet.* 27:399–405.
5. Andersen, L. B., Ballester, R., Marchuk, D. A., Chang, E., Gutmann, D. H., Saulino, A. M., Camonis, J., Wigler, M., and Collins, F. S. (1993). "A conserved alternative splice in the von Recklinghausen neurofibromatosis (NF1) gene produces two neurofibromin isoforms, both of which have GTPase-activating protein activity." *Mol. Cell. Biol.* 13:487–495.
6. Zhu, Y., and Parada, L. F. (2001). "A particular GAP in mind." *Nat. Genet.* 27:354–355.
7. Ohno, M., Frankland, P. W., Chen, A. P., Costa, R. M., and Silva, A. J. (2001). "Inducible, pharmacogenetic approaches to the study of learning and memory." *Nat. Neurosci.* 4:1238–1243.
8. Ingram, D. A., Hiatt, K., King, A. J., Fisher, L., Shivakumar, R., Derstine, C., Wenning, M. J., Diaz, B., Travers, J. B., Hood, A., Marshall, M., Williams, D. A., and Clapp, D. W. (2001). "Hyperactivation of p21(ras) and the hematopoietic-specific Rho GTPase, Rac2, cooperate to alter the proliferation of neurofibromin-deficient mast cells in vivo and in vitro." *J. Exp. Med.* 194:57–69.
9. Tong, J., Hannan, F., Zhu, Y., Bernards, A., and Zhong, Y. (2002). "Neurofibromin regulates G protein-stimulated adenylyl cyclase activity." *Nat. Neurosci.* 5:95–96.
10. Impey, S., Obrietan, K., Wong, S. T., Poser, S., Yano, S., Wayman, G., Deloulme, J. C., Chan, G., and Storm, D. R. (1998). "Cross talk between ERK and PKA is required for Ca^{2+} stimulation of CREB-dependent transcription and ERK nuclear translocation." *Neuron* 21:869–883.
11. Roberson, E. D., English, J. D., Adams, J. P., Selcher, J. C., Kondratick, C., and Sweatt, J. D. (1999). "The mitogen-activated protein kinase cascade couples PKA and PKC to cAMP response element binding protein phosphorylation in area CA1 of hippocampus." *J. Neurosci.* 19:4337–4348.
12. Dufresne, S. D., Bjorbaek, C., El-Haschimi, K., Zhao, Y., Aschenbach, W. G., Moller, D. E., and Goodyear, L. J. (2001). "Altered extracellular signal-regulated kinase signaling and glycogen metabolism in skeletal muscle from p90 ribosomal S6 kinase 2 knockout mice." *Mol. Cell. Biol.* 21:81–87.
13. Harum, K. H., Alemi, L., and Johnston, M. V. (2001). "Cognitive impairment in Coffin-Lowry syndrome correlates with reduced RSK2 activation." *Neurology* 56:207–214.
14. Greenough, W. T., Klintsova, A. Y., Irwin, S. A., Galvez, R., Bates, K. E., and Weiler, I. J. (2001).

"Synaptic regulation of protein synthesis and the fragile X protein." *Proc. Natl. Acad. Sci. USA* 98:7101–7106.

15. Jiang, Y. H., Armstrong, D., Albrecht, U., Atkins, C. M., Noebels, J. L., Eichele, G., Sweatt, J. D., and Beaudet, A. L. (1998). "Mutation of the Angelman ubiquitin ligase in mice causes increased cytoplasmic p53 and deficits of contextual learning and long-term potentiation." *Neuron* 21:799–811.

16. Hagerman, R. J., and Hagerman, P. J. (2001). "Fragile X syndrome: a model of gene-brain-behavior relationships." *Mol. Genet. Metab.* 74:89–97.

17. Bardoni, B., Schenck, A., and Mandel, J. L. (2001). "The Fragile X mental retardation protein." *Brain Res. Bull.* 56:375–382.

18. Zhang, Y. Q., Bailey, A. M., Matthies, H. J., Renden, R. B., Smith, M. A., Speese, S. D., Rubin, G. M., and Broadie, K. (2001). "Drosophila fragile X-related gene regulates the MAP1B homolog Futsch to control synaptic structure and function." *Cell* 107:591–603.

19. Gu, Y., McIlwain, K., Weeber, E. J., Yamagata, T., Xu, B., Antalffy, B., Reye, C., Yuva-Paylor, L., Armstrong, D., Zoghbi, H., Sweatt, J. D., Paylor, R., and Nelson, D. (2002). "Impaired conditioned fear and enhanced long-term potentiation in Fmr2 knockout mice." *J. Neurosci.* 22(7):1753–1763.

20. Oike, Y., Hata, A., Mamiya, T., Kaname, T., Noda, Y., Suzuki, M., Yasue, H., Nabeshima, T., Araki, K., and Yamamura, K. (1999). "Truncated CBP protein leads to classical Rubinstein-Taybi syndrome phenotypes in mice: implications for a dominant-negative mechanism." *Hum. Mol. Genet.* 8:387–396.

21. Hegde, A. N., Inokuchi, K., Pei, W., Casadio, A., Ghirardi, M., Chain, D. G., Martin, K. C., Kandel, E. R., and Schwartz, J. H. (1997). "Ubiquitin C-terminal hydrolase is an immediate-early gene essential for long-term facilitation in Aplysia." *Cell* 89:115–126.

22. Chain, D. G., Hegde, A. N., Yamamoto, N., Liu-Marsh, B., and Schwartz, J. H. (1995). "Persistent activation of cAMP-dependent protein kinase by regulated proteolysis suggests a neuron-specific function of the ubiquitin system in Aplysia." *J. Neurosci.* 15:7592–7603.

23. Shahbazian, M. D., Antalffy, B., Armstrong, D. L., and Zoghbi, H. Y. (2002). "Insight into Rett syndrome: MeCP2 levels display tissue- and cell-specific differences and correlate with neuronal maturation." *Hum. Mol. Genet.* 11:115–124.

24. Bellugi, U., Adolphs, R., Cassady, C., and Chiles, M. (1999). "Towards the neural basis for hypersociability in a genetic syndrome." *Neuroreport* 10:1653–1657.

25. Donnai, D., and Karmiloff-Smith, A. (2000). "Williams syndrome: from genotype through to the cognitive phenotype." *Am. J. Med. Genet.* 97:164–171.

26. Korenberg, J. R., Chen, X. N., Hirota, H., Lai, Z., Bellugi, U., Burian, D., Roe, B., and Matsuoka, R. (2000). "VI. Genome structure and cognitive map of Williams syndrome." *J. Cogn. Neurosci.* 12 Suppl 1:89–107.

27. Meng, Y., Zhang, Y., Tregoubov, V., Janus, C., Cruz, L., Jackson, M., Lu, W. Y., MacDonald, J. F., Wang, J. Y., Falls, D. L., and Jia, Z. (2002). "Abnormal spine morphology and enhanced LTP in LIMK-1 knockout mice." *Neuron* 35:121–133.

28. Bienvenu, T., des Portes, V., McDonell, N., Carrie, A., Zemni, R., Couvert, P., Ropers, H. H., Moraine, C., van Bokhoven, H., Fryns, J. P., Allen, K., Walsh, C. A., Boue, J., Kahn, A., Chelly, J., and Beldjord, C. (2000). "Missense mutation in PAK3, R67C, causes X-linked nonspecific mental retardation." *Am. J. Med. Genet.* 93:294–298.

29. Schmid, R. S., Pruitt, W. M., and Maness, P. F. (2000). "A MAP kinase-signaling pathway mediates neurite outgrowth on L1 and requires Src-dependent endocytosis." *J. Neurosci.* 20:4177–4188.

30. Kutsche, K., Yntema, H., Brandt, A., Jantke, I., Nothwang, H. G., Orth, U., Boavida, M. G., David, D., Chelly, J., Fryns, J. P., Moraine, C., Ropers, H. H., Hamel, B. C., van Bokhoven, H., and Gal, A. (2000). "Mutations in ARHGEF6, encoding a guanine nucleotide exchange factor for Rho GTPases, in patients with X-linked mental retardation." *Nat. Genet.* 26:247–250.

31. Allen, K. M., Gleeson, J. G., Bagrodia, S., Partington, M. W., MacMillan, J. C., Cerione, R. A., Mulley, J. C., and Walsh, C. A. (1998). "PAK3 mutation in nonsyndromic X-linked mental retardation." *Nat. Genet.* 20:25–30.

32. Ridley, A. J. (2001). "Rho family proteins: coordinating cell responses." *Trends Cell. Biol.* 11:471–477.

33. King, A. J., Sun, H., Diaz, B., Barnard, D., Miao, W., Bagrodia, S., and Marshall, M. S. (1998). "The protein kinase Pak3 positively regulates Raf-1 activity through phosphorylation of serine 338." *Nature* 396:180–183.

34. Billuart, P., Bienvenu, T., Ronce, N., des Portes, V., Vinet, M. C., Zemni, R., Roest Crollius, H., Carrie, A., Fauchereau, F., Cherry, M., Briault, S., Hamel, B., Fryns, J. P., Beldjord, C., Kahn, A., Moraine, C., and Chelly, J. (1998). "Oligophrenin-1 encodes a rhoGAP protein involved in X-linked mental retardation." *Nature* 392:923–926.

35. Altafaj, X., Dierssen, M., Baamonde, C., Marti, E., Visa, J., Guimera, J., Oset, M., Gonzalez, J. R., Florez, J., Fillat, C., and Estivill, X. (2001). "Neurodevelopmental delay, motor abnormalities and cognitive deficits in transgenic mice overexpressing Dyrk1A (minibrain), a murine model of Down's syndrome." *Hum. Mol. Genet.* 10:1915–1923.

36. Siarey, R. J., Carlson, E. J., Epstein, C. J., Balbo, A., Rapoport, S. I., and Galdzicki, Z. (1999). "Increased synaptic depression in the Ts65Dn mouse, a model for mental retardation in Down syndrome." *Neuropharmacology* 38:1917–1920.

37. Thiels, E., Urban, N. N., Gonzalez-Burgos, G. R., Kanterewicz, B. I., Barrionuevo, G., Chu, C. T., Oury, T. D., and Klann, E. (2000). "Impairment of long-term potentiation and associative memory in mice that overexpress extracellular superoxide dismutase." *J. Neurosci.* 20:7631–7639.

38. Rampon, C., Tang, Y. P., Goodhouse, J., Shimizu, E., Kyin, M., and Tsien, J. Z. (2000). "Enrichment induces structural changes and recovery from nonspatial memory deficits in CA1 NMDAR1-knockout mice." *Nat. Neurosci.* 3:238–244.

39. Costa, R. M., Federov, N. B., Kogan, J. H., Murphy, G. G., Stern, J., Ohno, M., Kucherlapati, R., Jacks, T., and Silva, A. J. (2002). "Mechanism for the learning deficits in a mouse model of neurofibromatosis type 1." *Nature* 415:526–530.

40. Jiang, Y. H., Armstrong, D., Albrecht, U., Atkins, C. M., Noebels, J. L., Eichele, G., Sweatt, J. D., and Beaudet, A. L. (1998). "Mutation of the Angelman ubiquitin ligase in mice causes increased cytoplasmic p53 and deficits of contextual learning and long-term potentiation." *Neuron* 21:799–811.

41. Gu, Y., McIlwain, K. L., Weeber, E. J., Yamagata, T., Xu, B., Antalffy, B. A., Reyes, C., Yuva-Paylor, L., Armstrong, D., Zoghbi, H., Sweatt, J. D., Paylor, R., and Nelson, D. L. (2002). "Impaired conditioned fear and enhanced long-term potentiation in Fmr2 knock-out mice." *J. Neurosci.* 22:2753–2763.

42. Mistry, D. J., Moorman, J. R., Reddy, S., and Mounsey, J. P. (2001). "Skeletal muscle Na currents in mice heterozygous for Six5 deficiency." *Physiol. Genomics* 6:153–158.

43. Gahtan, E., Auerbach, J. M., Groner, Y., and Segal, M. (1998). "Reversible impairment of long-term potentiation in transgenic Cu/Zn-SOD mice." *Eur. J. Neurosci.* 10:538–544.

44. Morris, C. A., and Mervis, C. B. (2000). "Williams syndrome and related disorders." *Annu. Rev. Genomics Hum. Genet.* 1:461–484.

45. Sweatt, J. D. (2001). "Protooncogenes subserve memory formation in the adult CNS." *Neuron* 31:671–674.

46. Weeber, E. J., and Sweatt, J. D. (2000). "Disruptions of signal transduction pathways in mental retardation: Angelman and Coffin-Lowry syndrome." *Recent Res. Devel. Neurochem.* 3:289–299.

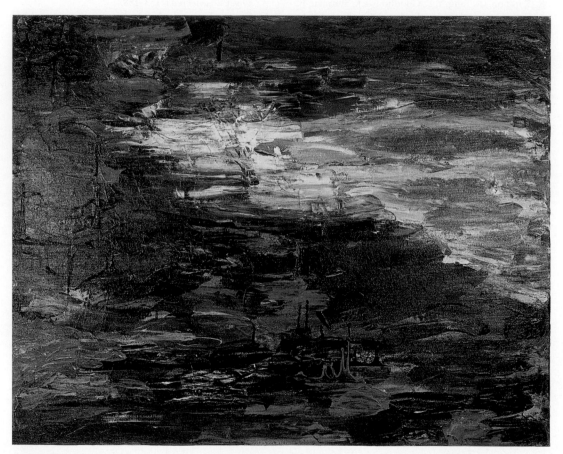

Alzheimer's Disease
J. David Sweatt, Acrylic on canvas, 2002

11

Aging-Related
Memory Disorders

Alzheimer's Disease

In the last chapter, we talked about human mental retardation syndromes—inherited deficiencies in learning and memory that manifest themselves from birth. In this chapter, we move to the other end of the developmental spectrum and will discuss aging-related memory dysfunction. In particular we will focus on Alzheimer's disease (AD) as an example of an inherited memory disorder that does not manifest itself until adulthood is reached. We will focus on inherited forms of AD *not* because they are the most prevalent but rather because they are the forms most tractable for experimental investigation at present. This is because inherited forms of AD,

being gene-based, lend themselves to investigation using genetically engineered mice. As we have seen throughout the book, the recent advent of the capacity for genetic engineering in animal models holds the promise of a watershed of new insights into all aspects of memory, including investigating aging-related memory dysfunction such as AD.

In this chapter, I will present an overview of the clinical and pathological manifestations of AD. I will discuss in particular the emerging hypothesis that amyloid beta (Aβ) is the proximal causative agent for AD. We also will discuss other important molecular events involved in AD pathogenesis, always with an eye toward how these events might impinge upon the molecular mechanisms for learning and memory that we have been discussing in detail throughout the book. I also will spend a little time going over new mouse models that are relevant to AD, in keeping with our motif of investigating rodent models and behavioral paradigms of relevance to memory.

I. AGING-RELATED MEMORY DECLINE

As most people over the age of 60 will attest, a decline in learning and memory is a part of the "normal" aging process (see reference 1 for a review). Most noticeable in humans is the decline in hippocampus-dependent forms of memory, the learning and remembering of new names, recent events, and even spatial information. For the most part, in normal individuals, these memory deficits are not debilitating, but they are quite noticeable because they are involved so directly in human conscious behavior.

These types of hippocampus-dependent memory dysfunction are recapitulated in aging rodents, as assessed using various learning paradigms that we have discussed throughout this book. Carol Barnes has been a leader in this area and, in fact, developed her maze learning task specifically to probe for memory deficits in aged animals, as was described in Chapter 2. In vivo recordings have also demonstrated deficiencies in hippocampal place field stabilization in aged rats (2). Thus, an aging-related decline in behavioral and cellular manifestations of hippocampus-dependent learning is well established in humans and other mammals.

Hippocampal LTP is similarly diminished in aged animals (3). The basis for these declines remains mysterious, although decreased synaptic inputs or diminished NMDA receptor function are possibilities, depending on the hippocampal region

under consideration (3, 4). In addition, Marina Lynch's group has executed a nice series of studies implicating excessive production or reactive oxygen species as a contributing factor in aging-related memory and synaptic plasticity dysfunction (5). Given the ambiguous nature of the molecular process we call 'aging," the biochemical mechanisms underlying aging-related memory decline are likely to remain enigmatic for some period of time. This does not diminish the importance of understanding them, but rather highlights their complexity.

Superimposed upon the normal aging process can be much more dramatic insults to the human capacity for hippocampus-dependent learning and memory. These can arise for a number of reasons—stroke, vascular problems, psychiatric disorders, Parkinson's disease, and Alzheimer's disease principally among them. These all can lead to dementia much more pronounced than ever occurs with normal aging. The focus of this chapter will be dementia of the Alzheimer's type.

Please keep in mind that "dementia" does not mean the same thing in the clinical realm that it does in general parlance. "Demented" is generally used by the lay public synonymously with "mad" or "insane." In clinical terms dementia refers to a specific and pronounced decline of cognitive function in humans—a decline in mentation. Among the symptoms of dementia are loss of learning and memory capacity, decline in reasoning ability, attention problems, language difficulties, and problems with perception.

AD is the most common of the tragically debilitating senile (i.e., age-related) dementias, and in the United States alone AD is projected to affect approximately 4 million people total in the next few years. In the United States, about one in ten people over the age of 65 have AD. If you live to age 85 you have about a one in two chance of developing AD. As human longevity increases worldwide, the ironic and at-present unavoidable consequence of that fact is that the prevalence of AD will similarly increase on a global scale. AD is projected to affect nearly 20 million people worldwide by 2025. These are sobering statistics given that at present there is no effective treatment for the disease.

II. WHAT IS AD?

Of the various dementing illnesses our understanding of AD has progressed the farthest at the molecular level. That is not to say that our molecular understanding of AD is good, but rather that we have at least a few clues as to what is happening. As we will discuss later, a number of specific genes involved with AD have been identified. These genes, when mutated, essentially invariably lead to an individual developing AD. We will discuss these genes and gene products in more detail later, but for now I raise the issue to make two points. First, even considering the already-identified genes for AD, we can still only account mechanistically for factors contributing to about 30% of AD cases. Second, among the known genes, there are heterogeneous mechanisms by which they lead one to arrive in the AD state. Thus, it appears certain that AD is, in fact, more than one disease. As our understanding of the molecular bases of

AD increases, it is likely that AD subtypes will be diagnosable and perhaps differentially treatable. For our purposes in this chapter, because of the present limited state of understanding, I will refer to AD monolithically.

Despite the clear molecular heterogeneity of AD, there are commonalities to AD that are defined clinically. A number of different schema have emerged for describing the progression of AD (see Table 1). The one that I will follow here is based on the system promulgated by Heiko and Eva Braak (6–9) that is based on histopathological criteria, specifically the development of neurofibrillary tangles in various brain regions and associated clinical symptomology.

A. Stages of AD

In the final stages (Stages V and VI), typically about 8–10 years after the initial diagnosis of AD, patients are completely bedridden and unable to care for themselves. There is complete dementia and an inability to communicate effectively. Perpetual confusion, incontinence, and an inability to execute the most basic cognitive functions are the hallmarks of this final stage of AD.

This final stage is preceded by a period of progressive loss of reasoning and cognitive ability (Stages III and IV). There is

TABLE 1   Staged Progression of AD

AD Stage	Areas First Affected	Symptoms
I, II	Trans-entorhinal region Entorhinal cortex Area CA1	Can be clinically silent: subtle loss of episodic memory and difficulty executing complex progressive tasks; anecdotal repetition; some spatial disorientation
III, IV	Entirety of hippocampus	Early-stage AD: loss of episodic memory, difficulty with spatial reasoning and recognition, difficulty with coherent speech and planning
V, VI	Neocortex	Fully developed AD: pronounced decline in cognition; frank dementia, can include psychosis or depression; ultimately a complete inability to communicate or care for themselves

profound anterograde episodic memory loss. In many cases, additional symptoms such as psychosis, delusional behavior, and depression are present. Reading and writing are essentially impossible, as is watching a movie or television program, because episodic and declarative memory are so impaired. Verbal communication becomes progressively incoherent. Recognition of known individuals progressively declines.

The earlier stages of AD (Stages I and II) typically read like a textbook case of hippocampal dysfunction.[1] Episodic memory formation is lost—a patient typically has no recollection of their ongoing experiences on a daily basis. Spatial disorientation is pronounced, both in the sense of navigation and in place recognition. For example, AD patients in this stage may regularly ask when they are "going home," when in fact they are at home already. The capacity to remember new individuals and other specific named items becomes increasingly difficult. The execution of complex serial tasks is affected, as is expected, if ordering of episodic events is impaired. Cooking, for

example, or other serial tasks, become difficult and then impossible to execute.

The increasing frequency over time of these types of hippocampal memory deficits are what lead patients and their family members to suspect that AD might be present and to go to a physician to have themselves checked out. These types of memory deficits are also the basis for the initial diagnosis of early AD by the clinician (see Box 1). I emphasize this because, while later stages of AD are a manifestation of a horrible dementing illness, the early stages of AD are a much more subtle derangement of normal hippocampus-dependent memory formation and hippocampal function.

In my opinion investigating the basis of hippocampus-dependent synaptic plasticity and learning has much to offer in the context of our understanding of the mechanisms of early AD. This perspective is somewhat out of the mainstream of AD research at present. Clearly later stages of AD involve extensive cell death across broad areas of the CNS. Understanding these processes is critical to understanding and potentially developing treatments for AD. However, ideally one would like to develop treatments that intervene *before* any extensive cell death begins to occur. Focusing on processes involved in early-stage AD provides the promise of early intervention. Understanding the basis for the more subtle disruptions in hippocampal function that are the hallmarks of early AD is a key to finding the first line of attack in developing new therapies.

This is why I have included a chapter on AD in this book devoted to hippocampus-dependent learning and memory. I think that it is important to promote our thinking of AD, at least in its early stages, as a memory disorder. This is in contrast to thinking of AD as a dementing illness with wide-ranging cognitive and perceptual effects. This clearly is the case in later stages of the disease and is an important area of investigation. However, as an adjunct to these lines of investigation, we also should consider how we can capitalize upon

---

[1]Consider the following description taken verbatim from "Diagnosis of Alzheimer's Disease" by John C. Morris (Khachaturian and Radebaugh *Alzheimer's Disease* CRC Press New York, 1996, p. 78), and compare it to the roles of hippocampal synaptic plasticity that we have been discussing throughout the book: "Probable AD begins insidiously, and it is often impossible to precisely date its onset. Several years may pass before the family recognizes that everyday functioning has been sufficiently compromised to the point that medical attention is sought. Forgetfulness is the typical presenting symptom. Common examples of memory deficits in this stage are the repetition of questions or statements and the misplacement of items without independent retrieval. Impaired acquisition of new information is manifested by inability to recall recent conversations or events, whereas highly learned material from years gone by may be remembered with seeming clarity. Minor geographic and temporal disorientation also may be early symptoms; the patient may need directions to find even familiar locations or ask for frequent reminders of the date. Poor judgment and impaired problem solving occur as part of the dysexecutive syndrome wherein patients lack insight (often being unaware of their deficits), have poor attention, and experience uncharacteristic difficulty in completing tasks that involve sequencing of information, such as operating an automatic coffee maker or balancing the checkbook."

BOX 1

DIAGNOSING AD

At present there is no definitive method for pre-mortem diagnosis of AD. Accepted practice is for AD to be diagnosed post-mortem by pathological examination of autopsy tissue. Histopathological analysis of post-mortem tissue uses criteria not appreciably different from those described by Alois Alzheimer himself in 1907 (10). The gross hallmarks are cortical atrophy, enlargement of the ventricles, and shrinkage of the hippocampus and surrounding areas of the medial temporal lobe.

Microscopic examination reveals diffuse neuronal death, and the presence of "senile plaques" and "neurofibrillary tangles." The plaques are a molecular admixture of amyloid peptides and other constituents, and they can be subdivided into two categories. *Neuritic plaques* contain a dense core of amyloid peptide aggregate and are surrounded by distressed neuronal processes. *Diffuse plaques* lack associated neuronal processes and exhibit a more diffuse deposition of amyloid. Plaques can be seen readily using silver stains or thioflavin stains—the advent of silver staining chemistry is, in fact, what allowed Alzheimer to make his landmark discovery (see figure).

Microscopy of post-mortem AD tissue also reveals the presence of neurofibrillary tangles in the cytoplasm of neurons in affected brain areas. Neurofibrillary tangles are insoluble deposits of hyperphosporylated tau protein (see text). An additional feature of AD is the presence of angiopathy, that is, pathology of the cerebral vasculature. Blood vessels in the AD patient exhibit amyloid deposition to varying degrees, an attribute that has been termed "hardening of the arteries."

Pre-mortem diagnosis of AD is an iffier proposition. Established criteria have been

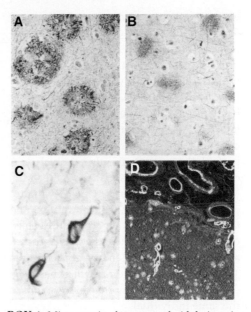

BOX 1 Microscopic features of Alzheimer's disease. (A) Several neuritic plaques within the cerebral cortex are seen on this silver stain. (B) Diffuse plaques predominate in this field of cerebral cortex. Silver stain. (C) Two neurofibrillary tangles are seen on silver stain. (D) A fluorescent stain (thioflavin S) reveals the ring-like profiles of amyloid within blood vessel walls in the meninges or coverings of the brain. The underlying cortical blood vessels also evidence amyloid angiopathy. Senile plaques in the cortex are also seen in this preparation. Reproduced from Khachaturian and Radebaugh (113).

published under the aegis of the NIH (78) that when adhered to can give about 90% accuracy versus post-mortem assessment of the same individual.

Clinical diagnosis of AD requires the availability of a spouse or other frequent companion for cross-reference. Inaccurate recollection on the part of the patient themselves is a great confound, so that an informed acquaintance needs to be available to give an objective description

Continued

BOX 1—cont'd

DIAGNOSING AD

of the patient's symptoms. Preliminary diagnosis of AD revolves around assessment of hippocampus-dependent memory function, for the most part. For example, a typical test battery involves giving a list of three words and then asking the patient to recall them at some later point in the interview (see reference 79). The general degree of orientation and attention on the part of the patient are also evaluated. A commonly utilized test battery is the "Mini Mental State" battery, which evaluates orientation, memory, concentration, and language usage (80). A slightly more detailed exam is the "Blessed" battery, also known as the Information-Memory-Concentration Test (81), performance on which has been correlated with post-mortem assessments in the same individual.

A thorough neurological exam is also requisite as part of the diagnostic process because diagnosis of AD is, in large part, an elimination of other possible explanations— a diagnosis by serial elimination. Other possibilities that need to be excluded are stroke, trauma, diffuse vascular insult, transient delirium due to metabolic imbalance, Parkinson's disease, psychosis, and "pseudodementia" associated with depression. Brain imaging is a necessary adjunct to assess specific anatomical pathologies such

as tumors and strokes. Although brain imaging techniques do not allow independent diagnosis of AD, specific metabolic changes in the temporal lobes associated with AD can be detected with PET scans (see reference 82).

The state of the art in diagnosing AD is steadily improving. The rapid expansion of our understanding of the genetic components contributing to AD will no doubt allow further refinements in pre-mortem diagnosis of AD. The irony of the present situation is that because no effective treatments for AD pathogenesis are available at present (see Box 2), a definitive diagnosis of AD is of little direct benefit to the patient. This might lead one to ask the question, "What's the point?" If nothing else, it helps the patient and their families prepare for what lies ahead. However, there also is a larger picture to be kept in mind. There are many ongoing clinical trials related to various aspects of AD, including trials related to the development of new AD treatments. Patients diagnosed with AD potentially will benefit themselves by participating in these trials, and definitely through their participation the greater society in which we all live will benefit. Diagnosis opens the door for this opportunity.

---

ongoing discoveries of the cellular and molecular basis of hippocampal function in order to improve our understanding of the earliest stages of AD. For the rest of the chapter, I will proceed with this perspective in mind—biasing the discussion toward early molecular events of relevance to the hippocampus and hippocampal synaptic plasticity.

B. Pathological Hallmarks of AD

It has been known for almost a century now (10) that AD clinical signs and symptoms are correlated with selective dysfunction (and ultimately death) of neurons in brain regions and neural circuits critical for memory and cognition (see Table 1). These include the hippocampus, amygdala, neocortex, anterior thalamus, the basal forebrain cholinergic system (see Box 2) and the mono-aminergic brain stem system (6, 11–15). Areas initially affected are the entorhinal and transentorhinal cortex, and parts of the hippocampus. This progresses to increasing hippocampal involvement and is followed by spread to the amygdala and limbic nuclei of the thalamus. It is accompanied by a worsening of initially affected areas. Final stages involve various areas of the cerebral cortex with subsequent cellular pathology in the association areas.

At the cellular level, a predictable sequence of damage to these brain regions occurs. A principal pathologic feature of AD brain are the presence of *senile plaques*

BOX 2

THE CHOLINERGIC HYPOTHESIS OF AD AND CURRENT PHARMACOTHERAPIES

In the mid to late 1970s and early 1980s, there were a series of landmark papers published describing a loss of cholinergic neurons in the brains of AD patients (11, 83, 84). This led to the formulation of the "cholinergic hypothesis" of AD (85–87), which briefly stated posited that loss of cholinergic function in the CNS was the basis for the dementia in AD. There was palpable optimism in the papers published during that period, which is poignant in retrospect. The feeling was that this might be the breakthrough in AD that would be analogous to the dopaminergic hypothesis of Parkinson's disease—perhaps treatment with cholinomimetics or acetylcholinesterase inhibitors might do for AD patients what L-DOPA had done for Parkinson's patients.

It is now clear that this is not going to be the case. AD has a complex pathophysiology, and the cholinergic treatment route is not nearly as efficacious as it was hoped to be. Nevertheless, augmenting cholinergic function does provide symptomatic ameliorative effects in a subpopulation of patients. In other words, augmenting acetylcholine function helps improve some of the cognitive effects in earlier stages of AD, for some patients. The efficacy of the treatment declines as the disease progresses. Acetylcholine-targeted treatments do not affect or slow the underlying pathogenesis of AD (see reference 88).

All of the currently available drugs prescribed for AD act to augment acetylcholine function in the CNS by inhibiting acetylcholinesterase, which is the enzyme that breaks down acetylcholine, converting it to acetate and choline. The specific drugs available at present are donepezil (Aricept), rivastigmine (Exelon), galantamine (Reminyl), and tacrine (Cognex).

Aside from providing a rationale for drug development, the selective loss of cholinergic neurons in AD raises an additional interesting point. How is it that cholinergic neurons get selectively targeted? Some AD-related process is clearly picking cholinergic neurons out of the diverse array of central neurons in a highly selective manner. Recent work from a number of groups has suggested a partial answer to this question. It turns out that amyloid beta peptide binds with extremely high affinity to CNS nicotinic acetylcholine receptors (see figure). This provides an insight into how cholinergic neurons might be targeted—amyloid beta peptide selectively

Continued

BOX 2—cont'd

THE CHOLINERGIC HYPOTHESIS OF AD AND CURRENT PHARMACOTHERAPIES

binds to cholinergic autoreceptors on their cell surface. The precise mechanisms for how this might lead to neuron loss or derangement is actively under investigation. Possibilities include direct effects of Aβ on the receptors themselves, which are ligand-gated ion channels (74), or elevated intracellular levels of Aβ in cholinergic neurons resulting from nicotinic receptor-mediated endocytosis (90, 91).

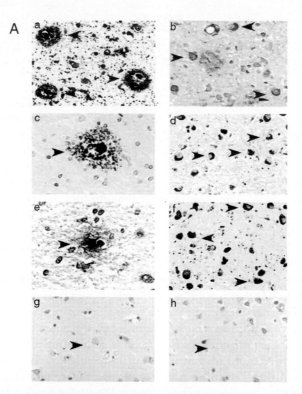

BOX 2   (A) Immunohistochemical detection of α7 nicotinic ACh Receptor (α7nAChR) in neuritic plaques of AD hippocampus. (a) Tissues were stained with a modified Bielschowsky silver stain technique. Arrowheads indicate areas of neuritic plaques. Tissues were then stained with the appropriate antibodies to either amyloid beta peptide or α7nAChR. (b) Arrowheads indicate neurofibrillary tangles. (c) Presence of $A\beta_{1-42}$ (arrowheads) in a dense core plaque. (d) Presence of $A\beta_{1-42}$ (arrowheads) in neurons. (e) Presence of α7nAChR (arrowheads) in a neuritic plaque. (f) Presence of α7nAChR (arrowheads) in neurons. (g) Lack of α4nAChR immunoreactivity in a plaque (arrowhead) in a section stained with an alpha4 nicotinic receptor-selective antibody. (h) Lack of N-methyl-D-aspartate R1 glutamate receptor immunoreactivity in a plaque (arrowhead) stained with an NMDAR antibody. Magnification: (a) × 20; (b–h) × 40. All 12 AD brain samples showed identical results, and representative data from two cases of sporadic AD are shown.

Continued

THE CHOLINERGIC HYPOTHESIS OF AD AND CURRENT PHARMACOTHERAPIES

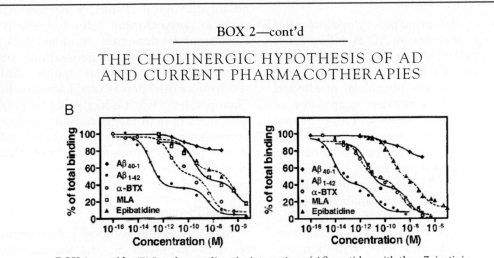

BOX 2, cont'd (B) In other studies, the interaction of Aβ peptides with the α7nicotinic ACh receptor was assessed by ligand receptor binding assay using the α7nAChR-selective ligand alpha-bungarotoxin. (Left-hand panel) ^{125}I-α-bungarotoxin (BTX) binding to α7 receptor-containing cell membranes was assessed. Amyloid beta peptide competes for bungarotoxin binding to the alpha-7 receptor with high affinity. (Right-hand panel) ^{125}I-Aβ$_{1-40}$ binding to α7 receptor-containing membrane was also assessed. Alpha-7 selective antagonists (BTX, MLA, and epibatidine) compete for ^{125}I-Aβ$_{1-40}$ binding with high affinity. Overall these data indicate a high-affinity interaction of amyloid beta peptide with the alpha7 nicotinic acetylcholine receptor. Mean data from at least three experiments are presented. Nonlinear regression data curve fit was performed by Prism. Reproduced from Wang et al. (89).

(Figure 1). Senile plaques exhibit several features. Plaque formation is associated with the accumulation of dystrophic neurites in the areas surrounding senile plaques. At the core of the senile plaque is a structure known as the *amyloid plaque* (10). An additional neuropathological feature of AD is *neurofibrillary tangles* (NFTs). Progression of the disease is marked by an increase in the number of amyloid plaques and neurofibrillary tangles in affected neurons and brain areas, accompanied ultimately by neuronal loss. In the next two sections, we will cover the molecular composition of NFTs and amyloid plaques. A number of the most important findings in the history of AD research were related to discovering the chemical nature of these materials.

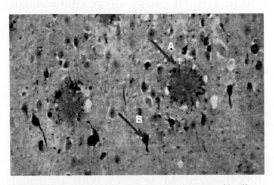

FIGURE 1 Amyloid plaques and neurofibrillary tangles, the two principal neuropathologic markers for AD. A indicates an amyloid plaque and B indicates a neurofibrillary tangle. See text for additional discussion. Figure courtesy of Poul Jørgensen, Claus Bus, Niels Pallisgaard, Marianne Bryder, and Arne Lund Jørgensen.

Neurofibrillary Tangles

One of the principal cytopathological diagnostic features of AD is NFTs. NFTs are located in the soma, dendrites, and dystrophic neurites (abnormal neuronal processes and axon terminals) of affected neurons. NFTs comprise aggregates of poorly soluble filaments, the principal component being hyperphosphorylated isoforms of the microtubule-associated protein *tau* (see reference 16 for a review and Figure 1). Hyperphosphorylated tau from human AD tissue can be phosphorylated at more than 20 different sites. Tau is a substrate for a variety of protein kinases including ERK and JNK MAP kinases, cyclin-dependent kinase 5 (cdk5) and Glycogen Synthase Kinase 3 (GSK3). The relevant kinases that phosphorylate tau in AD and other pathologic states are currently under investigation, but all these kinases are viable candidates for mediating increased tau phosphorylation in AD. Similarly, the basis for aberrant kinase activation (or aberrant phosphatase inhibition) in AD is an area of ongoing investigation.

Current hypotheses invoke the idea that hyperphosphorylation of tau has two effects. First, it causes dissociation of tau from the microtubule cytoskeleton and hence leads to cytoskeletal derangement. Second, hyperphosphorylated tau aggregates into a cytopathologic feature known as paired helical filaments (PHFs). These intracellular protein aggregates themselves may be cytotoxic, by mechanisms yet to be discerned (see reference 17 for a review). Thus, the combination of architectural derangement and neuronal inclusions is hypothesized to lead to both neuronal dysfunction and ultimately neuron death. It should not escape our attention that we discussed many of the identified tau kinases in Chapters 6 and 7 in terms of their involvement in synaptic plasticity and memory formation.

The neurofibrillary tangle is a cytopathological feature associated with several neuropathological disorders besides AD, such as amyotrophic lateral sclerosis/ Parkinsonism dementia complex, Pick's disease, corticobasal degeneration, and progressive supranuclear palsy. This spectrum of disorders is now known as the "Tauopathies" (17). It is likely that NFTs are a hallmark of neurodegeneration; however, as mentioned previously, the causative role that hyperphosphorylated tau and NFTs play in neurodegeneration is not well understood.

Amyloid Plaques

Senile plaques are composed of dystrophic neurites displayed around extracellular deposits of amyloid. A key breakthrough, and perhaps the key breakthrough, in understanding the molecular pathology of AD came with the identification of the chemical structure of amyloid by George Glenner in 1984 (18). This work along with subsequent studies (19) made clear that AD-associated amyloid in both the vascular system and in amyloid plaques is comprised of aggregates of a peptide termed amyloid beta (Aβ) peptide.

"Amyloid beta peptide" is actually a mixture of peptides in vivo. Aβ comprises peptides with a length of 40 to 43 amino acids, all of which are identical except for the carboxy-terminal 3 amino acids. The sequence of the longest (43 amino acid) peptide is

DAEFR(G)HDSGY(F) EVH(R)HQKLVFF
AEDVGSNKGA I IGLMVGGVV IAT

This is the human amino acid sequence. In keeping with our focus on rodent models, I also have included in parentheses the rat sequence, which differs only at the three indicated amino acids. Current work focuses on the 42-amino acid variant as a principal culprit in AD, as we will return to later.

Aβ42, being a fairly small peptide, can assume a number of different conformations in solution and even in protein crystals. One three-dimensional structure of an Aβ peptide that has been determined

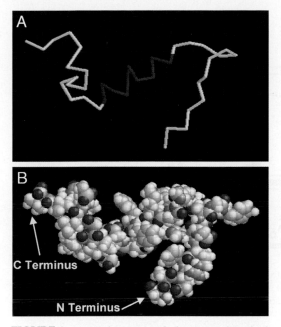

FIGURE 2 A crystal structure of a fragment of amyloid beta peptide. These two panels show a peptide backbone (A) and spacefill (B) rendering of amino acids 1–39 of amyloid beta peptide. Figures rendered using Rasmol and file 1BA6 from the Brookhaven National Protein Database. Note that amyloid beta peptide can assume many different conformations, and this particular structure is only representative of one known conformation of the peptide. In panel A, the shaded region indicates a central alpha-helical domain. Both panels are the same perspective of the molecule. The amino terminus of the molecule is at the lower right. Data for image is published in Watson et al. (111).

is shown in Figure 2 for your reference. However, Aβ42 is highly "fibrillogenic," that is, it is subject to not remaining as a monomer in solution but rather to forming oligomers, multimers, and aggregates. These polymerized forms of Aβ42, in complex with Aβ40, make up the amyloid plaques that are characteristic of AD. Exactly which state of Aβ (monomer versus multimer versus aggregate) is involved in AD pathogenesis is an area of much debate at present.

Work subsequent to the discovery of the sequence of Aβ revealed that Aβ is derived from β-amyloid precursor proteins (APPs; 20), yet another finding that has catalyzed progress in understanding the cellular and

molecular underpinnings of AD. APPs are type I integral membrane proteins that are expressed at the cell surface (see Figure 3). The APP gene is located on chromosome 21 and contains 19 exons—over ~400 kb of DNA (21). Several alternatively spliced mRNAs encode APP in neurons and, to a lesser extent, glia. The 695 amino acid splice variant (APP695) is expressed exclusively in neurons—the APP751 and APP770 variants are more widely expressed.

In axons of the peripheral and central nervous system, APP is transported by the fast anterograde system to nerve terminals, where Aβ peptides are generated and released into the extracellular space by mechanisms that are not clear at present (22, 23). Aβ peptide is a normal constituent of the extracellular milieu and is present in your brain and CSF as you are reading this sentence. Only when it is aberrantly over-produced (or underdegraded) do amyloid plaques form. The normal physiologic role of Aβ peptide and its precursor APP are completely unknown at present. Not surprisingly, almost all the work in this area has focused on the role of these proteins in AD pathogenesis.

Given that the overproduction of Aβ appears to be such a critical factor in the development of AD, much important effort has been invested in understanding the production of this peptide. APPs are subject to alternative proteolytic processing by a family of "secretase" activities that are still being defined at the molecular level (24–26). The three relevant secretases for processing APP and other similar proteins (the developmental regulator Notch is another example) are termed alpha, beta, and gamma secretase (see Figure 3). The α-secretase cleaves APP within the Aβ sequence to release the N-terminal ectodomain of APP (APPsα); thus, α-secretase cleavage within the Aβ domain *precludes* production of Aβ peptides. The alpha-secretase activity, therefore, dictates a route of APP processing distinct from the amyloidogenic, AD-related process.

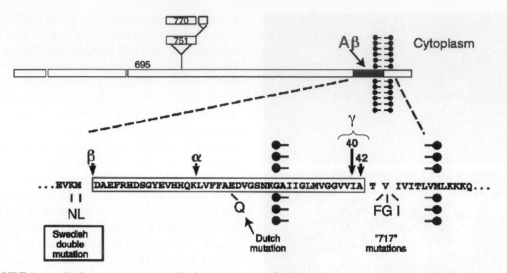

FIGURE 3 Amyloid precursor protein. The basic structure of APP is shown (upper section), along with several known mutations and the sites of alpha, beta, and gamma secretase cleavage (marked α, β, and γ, lower section). See text for additional discussion. Adapted from Price, Sisodia, and Borchelt (112).

However, the actions of the beta and gamma secretases lead to production of Aβ peptides (reviewed in reference 27). The γ-secretase is unusual because it cleaves proteins, including APP, within the lipid bilayer. That is, this protease actually acts to cut the APP at its alpha-helical trans-membrane domain while it is still in the membrane. The β-secretase is more pedestrian, cleaving the APP in a soluble domain. However, even the β-secretase has the unusual attribute that it is an ecto-protease, that is, it acts upon the extracellular domain of the APP molecule.

The β-secretase has been identified and termed BACE for Beta-site APP Cleaving Enzyme (28; reviewed in Vassar and Citron, 29).This important discovery was made by Mark Citron's group at Amgen. BACE is a single-transmembrane domain aspartyl protease that can cleave APP at several sites including the one responsible for generating Aβ peptide. BACE also cleaves other proteins. Knockout mice deficient in BACE produce essentially no amyloid beta peptide (30). These knockout mice also have no discernable behavioral or developmental phenotype, a good sign in terms of the possibility of utilizing BACE inhibitors as a potential AD therapy.

What about the γ-secretase? There is a clear and compelling candidate for the γ-secretase; a family of proteins termed the presenilins (PSs). There are two homologous human PS genes, presenilin 1 (PS1) and presenilin 2 (PS2). As might be expected for an enzyme capable of proteolyzing a trans-membrane alpha helix, PSs have multiple transmembrane domains (see reference 31). These proteins also undergo proteolysis themselves as part of their conversion to the active state. Presenilins are hypothesized to be *the* gamma secretase, although there is some discussion in the literature that PSs might instead act indirectly to promote gamma secretase activity. Certainly other proteins such as nicastrin are necessary in addition to presenilins in order to achieve full gamma-secretase activity.

Presenilins act not only on APP but also on other proteins such as Notch, a general role referred to as Regulated Intramembrane Proteolysis (RIP; reviewed in reference 32). PS-mediated RIP is involved in a variety of cellular signaling processes that are important in neuro-development and homeostasis. For our purposes here we will focus on the role of Presenilins in regulating the production of Aβ peptides in AD.

The APP fragments produced by the combined activities of the beta- and gamma-secretases are generally 40 or 42–43 amino acids in length. There is some variability in the site of cleavage of the gamma secretase—it can cleave APP at any of three sites. Aβ40 comprises ~90% of the Aβ population while the rest is usually made up of Aβ42(43) (33). The minor Aβ species (42/43) is highly fibrillogenic, readily aggregates, and is neurotoxic (34–39).

C. Aβ42 as the Cause of AD

Briefly stated, decades of work indicate that Aβ42 is the likely causative agent of AD. This idea is commonly referred to as the amyloid hypothesis of AD (see Hardy and Selkoe, 31, for a review). The essential findings supporting this hypothesis follow:

1. As we have already discussed, amyloid senile plaque number (i.e., Aβ deposition) in the neocortex is the primary criterion for the post-mortem diagnosis of Alzheimer's disease (40–43). The initial deposits in senile plaques are the Aβ42 and Aβ43 peptides (39).

Moreover, Aβ burden is an early indiator of cognitive decline in AD. Post-mortem studies of total Aβ (nonaggregate and aggregates in diffuse or mature senile plaques combined) in the brains of recently deceased patients correlate with recent pre-morbid Clinical Dementia Rating scale values for those individuals. Quantitative histopathological studies have shown that the number of senile plaques correlates with dementia scores in AD patients (44). This is true even for patients not yet in advanced stages of the disease. These findings support the idea that extracellular Aβ levels are elevated in at-risk individuals even prior to gross plaque deposition and severe cognitive impairment.

2. Recent studies from animal and in vitro models have made clear the capacity of aberrant Aβ production to elicit pathological features of AD. For example,

animals genetically engineered to over-produce Aβ exhibit some of the pathological features of AD, such as amyloid plaque production (see references 45 and 46 and Figure 4). In vitro studies have shown that Aβ can elicit cytotoxic effects as well.

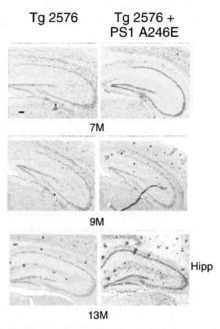

FIGURE 4 PS1 A246E FAD mutant transgene greatly accelerates amyloid plaque pathology of Tg2576 transgenic mice. Brain sections of the hippocampus of transgenic mice co-expressing APP K670N/M671L (the Tg 2576 line) and PS1 A246E FAD mutant transgenes were immunostained with Aβ specific mAb 6E10 and compared to that of age-matched Tg2576 transgenic animals. Panels are hippocampi of mice 7, 9, and 13 months of age. At all ages examined, both the density and the size of plaques in heterozygous doubly transgenic mice far exceeded that of heterozygous APP mice at comparable ages. Consistent plaque deposits were detected in 7-month-old heterozygous doubly transgenic mice when the APP transgenic mice were free of plaques. At 9 months of age, while APP transgenic mice exhibit occasional diffuse Aβ plaques, doubly transgenic mice showed numerous Aβ deposits in various regions of the brain, including cerebral cortex (data not shown) and hippocampus. Aβ load was further enhanced in 13-month-old doubly transgenic mice, and multiple brain areas were covered with plaques. Wild-type human PS1 transgene does not accelerate plaque deposition when co-expressed with the mutant APP transgene (data not shown). Littermates that express PS1 A246E alone do not develop detectable amyloid plaques up to 14 months of age (data not shown). Data courtesy of Dineley et al. (74).

3. The genetics of AD also support the hypothesis. Familial AD (FAD) is associated with the inheritance of specific genes, be they mutated genes or the presence of specific allele types. All known FAD gene products directly or indirectly impinge upon Aβ peptide production, resulting in increased Aβ levels in the CNS—we will return to this in more detail in the next section (see Box 3 as well).

If Aβ causes AD, how does this happen? The basic mechanisms underlying Aβ-mediated neuronal dysfunction and neuronal loss are unknown and, of course, a topic of much vigorous investigation. A number of scenarios are in play at present. A variety of evidence suggests the involvement of senile plaque components in triggering inflammatory responses that culminate in neuronal death. Plaque structures appear to act as irritants and initiate inflammatory responses. For example, hypertrophic astrocytes and activated microglia often surround plaques (47), and these responses likely lead to localized cell death. The overproduction of reactive oxygen species by inflammatory process or even direct chemical catalysis by the Aβ peptide, with resulting oxidative toxicity, is another hypothesis. A large number of research groups are working in the general area of testing for effects of Aβ as causing altered activation of cellular signaling processes such as protein kinases and phosphatases. The idea is that derangement of these signaling cascades can lead to both derangements of synaptic physiology and altered phosphorylation of proteins such as tau, that are known to be associated with cell death. Another idea is that Aβ peptide binds to cell-surface receptors in order to trigger its deleterious effects. My laboratory and a number of others are currently working on the idea that neuronal nicotinic acetylcholine receptors are targets of Aβ peptide (see Box 2). Misregulation of these surface ion channels could lead to both synaptic and cellular derangement; additionally, this mechanism could provide an explanation for the selective loss of cholinergic fibers and their targets in AD.

Even though the processes that Aβ peptide triggers still remain mysterious, a parsimonious explanation consistent with most of the available data is the idea that amyloid beta peptide causes AD. In the next section, we will review some of the strongest evidence available supporting this idea—findings that gene mutations known to invariably cause AD in humans occur in genes directly linked to the production of amyloid beta peptide.

BOX 3

Aβ PEPTIDE IMMUNIZATION AS A POTENTIAL THERAPY FOR AD

In 1999, Shenk et al. discovered that immunization with amyloid β peptide protects against amyloid β plaque deposition in a mutant mouse model for Alzheimer's disease (92). In these studies they used the "PDAPP" transgenic mouse expressing human APP mutated at amino acid 717. The approach was a fairly straightforward application of traditional immunization—they injected the Aβ peptide into the animals, using an adjuvant carrier to boost the immune response.

BOX 3—cont'd

Aβ PEPTIDE IMMUNIZATION AS A POTENTIAL THERAPY FOR AD

In this first study, the investigators documented significant prevention of plaque formation in the immunized mice. This was a very exciting finding concerning a new potential therapy for AD—immunization with Aβ, letting the body's normal immune response do the rest.

How does the immunization effect a decrease in amyloid plaque formation? These immunization procedures produce active anti-Aβ antibodies in the bloodstream, a fraction of which apparently can penetrate into the CNS. The idea is that microglia in the CNS clear the antibody- Aβ complexes, reducing Aβ burden. Alternatively, decreased Aβ in the bloodstream resulting from immune clearance outside the brain may result in lowered CNS Aβ levels, by passive diffusion of the Aβ peptide out of the CNS.

A year later two groups continued these efforts and published further exciting and encouraging results. Janus et al. (93) and Morgan et al. (94) both reported ameliorative effects of the immunization protocol on the development of aging-related deficits in learning and memory in AD mouse models as well. This took the observations to the next level, demonstrating important symptomatic relief, as least as assessed using the tools available currently. Also encouraging was that similar results were obtained using a variation of the immunization approach. "Passive" immunization involves the perfusion of previously isolated and purified antibodies into the test subject. Like the active immunization studies described previously, passive immunization with anti-Aβ antibodies similarly improves memory performance in AD model mice (95, 96).

Overall these findings precipitated great hope that an immunization approach might prove of practical utility in humans. Work in this area is unfortunately at somewhat of a standstill at present. Pilot immunization studies in normal humans indicated no deleterious effects of Aβ immunization. However, in the initial study of immunization therapy using human AD patients, a small number of study subjects developed brain inflammation. This side effect, while perhaps not entirely unexpected, necessitated a halt of the study and, at present, a moratorium on this specific line of human studies.

The potential of immunotherapy as an effective treatment for Alzheimer's disease is one of the most exciting developments in the recent history of Alzheimer's disease research, offering real hope for effective therapy in the aging human. However, at present it is clear that significant work lies ahead in evaluating whether the approach will be adaptable to the human clinically.

There is an additional reason to highlight these studies, independent of their significance as a potential new therapeutic approach. As we discussed in the main text, much work is currently underway aimed at testing various predictions of the amyloid beta hypothesis of AD. The behavioral studies with Aβ immunization test one key prediction of this hypothesis— the block prediction. The observation that decreasing Aβ burden in the CNS ameliorates behavioral deficiencies is strong support for the hypothesis that Aβ is a causative agent in the memory defects associated with early AD.

III. GENES—FAMILIAL AND LATE-ONSET AD

AD is broadly divided into two types. The first and relatively better understood category is early-onset familial AD, which I will abbreviate as FAD. FAD is relatively rare, accounting in aggregate for a few percent of total AD cases (see reference 48 for a review). FAD is inherited in an autosomal dominant fashion and is highly penetrant, meaning that if you inherit a single copy of the gene you are highly likely to develop AD before age 60. So far, FAD-causing mutations have been identified in the human genes for APP, PS1, and PS2.

The second category of AD is late-onset AD, commonly abbreviated LOAD. LOAD is associated with several risk factors, the most common of which are age and the inheritance of specific genes. The LOAD-related genetic factor that has been unambiguously demonstrated to date is the inheritance of the epsilon4 (ε4) allele type of Apolipoprotein E (ApoE4; see references 49–51). ApoE alleles vary normally among individuals. If you inherit the ε4 allele, you have an increased *likelihood* of developing LOAD. Interestingly, if you inherit the less common ε2 allele, there is a small protective effect against AD.

The existence of inherited factors in AD, of course, indicates that subtypes of the disease do in fact have a genetic component. This is not as obvious as it might at first sound, given that even FAD patients do not develop AD until age 40 or so at the earliest. Thus, even the inherited forms of AD are time-dependent and multifactorial.

One mystery for FAD is how an inherited disorder, present from conception, can take so long to develop clinical manifestations. FAD may require a second (albeit common) environmental insult, perhaps even one that can accumulate over time. An alternative model is that the kinetics of the underlying biochemistry are extremely slow. Finally, it may be that the underlying process is one for which appreciable compensatory capacity exists relative to the rate of insult accumulation (see Box 4). At present, these temporal aspects of AD development remain inexplicable.

One commonality across all forms of AD is the involvement of the metabolism of APP and its products. All the FAD autosomal dominant mutations, and the inheritance of the ApoE-ε4 allele, result in altered metabolism of the amyloid precursor protein (APP). These inherited factors moreover have in common that their major consequence is elevated production of Aβ42 in the CNS. In the following sections, I will briefly review how this is thought to happen.

A. APP Mutations

There are two categories of mutations in APP that lead to early-onset familial AD (see Figure 3). One is the so-called "Swedish double mutation," named for the Swedish kindred in which it was first identified. The Swedish mutation is a K670M, N671L double mutation in the APP gene (52, 53). This double mutation results in higher levels of secreted Aβ peptides in the CNS. The second type of AD-associated APP mutations results in a higher fraction of the longer Aβ peptides being produced. These are the missense mutations at residue 717 in the APP gene (38, 53, 54). Both categories of mutations affect the endoproteolytic cleavage pattern during APP processing, promoting the β- and γ-secretase cleavage activities over the α-secretase (55, 56). A final type of APP mutation, commonly referred to as the "Dutch" type of mutation, does not cause AD per se. These are mutations in and around amino acid 693 in the APP sequence. These mutations also elicit overproduction of amyloid but result in variations a syndrome known as Dutch-type hereditary cerebral hemorrhage with amyloidosis, a vascular disorder.

BOX 4

THE NUN STUDY

One of the most interesting studies ever published on the epidemiology of AD is the "Nun Study." In pursuing this work, David Snowdon undertook an amazingly sophisticated scientific and personal mission in order to help understand the epidemiologic factors involved in AD (97). He did this with the help and commitment of 678 Catholic Sisters of the "School Sisters of Notre Dame" Order, an order devoted to education, teaching, and service. They took as one of their missions to help us all learn about AD, by opening their personal lives and histories to prying scientific eyes, and by donating their brains for scientific study post-mortem.

David Snowdon and his colleagues had the insight to assess a large group of Catholic nuns as an epidemiologic cohort. This is about as scientifically well-controlled a group of humans as is imaginable, practically speaking. Most of them have lived their entire adult lives alongside their Sisters, eating the same foods and living in the same environment. Detailed personal histories are available, including very early records from when they joined the order in their late teens. Confounding vices, such as illicit drug use, are understandably of minimal concern with a group of this sort. A constant and comparable level of health care applies across the group as well. Comparison within this group to assess who develops AD and who doesn't allows new insights into individual attributes that correlate with a risk of AD.

An additional important component of the Nun Study is that each nun wrote a brief autobiography before taking her final vows to join the order. These writing samples were obtained on average from study participants when they were in their late teens or early twenties. This served as a critical point of reference concerning language usage by each of the study participants. One astounding finding from the Nun Study came from comparing language usage in their youth with their development of AD later in life. In brief, this type of analysis convincingly demonstrated that complex cognitive skills and abilities at a relatively young age correlate with a *decreased* likelihood of developing AD in late adulthood. These findings are in general agreement with a number of prior studies correlating college-level education or higher with a decreased incidence of AD.

It is not clear how a high level of cognitive ability in youth might relate mechanistically to developing late-onset AD. Three general possibilities have been suggested. First, AD may in fact start developing at a young age, manifesting subtle effects even in individuals in their late teens. Second, the two findings may be correlative but not causally related—for example the same genes that predispose one to AD may also impinge negatively upon cognitive function, for reasons unrelated to AD pathology. Finally, higher baseline abilities in cognitive function may allow a "reserve" of brain capacity, helping delay the detectable onset of AD. Which of these possibilities is relevant will hopefully become clear as the molecular underpinnings of AD are determined.

B. Presenilin Mutations

As you might have guessed from the name, the presenilin gene that likely codes for the APP-processing endoprotease was first identified as an AD candidate gene and termed presenilin on that basis (reviewed in reference 48). Only later was it identified as a strong candidate for being the actual gamma secretase that helps process APP into Aβ. Mutations in both the PS-1 and PS-2 genes (PSEN-1 and -2 in the human) result in early onset FAD, but PS-1 mutations result in a slightly earlier onset of FAD than PS-2 mutations.

Most of the known FAD-causing mutations that have been identified to date, several dozen distinct mutations, are mutations in PS-1 (see reference 31). These mutations in PS-1 and PS-2 have in common fact that they lead to alterations in APP processing. Transgenic mouse studies indicate that PS1 FAD mutations do not inactivate normal PS1 activity (57) but rather alter APP processing in a way as to enhance Aβ42 synthesis (57–59). The net result is that the ratio of secreted Aβ42(43) to Aβ40 in individuals with PS-1 or PS-2 mutations are elevated relative to unaffected family members (52). Furthermore, in transfected mammalian cells and the brains of transgenic (Tg) mice that coexpress APP and mutant PS1 variants, levels of secreted Aβ42 are also elevated (see reference 59 and Figure 4). These observations are consistent with changes in APP metabolism, due to altered secretase cleavage patterns, resulting in an increased burden of extracellular Aβ peptide. In essence, PS-1 and PS-2 mutations that lead to AD are "gain of function" mutations, leading to elevated Aβ peptide production.

Mutations in the APP and PSEN1/2 genes account for only about 5% of AD cases. Moreover, they account for only about 40% or so of autosomal dominant AD cases—that is, those that are clearly and proximally caused by inherited mutations. Clearly much is left to be learned from pursuing the identification of new AD genes. One promising category of genes left to be identified are those encoding for the enzymes that break down Aβ. Recent exciting work indicates that various groups are closing in on this culprit. Specifically, it appears to be the case that Insulin Degrading Enzyme or a gene near it on chromosome 10 may be involved in regulating Aβ levels and thus linked to LOAD (60–62).

C. ApoE4 Alleles in AD

Current estimates are that the ApoE ε4 allele is a contributing factor to about 20% of AD cases. The basis for ApoE alleles contributing to AD is much less clear than the APP and PSEN mutations (51). For one thing, the ApoE ε4 allele is neither necessary nor sufficient to cause AD. It is a contributing risk factor, when present, which decreases the average age of onset of AD and presumably by this mechanism increases the incidence of AD in that population.

One unifying attribute, which at least allows for a consistent model in the context of the APP and PSEN mutations, is that the presence of the ApoE ε4 allele clearly leads to elevated Aβ burden in the CNS. This not only is true both in the human brain (63) and in emerging mouse models for AD (64) but also gives a unifying model across the known genetic factors contributing to AD: elevation of Aβ in the CNS.

How ApoE might do this is the unclear part (reviewed in reference 51). The initial discovery of a role for ApoE in AD grew out of studies of a direct interaction of ApoE with Aβ, so direct effects on amyloid deposition are a clear possibility (49, 65, 66, reviewed in reference 67). ApoE also has classically been studied in terms of cholesterol handling, and this role might somehow play a part. However, more recent work has demonstrated that ApoE also binds directly to a number of neuronal cell surface receptors, and effects via this mechanism might also contribute to AD pathogenesis (see reference 68 for a review). In the next section, I will provide a brief overview of the ApoE system in order to give some context for how ApoE isoforms and their receptors might contribute to AD pathogenesis.

IV. APOLIPOPROTEIN E IN THE NERVOUS SYSTEM

Lipoproteins are complexes of carrier proteins and lipids, including cholesterol, that in the cardiovascular and digestive systems are involved in the trafficking of dietary lipids. Apolipoprotein E is a component of lipoproteins and mediates the uptake of these lipoprotein particles into target tissues. In the liver, ApoE is incorporated into very low density lipoproteins (VLDLs), which carry triglycerides and cholesterol to peripheral tissues, mainly muscle and adipose tissue. In the gut, ApoE becomes a component of chylomicrons and mediates the transport of dietary fat to the liver. In macrophages, the scavenger cells of the immune system, ApoE is involved in the resecretion of absorbed cholesterol. However, ApoE is also expressed in cells of the nervous system, predominantly in astrocytes. The role of ApoE secretion and its binding to the ApoE receptors (ApoERs) that are present on the surface of neurons is unclear at this point.

ApoE occurs in three major isoforms in the general human population, ApoE2, ApoE3, and ApoE4. As described earlier, the ApoE4 isoform, also known as ApoE ε4, is associated with AD.

There are a variety of ApoE receptors that are expressed on the surface of neurons that may be involved in the pathological process by which ApoE contributes to AD. Two members of this neuronal family of ApoE receptors warrant particular attention: the very low density lipoprotein receptor (VLDLR) and the Apolipoprotein E receptor 2 (ApoER2). Both receptors participate in neuronal signaling pathways related to memory formation. These receptors bind not only ApoE but also the signaling molecule Reelin, a large protein of approximately 400 kDa that is secreted by interneurons dispersed throughout the neocortex and the hippocampus.

The ApoE/Reelin receptors ApoER2 and VLDLR couple to the adaptor protein Dab1, which is essential to ApoE/Reelin signaling. As I mentioned in Chapter 6, these receptors couple via Dab1 to the src pathway and potentially via this mechanism contribute to NMDA receptor regulation.

In a recent series of experiments, we found that mice lacking the ApoE/Reelin receptors VLDLR and ApoER2 have pronounced defects in memory formation and hippocampal long-term potentiation (69). Furthermore, Reelin greatly enhances LTP in hippocampal slices. Our results thus reveal a role for ApoE receptors in synaptic function and in the formation of long-term memory. These data are also consistent with a hypothetical model in which the promotion of memory dysfunction by ApoE4 might involve an impairment of this ApoE receptor-dependent signaling pathway—how this might be involved in AD is a current line of investigation in several laboratories.

V. MOUSE MODELS FOR AD

Progress in understanding AD and developing new therapies for AD hinges upon the availability of suitable model systems for investigating the disease in the laboratory. In this vein, the application of transgenic animal technology to the pursuit of investigating AD appears to be a critically important endeavor. There are several considerations that factor into the critical role of genetic engineering in developing suitable laboratory models for AD. First, AD is an exclusively human disorder—no naturally occurring animal homologues that we can study in the lab appear to exist. AD is not transmissible, at least as far as we know, so one cannot attempt to mutate already occurring pathogens in order to generate new models. No environmental factor has yet been identified that is capable of producing AD or even aspects of the disease. Chemical or anatomical lesions to the CNS are unable to mimic the condition adequately. The only identified basis for AD is genetic. Thus, genetic engineering is the only practical route available for modeling AD in vivo.

Mouse models for AD fortunately are becoming increasingly available (see Table 2). These mouse models capitalize on the important studies, described earlier, that have identified human AD-causing mutations. Current mouse models are transgenic mouse models expressing mutated forms of human genes (reviewed in references 27, 70, and 71). The engineered animals generally use neuron-selective promoters to drive expression of the transgenes in the CNS. Currently available lines that model AD are all derived from transgenic animals expressing mutated human APP either alone or in combination with mutated human PS-1. Transgenic lines expressing ApoE alleles are still at a relatively early stage of development.

One prominent transgenic mouse model for AD expresses a human splice-variant of APP containing the "Swedish" double mutation. This specific mutation and splice variant was identified in a large family with FAD (45, 53). This model is variously referred to as the "Swedish" mouse (after the mutation), the "Mayo" mouse (after the patent holders), the "Hsiao" mouse (after Karen Hsiao Ashe, who made the mouse), or the "Tg2576" mouse (after the mouse line number). I will refer to it as the Tg2576 mouse. Since Karen Hsiao got married and changed her last name to Ashe, my preferred eponym is out of date.

The other major mouse line that has been extensively characterized so far is the "PDAPP" line. The name derives from the fact that it is a line expressing the human APP transgene (mutated at position 717) driven by a PDGF promoter. Other lines under development and characterization include another 717 APP mutant line, a mixture variation combining both the Swedish and 717 mutations, APP mutants combined with PS-1 mutants, and APP mutants combined with tau mutants. These mutant lines along with a few other related knockout mouse lines, and selected references, are given in Table 2.

For illustrative purposes, I will discuss some of the attributes of the Tg2576 line. I choose to focus on the Tg2576 line for two reasons. First, it is one of the lines that we have worked with in my lab, so I am most familiar with it. Second, its properties seem to be fairly representative of the various mouse lines under investigation at present. In particular, the Tg2576 line and the other major line, the PDAPP line, appear to have similar molecular and behavioral characteristics.

A. The Tg2576 Mouse

The Tg2576 strain is a mouse model for AD in which the transgene is the human 695 splice-variant of APP that contains the double mutation K670M, N671L driven by a hamster prion protein gene promoter (expression is predominantly in neurons). The brains of these animals contain about five times more transgenic mutant human APP than endogenous mouse APP. Transgenic APP expression appears to remain unchanged between 2 and 14 months of age. They exhibit about a fivefold increase in $A\beta40$ and a 10- to 15-fold increase in $A\beta42/43$ over levels measured in nontransgenic littermates. Similar to observations in AD brain, and consistent with the notion that elevated $A\beta$ is potentially toxic to brain cells, senile plaques in the brains of these mice are associated with signs of cellular inflammatory responses.

TABLE 2   Selected Mouse Models for AD

AD Models		Phenotypes			
Mouse model	Transgene	Plaques?	NFT's?	Cell Death?	Memory Deficits?
Tg2576 (APP$_{swe}$)	Human APP K670N/M671L	Yes	Minimal	Minimal	Fear conditioning (74)
	695 AA splice variant prion promotor				Water maze (73) Forced alternation (75)
PDAPP	Human APP V717F PDGF promotor	Yes	Partial (98)	Minimal	Water maze Spatial series (99) Object recognition (95) Holeboard (95)
Tg2576+JNPL3	APPswe P301L Tau	Yes	Yes (100)	Minimal	?
TgLRND8	Human APP 670N/671L + V717F	Yes	Minimal	Minimal	Water maze (93, 101)
	(+M146L L286V PS-1 mutant)	Plaques accelerated			
PS-1	Several–M146L, L286V	Minimal	Minimal	Minimal	No (74)
APP + PS-1	Tg2576 + A246E PS-1	Yes	Minimal	Minimal	Exacerbated relative to Tg2576 alone (74, 102)
V717I	Human APP V717I	Yes	Minimal	Minimal	Object recognition
V717I	Crossed with PS-1 knockout	No			Similar (103)

Relevant Molecules	Model Type	Phenotype
PS-1	Knockout	+/− developmental defects, −/− lethal; Forebrain:decreased hippocampal neurogenesis (104, 105)
ApoE	Knockout	Memory and LTP deficits (106, 107)
APP	Knockout	Hippocampal gliosis (108)
PS-2	Knockout	Modest phenotype (109)
ApoE4	Transgenic	No learning phenotype, accelerated plaque disposition when combined with APP V717F(66, 110)

Tg2576 mice exhibit many behavioral and pathological features of AD including elevated production of Aβ peptides, age-dependent accumulation of amyloid fibrils, and plaque formation with subsequent age-dependent hippocampal learning and memory deficits (45, 46, 70, 72–75). This mouse model demonstrates a correlation between hippocampal dysfunction at both the cellular and behavioral levels versus its increased burden of extracellular Aβ42(43), as I will describe briefly next.

At 6 months of age and older, mice exhibit a deficit in spatial memory (Morris water maze). In addition to impairment in spatial memory at 14–16 months of age, mice also exhibit a working memory deficit as measured using a forced-alternation paradigm (75, 76). Tg2576 mice also exhibit deficits in contextual fear conditioning (see references 74 and 76 and Figure 5). Several

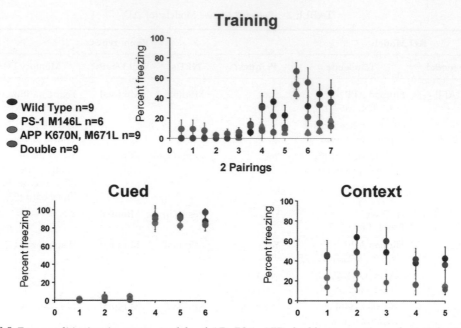

FIGURE 5 Fear conditioning in mouse models of AD. PS-1, APP, doubly transgenic, and control mice were subjected to a standard fear conditioning paradigm in which the animals learn to associate neutral stimuli with an aversive one. The mice were placed in a novel context (fear-conditioning box) and exposed to two pairings of a white-noise cue and mild foot shock. Fear learning was assessed 24 hours later by measuring freezing behavior in response to re-presentation of the context or of the auditory cue within a completely different context. At 5 months of age, there were no apparent differences in the freezing behavior of the different mouse genotypes during the two-pairing training phase of fear conditioning (top). In the contextual test for fear learning, the APP and doubly transgenic animals exhibited decreased freezing behavior compared to both the control littermates and PS-1 transgenic group (lower right). One-way ANOVA and Tukey post hoc analysis detected a significant difference in freezing behavior at the 1- through 4-minute time epochs compared to control littermates and at the 1-, 2-, 3-, and 5-minute epochs compared to the PS-1 transgenic group [min 1: $F(3,60) = 5.60$; min 2: $F = 7.68$; min 3: $F = 8.51$; min 4: $F = 4.26$; min 5: $F = 4.35$; $p < .05$ all groups]. Analysis of overall freezing behavior indicates that APP and doubly transgenic animals freeze significantly less than control and PS-1 transgenic animals [Tukey's multiple comparison test: $F(5,16) = 27.97$; control versus APP, control versus doubly, APP versus PS-1, doubly versus PS-1 all $p < .001$]. These data indicate that APP and doubly transgenic animals have a deficit in contextual fear learning. These same animals did not exhibit a deficit in cued fear conditioning (lower left). One-way ANOVA and Tukey post hoc analysis determined that all animals displayed similar and significant freezing in the cued test for associative learning, indicating that the impairment in contextual fear learning exhibited by the APP and doubly transgenic animal groups is not the result of an inability to freeze or to detect the aversive foot-shock stimulus ($p < .001$, all groups). Therefore, 5-month-old APP and doubly transgenic mice appear to have a selective hippocampus-dependent impairment in associative learning following two pairings of conditioned and unconditioned stimuli for fear conditioning. Adapted from Dineley et al. (74; see also reference 76).

AD-like pathologies are not present in these mice. For example, there is no neuronal loss in CA1 or other brain areas (37). Thus, these mice do not model AD-associated neuronal loss. Nonetheless, the age-dependent amyloidogenesis and working memory deficits are powerful correlates of AD and make this animal model an attractive launching point for investigations into the cellular signaling processes underlying neuronal dysfunction induced by an increased burden of extracellular A-beta.

It has also been reported that accompanying the behavioral deficits in working memory, Tg2576 mice exhibit disruptions of LTP in both the Schaffer collateral and perforant pathways of the hippocampus. Synaptic transmission and paired-pulse facilitation appear normal (indicating that Ca^{2+}-dependent synaptic vesicle release is normal), and there is no decrease in the number of CA1 neurons or synaptic density in the dentate gyrus (75). Thus, in Tg2576 mice, selective impairments in synaptic plasticity correlate with deficits in cognitive abilities.

Our take-home message from all of this is that the Tg2576 mouse strain exhibits learning deficits and alterations in synaptic plasticity with no neuronal cell loss. In that respect, it, along with all other available mouse strains modeling AD, does not recapitulate one of the major hallmarks of late-stage AD—cell death. However, these mouse lines accurately model amyloidosis and likely model early-stage AD. The lack of cell death in all these lines has an important implication as well. Because there is no appreciable cell loss nor pronounced alterations in neuronal morphology, the impairment that leads to the memory phenotype is likely in the normal cellular signaling cascades involved in learning and synaptic plasticity.

What is the site of derangement in neuronal signaling that underlies the Tg2576 mouse phenotype? Ongoing work by Kelly Dineley in my lab, done in collaboration with a number of investigators including Karen Hsiao and Hui Zheng, suggests the hypothesis that the increased burden of extracellular Aβ peptide in Tg2576 mice leads to derangement of hippocampal ERK MAPK activity (77). These derangements potentially result in subsequent learning and memory deficits in a fashion reminiscent of the various human mental retardation syndromes that we discussed in the last chapter. However, this is just one specific finding among a multitude of identified derangements in mouse lines modeling AD. I note the finding because, in my mind, it presents an interesting example of a potential AD-associated derangement in one of the principal memory-associated signal transduction pathway that we have been discussing throughout the book.

Crossing PS1 transgenic mice carrying the A246E FAD mutation with Tg2576 mice causes acceleration of CNS amyloid accumulation and plaque formation (see Figure 4 and Table 2). The doubly transgenic animals also have exacerbated associative learning deficits relative to the Tg2576 transgenic mice. These data indicate that, as might be expected, there is an interaction of the APP and PS-1 gene products in vivo. The point in raising this observation is twofold. First, over time their will likely be improvement in modeling AD in mice through these kinds of mix-and-match genetic experiments. Second, this result illustrates a use of genetically engineered mouse models of AD that is independent of their utility as a model for human disease per se. That is, the emergence of these various transgenic mouse lines will allow the testing of various specific predictions of current working models for how the various gene products identified as relevant to amyloid beta peptide production interact in the living animal.

Overall, the studies published so far indicate cause for optimism that transgenic mouse models for AD will be of great utility both in studying the biochemistry and physiology of the disease and in assessing potential new treatment avenues for AD (see Box 3). Important work in the near future will allow further evaluation and optimization of mouse models for investigating AD. In addition, as we obtain further basic information concerning human AD (for example, identification of additional genetic factors predisposing us to AD), further enhancement of progress in mouse models is likely.

These practical considerations should not completely overshadow the additional important implications of transgenic mouse experiments, however. The transgenic mouse studies to date can be looked at as experiments testing predictions of the amyloid beta hypothesis of AD. The measure experiments using human AD tissues identified an association of Aβ with

AD. Transgenic mouse experiments are the mimic experiments. Thus far, studies of transgenic mice overexpressing Aβ peptide certainly indicate that Aβ is sufficient to cause many of the pathological hallmarks and cognitive features of early AD. These are important experimental results in their own right.

VI. SUMMARY

In this chapter, I have promoted viewing Alzheimer's disease as a memory disorder, as opposed to thinking of AD as a generalized neuropathologic dementia. The basic hypothesis is that, for early stages of AD, which are characterized not by generalized dementia but rather by much more subtle deficits in memory consolidation, there will be derangements of the normal signal transduction machinery that underlies memory. This viewpoint sets me apart from most investigators in the AD field. However, I am optimistic that this will be a fruitful avenue of pursuit because the idea is based upon the tremendous advances that have been made in the last decade in our understanding of the basic biochemistry of memory. If this is the case, it also means that AD is likely the area where recent progress in understanding the basic science of memory will translate into an improvement in capacity to attack a clinical disorder of great significance.

Interestingly, as was described in the chapter, several studies have indicated that Aβ peptide overproduction in the CNS can elicit cognitive deficits in rodents in the absence of neuronal loss or even Aβ deposition into plaques. These findings are consistent with the idea that memory deficits in early stages of AD may be due to disruption of the neuronal signal transduction machinery that normally subserves memory formation.

We also talked about the great strides that have been made in identifying the genetic factors contributing to AD. Specifically, we talked about APP, presenilin, and ApoE4 and how mutations or isoforms of these gene products can cause or predispose one to developing AD. I also provided an overview of new mouse models for AD that capitalize upon the human findings in order to allow the generation of model systems of utility in the basic science research laboratory.

The principal unifying theme of the chapter is the amyloid beta hypothesis of AD. To my eye at least, there is a reassuring convergence of many different sorts of data that support the Aβ hypothesis of AD. While I did not organize the chapter around evaluating this hypothesis directly, evaluating the contents of the chapter with this question in mind is a useful exercise. Students in particular might find it useful to recast the section on mouse models of AD in terms of evaluating the block, mimic, and measure predictions of the Aβ hypothesis.

More than most other areas of contemporary neuroscience research, it seems to me that the AD field is at the intersection of basic and clinical research—a critically important clinical problem in search of answers that only basic science can provide. AD is a disease of human memory. The complexity of AD pathogenesis is rooted in the complexity of memory itself. Hopefully advances in understanding the basic science of memory will soon translate into tangible improvements in treating AD.

References

1. Barnes, C. A. (1988) "Aging and the physiology of spatial memory." *Neurobiol. Aging* 9:563–568.
2. Barnes, C. A., Suster, M. S., Shen, J., and McNaughton, B. L. (1997). "Multistability of cognitive maps in the hippocampus of old rats." *Nature* 388:272–275.
3. Barnes, C. A., Rao, G., and Houston, F. P. (2000). "LTP induction threshold change in old rats at the perforant path—granule cell synapse." *Neurobiol. Aging* 21:613–620.
4. Barnes, C. A., Rao, G., and Shen, J. (1997). "Age-related decrease in the N-methyl-D-spartateR-mediated excitatory postsynaptic potential in hippocampal region CA1." *Neurobiol. Aging* 18:445–452.

5. Lynch, M. A. (1998). "Analysis of the mechanisms underlying the age-related impairment in long-term potentiation in the rat." *Rev. Neurosci.* 9:169–201.

6. Braak, H., Braak, E., and Bohl, J. (1993). "Staging of Alzheimer-related cortical destruction." *Eur. Neurol.* 33:403–408.

7. Nagy, Z., Hindley, N. J., Braak, H., Braak, E., Yilmazer-Hanke, D. M., Schultz, C., Barnetson, L., Jobst, K. A., and Smith, A. D. (1999). "Relationship between clinical and radiological diagnostic criteria for Alzheimer's disease and the extent of neuropathology as reflected by 'stages': a prospective study." *Dement. Geriatr. Cogn. Disord.* 10:109–114.

8. Braak, E., and Braak, H. (1997). "Alzheimer's disease: transiently developing dendritic changes in pyramidal cells of sector CA1 of the Ammon's horn." *Acta. Neuropathol. (Berl)* 93:323–325.

9. Braak, H., and Braak, E. (1998). "Evolution of neuronal changes in the course of Alzheimer's disease." *J. Neural. Transm. Suppl.* 53:127–140.

10. Alzheimer, A. (1907). "Uber eine eigenartige Erkrankung der Hirnrinde." *Allgemeine Zeitschrift fur Psychiatrie und Psychisch-gerichtliche Medizin* 64:146–148.

11. Whitehouse, P. J., Price, D. L., Struble, R. G., Clark, A. W., Coyle, J. T., and Delon, M. R. (1982). "Alzheimer's disease and senile dementia: loss of neurons in the basal forebrain." *Science* 215:1237–1239.

12. Braak HaB, E. (1994). In: *Neurodegenerative diseases*, edited by Caine DB. Philadelphia: Saunders; 585–613.

13. Zweig, R. M., Ross, C. A., Hedreen, J. C., Steele, C., Cardillo, J. E., Whitehouse, P. J., Folstein, M. F., and Price, D. L. (1988). "The neuropathology of aminergic nuclei in Alzheimer's disease." *Ann. Neurol.* 24:233–242.

14. Hyman, B. T., Van Horsen, G. W., Damasio, A. R., and Barnes, C. L. (1984). "Alzheimer's disease: cell-specific pathology isolates the hippocampal formation." *Science* 225:1168–1170.

15. Hyman, B. T., Van Hoesen, G. W., Kromer, L. J., and Damasio, A. R. (1986). "Perforant pathway changes and the memory impairment of Alzheimer's disease." *Ann. Neurol.* 20:472–481.

16. Spillantini, M. G., and Goedert, M. (1998). "Tau protein pathology in neurodegenerative diseases." *Trends Neurosci.* 21:428–433.

17. Taylor, J. P., Hardy, J., and Fischbeck, K. H. (2002). "Toxic proteins in neurodegenerative disease." *Science* 296:1991–1995.

18. Glenner, G. G., and Wong, C. W. (1984). "Alzheimer's disease: initial report of the purification and characterization of a novel cerebrovasular amyloid protein." *Biochem. Biophys. Res. Commun.* 120:885–890.

19. Masters, C. L., Simms, G., Weinman, N. A., Multhaup, G., McDonald, B. L., and Beyreuther, K. (1985). "Amyloid plaque core protein in Alzheimer disease and Down syndrome." *Proc. Natl. Acad. Sci. USA* 82:4245–4249.

20. Kang, J., Lemaire, H. G., Unterbeck, A., Salbaum, J. M., Masters, C. L., Grzeschik, K. H., Multhaup, G., Beyreuther, K., and Muller-Hill, B. (1987). "The precursor of Alzheimer's disease amyloid A4 protein resembles a cell-surface receptor." *Nature* 325:733–736.

21. Lamb, B. T., Sisodia, S. S., Lawler, A. M., Slunt, H. H., Kitt, C. A., Kearns, W. G., Pearson, P. L., Price, D. L., and Gearhart, J. D. (1993). "Introduction and expression of the 400 kilobase amyloid precursor protein gene in transgenic mice [corrected]." *Nat. Genet.* 5:22–30.

22. Koo, E. H., Sisodia, S. S., Archer, D. R., Martin, L. J., Weidemann, A., Beyreuther, K., Fischer, P., Masters, C. L., and Price, D. L. (1990). "Precursor of amyloid protein in Alzheimer disease undergoes fast anterograde axonal transport." *Proc. Natl. Acad. Sci. USA* 87:1561–1565.

23. Buxbaum, J. D., Thinakaran, G., Koliatsos, V., O'Callahan, J., Slunt, H. H., Price, D. L., and Sisodia, S. S. (1998). "Alzheimer amyloid protein precursor in the rat hippocampus: transport and processing through the perforant path." *J. Neurosci.* 18:9629–9637.

24. Haass, C., and Selkoe, D. J. (1993). "Cellular processing of beta-amyloid precursor protein and the genesis of amyloid beta-peptide." *Cell* 75:1039–1042.

25. Sahasrabudhe, S. R., Spruyt, M. A., Muenkel, H. A., Blume, A. J., Vitek, M. P., and Jacobsen, J. S. (1992). "Release of amino-terminal fragments from amyloid precursor protein reporter and mutated derivatives in cultured cells." *J. Biol. Chem.* 267:25602–25608.

26. Sisodia, S. S. (1992). "Beta-amyloid precursor protein cleavage by a membrane-bound protease." *Proc. Natl. Acad. Sci. USA* 89:6075–6079.

27. Wong, P. C., Cai, H., Borchelt, D. R., and Price, D. L. (2002). "Genetically engineered mouse models of neurodegenerative diseases." *Nat. Neurosci.* 5:633–639.

28. Vassar, R., Bennett, B. D., Babu-Khan, S., Kahn, S., Mendiaz, E. A., Denis, P., Teplow, D. B., Ross, S., Amarante, P., Loeloff, R., Luo, Y., Fisher, S., Fuller, J., Edenson, S., Lile, J., Jarosinski, M. A., Biere, A. L., Curran, E., Burgess, T., Louis, J. C., Collins, F., Treanor, J., Rogers, G., and Citron, M. (1999). "Beta-secretase cleavage of Alzheimer's amyloid precursor protein by the transmembrane aspartic protease BACE." *Science* 286:735–741.

29. Vassar, R., and Citron, M. (2000). "Abeta-generating enzymes: recent advances in beta- and gamma-secretase research." *Neuron* 27:419–422.

30. Luo, Y., Bolon, B., Kahn, S., Bennett, B. D., Babu-Khan, S., Denis, P., Fan, W., Kha, H., Zhang, J., Gong, Y., Martin, L., Louis, J. C., Yan, Q., Richards, W. G., Citron, M., and Vassar, R. (2001). "Mice deficient in BACE1, the Alzheimer's

beta-secretase, have normal phenotype and abolished beta-amyloid generation." *Nat. Neurosci.* 4:231–232.

31. Hardy, J., and Selkoe, D. J. (2002). "The amyloid hypothesis of Alzheimer's disease: progress and problems on the road to therapeutics." *Science* 297:353–356.

32. Ebinu, J. O., and Yankner, B. A. (2002). "A RIP tide in neuronal signal transduction." *Neuron* 34:499–502.

33. Mann, D. M., Iwatsubo, T., Ihara, Y., Cairns, N. J., Lantos, P. L., Bogdanovic, N., Lannfelt, L., Winblad, B., Maat-Schieman, M. L., and Rossor, M. N. (1996). "Predominant deposition of amyloid-beta 42(43) in plaques in cases of Alzheimer's disease and hereditary cerebral hemorrhage associated with mutations in the amyloid precursor protein gene." *Am. J. Pathol.* 148:1257–1266.

34. Pike, C. J., Walencewicz, A. J., Glabe, C. G., and Cotman, C. W. (1991). "Aggregation-related toxicity of synthetic beta-amyloid protein in hippocampal cultures." *Eur. J. Pharmacol.* 207:367–368.

35. Roher, A. E., Lowenson, J. D., Clarke, S., Wolkow, C., Wang, R., Cotter, R. J., Reardon, I. M., Zurcher-Neely, H. A., Heinrikson, R. L., Ball, M. J., and Greenberg, B. D. (1993). "Structural alterations in the peptide backbone of beta-amyloid core protein may account for its deposition and stability in Alzheimer's disease." *J. Biol. Chem.* 268:3072–3083.

36. Yankner, B. A., Dawes, L. R., Fisher, S., Villa-Komaroff, L., Oster-Granite, M. L., and Neve, R. L. (1989). "Neurotoxicity of a fragment of the amyloid precursor associated with Alzheimer's disease." *Science* 245:417–420.

37. Yankner, B. A. (1996). "Mechanisms of neuronal degeneration in Alzheimer's disease." *Neuron* 16:921–932.

38. Suzuki, N., Cheung, T. T., Cai, X. D., Odaka, A., Otvos, L. Jr, Eckman, C., Golde, T. E., and Younkin, S. G. (1994). "An increased percentage of long amyloid beta protein secreted by familial amyloid beta protein precursor (beta APP717) mutants." *Science* 264:1336–1340.

39. Saido, T. C., Iwatsubo, T., Mann, D. M., Shimada, H., Ihara, Y., and Kawashima, S. (1995). "Dominant and differential deposition of distinct beta-amyloid peptide species, A beta N3(pE), in senile plaques." *Neuron* 14:457–466.

40. Khachaturian, Z. S. (1985). "Diagnosis of Alzheimer's disease." *Arch. Neurol.* 42:1097–1105.

41. Mirra, S. S., Heyman, A., McKeel, D., Sumi, S. M., Crain, B. J., Brownlee, L. M., Vogel, F. S., Hughes, J. P., van Belle, G., and Berg, L. (1991). "The Consortium to Establish a Registry for Alzheimer's Disease (CERAD). Part II. Standardization of the neuropathologic assessment of Alzheimer's disease." *Neurology* 41:479–486.

42. Mirra, S. S., Hart ,M. N., and Terry, R. D. (1993). "Making the diagnosis of Alzheimer's disease. A primer for practicing pathologists." *Arch. Pathol. Lab. Med.* 117:132–144.

43. Mirra, S. S., Gearing, M., and Nash, F. (1997). "Neuropathologic assessment of Alzheimer's disease." *Neurology* 49:S14–16.

44. Roth, M., Tomlinson, B. E., and Blessed, G. (1966). "Correlation between scores for dementia and counts of 'senile plaques' in cerebral grey matter of elderly subjects." *Nature* 209:109–110.

45. Hsiao, K., Chapman, P., Nilsen, S., Eckman, C., Harigaya, Y., Younkin, S., Yang, F., and Cole, G. (1996). "Correlative memory deficits, Abeta elevation, and amyloid plaques in transgenic mice." *Science* 274:99–102.

46. Hsiao, K. (1998). "Transgenic mice expressing Alzheimer amyloid precursor proteins." *Exp. Gerontol.* 33:883–889.

47. McGeer, P. L., and McGeer, E. G. (1998). "Mechanisms of cell death in Alzheimer disease—immunopathology." *J. Neural. Transm. Suppl.* 54:159–166.

48. Tanzi, R. E., and Bertram, L. (2001). "New frontiers in Alzheimer's disease genetics." *Neuron* 32:181–184.

49. Strittmatter, W. J., Saunders, A. M., Schmechel, D., Pericak-Vance, M., Enghild, J., Salvesen, G. S., and Roses, A. D. (1993). "Apolipoprotein E: high-avidity binding to beta-amyloid and increased frequency of type 4 allele in late-onset familial Alzheimer disease." *Proc. Natl. Acad. Sci. USA* 90:1977–1981.

50. Strittmatter, W. J., and Roses, A. D. (1996). "Apolipoprotein E and Alzheimer's disease." *Annu Rev. Neurosci.* 19:53–77.

51. Strittmatter, W. J. (2001). "Apolipoprotein E and Alzheimer's disease: signal transduction mechanisms." *Biochem. Soc. Symp.* 101–109.

52. Scheuner, D., Eckman, C., Jensen, M., Song, X., Citron, M., Suzuki, N., Bird, T. D., Hardy, J., Hutton, M., Kukull, W., Larson, E., Levy-Lahad, E., Viitanen, M., Peskind, E., Poorkaj, P., Schellenberg, G., Tanzi, R., Wasco, W., Lannfelt, L., Selkoe, D., and Younkin, S. (1996). "Secreted amyloid beta-protein similar to that in the senile plaques of Alzheimer's disease is increased in vivo by the presenilin 1 and 2 and APP mutations linked to familial Alzheimer's disease." *Nat. Med.* 2:864–870.

53. Mullan, M., Crawford, F., Axelman, K., Houlden, H., Lilius, L., Winblad, B., and Lannfelt, L. (1992). "A pathogenic mutation for probable Alzheimer's disease in the APP gene at the N-terminus of beta-amyloid." *Nat. Genet.* 1:345–347.

54. Goate, A., Chartier-Harlin, M. C., Mullan, M., Brown, J., Crawford, F., Fidani, L., Giuffra, L., Haynes, A., Irving, N., James, L., Mant, R., Newton, P., Rooke, K., Roques, C. T., Pericak-Vance, M., Roses, A., Williamson, R., Rossor, M., Owen, M., and Hardy, J. (1991). "Segregation of a missense mutation in the

amyloid precursor protein gene with familial Alzheimer's disease." *Nature* 349:704–706.

55. Thinakaran, G., Borchelt, D. R., Lee, M. K., Slunt, H. H., Spitzer, L., Kim, G., Ratovitsky, T., Davenport, F., Nordstedt, C., Seeger, M., Hardy, J., Levey, A. I., Gandy, S. E., Jenkins, N. A., Copeland, N. G., Price, D. L., and Sisodia, S. S. (1996). "Endoproteolysis of presenilin 1 and accumulation of processed derivatives in vivo." *Neuron* 17:181–190.

56. Perez, R. G., Squazzo, S. L., and Koo, E. H. (1996). "Enhanced release of amyloid beta-protein from codon 670/671 "Swedish" mutant beta-amyloid precursor protein occurs in both secretory and endocytic pathways." *J. Biol. Chem.* 271:9100 9107.

57. Qian, S., Jiang, P., Guan, X. M., Singh, G., Trumbauer, M. E., Yu, H., Chen, H. Y., Van de Ploeg, L. H., and Zheng, H. (1998). "Mutant human presenilin 1 protects presenilin 1 null mouse against embryonic lethality and elevates Abeta1-42/43 expression." *Neuron* 20:611–617.

58. Citron, M., Oltersdorf, T., Haass, C., McConlogue, L., Hung, A. Y., Scubert, P., Vigo-Pelfrey, C., Lieburburg, I., and Selkoe, D. J. (1992). "Mutation of the beta-amyloid precursor protein in familial Alzheimer's disease increases beta-protein production." *Nature* 360:672–674.

59. Borchelt, D. R., Wong, P. C., Sisodia, S. S., and Price, D. L. (1998). "Transgenic mouse models of Alzheimer's disease and amyotrophic lateral sclerosis." *Brain Pathol.* 8:735–757.

60. Bertram, L., Blacker, D., Mullin, K., Keeney, D., Jones, J., Basu, S., Yhu, S., McInnis, M. G., Go, R. C., Vekrellis, K., Selkoe, D. J., Saunders, A. J., and Tanzi, R. E. (2000). "Evidence for genetic linkage of Alzheimer's disease to chromosome 10q." *Science* 290:2302–2303.

61. Ertekin-Taner, N., Graff-Radford, N., Younkin, L. H., Eckman, C., Baker, M., Adamson, J., Ronald, J., Blangero, J., Hutton, M., and Younkin, S. G. (2000). "Linkage of plasma Abeta42 to a quantitative locus on chromosome 10 in late-onset Alzheimer's disease pedigrees." *Science* 290:2303–2304.

62. Myers, A., Holmans, P., Marshall, H., Kwon, J., Meyer, D., Ramic, D., Shears, S., Booth, J., DeVrieze, F. W., Crook, R., Hamshere, M., Abraham, R., Tunstall, N., Rice, F., Carty, S., Lillystone, S., Kehoe, P., Rudrasingham, V., Jones, L., Lovestone, S., Perez-Tur, J., Williams, J., Owen, M. J., Hardy, J., and Goate, A. M. (2000). "Susceptibility locus for Alzheimer's disease on chromosome 10." *Science* 290:2304–2305.

63. Schmechel, D. E., Saunders, A. M., Strittmatter, W. J., Crain, B. J., Hulette, C. M., Joo, S. H., Pericak-Vance, M. A., Goldgaber, D., and Roses, A. D. (1993). "Increased amyloid beta-peptide deposition in cerebral cortex as a consequence of apolipoprotein E genotype in late-onset Alzheimer disease." *Proc. Natl. Acad. Sci. USA* 90:9649–9653.

64. Brendza, R. P., Bales, K. R., Paul, S. M., and Holtzman, D. M. (2002). "Role of apoE/Abeta interactions in Alzheimer's disease: insights from transgenic mouse models." *Mol. Psychiatry* 7:132–135.

65. Corder, E. H., Saunders, A. M., Strittmatter, W. J., Schmechel, D. E., Gaskell, P. C., Small, G. W., Roses, A. D., Haines, J. L., and Pericak-Vance, M. A. (1993). "Gene dose of apolipoprotein E type 4 allele and the risk of Alzheimer's disease in late onset families." *Science* 261:921–923.

66. Holtzman, D. M., Bales, K. R., Tenkova, T., Fagan, A. M., Parsadanian, M., Sartorius, L. J., Mackey, B., Olney, J., McKeel, D., Wozniak, D., and Paul, S. M. (2000). "Apolipoprotein E isoform-dependent amyloid deposition and neuritic degeneration in a mouse model of Alzheimer's disease." *Proc. Natl. Acad. Sci. USA* 97:2892–2897.

67. Holtzman, D. M. (2001). "Role of apoe/Abeta interactions in the pathogenesis of Alzheimer's disease and cerebral amyloid angiopathy." *J. Mol. Neurosci.* 17:147–155.

68. Herz, J., Beffert, U. (2000)."Apolipoprotein E receptors: linking brain development and Alzheimer's disease." *Nat. Rev. Neurosci.* 1:51–58.

69. Weeber, E. J., Beffert, U., Jones, C., Christian, J. M., Forster, E., Sweatt, J. D., and Herz, J. (2002). "Reelin and ApoE receptors cooperate to enhance hippocampal synaptic plasticity and learning." *J. Biol. Chem.* 277(42):39944–39952

70. Chapman, P. F., Falinska, A. M., Knevett, S. G., and Ramsay, M. F. (2001). "Genes, models and Alzheimer's disease." *Trends Genet.* 17:254–261.

71. Janus, C., and Westaway, D. (2001). "Transgenic mouse models of Alzheimer's disease." *Physiol. Behav.* 73:873–886.

72. Irizarry, M. C., McNamara, M., Fedorchak, K., Hsiao, K., and Hyman, B. T. (1997). "APPSw transgenic mice develop age-related A beta deposits and neuropil abnormalities, but no neuronal loss in CA1." *J. Neuropathol. Exp. Neurol.* 56:965–973.

73. Westerman, M. A., Cooper-Blacketer, D., Mariash, A., Kotilinek, L., Kawarabayashi, T., Younkin, L. H., Carlson, G. A., Younkin, S. G., and Ashe, K. H. (2002). "The relationship between Abeta and memory in the Tg2576 mouse model of Alzheimer's disease." *J. Neurosci.* 22:1858–1867.

74. Dineley, K. T., Xia, X., Bui, D., Sweatt, J. D., and Zheng, H. (2002). "Accelerated plaque accumulation, associative learning deficits, and up-regulation of alpha 7 nicotinic receptor protein in transgenic mice co-expressing mutant human presenilin 1 and amyloid precursor proteins." *J. Biol. Chem.* 277:22768–22780.

75. Chapman, P. F., White, G. L., Jones, M. W., Cooper-Blacketer, D., Marshall, V. J., Irizarry, M., Younkin, L., Good, M. A., Bliss, T. V., Hyman, B. T., Younkin, S. G., and Hsiao, K. K. (1999). "Impaired

synaptic plasticity and learning in aged amyloid precursor protein transgenic mice." *Nat. Neurosci.* 2:271–276.

76. Corcoran, K. A., Lu, Y., Turner, R. S., and Maren, S. (2002). "Overexpression of hAPPswe impairs rewarded alternation and contextual fear conditioning in a transgenic mouse model of Alzheimer's disease." *Learn. Mem.* 9:243–252.

77. Dineley, K. T., Westerman, M., Bui, D., Bell, K., Ashe, K. H., and Sweatt, J. D. (2001). "Beta-amyloid activates the mitogen-activated protein kinase cascade via hippocampal alpha7 nicotinic acetylcholine receptors: in vitro and in vivo mechanisms related to Alzheimer's disease." *J. Neurosci.* 21:4125–4133.

78. McKhann, G., Drachman, D., Folstein, M., Katzman, R., Price, D., and Stadlan, E. M. (1984). "Clinical diagnosis of Alzheimer's disease: report of the NINCDS-ADRDA Work Group under the auspices of Department of Health and Human Services Task Force on Alzheimer's Disease." *Neurology* 34:939–944.

79. Kuslansky, G., Buschke, H., Katz, M., Sliwinski, M., and Lipton, R. B. (2002). "Screening for Alzheimer's disease: the memory impairment screen versus the conventional three-word memory test." *J. Am. Geriatr. Soc.* 50:1086–1091.

80. Folstein, M. F., Folstein, S. E., and McHugh, P. R. (1975). ""Mini-mental state." A practical method for grading the cognitive state of patients for the clinician." *J. Psychiatr. Res.* 12:189–198.

81. Blessed, G., Tomlinson, B. E., and Roth, M. (1968). "The association between quantitative measures of dementia and of senile change in the cerebral grey matter of elderly subjects." *Br. J. Psychiatry* 114:797–811.

82. Kumari, V., Mitterschiffthaler, M. T., and Sharma, T. (2002). "Neuroimaging to predict preclinical Alzheimer's disease." *Hosp. Med.* 63:341–345.

83. Whitehouse, P. J., Price, D. L., Clark, A. W., Coyle, J. T., and DeLong, M. R. (1981). "Alzheimer disease: evidence for selective loss of cholinergic neurons in the nucleus basalis." *Ann. Neurol.* 10:122–126.

84. Davies, P., and Maloney, A. J. (1976). "Selective loss of central cholinergic neurons in Alzheimer's disease." *Lancet* 2:1403.

85. Davies, P. (1983). "The neurochemistry of Alzheimer's disease and senile dementia." *Med. Res. Rev.* 3:221–236.

86. Coyle, J. T., Price, D. L., and DeLong, M. R. (1983). "Alzheimer's disease: a disorder of cortical cholinergic innervation." *Science* 219:1184–1190.

87. Bartus, R. T., Dean, R. L. 3rd, Beer, B., and Lippa, A. S. (1982). "The cholinergic hypothesis of geriatric memory dysfunction." *Science* 217:408–414.

88. Frolich, L. (2002). "The cholinergic pathology in Alzheimer's disease—discrepancies between clinical experience and pathophysiological findings." *J. Neural Transm.* 109:1003–1013.

89. Wang, H. Y., Lee, D. H., D'Andrea, M. R., Peterson, P. A., Shank, R. P., and Reitz, A. B. (2000). "beta-Amyloid(1-42) binds to alpha7 nicotinic acetylcholine receptor with high affinity. Implications for Alzheimer's disease pathology." *J. Biol. Chem.* 275:5626–5632.

90. Nagele, R. G., D'Andrea, M. R., Anderson, W. J., and Wang, H. Y. (2002). "Intracellular accumulation of beta-amyloid(1-42) in neurons is facilitated by the alpha 7 nicotinic acetylcholine receptor in Alzheimer's disease." *Neuroscience* 110:199–211.

91. Nordberg, A., Hellstrom-Lindahl, E., Lee, M., Johnson, M., Mousavi, M., Hall, R., Perry, E., Bednar, I., and Court, J. (2002). "Chronic nicotine treatment reduces beta-amyloidosis in the brain of a mouse model of Alzheimer's disease (APPsw)." *J. Neurochem.* 81:655–658.

92. Schenk, D., Barbour, R., Dunn, W., Gordon, G., Grajeda, H., Guido, T., Hu, K., Huang, J., Johnson-Wood, K., Khan, K., Kholodenko, D., Lee, M., Liao, Z., Lieberburg, I., Motter, R., Mutter, L., Soriano, F., Shopp, G., Vasquez, N., Vandevert, C., Walker, S., Wogulis, M., Yednock, T., Games, D., and Seubert, P. (1999). "Immunization with amyloid-beta attenuates Alzheimer-disease-like pathology in the PDAPP mouse." *Nature* 400:173–177.

93. Janus, C., Pearson, J., McLaurin, J., Mathews, P. M., Jiang, Y., Schmidt, S. D., Chishti, M. A., Horne, P., Heslin, D., French, J., Mount, H. T., Nixon, R. A., Mercken, M., Bergeron, C., Fraser, P. E., St George-Hyslop, P., and Westaway, D. (2000). "A beta peptide immunization reduces behavioural impairment and plaques in a model of Alzheimer's disease." *Nature* 408:979–982.

94. Morgan, D., Diamond, D. M., Gottschall, P. E., Ugen, K. E., Dickey, C., Hardy, J., Duff, K., Jantzen, P., DiCarlo, G., Wilcock, D., Connor, K., Hatcher, J., Hope, C., Gordon, M., and Arendash, G. W. (2000). "A beta peptide vaccination prevents memory loss in an animal model of Alzheimer's disease." *Nature* 408:982–985.

95. Dodart, J. C., Bales, K. R., Gannon, K. S., Greene, S. J., DeMattos, R. B., Mathis, C., DeLong, C. A., Wu, S., Wu, X., Holtzman, D. M., and Paul, S. M. (2002). "Immunization reverses memory deficits without reducing brain Abeta burden in Alzheimer's disease model." *Nat. Neurosci.* 5:452–457.

96. Bard, F., Cannon, C., Barbour, R., Burke, R. L., Games, D., Grajeda, H., Guido, T., Hu, K., Huang, J., Johnson-Wood, K., Khan, K., Kholodenko, D., Lee, M., Lieberburg, I., Motter, R., Nguyen, M., Soriano, F., Vasquez, N., Weiss, K., Welch, B., Seubert, P., Schenk, D., and Yednock, T. (2000). "Peripherally administered antibodies against amyloid beta-peptide enter the central nervous system and reduce pathology in a mouse model of Alzheimer disease." *Nat. Med.* 6:916–919.

97. Snowdon, D. A., Kemper, S. J., Mortimer, J. A., Greiner, L. H., Wekstein, D. R., and Markesbery, W. R. (1996). "Linguistic ability in early life and cognitive function and Alzheimer's disease in late life. Findings from the Nun Study." *JAMA* 275:528–532.

98. Masliah, E., Sisk, A., Mallory, M., and Games, D. (2001). "Neurofibrillary pathology in transgenic mice overexpressing V717F beta-amyloid precursor protein." *J. Neuropathol. Exp. Neurol.* 60:357–368.

99. Chen, G., Chen, K. S., Knox, J., Inglis, J., Bernard, A., Martin, S. J., Justice, A., McConlogue, L., Games, D., Freedman, S. B., and Morris, R. G. (2000). "A learning deficit related to age and beta-amyloid plaques in a mouse model of Alzheimer's disease." *Nature* 408:975–979.

100. Lewis, J., Dickson, D. W., Lin, W. L., Chisholm, L., Corral, A., Jones, G., Yen, S. H., Sahara, N., Skipper, L., Yager, D., Eckman, C., Hardy, J., Hutton, M., and McGowan, E. (2001). "Enhanced neurofibrillary degeneration in transgenic mice expressing mutant tau and APP." *Science* 293:1487–1491.

101. Chishti, M. A., Yang, D. S., Janus, C., Phinney, A. L., Horne, P., Pearson, J., Strome, R., Zuker, N., Loukides, J., French, J., Turner, S., Lozza, G., Grilli, M., Kunicki, S., Morissette, C., Paquette, J., Gervais, F., Bergeron, C., Fraser, P. E., Carlson, G. A., George-Hyslop, P. S., and Westaway, D. (2001). "Early-onset amyloid deposition and cognitive deficits in transgenic mice expressing a double mutant form of amyloid precursor protein 695." *J. Biol. Chem.* 276:21562–21570.

102. Arendash, G. W., King, D. L., Gordon, M. N., Morgan, D., Hatcher, J. M., Hope, C. E., and Diamond, D. M. (2001). "Progressive, age-related behavioral impairments in transgenic mice carrying both mutant amyloid precursor protein and presenilin-1 transgenes." *Brain Res.* 891:42–53.

103. Dewachter, I., Reverse, D., Caluwaerts, N., Ris, L., Kuiperi, C., Van den Haute, C., Spittaels, K., Umans, L., Serneels, L., Thiry, E., Moechars, D., Mercken, M., Godaux, E., and Van Leuven, F. (2002). "Neuronal deficiency of presenilin 1 inhibits amyloid plaque formation and corrects hippocampal long-term potentiation but not a cognitive defect of amyloid precursor protein [V717I] transgenic mice." *J. Neurosci.* 22:3445–3453.

104. Shen, J., Bronson, R. T., Chen, D. F., Xia, W., Selkoe, D. J., and Tonegawa, S. (1997). "Skeletal and CNS defects in Presenilin-1-deficient mice." *Cell* 89:629–639.

105. Feng, R., Rampon, C., Tang, Y. P., Shrom, D., Jin, J., Kyin, M., Sopher, B., Miller, M. W., Ware, C. B., Martin, G. M., Kim, S. H., Langdon, R. B., Sisodia, S. S., and Tsien, J. Z. (2001). "Deficient neurogenesis in forebrain-specific presenilin-1 knockout mice is associated with reduced clearance of hippocampal memory traces." *Neuron* 32:911–926.

106. Veinbergs, I., Jung, M. W., Young, S. J., Van Uden, E., Groves, P. M., and Masliah, E. (1998). "Altered long-term potentiation in the hippocampus of apolipoprotein E-deficient mice." *Neurosci. Lett.* 249:71–74.

107. Krzywkowski, P., Ghribi, O., Gagne, J., Chabot, C., Kar, S., Rochford, J., Massicotte, G., and Poirier, J. (1999). "Cholinergic systems and long-term potentiation in memory-impaired apolipoprotein E-deficient mice." *Neuroscience* 92:1273–1286.

108. Dawson, G. R., Seabrook, G. R., Zheng, H., Smith, D. W., Graham, S., O'Dowd, G., Bowery, B. J., Boyce, S., Trumbauer, M. E., Chen, H. Y., Van der Ploeg, L. H., and Sirinathsinghji, D. J. (1999). "Age-related cognitive deficits, impaired long-term potentiation and reduction in synaptic marker density in mice lacking the beta-amyloid precursor protein." *Neuroscience* 90:1–13.

109. Herreman, A., Hartmann, D., Annaert, W., Saftig, P., Craessaerts, K., Serneels, L., Umans, L., Schrijvers, V., Checler, F., Vanderstichele, H., Baekelandt, V., Dressel, R., Cupers, P., Huylebroeck, D., Zwijsen, A., Van Leuven, F., and De Strooper, B. (1999). "Presenilin 2 deficiency causes a mild pulmonary phenotype and no changes in amyloid precursor protein processing but enhances the embryonic lethal phenotype of presenilin 1 deficiency." *Proc. Natl. Acad. Sci. USA* 96:11872–11877.

110. Huber, G., Marz, W., Martin, J. R., Malherbe, P., Richards, J. G., Sueoka, N., Ohm, T., and Hoffmann, M. M. (2000). "Characterization of transgenic mice expressing apolipoprotein E4(C112R) and apolipoprotein E4(L28P; C112R)." *Neuroscience* 101:211–218.

111. Watson, A. A., Fairlie, D. P., and Craik, D. J. (1998). "Solution structure of methionine-oxidized amyloid beta-peptide (1-40). Does oxidation affect conformational switching?" *Biochemistry* 37:12700–12706.

112. Price, D. L., Sisodia, S. S., and Borchelt, D. R. (1998). "Genetic neurodegenerative diseases: the human illness and transgenic models." *Science* 282:1079–1083.

113. Khachaturian, Z. S., and Radebaugh, T. S. (1996). *Alzheimer's disease : cause(s), diagnosis, treatment, and care.* Boca Raton: CRC Press.

Through the Glass Darkly
J. David Sweatt, Acrylic on canvas, 2002

12

The Chemistry
of Perpetual Memory

Almost no human has a good intuitive grasp of the ephemeral nature of bio-molecules. Proteins and metabolic inter-mediates turn over at amazingly fast rates in a mammalian cell, including in a neuron in the CNS. Biochemical bonds are generally quite labile things, and the ongoing breakdown and resynthesis of the constituent molecules of the cells of your body occurs at what is, relatively speaking, breakneck speed. It is difficult to truly grasp this fact in the face of what appears to be such stability and consistency of both our bodies and our minds.

Neuroscientists are not immune to this lack of intuition. The apparent stability of synapses, cells, behavioral patterns, and CNS morphology in our everyday experi-ments tends to deceive us in our thinking about neuronal function. LTP is long-lasting and stable over the course of a day. Memories are measurably preserved over a significant fraction of an animal's life-time. This constancy and durability of CNS-based phenomena obscures the underlying rapid turnover of most of the constituent molecules that provide their molecular underpinnings.

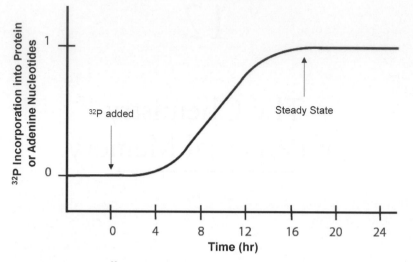

FIGURE 1   Hypothetical graph of ^{32}P-PO$_4$ reaching steady state. Steady-state is the point at which the rate of incorporation of the radioactive label equals the rate of breakdown of phosphate bonds in labeled proteins, RNA, or DNA. Isotopic equilibrium is the point at which all phosphate-containing molecules throughout the cell have achieved steady-state labeling. See text for additional discussion.

I come from a background in signal transduction, where issues of molecular turnover are dealt with on a more daily basis. I will use one example from my own experiments to illustrate my point of rapid molecular turnover in cells, although the biochemistry and signal transduction literature is full of thousands of similar examples.

Biochemists are fond of using radioactive tracer compounds to track specific molecular events in cells. A typical experimental design is, for example, to introduce 32-P labeled inorganic phosphate (^{32}PO$_4^-$) into the culture medium surrounding a neuron maintained in vitro. It is then taken up and incorporated into phosphate-containing molecules in the cell. This radioactive label can then be used to measure the extent of phosphate incorporation into cellular proteins by measuring their level of radioactivity. This is a direct measure of protein phosphorylation by kinases in the cell, or, more accurately stated, it is a direct measure of the steady-state ratio of kinase to phosphatase activity acting on a specific substrate at a specific time point.

The control experiment that one has to do in order to validate this type of approach is to demonstrate that the ^{32}P isotope has reached *isotopic equilibrium* in the cell. This simply means that the ^{32}P-PO$_4$ must have completely dispersed itself throughout all the relevant pools of phosphate that already existed in the cell, which are, of course, not initially radioactive. One needs to know that a change in radioactive content is truly a reflection of a change in phosphate content in, for example, a substrate protein. One demonstrates this by showing experimentally that the ^{32}P has reached isotopic equilibrium, that is that the labeled compound has come to a random distribution throughout all the nonradioactive phosphate that was previously there.[1] Thus, a change in ^{32}P content is truly a reflection of a change in phosphate content in a protein.

There are several ways to demonstrate that the cells under study have reached

---

[1]DNA is likely not at equilibrium in these types of experiments.

isotopic equilibrium in the pool of molecules you are investigating. The simplest, if you are interested in protein phosphorylation, is to show that the total $^{32}PO_4$ in cellular proteins has reached a plateau level (see Figure 1). This means that the incorporation of label into cellular proteins has achieved a steady-state level—the rate of increase in label in proteins has now been matched by the rate of decrease in label in proteins. The radiolabel has reached equilibrium and is no longer showing either a net increase or a net decrease. One can also specifically measure the $^{32}PO_4$ content of cellular ATP, ADP, and AMP and show that they are at a steady-state level as well. This means that the phosphates in the alpha, beta, and gamma positions of all these adenine nucleotides has undergone turnover at least once and that the net rate of ^{32}P incorporation is matched by the net rate of ^{32}P loss.

To further refine the control experiment, you can show that if the cell is stimulated with a neurotransmitter, for example, there is no additional increase in overall phosphate content in all the cellular proteins or in cellular ATP. This means there is no hidden pool of phosphate in the cell that is accessed only under the conditions of stimulation.

I did these types of experiments as part of studies I did in Eric Kandel's lab when we were studying substrate protein phosphorylation in *Aplysia* sensory neurons, which we maintained in vitro and labeled with $^{32}PO_4$ (1). How long does it take for ^{32}P-phosphate to reach isotopic equilibrium in an *Aplysia* sensory neuron? The answer is: less than 24 hours, a number that is typical for neurons in culture, and mammalian cells in general, when maintained at 37°C.

But think about the implications of this number. It means that essentially every phosphate bond at all three positions in the entire cellular ATP pool, and essentially every phosphate moiety in every cellular phosphate-containing protein, has been broken down and resynthesized in a 1-day

time period! As a first approximation *every* day *all* the phospho-proteins in your brain have had their phosphate removed and replaced. Any researchers who are considering protein phosphorylation as a mechanism that contributes to information storage for any appreciable period of time must remember that there is continual breakdown and resynthesis of the basic molecular structure underlying the memory.

This high rate of turnover is not limited to phosphorylation events. Protein constituents of neurons are broken down and resynthesized at a rapid rate as well. Andrew Varga in my laboratory has been investigating the turnover of the Kv4.2 potassium channel that we discussed in Chapters 5 and 6 and found that its half-life in a cell is about 4 hours. This means that roughly speaking the entire cellular content of this potassium channel is broken down and resynthesized over a 1-day period. Studies of AMPA receptors done in Rick Huganir's lab have shown that the half-life for this protein in neurons is approximately 30 hours (see reference 2 and Figure 2). These investigations specifically measured the GluR1 cell surface pool, along with the total cellular GluR1. The implication of this finding is that neuronal cell surface AMPA receptors are completely broken down and resynthesized from scratch over the course of a week.

A rapid rate of protein turnover is the rule rather than the exception. This is illustrated by the simple experiment shown in Figure 3. In this experiment, guinea pig hippocampal slices were prepared and labeled in vitro with ^{35}S-methionine for just 30 minutes. Thus, any protein that is labeled with ^{35}S was synthesized *de novo* from precursor amino acids over the course of this 0.5-hour time frame, or even less because the precursor methionine was added to the extracellular medium and had to cross the cell membrane and be incorporated into methionyl-tRNA before it could be incorporated into a cellular protein. After the labeling period, area CA1

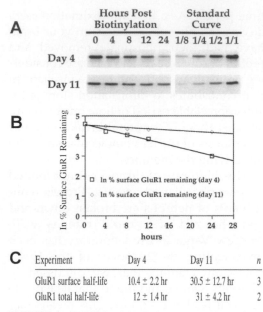

A

	Hours Post Biotinylation					Standard Curve			
	0	4	8	12	24	1/8	1/4	1/2	1/1
Day 4									
Day 11									

B

C

Experiment	Day 4	Day 11	n
GluR1 surface half-life	10.4 ± 2.2 hr	30.5 ± 12.7 hr	3
GluR1 total half-life	12 ± 1.4 hr	31 ± 4.2 hr	2

FIGURE 2   Half-life of AMPA receptors. Shown here is the half-life of cell-surface GluR1 in spinal cord neuronal cultures at day 4 and day 11 in vitro. Cell-surface molecules were selectively labeled by reacting them with biotin. Plates of spinal cord neurons were biotinylated at day 4 and day 11 and recultured for 0–24 hr, at which time cell extracts were harvested, sonicated, and frozen. Subsequently, these samples were thawed and incubated with streptavidin-linked beads, and the streptavidin-precipitated material was loaded onto gels. (Streptavidin selectively binds biotinylated proteins with very high affinity.) (A) A standard curve including serial dilutions of the $t = 0$ streptavidin-precipitated material was included on each gel for purposes of quantitation. After transfer, gels were probed with a GluR1-rective antibody in order to quantitate the amount of glutamate receptor remaining from the initial labeling with biotin. (B) The natural log of the percent of remaining surface GluR1 was plotted against time, and half-lives were calculated from the regression slopes of the resulting lines. (C) Half-life and percent of receptor on surface experiments is summarized. A paired t test demonstrated a significant increase in the half-life of surface GluR1 from day 4 to day 11 ($p < .05$). Data and figure legend adapted from Mammen, Huganir, and O'Brien (2).

was dissected out, and cellular proteins were separated on the basis of charge and molecular weight using two-dimensional gel electrophoresis. As you can see in Figure 3, at least a couple hundred different protein spots were labeled sufficiently to be detectable using autoradiography of this 2-D gel. Thus, hundreds of proteins in hippocampal area CA1 are being synthesized at a sufficiently rapid rate that they show up using this brief period of pulse-labeling. It is reasonable to infer that, because the cell is at steady state, (i.e., the cells are not growing larger), the rate of breakdown of these same proteins is matching their high rate of synthesis. These data are just a specific example from the hippocampus of what is generally known about protein synthesis—protein half-lives in the cell range from about 2 minutes to about 20 hours, and half-lives of proteins typically are in the 2- to 4-hour time range.

Okay, you say, that's fine for proteins, but what about "stable" things like the plasma membrane and the cytoskeleton? Neuronal membrane phospholipids turn over with half-lives in the minutes-to-hours range as well (3, 4). The vast majority of actin microfilaments in dendritic spines of hippocampal pyramidal neurons turn over with astonishing rapidity—the average turnover time for an actin microfilament in a dendritic spine is 44 *seconds* (see reference 5 and Figure 4).

The bottom line of all this is that if you are thinking of a single phosphorylation event or the synthesis of a new protein or the insertion of a membrane receptor or ion channel or even the formation of a new synapse as being capable of storing memory for any appreciable period of time, you must readjust your thinking. As a first approximation, the entirety of the functional components of your whole CNS have been broken down and resynthesized over a 2-month time span. This should scare you. Your apparent stability as an individual is a perceptual illusion.

These considerations apply equally well to anatomical structures. Direct measurements of fractional breakdown rates of skeletal muscle protein indicate that your muscle mass is broken down and resynthesized at about 3–4%/day (6). That's equivalent to a complete turnover of what you think of as your "body" in about a month. Development puts everything in

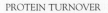

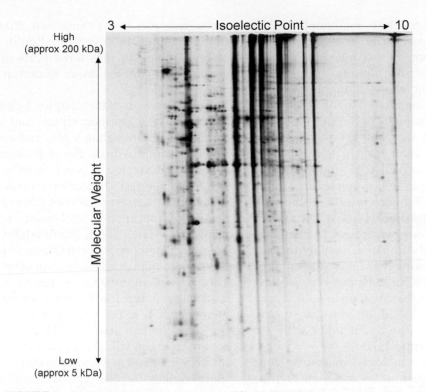

FIGURE 3 Rapid rate of protein turnover. In this experiment (Sweatt and Kandel, unpublished), two-dimensional gel analysis of ^{35}S-methionine-labeled proteins from area CA1 of guinea pig hippocampus reveals rapid and extensive labeling of proteins over a very short time period. This implies a fairly rapid breakdown and resynthesis of the labeled proteins. See text for additional explanation of the experiment.

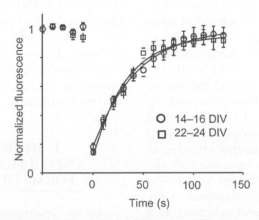

FIGURE 4 Rapid basal actin turnover in dendritic spines. The turnover of actin in dendritic spines from neurons grown for 14–16 days in vitro (DIV) was indistinguishable from those grown for 22–24 DIV. Under both conditions, actin microfilaments undergo essentially complete breakdown and re-formation about every 2 minutes. Actin turnover was assessed using fluorescent actin and monitoring recovery from photobleaching. Adapted from Star, Kwiatkowski, and Murthy (5).

its right place, but maintaining that anatomical structure is an active process, and the component molecules are turning over with surprising rapidity.

In pursuing these thoughts, we are bumping up against one of the philosophical discussions concerning the scientific approach that has arisen repeatedly throughout human history. Is the human brain really capable of understanding itself? The fact of the complete turnover of cellular signaling constituents on the time frame we are talking about flies completely in the face of our perception. The facts are at odds with the apparent stability that we perceive in ourselves and others. Our memories last. Our behavior is consistent. Our facial features stay the same. However, our intuition based on our day-to-day perceptions is directly at odds with the available experimental data.

The memory biologist must overcome this cognitive dissonance and come to grips with the rapid turnover of individual molecular components in the nervous system, to be able to begin to understand memory storage in earnest. In this chapter, we will think about memory processes from this perspective. We will think about them as chemical reactions that subserve persisting changes of varying durations. We will develop a generalized chemical categorization of the types of chemical reactions that underlie memory storage. I will describe three types of memory-storing reactions: short-term reactions mediated by transient changes in second messenger levels, long-term reactions mediated by species with long half-lives, and ultralong-term or mnemogenic reactions that can store memory indefinitely, even in the face of ongoing turnover of the molecules involved. Using this framework, I will give some specific examples of the various types of chemical reactions that may and must underlie memory storage in biological systems.

In this chapter, I will use examples from both invertebrate and mammalian learning systems, picking and choosing with relish those examples that I think best illustrate the principles involved. I should note before setting out that some parts of this chapter are adapted from Roberson and Sweatt (7).

In the first part of this chapter, I also will go outside the hippocampus, and even outside the mammalian CNS, and choose several examples from the *Aplysia* model system. Introducing a whole new model system in the last chapter of a book may seem odd. However, in many ways, the details of the specific molecular mechanisms underlying short, intermediate, and long-term memory are better understood in this system than in any mammalian system. This is particularly true as relates to the mechanisms for transitioning from one memory phase to the next while preserving the same cellular read-out. Thus, because we are trying to talk about specific *chemical reactions* involved in memory in this chapter, more details of the specific molecules involved is quite helpful.

Also, *Aplysia* has a long, storied, Nobel Committee-approved status in the memory field. In a sense, no book on memory mechanisms would be complete without some, at least passing, reference to studies using this preparation. In the next few sections, I will give a brief introduction to the *Aplysia* model to set the framework for the more detailed chemical description that will follow (see references 8–11 for reviews). I also will later in the chapter draw additional parallels to hippocampal molecular information storage processes where appropriate.

I. SHORT-, LONG-, AND ULTRALONG-TERM FORMS OF LEARNING

As we discussed in the first chapter, essentially all forms of learning exhibit themselves in either short- or long-term forms. Indeed, with only a few exceptions, the duration of the memory for a learned event depends on the number of times an animal experiences the behavior-modifying stimulus. A single sensitizing stimulation may elicit sensitization that lasts only a few minutes, whereas repeated stimulation results in sensitization lasting hours to days (See Figure 4 in Chapter 1). Repeated presentations of multiple training trials can elicit sensitization lasting for even more prolonged periods, in many cases memories that last a significant fraction of the animal's lifetime. Thus, the acquisition of memory is a *graded* phenomenon. As we have discussed many times in reference to LTP, it is intriguing to wonder how repeated presentations of the identical stimulus can uniquely elicit a long-lasting behavioral alteration, especially when one considers that the behavioral output (e.g., enhanced responsiveness) is identical in the short- and long-lasting forms.

II. USE OF INVERTEBRATE PREPARATIONS TO STUDY SIMPLE FORMS OF LEARNING

Starting in the 1960s the answers to intriguing questions such as this began to be worked out at the cellular and biochemical level. Part of this watershed of new insight into the basis of learning and memory came about as a result of the insight to capitalize on easily studied, simple forms of learning in special preparations that lent themselves to experimental investigation at the cellular level. In particular, the work of Eric Kandel and his colleagues allowed enormous progress in our understanding of the cellular basis of behavior, and learning and memory specifically. Kandel, along with Jimmy Schwartz, Vince Castellucci, Jack Byrne, Tom Carew, Bob Hawkins, and many others have used the simple marine mollusk *Aplysia californica* to great effect to study the behavioral attributes and cellular and molecular mechanisms of learning and memory.

Much (but by no means all) of the work in *Aplysia* has been geared toward understanding the basis of sensitization in this animal. *Aplysia* has on its dorsum a respiratory gill and siphon complex, which is normally extended when the animal is in the resting state. If the gill or siphon is lightly touched (or experimentally squirted with a Water-Pic), a defensive withdrawal reflex is elicited to protect the gill from potential damage. This defensive withdrawal reflex can undergo both habituation (by repeated modest stimuli) and sensitization. Sensitization occurs when the animal receives an aversive stimulus, for example a tail shock. After sensitizing stimulation, the animal exhibits a more robust, longer-lasting gill-withdrawal in response to the identical light touch or water squirt. Acquisition of this sensitization response is graded; repetitive sensitizing stimuli can give sensitization lasting minutes to hours (one to a few shocks), or weeks (repeated training trials over a few days).

Progress in beginning to understand this memory system came by way of mapping certain aspects of the neuronal circuitry underlying the defensive withdrawal reflex and the associated modulatory inputs from the tail. One appeal of the *Aplysia* experimental system was the relatively simple nervous system in the animal, allowing the tracing of significant parts of the circuitry underlying the behavior using electrophysiology techniques. This circuit tracing was greatly facilitated by the enormous (relatively speaking) size of the neurons in *Aplysia*, allowing for easy microelectrode recording from specific, identified neurons in the animal's CNS. Ironically, the critical locus for the memory of sensitization resides for the most part in the smallest neurons in the animal.

A greatly simplified diagram of the circuitry underlying sensitization of the gill- and siphon-withdrawal reflex in *Aplysia* is given in Figure 5. The touch to the gill and siphon complex stimulates siphon sensory neurons, which make direct and indirect (via interneurons) connections to gill motor neurons. The gill motor neurons stimulate muscles in the gill-and-siphon complex that mediate the defensive

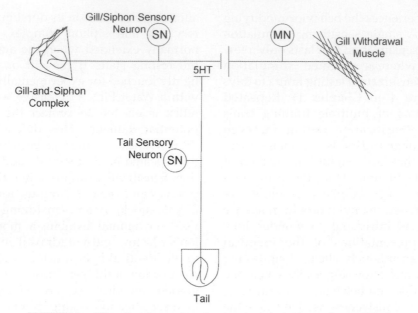

FIGURE 5   Gill and siphon reflex circuitry in *Aplysia*. A greatly simplified description of the gill-and-siphon withdrawal circuitry underlying *Aplysia* sensitization is shown. See explanation in text. Abbreviations used in diagram are sensory neurons (SN), motor neuron (MN), and serotonin (5HT).

BOX 1

CENTRAL PATTERN GENERATORS

Some of the most striking examples of the use of invertebrate models to investigate the neural mechanisms underlying behavior come from studies of *fixed pattern generators*, also known as *central pattern generators*. There are many examples of animals utilizing fixed patterns of movement, for example in cases where ongoing repetitive movements are utilized subconsciously (walking for example), or where a rapid but fixed response pattern is required (such as dodging an oncoming object that you don't see until the last second).

Crabs and lobsters have been widely used to study one example of repetitive subconscious movements. The *stomatogastric ganglion* in crustaceans such as these controls a stereotyped pattern of muscle contractions in the animals' digestive systems.

The muscle movement pattern is a highly synchronized, coordinated response to food ingestion that serves to provide the smooth movement of foodstuffs down the digestive tract. Many details of the neuronal circuitry and coordinated firing of individual neurons have been worked out for this system, along with an impressive dissection of the underlying cellular physiology.

In some cases the stereotyped behaviors can be quite elaborate, involving extended, multicomponent patterns of movement in the entire animal. One such example is a defensive escape response exhibited by the opisthobranch mollusc *Tritonia* (see Figures). Predatory starfish feed upon *Tritonia*, and a starfish touching *Tritonia* leads to the animal exhibiting a stereotyped response of defensive withdrawal and escape swimming.

BOX 1—cont'd

CENTRAL PATTERN GENERATORS

Again, this pattern of behavior is mediated by the highly coordinated firing of an elaborate network of neurons in the animal's nervous system. Much of the circuitry and cellular physiology of this central pattern generator was worked out in the late Peter Getting's laboratory.

Why do I bring this up in the context of general theories of the chemistry of memory? Because these are classic examples of

hard-wired behavioral responses. They are seemingly immutable in the absence of injury to the animal or its nervous system. Nevertheless, even highly stable behavioral patterns are mediated by neurons whose molecular constituents are undergoing constant turnover. Self-perpetuating chemical reactions, not anatomy, provide the constancy of behavioral output in these "fixed" patterns.

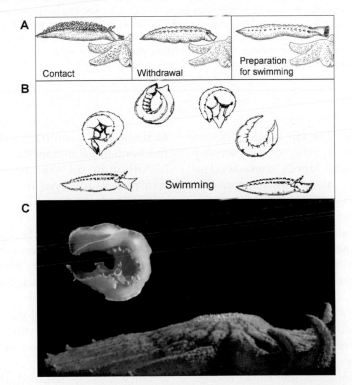

BOX 1   Escape swimming in *Tritonia*, a fixed-action pattern consisting of four stages. (A and B) Stages of *Tritonia* escape. (1) Contact and withdrawal—The relaxed animal with branchial tufts and rhinopores extended contacts a predator. After contact with a starfish the animal withdraws reflexly and bends ventrally. (2) Preparation for swimming—The animal elongates and enlarges the oral veil while bending slightly in the dorsal direction. (3) Swimming—The animal first makes vigorous ventral flexion and then vigorous dorsal flexion. This cycle is repeated several times (adapted from a figure by Tom Prentis). (4) Termination—After a final dorsal flexion the animal returns to an unflexed position with the extremities still withdrawn, oral veil and tail enlarged. One to five dorsal flexions occur before the animal regains its original relaxed posture. (C) Escape response (photograph by Bill Frost).

Continued

BOX 1—cont'd

CENTRAL PATTERN GENERATORS

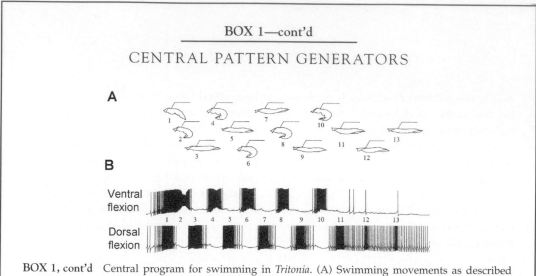

BOX 1, cont'd Central program for swimming in *Tritonia*. (A) Swimming movements as described previously. (B) Intracellular recordings from neurons in the *Tritonia* CNS. The top record represents a cell that drives the animal's downward (ventral) flexion; the lower record shows the cell that drives the upward (dorsal) flexion. The numbers between records correspond to the numbers in A and show the types of recordings obtained during the corresponding phases of the swimming movement. From Willows (24). Copyright by Scientific American.

withdrawal reflex. The tail shock impinges upon this circuit by way of tail sensory neurons that make direct contacts (and interneurons that make indirect contacts) with the presynaptic terminals of the siphon sensory neurons.

It was soon realized that plasticity at the siphon sensory neuron/gill motor neuron synapse is one critical locus contributing to sensitization in the animal—one of the first demonstrations of the importance of synaptic plasticity in learning and memory. A predominant component of plasticity at this synapse is increased neurotransmitter release from the gill-and-siphon sensory neurons. Thus, tail shock and the attendant activity in tail sensory neurons and associated interneurons leads to the release of modulatory neurotransmitters onto the siphon sensory neuron presynaptic terminal, increasing the release of neurotransmitter from these cells and augmenting the defensive withdrawal reflex. These observations highlighted the role of presynaptic

facilitation of neurotransmitter release as a mechanism for memory in this system.

Although all the modulatory neurotransmitters involved in presynaptic facilitation in *Aplysia* sensory neurons are not yet identified, one important player is serotonin. Serotonin is released onto a subset of the siphon sensory neurons by a serotonergic tail sensory neuron stimulated by tail shock. In fact, serotonin application to siphon sensory neurons elicits the vast majority of the physiologic responses contributing to presynaptic facilitation of neurotransmitter release and sensitization in the animal.

Once it was realized that facilitation of neurotransmitter release from siphon sensory neurons (hereafter referred to simply as sensory neurons) was an important component of sensitization in the animal, and that serotonin could mimic the effects of sensitizing stimulation on sensory neuron physiology, it became clear that an effective model system for studying sensitization in

Aplysia was to study the cascade of events elicited by serotonin application to sensory neurons. This model system has been exploited to characterize the cellular, electrophysiologic, and biochemical mechanisms operating to achieve enduring presynaptic facilitation in these cells.

As mentioned earlier, sensitization in *Aplysia* exhibits both short-term and long-term forms. Similarly, in sensory neurons, serotonin application can lead to either short-term or long-term facilitation of neurotransmitter release. Single (5-minute) applications of serotonin give facilitation that lasts only a few minutes; repeated (5 × 5 minutes over the course of an hour) applications give facilitation lasting at least 24 hours. This is, of course, very reminiscent of the durations of behavioral sensitization in response to single or multiple presentations of tail shock stimuli. One very active area of *Aplysia* research over the last 20 years has been dissecting the biochemical cascades operating to cause these short- and long-term effects, in particular trying to understand how the different durations of effects are achieved. In the following sections, I will briefly describe the molecular mechanisms that have been discovered to play a role in short-term, intermediate-term, and long-term facilitation of neurotransmitter release in *Aplysia* sensory neurons.

III. SHORT-TERM FACILITATION IN *APLYSIA* IS MEDIATED BY CHANGES IN THE LEVELS OF INTRACELLULAR SECOND MESSENGERS

What happens when serotonin is applied to sensory neurons? Serotonin binds to receptors in the neuron's cell surface membrane that are coupled to adenylyl cyclase and phospholipase C, which generate cAMP and DAG, respectively. When a sensory neuron sees a single pulse

of serotonin, adenylyl cyclase and phospholipase C are activated, cAMP and DAG levels increase, and the activities of PKA and PKC are greatly enhanced. As long as serotonin is present, these enzymatic activities remain elevated. However, after serotonin is removed, metabolic enzymes in the sensory neuron return the cell to its resting state. In this case, phosphodiesterase breaks down cAMP, diacylglycerol lipase breaks down DAG, and protein phosphatases dephosphorylate the protein kinase substrates. Thus, the duration of facilitation in response to a single application of serotonin is determined by the amount of time serotonin is present, the rate of breakdown of the second messengers, and the rate of reversal of the effects of the protein kinases after serotonin is removed. After a single application of serotonin, these effects are rapidly reversed (usually within a few minutes); therefore, a single application of serotonin gives only short-lasting facilitation.

Thus, Reaction Category 1: Altered Levels of Second Messengers

Thus, *Aplysia* short-term facilitation of neurotransmitter release provides an example of our first category of memory-forming chemical reaction: transient, stimulus-mediated changes. In this case, the duration of the memory is essentially dependent upon continued release of 5HT onto the neuron.

It is an interesting thought experiment to consider the effects in this system if the breakdown enzymes were removed. Over time, second messengers and phosphorylated proteins would accumulate, eventually driving the system to saturation. Then, whenever a sensory neuron received a serotonin signal, it would be unable to modulate its intracellular milieu appropriately, and no alteration in synaptic efficacy could be achieved. This thought experiment illustrates an important point; the capacity to dynamically regulate the

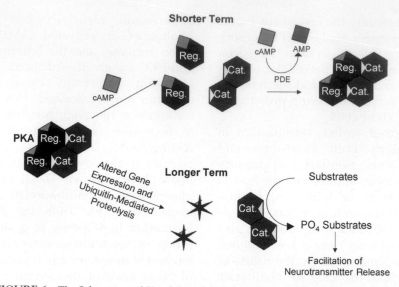

FIGURE 6   The Schwartz and Kandel model of short-term and long-term regulation of
PKA in *Aplysia* sensory neurons. This is a mechanism for short- and intermediate-term
facilitation of neurotransmitter release. See references 8 and 9 and explanation of pathway
in text. PKA shown as tetramer of two regulatory (Reg.) and two catalytic (Cat.) subunits.
The catalytic site is shown in yellow. PDE = Phosphodiesterase.

molecular messengers in a system is critical to the synaptic plasticity that underlies learning.

IV. INTERMEDIATE-TERM FACILITATION IN *APLYSIA* INVOLVES ALTERED GENE EXPRESSION AND PERSISTENT PROTEIN KINASE ACTIVATION—A SECOND CATEGORY OF REACTION

What happens when the sensory neuron sees repeated applications of serotonin, which elicits long-lasting synaptic facilitation? Repeated applications of serotonin lead to sustained elevations of second messengers, and this sustained elevation elicits activation of a unique and elaborate cascade of biochemical events. Although many mechanistic details have not yet been worked out, several key steps in this cascade have been identified. The long-lasting elevation of cAMP leads to PKA activation and subsequent phosphorylation of the transcription factor CREB. Activation of the ERK MAP kinase cascade is also likely involved as a modulator of CREB activation, specifically acting through disinhibition via repression of negative regulators of CREB. Through mechanisms that are still being investigated, CREB activation leads to regulation of protein breakdown. Specifically, the ubiquitin system is recruited to cause the proteolytic degradation of one subunit of PKA, the PKA regulatory subunit.

An understanding of the consequences of the loss of PKA regulatory subunits becomes clear upon review of the normal control of this enzyme. The cAMP-dependent protein kinase is, of course, a tetramer comprising two regulatory and two catalytic subunits (Figure 6). The two identical regulatory subunits each contain one cAMP binding site; when cAMP binds, the regulatory subunits dissociate from the two (identical) catalytic subunits. The free catalytic subunits are then enzymatically competent and able to phosphorylate their downstream effector proteins. Therefore, proteolytic loss of regulatory subunits results in a decrease in the overall ratio of regulatory to catalytic subunits, promoting an excess of free, active catalytic subunits, and an increase in the phosphorylation of PKA substrates.

In this manner, PKA is *persistently activated*. Even after cAMP returns to its resting level after serotonin is removed, the excess catalytic subunits remain free of regulatory subunits and active in the sensory neuron. By this clever mechanism, a chain of events is set in motion whereby a biochemical effect that outlasts the initial, triggering elevation of the second messenger cAMP is established in the cell. The PKA will remain activated until compensatory resynthesis of new regulatory subunits occurs, or until the catalytic subunit is degraded. Interestingly, although the mechanism has not yet been worked out, recent evidence indicates that the DAG-responsive effector PKC also is persistently activated after serotonin stimulation of sensory neurons.

Persistent kinase activation is one powerful mechanism contributing to long-lasting facilitation of neurotransmitter release in sensory neurons. Available evidence indicates that the persistent activation of PKA underlies an intermediate stage of facilitation, lasting on the order of many hours after the triggering applications of serotonin are finished. Interestingly, pioneering work on this mechanism was performed using sensitization training in animals, emphasizing the strong likelihood of this mechanism contributing to the underlying cellular basis for the change in the animal's behavior in vivo.

Thus, We Have Reaction Category 2: Generation of Long Half-Life Molecules

Aplysia intermediate-term facilitation of neurotransmitter release provides an example of our second category of memory-forming chemical reaction: generation of long half-life signaling molecules. In this case, the duration of the memory is essentially

dependent upon the half-life of the free PKA catalytic subunit. Reversal of the persisting event is dependent upon the half-life of the protein or the rate of synthesis of regulatory subunit. Later in the chapter, I will highlight a few corresponding types of molecular memory traces that have been observed in hippocampal synaptic plasticity, which we have already covered in great detail in Chapter 7.

Before proceeding to Reaction Category 3, it is worth noting how the short- and intermediate-term mechanisms manage to achieve the same final common output of increased synaptic strength. The elegant solution to this problem is inherent in the mechanisms themselves. As both short-term mechanisms and longer-term mechanisms result ultimately in activation of the same kinases, PKA and PKC, the final read-out is the same: increased phosphorylation of PKA and PKC substrates. Only the mechanisms to achieve the kinase activation are distinct and of different durations.

The substrates affected by PKA and PKC are varied (see Box 2), involving proteins controlling both the electrical properties of the sensory neuron cell membrane and the mechanisms involved in the process of neurotransmitter release. The overall result, though, is an orchestrated set of changes leading ultimately to increased neurotransmitter release from the sensory neuron.

V. LONG-TERM SYNAPTIC FACILITATION IN *APLYSIA* INVOLVES CHANGES IN GENE EXPRESSION AND RESULTING ANATOMICAL CHANGES

After the persistent kinase activation has decayed, what then maintains the strengthened connection between the siphon sensory neurons and their follower motor neurons? Strikingly, continued augmentation of the defensive withdrawal reflex is based on *morphological* changes in

BOX 2

EFFECTORS OF PKA AND PKC IN *APLYSIA* PRESYNAPTIC FACILITATION

In attempting to understand how presynaptic facilitation in *Aplysia* sensory neurons occurs, it is worth considering the mechanisms normally operating to produce *baseline* neurotransmitter release (see figure). First, stimulation of siphon sensory neuron nerve endings in the gill and siphon complex (e.g., by light touch) leads to membrane depolarization and generation of an action potential. Invasion of the action potential into the presynaptic terminal causes the opening of voltage-gated calcium channels, which are open for a period of time proportional to the duration of the action potential. Of course, the invasion of multiple action potentials will also elicit additional calcium influx. This calcium signal triggers activation of the molecular machinery leading to fusion of neurotransmitter-containing vesicles with the sensory neuron presynaptic membrane, resulting in release of neurotransmitter into the synaptic cleft.

By and large, presynaptic facilitation is achieved by modulation of three sites in the cascade of events resulting in neurotransmitter release. One site is closure of *"S"-channels*, or serotonin-sensitive potassium channels. A second site is modulation of *Ikv*, or *voltage-sensitive potassium channels*. Finally, there is modulation of the responsiveness of the neurotransmitter release machinery to the action potential-associated calcium influx. In the remainder of the section, I will briefly describe the impact of the alterations of each of these sites.

S CHANNELS

The S channel achieved fame as one of the first ion channels discovered to be modulated by a phosphorylation event (23). The S channel is what is referred to as a "leak" potassium channel; that is, it is normally open at rest and thus contributes to establishing the resting membrane

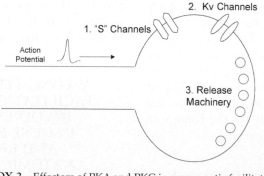

BOX 2 Effectors of PKA and PKC in presynaptic facilitation. See reference 9 for additional information.

BOX 2—cont'd

EFFECTORS OF PKA AND PKC IN *APLYSIA* PRESYNAPTIC FACILITATION

potential. The cAMP-dependent protein kinase phosphorylates and closes the S channel. Closure of this channel has several effects on the electrical properties of the sensory neuron cell membrane. First, as the channels are closed, there is less resting potassium current flowing across the membrane, resulting in a modest depolarization of the membrane. This brings the resting membrane potential closer to the *threshold* for action potential generation and increases the likelihood of action potential firing. In addition, the closure of S channels leads to decreased *spike-frequency accommodation*, such that the cell is more likely to fire multiple action potentials with prolonged stimulation. Finally, the S channel makes a modest contribution to repolarizing the membrane after an action potential, so closure of voltage-gated calcium channels contributes to a *prolongation* of the action potential duration, allowing increased duration of calcium influx through voltage-gated calcium channels. (In fact, an additional component of the effect of serotonin is a direct effect on these calcium channels, augmenting their responsiveness to depolarization.) Thus, closure of the S channel overall leads to increased likelihood of triggering one or more action potentials and to increased calcium influx in response to the action potential.

IKv

The work of Jack Byrne's laboratory has been instrumental in the discovery of the modulation of this channel as a mechanism

for presynaptic facilitation in *Aplysia* sensory neurons (9). Ikv is a voltage-sensitive potassium channel that opens in response to the membrane depolarization caused by the arrival of the action potential. After opening, the potassium current flowing through this channel contributes substantially to returning the membrane potential to its resting level. Therefore, in contrast to the S channel, the voltage-sensitive potassium channel Ikv is a major player in repolarizing the cell membrane after the arrival of an action potential, and modulation of this channel is a potent mechanism for prolonging action potential duration. Both the PKA and PKC cascade impinge upon this mechanism, leading to inhibition of Ikv function, action potential prolongation, and an attendant increase in calcium influx with each action potential.

MODULATION OF THE RELEASE MACHINERY

A third, less well-understood mechanism recruited by the PKA and PKC pathways is direct augmentation of the responsiveness of the neurotransmitter release machinery to the action-potential-associated calcium influx. Even though the effect recruited by serotonin to contribute to presynaptic facilitation is quite robust, at present the incompleteness of our understanding of the release process itself precludes a mechanistic description of this component. This is, however, a very active area of research, and hopefully elucidation of this important mechanism will be forthcoming.

the circuit. Sensitization lasting on the order of 24 hours or more is mediated by an actual increase in the number of synaptic contacts between siphon sensory neurons and follower motor neurons. Thereby stimulation of the siphon sensory neuron elicits a greater response in gill withdrawal because a greater number and density of excitatory connections are made between the two cells. Studies into long-term effects of serotonin on sensory neurons strongly suggests that these morphological changes are a result of a pathway involving cAMP- and MAPK-mediated changes in gene expression, resulting in increased synthesis of some proteins, down-regulation of others, and an overall remodeling of the zones of contact between sensory and motor neurons. The dissection of these molecular cascades is an active area of research at present. Future work hopefully will allow the definition of all the components of the complex molecular machinery involved.

With the discovery that morphological changes underlie long-lasting facilitation of neurotransmitter release and behavioral sensitization in the animal, the field has in a sense come full circle. I say this because pioneering work in *Aplysia* demonstrated that long-lasting *habituation* of the gill-and-siphon withdrawal response was associated with a *decreased* number of synaptic contacts between siphon sensory neurons and gill motor neurons. Both long-term inhibition and enhancement of behavior therefore have in common an underlying anatomical basis. Although our understanding of the molecular mechanisms underlying these types of anatomical changes is marginal at present, these observations about long-term sensitization and long-term habituation serve to illustrate that structural rearrangements of synaptic connections are likely to be a powerful and general mechanism underlying long-lasting behavioral changes.

However, remember the discussion that started this chapter. There is nothing inherently stable about morphological changes or increased synaptic contacts. All the component molecules that make up these structures are being continually broken down and resynthesized. How does the cell solve the problem of maintaining a change in the face of continual loss and replacement of its component molecules?

The answer to this question is based in a specific category of chemical reactions that Eric Roberson and I have referred to as *mnemogenic* chemical reactions (7).

The essential descriptor of a mnemogenic chemical reaction is given in Equation 1.

$$X + X^{\bullet} \rightarrow X^{\bullet} + X^{\bullet} \qquad (1)$$

In this reaction, X is a molecule that can exist in either a basal state (X) or an activated or modified form ($X^{\bullet}$). The initiation of a learning event triggers activation of X by conversion into the $X^{\bullet}$, or activated form.

$$X \xrightarrow{\text{trigger}} X^{\bullet} \qquad (2)$$

This activated $X^{\bullet}$ leads to manifestation of the memory phenotype, affecting either directly or indirectly some biochemical process regulating neuronal function (e.g., synaptic strength or neuronal excitability).

The unique feature of the mnemogenic reaction is that the activated molecule, $X^{\bullet}$, can react with an inactive molecule of X and convert it to the $X^{\bullet}$ form. This is how levels of $X^{\bullet}$ are sustained despite molecular turnover. Although the nucleus synthesizes only the inactive form, the activated species at the synapse catalyzes its activation; thus, more active $X^{\bullet}$ is created, perpetuating the reaction.

In the next section, we will return to several specific examples of mnemogenic chemical reactions that have been identified in mammalian systems. However, before proceeding, I will give a specific molecular example of the general category that has been identified as potentially maintaining long-lasting synaptic facilitation in *Aplysia*. This example is based on seminal work in this area by Arnold Eskin, Jack Byrne, and their colleagues (12, 13).

How is an increased number of synaptic contacts maintained in the face of continual breakdown and resynthesis of the synaptic molecular infrastructure? Eskin, Byrne, and co-workers have found that long-term facilitation is associated with increased expression of a tolloid/bone morphogenetic protein referred to as *Aplysia* TBL-1 (Tolloid/*B*one morphogenetic protein— Like protein—1). TBL-1 is, among other things, a protease that is involved in growth factor processing. The current hypothesis is that TBL-1 is induced with serotonin treatment and secreted into the extracellular space, where it converts pro-TGFβ into active TGFβ (Transforming Growth Factor Beta). TGFβ can then bind to its receptors on the cell surface, and activate signal transduction cascades that, like serotonin, lead to increased expression of TBL-1 (see Figure 7). In this way, a self-reinforcing loop is established and can persist beyond the breakdown and resynthesis of individual component molecules. The increased number of synaptic connections is maintained in this model by having the component molecules for synapse maintenance synthesized in parallel with the TBL-1—a conceptually straightforward mechanism for this is to simply have them read out from the same gene promoters that regulate TBL-1 expression.

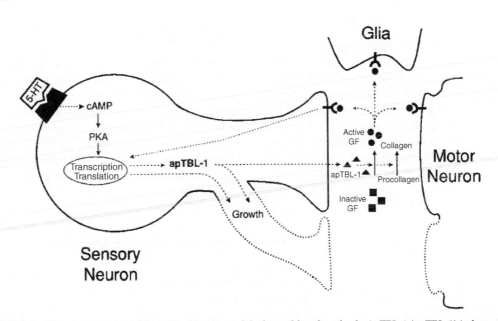

FIGURE 7   This figure presents the Eskin/Byrne model of possible roles of aplysia TBL-1 (apTBL-1) in long-term presynaptic facilitation in *Aplysia* sensory neurons. A sensory neuron, motor neuron, and glial cell are represented schematically. The growth processes of sensory neurons and motor neurons are drawn with dotted lines. 5-HT increases the transcription of the apTBL-1 gene. apTBL-1 protein might remain in the cytoplasm by alternative translation and might play a role as a protease to modify the cytoskeleton structure in the growth process within the sensory neuron. apTBL-1 also might be secreted to modify the extracellular matrix (procollagen) or activate TGF-β-like growth factors. The activated growth factors could bind to Ser/Thr kinase receptors and trigger the signal transduction cascade, leading to the regulation of cell growth. The activated growth factors also might modify the motor neurons to complement the morphological changes in the sensory neurons, or they might activate glial cells to secrete extracellular matrix components that might then help stabilize the morphological changes. Some of the same events elicited by the activation of TGF-β also could be caused by modification of the extracellular matrix component collagen. Figure and legend reproduced from Liu et al. (13).

This process is an example of a mnemogenic chemical reaction, specifically a variant that Eric Roberson and I have termed a *circular mnemogenic reaction*. Mnemogenic reactions are not limited to a single molecule catalyzing production or activation of itself. Interacting sets of molecules can act in series to establish a regenerative molecular circuit. In this case, the reactions have the following forms, where $X^{\bullet}$ catalyzes activation of Y, and $Y^{\bullet}$ in turn catalyzed activation of X:

$$X^{\bullet} + Y \rightarrow X^{\bullet} + Y^{\bullet}$$

$$X + Y^{\bullet} \rightarrow X^{\bullet} + Y^{\bullet}$$

By summing these partial reactions and rearranging to the form of equation 1, we see that this system creates a sort of double mnemogenic reaction:

$$X + X^{\bullet} + Y + Y^{\bullet} \rightarrow X^{\bullet} + X^{\bullet} + Y^{\bullet} + Y^{\bullet}$$

Other examples of mnemogenic reaction systems such as this have recently been elaborated based on computer modeling of signal transduction mechanisms operating in synaptic plasticity (14). In the case of the *Aplysia* TBL-1/TGFβ system, the interacting cascades produce a bistable molecular state of a synapse that is capable of perpetual memory storage.

VI. THREE ATTRIBUTES OF CHEMICAL REACTIONS MEDIATING MEMORY

What do these examples of memory mechanisms in *Aplysia* tell us about the chemical reactions that support them? First, there must be chemical reactions with different time courses that mediate short-term, long-term, and ultralong-term memory. Second, because manifestation of the memory phenotype between shorter-term and longer-term memories is seamless, the various chemical reactions are likely to converge on common effectors. And finally, there must be some unique mechanism to mediate those ultralong-term memories that defeats the problem of molecular turnover.

A. Long-Term Memory in Mammals

As is nicely illustrated by studies in *Aplysia* described previously, because synapses mediate the neuron-neuron communication that underlies an animal's behavior, changes in behavior are ultimately subserved by alterations in the nature, strength, or number of interneuronal synaptic contacts in the animal's nervous

---

BOX 3

FORGETTING

Given the continual turnover of the molecular constituents of our CNS, it's amazing that we can remember anything at all for any period of time. With this in mind, the emerging recognition of the error-proneness of human memory may come as no surprise.

Daniel Schacter has delineated and categorized the flawed nature of human memory in his recent book *The Seven Sins of Memory* (25). Forgetting and memory lability come part and parcel with molecular turnover. Even an extremely low error rate as one molecule passes along its

BOX 3—cont'd

FORGETTING

information to its successor will accumulate significant retention errors over the course of a lifetime. After all, a long-lived protein in a neuron has a half-life of about 24 hours. It will be broken down and resynthesized from scratch about 50 times over the course of a single year.

Although it is a stretch to go from molecules to cognitive psychology, it is entertaining to think of "sins" for which protein turnover may be the underlying culprit. The easiest example is *transience*. Transience is simply the diminution of a particular memory over time. Your memory for recent events is more robust and detailed for recent events than for those from farther in your past. Memory has a half-life because the molecules that store it have a half-life. In the case of those memories stored using a mnemogenic, self-perpetuating reaction, the memory half-life is basically determined by the error rate of the underlying mnemogenic reaction as it replicates itself.

Misattribution is a memory sin wherein an association is erroneous for example

you think you remember that Kim told you something when actually it was Eric. At the time Eric told you the story and shortly thereafter you obviously knew the source—over time the molecules subserving that particular association have been erroneously resynthesized in a configuration that has wired the memory up with Kim.

A final "sin," *persistence*, is the mirror image of transience. Persistence is basically remembering things you would prefer to forget, or would be better off forgetting. Persistence stands as testament to the robustness of the mnemogenic reaction—once it has been set in motion the molecular positive feedback cycle may difficult to break. This may be particularly true for highly emotional experiences—as we discussed in Chapter 6, many modulatory influences can enter into play in the initial establishment of highly emotional memories. A mnemogenic reaction that is established at a level high above the threshold needed for its maintenance will be particularly unsusceptible to subsequent erasure through active or passive processes.

system. As we discussed in Chapter 1, one of the great unifying theories to emerge out of neuroscience research in the last century was that synaptic plasticity subserves learning and memory. In the next section we will identify several examples of biochemical mechanisms operating in mammalian hippocampal long-term synaptic potentiation that fall into one of the three categories outlined before as general descriptors of the classes of chemical reactions involved in memory formation.

B. Long Half-Life Reactions

For an example of a long half-life biochemical reaction involved in LTP, we will focus on PKC. This is because, as described in Chapter 7, several of the mechanisms for persistent PKC activation that have been identified based on in vitro studies of the enzyme are now known to contribute to the persistent activation of PKC in LTP. For example, PKC was originally identified as an enzyme activated by calcium-dependent proteolysis, and proteolytic activation of classical PKC isoforms in TEA-induced NMDA receptor-independent LTP has been observed. In addition, as described in Chapter 7, Todd Sacktor has shown up-regulation, most likely mediated by increased synthesis, of an autonomously active truncated form of PKC-zeta in LTP. Oxidative activation of PKC renders the enzyme autonomously active, and this mechanism is likely to contribute to the persistent activation of PKC in the maintenance phase of LTP. Thus, all these mechanisms: proteolysis, increased synthesis, and oxidation, act on PKC to render it persistently activated in LTP. These reactions are examples of long half-life chemical reactions where decay depends on the breakdown of the persistently activated protein.

In this context, another interesting finding is that there is increased autophosphorylation of PKC in LTP. PKC C-terminal autophosphorylation, such as is observed in LTP, preserves the enzyme against down-regulation and is correlated with PKC binding to actin microfilaments. Thus, the probable role of PKC autophosphorylation in LTP is to preserve the persistently activated enzyme from proteolytic down-regulation and to maintain its localization to the appropriate synaptic region of the neuron. Thus, the generation of a long-lasting signal in LTP (i.e., persistent PKC activation) depends on two mechanisms: generation of autonomous PKC and protection from down-regulation. These two mechanisms act in concert to provide a persistent signal in the cell.

It is worth noting that PKC autophosphorylation is intramolecular and, therefore, cannot be self-perpetuating. This means that the persistence of the autonomous activity will be limited by the half-life of the persistently activated PKC. Thus, while PKC activation in LTP is a persistent and long half-life reaction, it is not an example of an effect rendered immune to molecular turnover.

C. Ultralong-Term Memory: Mnemogenic Chemical Reactions

A variety of chemical reactions identified in mammalian cells qualify as mnemogenic. The first examples of reactions that qualify as mnemogenic were independently proposed by Francis Crick and John Lisman (15, 16 and see later discussion). Crick and Lisman focused on reactions that were enzymatic in nature, involving covalent modifications of inactive precursors (X) by activated forms of the enzyme ($X^\bullet$). This sort of reaction has been formalized and investigated experimentally in the context of the generation of autonomously active CaMKII by intersubunit autophosphorylation.

CaMKII is synthesized in the inactive state and is normally regulated by calcium and calmodulin. As we discussed in detail in Chapter 7, while CaMKII can be transiently activated by calcium/calmodulin, CaMKII can also be triggered to undergo autophosphorylation by this same stimulus. After this occurs, the phosphorylated form of CaMKII is autonomously active, even in the absence of the calcium/calmodulin trigger (17). The critical feature of CaMKII is that the activated ($X^\bullet$) form can phosphorylate the inactive (X) form of CaMKII in an intermolecular "mnemogenic" reaction. Thus, CaMKII theoretically remains autonomously active despite protein turnover.

Because this type of mnemogenic reaction has received considerable attention, I refer the reader to a recent treatment of this topic for additional details (18). I would be remiss if I did not point out, however, that to date there has been no direct experimental demonstration of CaMKII being rendered permanently active in a cell. It is likely that the necessary subunit turnover does not occur intracellularly. Regardless of the mechanistic basis for reversal of the activation, examples of autonomously active CaMKII that have been reported thus far in the literature have been observed to last only 1 to 2 hours. Thus, in real life, autonomous CaMKII probably falls into the category of a long half-life reaction, as opposed to generation of a self-perpetuating species. Nevertheless, the theoretical capacity of CaMKII to undergo self-perpetuating activation independent of subunit turnover makes this a good theoretical example of a mnemogenic chemical reaction.

Enzymatic mnemogenic reactions need not be based on phosphorylation reactions. For example, any reaction wherein a zymogen is cleaved into its final active product by that product is a mnemogenic reaction (19). In essence the active conformation of the enzyme serves to store the necessary information for converting the inactive precursor to the active product. Finally, as noted previously in discussing PKC autophosphorylation in LTP, only intermolecular (or intersubunit) reactions can be mnemogenic. Intramolecular reactions are unable to undergo self-perpetuation due to their self-delimiting nature.

There are a variety of other examples of mnemogenic reactions that can be found outside the realm of neuronal plasticity. Although the involvement of these other reactions in memory per se is unlikely, it nevertheless is instructive to consider them as examples of the diverse possibilities for types of mnemogenic reactions in neurons. Also, consideration of these other examples helps to illustrate that the mnemogenic chemical reaction solves a more general biological problem of maintaining long-lasting change. The mnemogenic reaction must be utilized in any example of lasting change persisting despite molecular turnover (e.g., in development, immunological memory, and certain pathological states).

Conformational mnemogenic reactions Prion proteins undergo a mnemogenic reaction that is not based on covalent modifications but rather on the self-promoted catalysis of a persisting conformational change (20). Prion proteins are hypothesized to exist in two conformations—the cellular form that is present normally in cells and a "scrapie" form that is an infectious particle and the cause of various neurodegenerative disorders. One molecule of the scrapie form catalyzes the conversion of a molecule of the cellular form into a second molecule of the scrapie form; a reaction of the type described by equation 1. Once converted to the scrapie conformation, the molecule is essentially irreversibly changed, and by promoting the generation of copies of itself, the scrapie conformation preserves itself against elimination by proteolytic cellular protein turnover.

Synthetic mnemogenic reactions Instead of eliciting an alteration in a pre-existing molecule of itself, a chemical species can participate in a mnemogenic reaction by promoting its own synthesis. Examples of this type of mnemogenic reaction are increasingly being found in the area of cellular differentiation, where transcription factors are being discovered to regulate their own synthesis as committed steps toward a final cellular phenotype. For example, the transcription factor myoD, a master control protein that elicits the conversion of a precursor cell into a differentiated myocyte, binds to an upstream regulatory sequence controlling its expression of its own gene (21). By this mnemogenic reaction, after a threshold level of myoD is reached in the cell, the cell is irreversibly committed to a lifetime of myoD protein expression and maintenance of the muscle phenotype. Interestingly, an extension of this concept is DNA itself, which catalyzes (indirectly) its own replication.

Autocrine mnemogenic reactions The example of the BMP-1/TGFβ loop in *Aplysia* long-term facilitation, which was described previously, is but one specific example of a general form of mnemogenic reaction. As described by Shvartzman et al. (22), many types of cells can participate in autocrine loops of this sort. Autocrine loop simply refs to the cell's making and secreting a ligand that binds to a receptor on the surface of that same cell—a receptor that when activated, promotes synthesis of its activating ligand. This positive feedback loop can be set to either turn a transient signal into a persisting change or to establish a permanent change. To date, autocrine loops of this sort have been thought of mostly in the context of carcinogenesis, where a transient exposure to an extracellular signal can result in the permanent transformation of a cell.

VII. SUMMARY: A GENERAL CHEMICAL MODEL FOR MEMORY

Learning and memory have always intrigued those interested in the functioning of the brain. The mammalian CNS has an amazing capacity to store and recall diverse types of information, and learned responses shape to a great degree an animal's behavior. How are memories formed and stored? Contemporary understanding of this issue highlights the importance of changes in synaptic strength (synaptic plasticity) as the means whereby the nervous system forms and stores memory. But by what means are changes in synaptic strength achieved? The fundamental answer to this question is not a mystery: changes in synaptic strength must of necessity be mediated by chemical changes (i.e., changes in the fundamental properties of the enzymes and other proteins comprising the synapse).

What sorts of chemical changes underlie memory formation and storage? Memory has as its defining characteristic persistence: an environmental stimulus causes a change that greatly outlasts the duration of the triggering signal. Therefore, at the chemical level, memory must have as its hallmark changes in protein function that are able to persist beyond initial, triggering events. Understanding biochemical reactions that

manifest this property will greatly increase our understanding of the mechanisms that must underlie memory. Though many papers have dealt with biochemical mechanisms potentially contributing to memory, few have focused on this essential, defining characteristic of the mechanism at the heart of memory.

In this chapter, my goal has been to identify and characterize the types and time courses of persisting biochemical reactions underlying learning and memory and, where possible, to highlight specific, well-documented examples from the literature. The types of biochemical reactions underlying information storage fall into three general classes:

Category 1 includes short-term changes that are mediated by the presence of extracellular or intracellular messenger molecules and that are subject to fairly rapid removal resulting from the specific breakdown or clearance mechanisms. The prototype example is the acute action of a neurotransmitter on cellular biophysical or synaptic properties. In this phase, the memory trace resides in the continued presence of the stimulus. The duration of the memory is dependent upon ongoing production of the signal (e.g., the continued release of neurotransmitter into the synaptic cleft).

Category 2 includes the intermediate- and long-term changes that are mediated by a transient signal producing a persisting chemical memory trace. The generation of the persisting species may be produced by direct covalent modification of a pre-existing molecule, the triggering of an enzymatic modification of a pre-existing molecule, increased synthesis of an active enzyme, or altered gene expression resulting in enzyme activation or synthesis. In general, the duration of the chemical trace is determined by the half-life of the activated protein. The half-life of the protein may be controlled by passive metabolic processes or alternatively may be regulated by specific control mechanisms. In some cases, the half-lives of the relevant species may be very long and capable of supporting a memory for hours, days, or even weeks. These memories cannot be stored indefinitely, however, because they remain susceptible in time to degradation of the trace molecule.

Category 3 includes lifelong changes that are mediated by mnemogenic chemical reactions. The mnemogenic reaction could be triggered by the transient signal of Category 1, the persisting signal of Category 2, or by a distinct and parallel mechanism. The mnemogenic reaction, being self-perpetuating, does not have a half-life in the normal sense, but it potentially can be reversed by a specific triggered mechanism. The activated mnemogenic species maintains the memory trace and results in the expression of memory by impinging on some biophysical, metabolic, or structural neuronal component.

While certainly lacking in specifics, the preceding general model serves as an organizing structure for thinking about various phases of memory from the perspective of their being subserved by specific subtypes of chemical reactions.

Returning to the conundrum raised in the beginning of this chapter: How are robust lifelong memories stored as a biochemical reaction when their constituent molecules are subject to molecular turnover? If memories are stored in a synapse (or any other cellular compartment), how does a sustaining chemical species necessary for the memory render itself immune to degradation or spontaneous decay? This problem is particularly profound when considering examples of lifelong memory that can be induced by a single, transient environmental stimulus. The generic answer to this question has historically been that long-term changes are mediated by "anatomical" or "structural" changes, somehow implying that these changes are somehow protected from degradation.

However, the same question of protein turnover applies to anatomical or structural changes. A structural feature does not "develop" and stay that way. It must be preserved (by being restored) on a minute-to-minute basis.

The erroneous assumption of structural stability has even been perpetuated in Hebb's Postulate:

> When an axon of cell A . . . excites cell B and repeatedly or persistently takes part in firing it, some growth process or metabolic change takes place in one or both cells so that A's efficiency as one of the cells firing B is increased.

Hebb's flaw was to make a distinction between a growth process and a metabolic change. A growth process *is* a metabolic change. A "structure" is built of rapidly turning-over molecular components. Thinking of a "structural" change or "anatomical" change as being somehow uniquely stable is an erroneous assumption. Preservation of memories is an active, ongoing process at the chemical level. A molecule of finite lifetime that is involved in memory storage must somehow pass along its acquired characteristics to a successor molecule before it is degraded and the information is lost. The future of memory research is to identify the mechanisms for the preservation of acquired molecular characteristics.

References

1. Sweatt, J. D., and Kandel, E. R. (1989). "Persistent and transcriptionally-dependent increase in protein phosphorylation in long-term facilitation of Aplysia sensory neurons." *Nature* 339:51–54.
2. Mammen, A. L., Huganir, R. L., and O'Brien, R. J. (1997). "Redistribution and stabilization of cell surface glutamate receptors during synapse formation." *J. Neurosci.* 17:7351–7358.
3. Chikhale, E. G., Balbo, A., Galdzicki, Z., Rapoport, S. I., and Shetty, H. U. (2001). "Measurement of myo-inositol turnover in phosphatidylinositol: description of a model and mass spectrometric method for cultured cortical neurons." *Biochemistry* 40:11114–11120.

4. Rapoport, S. I. (2001). "In vivo fatty acid incorporation into brain phosholipids in relation to plasma availability, signal transduction and membrane remodeling." *J. Mol. Neurosci.* 16:243–261; discussion 279–284.

5. Star, E. N., Kwiatkowski, D. J., and Murthy, V. N. (2002). "Rapid turnover of actin in dendritic spines and its regulation by activity." *Nat. Neurosc.* 5:239–246.

6. Zhang, X. J., Chinkes, D. L., Sakurai, Y., and Wolfe, R. R. (1996). "An isotopic method for measurement of muscle protein fractional breakdown rate in vivo." *Am. J. Physiol.* 270:E759–767.

7. Roberson, E. D., and Sweatt, J. D. (1999). "A biochemical blueprint for long-term memory." *Learn. Mem.* 6:381–388.

8. Bailey, C. H., Bartsch, D., and Kandel, E. R. (1996). "Toward a molecular definition of long-term memory storage." *Proc. Natl. Acad. Sci. USA* 93:13445–13452.

9. Byrne, J. H., and Kandel, E. R. (1996). "Presynaptic facilitation revisited: state and time dependence." *J. Neurosci.* 16:425–435.

10. Frost, W. N., and Kandel, E. R. (1995). "Structure of the network mediating siphon-elicited siphon withdrawal in Aplysia." *J. Neurophysiol.* 73:2413–2427.

11. Kandel, E. R. (1976). Cellular basis of behavior : an introduction to behavioral neurobiology. San Francisco: W. H. Freeman.

12. Zhang, F., Endo, S., Cleary, L. J., Eskin, A., and Byrne, J. H. (1997). "Role of transforming growth factor-beta in long-term synaptic facilitation in Aplysia." *Science* 275:1318–1320.

13. Liu, Q. R., Hattar, S., Endo, S., MacPhee, K., Zhang, H., Cleary, L. J., Byrne, J. H., and Eskin, A. (1997). "A developmental gene (Tolloid/BMP-1) is regulated in Aplysia neurons by treatments that induce long-term sensitization." *J. Neurosci.* 17:755–764.

14. Weng, G., Bhalla, U. S., and Iyengar, R. (1999). "Complexity in biological signaling systems." *Science* 284:92–96.

15. Crick, F. (1984). "Memory and molecular turnover." *Nature* 312:101.

16. Lisman, J. E. (1985). "A mechanism for memory storage insensitive to molecular turnover: a bistable autophosphorylating kinase." *Proc. Natl. Acad. Sci. USA* 82:3055–3057.

17. Miller, S. G., and Kennedy, M. B. (1986). "Regulation of brain type II Ca^{2+}/calmodulin-dependent protein kinase by autophosphorylation: a Ca^{2+}-triggered molecular switch." *Cell* 44:861–870.

18. Lisman, J. E., Fallon, J. R. (1999). "What maintains memories?" *Science* 283:339–340.

19. Slee, E. A., Harte, M. T., Kluck, R. M., Wolf, B. B., Casiano, C. A., Newmeyer, D. D., Wang, H. G., Reed, J. C., Nicholson, D. W., Alnemri, E. S., Green, D. R., and Martin, S. J. (1999). "Ordering the cytochrome c-initiated caspase cascade: hierarchical activation of caspases-2, -3, -6, -7, -8, and -10 in a caspase-9-dependent manner." *J. Cell. Biol.* 144:281–292.

20. Li, L., and Lindquist, S. (2000). "Creating a protein-based element of inheritance." *Science* 287:661–664.

21. Thayer, M. J., Tapscott, S. J., Davis, R. L., Wright, W. E., Lassar, A. B., and Weintraub, H. (1989). "Positive autoregulation of the myogenic determination gene MyoD1." *Cell* 58:241–248.

22. Shvartsman, S. Y., Hagan, M. P., Yacoub, A., Dent, P., Wiley, H. S., and Lauffenburger, D. A. (2002). "Autocrine loops with positive feedback enable context-dependent cell signaling." *Am. J. Physiol. Cell. Physiol.* 282:C545–559.

23. Shuster, M. J., Camardo, J. S., Siegelbaum, S. A., and Kandel, E. R. (1985). "Cyclic AMP-dependent protein kinase closes the serotonin-sensitive K^+ channels of Aplysia sensory neurones in cell-free membrane patches." *Nature* 313:392–395.

24. Willows, A. O. (1971). "Giant brain cells in mollusks." *Sci. Am.* 224:68–75.

25. Schacter, D. L. "The seven sins of memory: how the mind forgets and remembers." Houghton Mifflin, Boston: 1–272.

Index